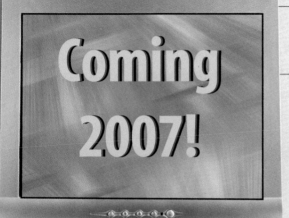

Leading
and
Managing
in
Nursing

FOURTH EDITION

Patricia S. Yoder-Wise

Texas Tech University Health Sciences Center
Lubbock, Texas

MOSBY

ELSEVIER

MOSBY
ELSEVIER

11830 Westline Industrial Drive
St. Louis, MO 63146

LEADING AND MANAGING IN NURSING,
FOURTH EDITION

ISBN-13: 978-0-323-03900-0
ISBN-10: 0-323-03900-6

Previous editions copyrighted 2003, 1999, and 1995.

ISBN-13: 978-0-323-03900-0
ISBN-10: 0-323-03900-6

Senior Editor: Yvonne Alexopoulos
Senior Developmental Editor: Danielle M. Frazier
Publishing Services Manager: Jeff Patterson
Senior Project Manager: Clay S. Broeker
Design Direction: Julia Dummitt

Printed in Canada

Last digit is the print number: 9 8 7 6 5 4 3 2

Contributors

Michael R. Bleich, PhD, RN, CNAA-BC, FAAN
Associate Dean and Professor, Clinical and
 Community Affairs
School of Nursing
University of Kansas
Kansas City, Kansas
Executive Director and Chief Operating Officer
KU Health*Partners*, Inc.
Kansas City, Kansas
Chapter 1: Managing, Leading, and Following

Mary Ellen Bonczek, BSN, RN, MPA,
 CNAA, BC
Senior Vice President and Chief Nurse Executive
New Hanover Regional Medical Center
Wilmington, North Carolina
Chapter 13: Staffing and Scheduling

Sharon A. Brigner, MS, RN
Senior Health Policy Analyst
National Committee to Preserve Social Security
 and Medicare
Washington, DC
Chapter 28: Leading Through Professional
 Associations

Karen S. Cox, RN, PhD, CNAA
Senior Vice President
Patient Care Services
Children's Mercy Hospitals and Clinics
Kansas City, Missouri
Chapter 10: Managing Information and
 Technology: Caring and Communicating with
 Computers

Karen Ann Dadich, RN, MN, CNS
Associate Professor
School of Nursing
Texas Tech University Health Sciences Center
Lubbock, Texas
Chapter 12: Care Delivery Strategies
Chapter 27: Career Management: Putting
 Yourself in Charge

Mary Ann T. Donohue, PhD, RN, APN, C
Administrative Director of Nursing for
 Professional Practice and Clinical Affairs
Hackensack University Medical Center
Hackensack, New Jersey
Chapter 22: Conflict: The Cutting Edge of
 Change

Michael L. Evans, PhD, RN, CNAA, FACHE
Vice President and Chief Learning Officer
The Center for Learning
Texas Health Resources
Arlington, Texas
Chapter 2: Developing the Role of Leader

Victoria N. Folse, PhD, APRN, BC, LCPC
Assistant Professor
School of Nursing
Illinois Wesleyan University
Bloomington, Illinois
Chapter 19: Managing Quality and Risk

Jennifer Jackson Gray, RN, PhD
Assistant Professor
School of Nursing
University of Texas at Arlington
Arlington, Texas
Chapter 25: Role Transition

Ginny Wacker Guido, JD, MSN, RN, FAAN
Associate Dean and Director, Graduate Studies
College of Nursing
University of North Dakota
Grand Forks, North Dakota
Chapter 4: Legal and Ethical Issues

Fran Hicks, RN, BS, MS, PhD, FAAN
Consultant
Woodland, Washington
Chapter 18: Collective Action

Cheri E. Hunt, RN, MHA
Chief Nursing Officer
Patient Care Services
Children's Mercy Hospital
Kansas City, Missouri
Chapter 10: Managing Information and
Technology: Caring and Communicating with
Computers

Karen Kelly, EdD, RN, CNAA, BC
Associate Professor and Coordinator, Continuing
Education
School of Nursing
Southern Illinois University at Edwardsville
Edwardsville, Illinois
Chapter 9: Power, Politics, and Influence

Colleen P. Kosiak, RN, MS, ARNP
Clinical Assistant Professor
School of Nursing
University of Kansas
Kansas City, Kansas
Chapter 1: Managing, Leading, and Following

Karren Kowalski, PhD, RN, CNAA, BC, FAAN
President
Kowalski Associates
Grant Project Director
Colorado Center for Nursing Excellence
Larkspur, Colorado
Chapter 17: Building Teams Through
Communication and Partnerships
Chapter 24: Managing Personal/Personnel
Problems

Mary Elizabeth Mancini, RN, PhD, CNA, FAAN
Professor and Associate Dean for Undergraduate
Nursing Programs
School of Nursing
University of Texas at Arlington
Arlington, Texas
Chapter 6: Healthcare Organizations
Chapter 7: Understanding and Designing
Organizational Structures

Kristi D. Menix, RN, EdD, CNAA, BC
Education Consultant
Former Assistant Professor and CNE Nurse
Planner
University of Texas at Tyler
Tyler, Texas
Chapter 16: Leading Change

Dorothy A. Otto, RN, MSN, EdD
Associate Professor
School of Nursing
University of Texas Health Science
Center-Houston
Houston, Texas
Chapter 3: Developing the Role of Manager
Chapter 8: Cultural Diversity in Health Care

Amy C. Pettigrew, RN, BSN, MSN, DNS
Associate Professor and Associate Director of the
Institute for Nursing Research/Scholarship of
Teaching and Learning
College of Nursing
University of Cincinnati
Cincinnati, Ohio
Chapter 26: Self-Management: Stress and Time

Cynthia Whittig Roach, RN, DSN
Associate Professor
Beth-El College of Nursing and Health Sciences
of the University of Colorado at Colorado
Springs
Colorado Springs, Colorado
Chapter 24: Managing Personal/Personnel
Problems

Trudi B. Stafford, RN, PhD(c)
Assistant Vice President
Patient Care
Memorial Hermann Southeast Hospital
Houston, Texas
Chapter 11: Managing Costs and Budgets

Darlene Steven, RN, BScN, BA, MHSA, PhD
Professor, Nursing
Graduate Coordinator, Masters of Public Health
Departments of Nursing and Masters of Public
Health
Lakehead University
Thunder Bay, Ontario
Canada
Chapter 15: Strategic Planning, Goal-Setting, and
Marketing

Diane M. Twedell, MS, RN, CNAA
Nurse Administrator, Education and Professional
  Development
Nursing Department
Mayo Clinic
Rochester, Minnesota
Chapter 14: Selecting, Developing, and Evaluating
  Staff
Chapter 25: Role Transition

Ana M. Valadez, RN, EdD, CNAA, BC, FAAN
Associate Dean for the Undergraduate Program
Professor in the Roberts' Practiceship
School of Nursing
Texas Tech University Health Sciences Center
Lubbock, Texas
Chapter 3: Developing the Role of Manager
Chapter 8: Cultural Diversity in Health Care

Rose Aguilar Welch, RN, EdD
Professor
School of Nursing
California State University, Dominguez Hills
Carson, California
Chapter 5: Making Decisions and Solving
  Problems

Patricia S. Yoder-Wise, RN, EdD, CNAA, FAAN
Texas Tech University Health Sciences Center
Lubbock, Texas
Chapter 16: Leading Change
Chapter 23: Delegation: An Art of Professional
  Practice
Chapter 27: Career Management: Putting
  Yourself in Charge
Chapter 29: Thriving for the Future

Margarete Lieb Zalon, PhD, RN, APRN, BC
Professor
Department of Nursing
University of Scranton
Scranton, Pennsylvania
Chapter 20: Translating Research into Practice
Chapter 21: Consumer Relationships

PHOTO CREDITS

Chapter 1 (opener), p. 3, courtesy Chuck Dresner,
photographer
Chapter 10 (opener), p. 191, courtesy Corometrics
Medical Systems, Wallingford, Connecticut
Chapter 25 (opener, top and bottom photos),
p. 515, courtesy Chuck Dresner, photographer
Chapter 26 (opener, right photo), p. 531, courtesy
Chuck Dresner, photographer

Acknowledgments

We are indebted to our reviewers, whose insightful comments and suggestions were invaluable in helping revise this book. The end result of their efforts, as in any peer-review process, is a stronger presentation. We are deeply grateful to the following people for their assistance:

Lynda H. Crawford, PhD, RN, CAE
Associate Dean of the Center for Non-Profit
    Management
Spertus Institute
Chicago, Illinois

Judy A. Davis, MS, MPH, APRN, BC, APN
Assistant Professor
West Suburban College of Nursing
Oak Park, Illinois

Mary L. Fisher, PhD, RN, CNAA, BC
Professor, Environments for Health
Indiana University School of Nursing
Consultant
St. Vincent Health Services
Indianapolis, Indiana

Nancy C. Grove, RN, BSN, MEd, MSN, PhD
Director and Associate Professor, Nursing
    Program
Coordinator, School Nurse Certificate Program
School of Nursing
University of Pittsburgh at Johnstown
Johnstown, Pittsburgh

Brenda Lea Hosley, RN, MSN, PhD
Associate Professor
Department of Nursing
Berea College
Berea, Kentucky

Debra A. Indorato, RD, LDN
Owner, Nutrition Therapist
Approach Nutrition and Fitness
Chesapeake, Virginia
Patient Services Manager
Morrison Healthcare Management
Norfolk, Virginia

Andrea N. Koepke, BSN, MAN, DSN
Director
School of Nursing
Anderson University
Anderson, Indiana

Ellen M. LaDieu, MS, RN
Nursing Faculty
AD Program
Excelsior College
Albany, New York

Mary Martelon, RN
Charge Nurse
Exempla Good Samaritan Medical Center
Lafayette, Colorado

Claudia Louth Mitchell, RN, BSN, MSN
Professor
Associate Degree Nursing Program
Santa Barbara City College
Santa Barbara, California

Desma Reno, MSN, RN, CS, GCNS
Assistant Professor
Department of Nursing
Southeast Missouri State University
Cape Girardeau, Missouri

Denise Top Rhine, RN, MEd, CEN
Professor, Associate Degree Nursing
Oakton Community College
Des Plains, Illinois

Barbara Scheirer, RN, MSN
Assistant Professor
School of Nursing
Grambling State University
Grambling, Louisiana

Christina Leibold Sieloff, PhD, RN, CAN, BC
Associate Professor
College of Nursing
Montana State University
Billings, Montana

Joyce Simones, RN, MS, EdD-C
Associate Professor
Department of Nursing Science
St. Cloud State University
St. Cloud, Minnesota

Georgianna Thomas, EdD, MSN, RN
Assistant Dean and Associate Professor
West Suburban College of Nursing
Oak Park, Illinois

Margaret Mary West, DNSc, RN
Associate Professor
Geisinger Site Coordinator
Nursing Education Center
Thomas Jefferson University
Danville, Pennsylvania

David Wilson, MS, RNC
Adjunct Faculty
Langston University School of Nursing
Southern Nazarene University
Staff Nurse, Urgent Care Center
The Children's Hospital at Saint Francis
Tulsa, Oklahoma

SPECIAL ACKNOWLEDGMENTS

Many people helped make this book a reality. All of the contributing authors to this book worked within very tight time frames to accomplish their work. To them I extend my deepest appreciation for being creative and responsive, making the necessary revisions, and sounding eager to hear from me whenever I emailed them. AOL, Federal Express, and Kinko's remain household words!

Special thanks go to our editor, Yvonne Alexopoulos and to our developmental editor, Danielle Frazier; for answering questions, providing the "latest" version of whatever we were talking about, and doing all sorts of tasks that kept us on track; to those who exceeded our wildest expectations of involvement (you know who you are); and to Robert Thomas Wise, my husband and best friend, for being such a great sounding board and consistent supporter. This time he even took a vacation by himself because I was too intent on the deadlines. What flexibility!

One final note: No learner can remain stagnant, that includes those of us who prepared the content in this book. We all learned more about leading and managing as we revised or created our work. The context in which nurses manage and lead is constantly changing, sometimes for the better, sometimes for the worse. The key to success is to keep learning, keep caring, and maintain our passion for nursing and the patients we serve. That, if nothing else, must be instilled in our leaders of tomorrow. Lead on . . . ¡Adelanté!

Patricia S. Yoder-Wise
RN, EdD, CNAA, FAAN
Texas Tech University Health Sciences Center
Lubbock, Texas

This book is dedicated to the
families and friends who supported all of us who created it,
to the faculty who use it to develop nursing's new leaders and managers,
and to the learners who have the vision and insight to
grasp today's reality and mold it into the
future of dynamic nursing leadership.

Lead on . . . ¡Adelanté!

Preface to the Instructor

Leading and managing are two essential expectations of all professional nurses, and they are more important than ever in today's rapidly changing healthcare system. To lead and manage successfully, nurses must possess not only knowledge and skills but also a caring and compassionate attitude. After all, leading and managing are both about people.

Volumes of information on leadership and management principles can be found in nursing, healthcare administration, business, and general literature. The numerous journals in each of these fields offer research and opinion articles focused on improving leaders' and managers' abilities. The first three editions of this text demonstrated that learners, faculty, and registered nurses in practice found that a text that synthesized applicable knowledge and related it to contemporary practice was useful. Unlike clinical nursing textbooks, which offer exercises and assignments designed to provide opportunities for learners to apply theory to patients, nursing leadership and management textbooks traditionally offered limited opportunities of this kind. We changed that tradition in 1995 by incorporating application exercises within the text and workbook section for learners. With the third edition, we changed that tradition yet again by linking this text to a Website where case studies exemplify a chapter's point and provide even more recent references. Today, the fourth edition again breaks a new pathway for learning, providing a web-based course that will be available through Evolve.

This book results from our continued strong belief in the need for a text that focuses on the nursing leadership and management issues of today and tomorrow in a distinctive way. We continue to find that we are not alone in this belief. Before the first edition, Mosby, primarily through the efforts of Darlene Como, solicited faculty members' and administrators' ideas to determine what they thought professional nurses most needed to know about leading and managing and what kind of text would best help them obtain the necessary knowledge and skills. Their comprehensive list of suggestions remains relevant in this edition. This edition incorporates many reviewers from both service and education to be sure that the text conveys important and timely information to users as they focus on the critical roles of leading, managing, and following. Additionally, we took seriously the various comments by faculty and learners, offered as I met them in person or heard from them by email.

CONCEPT AND PRACTICE COMBINED

Innovative in both content and presentation, *Leading and Managing in Nursing* merges theory, research, and practical application in key leadership and management areas. Our overriding concern in this edition remains to create a text that, while well grounded in theory and concept, presents the content in a way that is real. Wherever possible, we use real-world examples from the continuum of today's healthcare settings to illustrate the concepts. Because each chapter contributor focuses on synthesizing the assigned content, you will find no lengthy quotations in these chapters. Instead, we have made every effort to make the content as engaging, inviting, and interesting as possible. Reflecting our view of the real world of nursing leadership and management today, the following themes pervade the text:

- Every role within nursing has the basic concern for safe, effective care for the people we exist for—our clients and patients.
- The focus of health care is shifting from the hospital to the community.
- Healthcare consumers and the healthcare workforce are becoming increasingly culturally diverse.
- Today, virtually every professional nurse leads, manages, and follows, regardless of title or position.
- Consumer relationships play a central role in the delivery of nursing and health care.

- Communication, collaboration, team-building, and other interpersonal skills form the foundation of effective nursing leadership and management.
- Change continues at a rapid pace in healthcare and society in general.
- Movement toward evidence-based practice is long overdue.

DIVERSITY OF PERSPECTIVES

Contributors are recruited from diverse settings, roles, and geographic areas, enabling them to offer a broad perspective on the critical elements of nursing leadership and management roles. To help bridge the gap often found between nursing education and nursing practice, some contributors were recruited from academia and others from practice settings. This blend not only contributes to the richness of this text but also conveys a sense of oneness in nursing. The historical "gap" between education and service must become a sense of a continuum and not a chasm.

AUDIENCE

This book is designed for undergraduate learners in nursing leadership and management courses, including those in BSN-completion courses and second-degree programs. In addition, we know that nurses in practice, who had not anticipated formal leadership and management roles in their careers, use this text to capitalize on their own real-life experiences as a way to develop greater understanding about leading and managing and the important role of following. Because today's learners are more visually oriented than past learners, we incorporated illustrations, boxes, and a functional full-color design to stimulate interest and maximize learning. In addition, numerous examples and The Challenge in each chapter remain to provide relevance to the real world of nursing.

ORGANIZATION

We organized this text around issues that are key to the success of professional nurses in today's constantly changing healthcare environment.

First, it is important to understand the concepts of leading and managing and how the theories and foci differ from each other. For example, headship (holding a formal position or title) does not always mean that person is demonstrating leadership. Next, nurses should understand key concepts as they relate to leading and managing. You will find key organizational information that ranges from a basic understanding about the kinds of organizations delivering care to the changing demands for quality, technology, and cost-effectiveness. Consumer relationships lead into considerations of how to deliver care and relationships with staff. Cultural diversity does not focus so much on understanding diversities of patients (appropriate for clinical textbooks) as it does on understanding and valuing diversities in employees (critical to leading and managing). The text then transitions from the critical elements of teams and how they interact to accomplish work to the individual expectations and influences we must have throughout our careers.

Because repetition plays a crucial role in how well learners learn and retain new content, some topics appear in more than one chapter and in more than one section. We have also made an effort to express a variety of different views on some topics, as is true in the real world of nursing.

DESIGN

The functional full-color design, still distinctive to this text, is used to emphasize and identify the text's many teaching/learning strategies, which are featured to enhance learning. Full-color photographs provide visual reinforcement of concepts, such as body language and the changes occurring in contemporary healthcare settings, while adding visual interest. Figures elucidate and depict concepts and activities described in the text graphically.

TEACHING/LEARNING STRATEGIES

The numerous teaching/learning strategies featured in this text are designed both to stimulate learners' interest and to provide constant reinforcement throughout the learning process. In addition, the visually appealing, full-color design itself serves a learning purpose. Color is used consistently throughout the text to help the reader identify the various chapter elements described in the following sections.

CHAPTER OPENER ELEMENTS

- The introductory paragraph briefly describes the purpose and scope of the chapter.
- Objectives articulate the chapter's learning goals, typically at the application level or higher.
- Questions to Consider stimulate learners to think about their personal viewpoint or experience with the topics and issues discussed in the chapter.
- The Challenge presents a contemporary nurse's real-world concern related to the chapter's focus.

ELEMENTS WITHIN THE CHAPTERS

Glossary Terms appear in bold type in each chapter. They are also listed in the "Terms to Know" at the end of the chapter. Definitions appear in the Glossary at the end of the text.

Exercises stimulate learners to think critically about how to apply chapter content to the workplace and other real-world situations. They provide experiential reinforcement of key leading and managing skills. Exercises are highlighted with a colored vertical rule and are numbered sequentially within each chapter to facilitate using them as assignments or activities.

Research Perspectives and *Literature Perspectives* illustrate the relevance and applicability of current scholarship to practice. Perspectives always appear in boxes with an "book" icon in the upper left corner.

Theory Boxes provide a brief description of relevant theory and key concepts.

Numbered boxes contain lists, tools such as forms and work sheets, and other information relevant to chapter content that learners will find useful and interesting.

END OF CHAPTER ELEMENTS

The Solution provides an effective method to handle the real-life situations set forth in *The Challenge*.

Chapter Checklists summarize key concepts from the chapter in both paragraph and itemized list form.

Tips offer practical guidelines for learners to follow in applying the information presented in each chapter.

Terms to Know are included as additional study/review aids.

References and *Suggested Readings* provide the learner with a list of key sources for further reading on topics found in the chapter.

OTHER TEACHING/ LEARNING STRATEGIES

The *Glossary* contains a comprehensive list of definitions of all boldfaced terms used in the chapters.

The *Application Activities* are a built-in, perforated tool to help learners assess and evaluate understanding of the content in the text.

COMPLETE TEACHING AND LEARNING PACKAGE

In addition to the text *Leading and Managing in Nursing*, Instructor Resources are provided online through Evolve (http://evolve.elsevier.com/Yoder-Wise/). These resources are designed to help instructors present the material in this text and include the following assets:

- **NEW!** Power Point Slides for each chapter with lecture notes where applicable (over 450 slides total)
- **UPDATED!** ExamView Test Bank with over 275 multiple-choice questions. Rationales are based on AONE Competencies and ANA Scope and Standards for Nurse Administrators. Answers are also provided.
- Instructor's Manual
  - Chapter Objectives
  - Chapter Outline
  - Terms to Know
  - Teaching Suggestions

- ○ Instructions for Text Chapter Exercises
- ○ Skills Checklist
- ○ Discussion/Essay Questions
- ○ Experiential Exercises and Learning Activities
- ○ Suggested Guest Speakers
- Case Studies for each chapter
- Image Collection (approximately 40 images)
- **COMING 2007!** Online Course with twenty-seven modules presented in a consistent organizational structure, including features such as an overview, critical questions, objectives, reading assignments, learning activities, and case studies

Student Resources can also be found online through Evolve (http://evolve.elsevier.com/Yoder-Wise/). These resources provide students with additional tools for learning and include the following assets:

- Sample Resumés
- WebLinks

Learner's Guide

As a professional nurse in today's changing health-care system, you will need strong leadership and management skills more than ever, regardless of your specific role. You will also need to be an independent, dependable follower. The fourth edition of *Leading and Managing in Nursing* not only provides the conceptual knowledge you will need but also offers practical strategies to help you hone the various skills so vital to your success as a leader and manager.

Because repetition is a key strategy in learning and retaining new information, you will find many topics discussed in more than one chapter. In addition, as in the real world of nursing, you will often find several different views expressed on a single topic. This repetition reinforces ideas and illustrates how one concept has multiple applications. Rather than referring you to another portion of the text, the key information is provided within the specific chapter. Because leading and managing are skills that require specific situation considerations, you can see why such a diversity of views exists.

To help you make the most of your learning experience, try the following strategy. Read the opening paragraph (on the title page of each chapter). This preview should create a context for your reading. The objectives suggest what your accomplishments should be by the time you conclude the chapter. Questions to consider form a way for you to think about your own relevant abilities and experiences. The Challenge allows you to "hear" a real-life situation and always poses the question, "What do you think you would do if you were this nurse?" (The Solution, at the end of the chapter, examines what one individual did in this situation and again asks you to think about how that fits for you and why.) The Introduction and subsequent content, like any text, provide critical information. For some learners, it is useful to skim those headings and the box content to gain an overall sense of the concepts inherent in the chapter. For others, reading and reflecting from the beginning of the chapter to the end might be useful. The material in boxes (boxes, tables, Research Perspectives and Literature Perspectives, and Theory Boxes) is designed to augment understanding of the content in the text narrative. The checklist at the end of each chapter highlights the key points the chapter presented, and tips illustrate ways to apply the content just studied. After you complete each chapter, stop and think about what the chapter conveyed. What does it mean for you as a leader, follower, and manager? How do the chapter's content and your interaction with it relate to the other chapters you have already completed? How might you briefly synthesize the content for a non-nurse friend? Reading the chapter, restating its key points in your own words, and completing the text exercises and workbook activities will go far to help you make the content truly your own.

We think you will find leading and managing to be an exciting, challenging field of study, and we have made every attempt to reflect that belief in the design and approach of this edition.

LEARNING AIDS

The fourth edition of *Leading and Managing in Nursing* continues to incorporate important tools to help you learn about leading and managing and apply your new knowledge to the real world. The next few pages graphically point out how to use these study aids to your best advantage.

The vivid full-color chapter opener *photographs* and other photographs throughout the text help convey each chapter's key message while providing a glimpse into the real world of leading and managing in nursing.

The *introductory paragraph* tells you what you can expect to find in the chapter. To help set the stage for your study of the chapter, read it first and then summarize in your own words what you expect to gain from the chapter.

The list of *Objectives* helps you focus on the key information you should be able to apply after having studied the chapter.

The *Questions to Consider* challenge you to think critically about issues in the chapter. You might want to write down your answers both before and after reading the chapter, and then compare them.

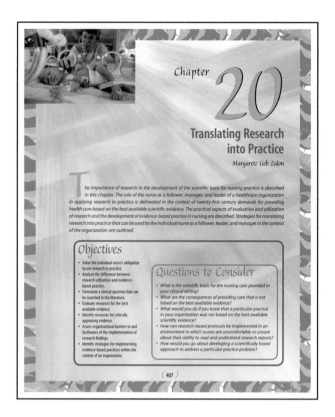

Chapter 20

Translating Research into Practice

Margarete Lieb Zalon

The importance of research in the development of the scientific basis for nursing practice is described in this chapter. The role of the nurse as a follower, manager, and leader of a healthcare organization in applying research to practice is delineated in the context of twenty-first century demands for providing health care based on the best available scientific evidence. The practical aspects of evaluation and utilization of research and the development of evidence-based practice in nursing are described. Strategies for translating research into practice that can be used by the individual nurse as a follower, leader, and manager in the context of the organization are outlined.

Objectives

- Value the individual nurse's obligation to use research in practice.
- Analyze the difference between research utilization and evidence-based practice.
- Formulate a clinical question that can be searched in the literature.
- Evaluate resources for the best available evidence.
- Identify resources for critically appraising evidence.
- Assess organizational barriers to and facilitators of the implementation of research findings.
- Identify strategies for implementing evidence-based practices within the context of an organization.

Questions to Consider

- What is the scientific basis for the nursing care provided in your clinical setting?
- What are the consequences of providing care that is not based on the best available evidence?
- What would you do if you knew that a particular practice in your organization was not based on the best available scientific evidence?
- How can research-based protocols be implemented in an environment in which nurses are uncomfortable or unsure about their ability to read and understand research reports?
- How would you go about developing a scientifically based approach to address a particular practice problem?

(407)

---

92   Part One   **Core Concepts**

The Challenge

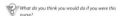

Vickie Lemmon, RN, MSN
Director of Clinical Strategies and Operations, Wellpoint, Inc., Ventura, California

Healthcare managers today are faced with numerous and complex issues that pertain to providing quality services for patients within a resource-scarce environment. Stress levels among staff can escalate when problems are not resolved, leading to a decrease in morale, productivity, and quality service. This was the situation I encountered in my previous job as Administrator for California Children Services (CCS). When I began my tenure as the new CCS Administrator, staff expressed frustration and dissatisfaction with staffing, workload, and team communications. This was evidenced by high staff turnover, lack of teamwork, customer complaints, unmet deadlines for referral and enrollment cycle times, and poor documentation. The team was in crisis, characterized by in-fighting, blaming, lack of respectful communication, and lack of commitment to program goals and objectives. I had not worked as a case manager in this program. It was hard for me to determine how to address the problems the staff presented to me. I wanted to be fair, yet felt that I did not have enough information to make immediate changes. My challenge was to lead this team to greater compliance with state-mandated performance measures.

What do you think you would do if you were this nurse?

INTRODUCTION

Problem-solving and decision-making are vital abilities for nursing practice. Not only are these processes involved in managing and delivering care but also they are essential for engaging in planned change. Myriad technologic, social, political, and economic changes have had a dramatic effect on health care and nursing. Increased patient acuity, shorter hospital stays, shortage of healthcare providers, increased technology, and the continuing shift from inpatient to ambulatory and home health care are some of the changes that require nurses to make rational and valid decisions that achieve results. Moreover, increased diversity in employment settings and types of healthcare providers demands efficient and effective decision-making and problem-solving. In addition to the focus on achieving people-oriented and cost-effective results, more emphasis is now placed on involving patients in decision-making and problem-solving and using multidisciplinary teams.

Professional nursing organizations have affirmed that competency in decision-making and problem-solving is essential to nursing practice. The reader can review select position and policy statements by referring to the Internet resources in

Table 5-1 (or conduct a search using the organization's name).

Nurses must possess the basic knowledge and skills required for effective problem-solving and decision-making. These competencies are especially important for nurses with leadership and management responsibilities.

Definitions

Problem-solving and *decision-making* are not synonymous terms. However, the processes for engaging in both behaviors are similar. Both skills require **critical-thinking**, which is a high-level cognitive process, and both can be improved with practice.

Decision-making is a purposeful and goal-directed effort that uses a systematic process to choose among options. Not all decision-making begins with a problem situation. Instead, the hallmark of decision-making is the identification and selection of options or alternatives. For example, the nurse manager of a home healthcare agency is strategizing ways to empower the nursing staff. The options under consideration include having the staff create the schedule, having them perform self-evaluations, or having them provide more input in the formulation of agency policy.

In *The Challenge*, practicing nurse leaders/managers offer their real-world views of a concern related to the chapter. Has a nurse you know had similar or dissimilar challenges?

Most chapters contain at least one *Research Perspective* or *Literature Perspective* box that you can identify by the "book" icon in the upper left corner. These boxes summarize articles of interest and point out their relevance and applicability to practice. Check the journal that the article came from to find a list of indexing terms to help you locate additional and even more recent articles on the same topic.

---

6   Part One   **Core Concepts**

Literature Perspective

Jooste, K. (2004). Leadership: a new perspective. *Journal of Nursing Management, 12,* 217-223.

In today's fast-paced, challenging, and fluid healthcare environment, nurses are in leadership roles at various levels within organizations. These nurses are impacted by many diverse influences, including professional, political, and economical forces. The role of the nurse leader is changing. The nurse leader of today needs to be a person of vision who creates a learning environment in which nurses are encouraged to manage their own activities.

Jooste has developed an "arch of leadership" (p. 220) that includes the concepts of clarity, commitment, self-image, price, and behavior as tools to identify effective leadership characteristics and aid in recognizing and resolving health-management problems. At the pillars, or ends of the arch, are the concepts of clarity and behavior. The first pillar in the arch, where everything begins, is clarity. The leader should develop a vision and ensure it is communicated to followers. Committed individuals take action and follow through to completion.

At the keystone (center) of the arch is self-image, and that involves inner leadership. Through enhanced self-awareness, understanding one's own assumptions and beliefs, taking action based on values and purpose, individuals can realize their own resources and potential. Price, more than an hourly rate or salary, has to

do with how employees are treated by management and administration. How employees perceive their value to management will in turn impact their satisfaction, loyalty, and behavior towards clients. The other pillar in the arch is the concept of behavior. A leader should develop a clear vision of the future and, by increasing followers' involvement in planning and decision-making, instill this vision in them.

There are challenges facing the nurse leader of the future. Leaders will need strong communication and negotiation skills to interact with multidisciplinary groups and informed patients. In this rapidly evolving healthcare environment, nurse leaders need to be aware of past change and anticipate future change to plan strategically and look creatively for ways to manage scarce resources, to retain staff in a time of shortages, and to maximize everyone's abilities.

IMPLICATIONS FOR PRACTICE

Nurse leaders have the opportunity to actively participate in shaping the future of health care and nursing practice using knowledge from the past and present. The future nurse leader will need new leadership skills and styles that are different from those used in the past to be successful in the environment of the future.

Think of leadership as being responsible for a ship sailing into uncharted waters that encounters unplanned and complex obstacles. The leader uses knowledge and skills from previous journeys to develop new strategies and responses to the obstacles, while inspiring the crew to engage fully in critical decision-making and draw on their own experiences, constantly re-evaluating plans to safely reach shore. Leadership should not involve coercion or manipulation of others; the constructive leader informs the followers of the goal or target to be attained so that solutions can be co-created. In the

event that leadership is misused, coercive relationships with followers form, often involving unethical decision-making and the withholding of information about the true goal to be achieved. In the scenario just presented, imagine the treacherous results of coercive leadership.

Management refers to persons holding top positions of authority (such as a Nurse Director or Chief Nursing Officer). Management here is defined as the work of any individual who guides others through a series of routines, procedure, or pre-defined practice guidelines. Management tasks are

---

Chapter 1   **Managing, Leading, and Following**   11

Theory Box—cont'd

LEADERSHIP THEORIES

THEORY/CONTRIBUTOR	KEY IDEA	APPLICATION TO PRACTICE
(1956), Stogdill (1963), and Likert (1961).	the factors in the work environment that influence outcomes.	centered leaders tend to be the leaders most able to achieve effective work environments and productivity.
Situational-Contingency Theories The situational-contingency theorists emerged in the 1960s and early to mid-1970s. These theorists believed that leadership effectiveness depends on the relationship among (1) the leader's task at hand, (2) his or her interpersonal skills, and (3) the favorableness of the work situation. Examples of theory development with this expanded perspective include Fiedler's (1967) Contingency Model, the Vroom and Yetton (1973) Normative Decision-Making Model, and House and Mitchell's (1974) Path-Goal theory.	Three factors are critical: (1) the degree of trust and respect between leaders and followers, (2) the task structure denoting the clarity of goals and the complexity of problems faced, and (3) the position power in terms of where the leader was able to reward followers and exert influence. Consequently, leaders were viewed as able to adapt their style according to the presenting situation. The Vroom-Yetton model was a problem-solving approach to leadership. Path-Goal theory recognized two contingent variables: (1) the personal characteristics of followers and (2) environmental demands. On the basis of these factors, the leader sets forth clear expectations, eliminates obstacles to goal achievements, motivates and rewards staff, and increases opportunities for follower satisfaction based on effective job performance.	The most important implications for leaders are that these theories consider the challenge of a situation and encourage an adaptive leadership style to complement the issue being faced. In other words, nurses must assess each situation and determine appropriate action based on the people involved.
Transformational Theories Transformational theories arose late in the last millennium when globalization and other factors caused organizations to fundamentally reestablish themselves. Many of these attempts were failures, but great attention was given to those leaders who effectively transformed structures, human resources, and profitability balanced with quality. Bass (1990), Bennis and Nanus (1985), and Tichy and Devanna (1986) are commonly associated with the study of transformational theory.	Transformational leadership refers to a process whereby the leader attends to the needs and motives of followers so that the interaction raises each to high levels of motivation and morality. The leader is a role model who inspires followers through displayed optimism, provides intellectual stimulation, and encourages follower creativity.	Transformed organizations are responsive to customer needs, are morally and ethically intact, promote employee development, and encourage self-management. Nurse leaders with transformational characteristics experiment with systems redesign, empower staff, create enthusiasm for practice, and promote scholarship of practice at the patient-side.

Most chapters contain a *Theory Box* to highlight and summarize pertinent theoretical concepts.

Every chapter contains numbered *Exercises* that challenge you to think critically about concepts in the text and apply them to real-life situations.

Key terms appear in boldface type throughout the chapter. (A list of all key terms used in the chapter appears at the end of the chapter, and the Glossary at the end of the text contains a list of their definitions.)

The *boxes* in every chapter highlight key information such as lists and contain forms, worksheets, and self-assessments to help reinforce chapter content.

nurse manager also can make a special effort to pair mentors and mentees who have different ethnic backgrounds. The use of a bilingual health professional interpreter can be an effective strategy when caring for non–English-speaking or limited English-speaking proficiency patients.

The current trend seems to be one of using interpreters rather than translators when speaking with non-English-speaking patients and clients. Why? Purnell and Paulanka (2003) advocate that trained healthcare providers as interpreters can decode words and provide the right meaning of the message. However, the authors also suggest being aware that interpreters might affect the reporting of symptoms, using their own ideas, or omitting information. It is important to allow time for translation and interpretation and to clarify information as needed. Purnell and Paulanka provided 21 guidelines for communicating with those who are non–English-speaking.

Exercise 8-5
During one of your group meetings, have everyone share one or two slang words that may have a different meaning for different groups of people. Following this meeting, have one in your group post a list of the words and meanings discussed in the meeting (similar to the list shown in Box 8-2). Allow everyone to continue to add slang words that patients or staff use that may create confusion or misunderstanding. Reviewing the list regularly allows staff to understand phrases and, in some instances, to gain a cultural perspective connected to the phrase.

INDIVIDUAL AND SOCIETAL FACTORS

Nurse managers must work with staff to foster respect of different lifestyles. To do this, nurse managers need to accept three key principles: **multiculturalism**, which refers to maintaining several different cultures; **cross-culturalism**, which

BOX 8-2

Slang Terms and Their Meanings

TERM	MEANING
"Circling the drain," Irish	Repeating behaviors with a downward outcome
"Pull up your socks," southern United States	Get on with it!
"Left to go up in the hollow," Appalachian	Death
"mija", Spanish	My daughter (from "mihija")
"I feel you," U.S. black	I sympathize with you
"Chill out; chillin," U.S. black	Relax; down time
"Running off," Appalachian	Diarrhea
"High blood," Appalachian	Hypertension
"Birds don't marry fishes," Japanese mother	Don't marry outside your race
"It's a disaster," various cultures	Chaos
"Fighting the fire within," white	Anger, hostility
"Lip lard," southern United States	Lipstick
"Lets leg it," England	Move on, walk faster
"Getting a husband is like catching a cold," common Ethiopian saying	Expected norm that every woman will get married at some point in her life
"Bakwas," India	Nonsense talk
"Vomiting the heart out and dripping the blood dry," Chinese	Making the ultimate sacrifice for a cause
"Puti," Philippines	White American
"Too little jam to spread over too much bread," United States	Not enough time, too many tasks
"Nip it in the bud", United States	Admonishment without embarrassment to keep information confidential
"On the down ramp of life," American	Aging and in decline

Others would identify collaboration, especially with other departments, to enhance quality patient outcomes. Truly effective care is the result of efforts by the total healthcare team. Effective collaboration includes honesty, directness, and listening to others' points of view. However, management is more complex than this.

THE MANAGEMENT ROLE

Management is a generic function that includes similar basic tasks in every discipline and in every society. However, before the nurse manager can be effective, he or she must be well-grounded in nursing practice. Drucker (1974), in his classic writings, identified five basic functions of a manager:

- Establishes objectives and goals for each area and communicates them to the persons who are responsible for attaining them
- Organizes and analyzes the activities, decisions, and relations needed and divides them into manageable tasks
- Motivates and communicates with the people responsible for various jobs through teamwork
- Analyzes, appraises, and interprets performance and communicates the meaning of measurement tools and their results to staff and superiors
- Develops people, including self

Table 3-1 shows how these basic management functions apply to the nurse manager.

Managers develop efforts that focus on the individual. Their aim is to enable the person to develop his or her abilities and strengths to the fullest and to achieve excellence. Thus, a manager has a role in helping people develop goals that are realistic. Goals should be set high enough, yet be attainable. Active participation, encouragement, and guidance from the manager and from the organization are needed for the individual's developmental efforts to be fully productive. Nurse managers who are successful in motivating staff are often providing an environment that facilitates accomplishment of goals, resulting in personal satisfactions.

The nurse manager must possess qualities similar to those of a good leader: knowledge, integrity, ambition, judgment, courage, stamina, enthusiasm, communication skills, planning skills, and administrative abilities. The arena of management versus leadership has been addressed by numerous authors, and although there are differences in points of view, there are some similarities between managers and leaders.

Managers address complex issues by planning, budgeting, and setting target goals. They meet their goals by organizing, staffing, controlling, and solving problems. By contrast, **leaders** set a direc-

Table 3-1 BASIC MANAGER FUNCTIONS AND NURSE MANAGER FUNCTIONS

Basic Manager Functions	Nurse Manager Functions
Establishes and communicates goals and objectives	Delineates objectives and goals for assigned area Communicates objectives and goals effectively to staff members who will help attain goals
Organizes, analyzes, and divides work into tasks	Assesses and evaluates activities on assigned area Makes sound decisions about dividing up daily work activities for staff
Motivates and communicates	Stresses the importance of being a good team player Provides positive reinforcement
Analyzes, appraises, and interprets performance and measurements	Completes performance appraisals of individual staff members Communicates results to staff and management
Develops people, including self	Addresses staff development continuously through mentoring and preceptorships Furthers self-development by attending educational programs and seeking specialty certification credentialing

Based on Drucker, P. F. (1974). *Management tasks, responsibilities and practices*. New York: Harper & Row.

The *tables* that appear throughout the text provide convenient capsules of information for your reference.

The numerous full-color *illustrations* visually reinforce key concepts.

Each chapter ends with these features:

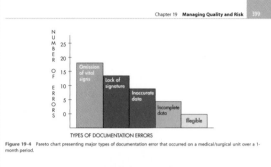

Figure 19-4 Pareto chart presenting major types of documentation error that occurred on a medical/surgical unit over a 1-month period.

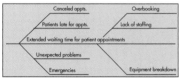

Figure 19-5 Fishbone diagram showing possible causes of extended waiting time for clinic patients.

quality of outcomes is to compare one agency's performance against that of similar organizations. In a process called **benchmarking**, a widespread search is conducted to identify the best performance against which to measure others. Through this process of comparing the best practices against your practice and process, your organization learns to identify desired standards of quality performance. Available data include all reported hospital-acquired infection rates in other institutions as well as specific data, such as postoperative infection rates in adult surgical intensive-care units of similar-size institutions. However, recent mandates in select states to publicly disclose nosocomial infection rates highlight potential issues with disclosure

of data. Specifically, simply reporting hospital infection rates is not enough to promote hand-hygiene practices and may do little to improve outcomes and reduce hospital-acquired infections. Unfortunately, the usefulness of the information from other institutions continues to be hampered by differences in terminology. Information technology plays a vital role in QI by increasing the efficiency of data entry and analysis. A consistent information system that trends high-risk procedures and systematic errors would provide a useful database regarding outcomes of care and resource allocation. The purpose of the National Quality Forum is designed to standardize measures so that true comparisons can be made.

The Solution

In a previous job, I had used multidisciplinary process improvement teams (PITs), which consisted of key stakeholders, to initiate process improvement. I chose to give this concept a try in this setting. Our team consisted of the Public Health Nurse (PHN) case managers, the CCS case workers, the billing and claims staff, the CCS Medical Director, clerical and support staff, and myself. I believed that a group approach to these problems would yield the most information and gain the greatest support for any changes that would be made. The team met weekly for an hour. We began by identifying our customers and key stakeholders and their expectations. This was extensive and took a few months to complete. Key stakeholders included the clients (children) and their parents, the providers (physicians and hospitals), pharmacies, vendors, schools, other insurance plans, the tax payers (in the form of the State and County), our own team members, and other agencies. The expectations for each stakeholder were listed, discussed for clarity, and recorded. During this exercise, the team learned a great deal about each person's job duties (there were a few surprises) and about the effect each person's job had on other team members' ability to do their job. As the team began understanding each person's job and issues, they focused less on blaming and more on how to change our processes.

Next, the team brainstormed (divergent thinking) a list of issues. The numerous issues were then grouped according to similarity, and duplicates were eliminated. Multivoting was then used to determine the three highest-priority issues. Our number one problem related to cycle time. When a client is referred to CCS, determination of eligibility, opening (or denying) the case, and authorizing care are key cycles. Patient care is often coordinated based on the client's eligibility, and delays in service can result when the process is not completed in a timely manner. The reasons for our failure to meet these deadlines seemed overwhelming and confusing. We needed a method to find the root-causes to improve our performance. We chose to use a fishbone diagram, also known as a cause-and-effect diagram (Figure 5-4). Our problem was "New referrals are not completed within 45 days." We categorized our known barriers on

the four "bones" of the fish, manpower, methods, machines, and materials. Once we had identified the factors contributing to our problem, we prioritized them and generated action plans for each major factor. These action plans were extensive and involved implementing training and education programs, re-designing work space for greater efficiency, purchasing more equipment, revising job descriptions, increasing provider outreach activities, and more. Performance data did not improve during the initial year of our PIT, and I chose not to share it with staff to avoid demoralizing them. My management team and I were taking a leap of faith that our process would eventually result in the desired outcome of meeting the performance metrics.

It took 18 months for CCS to "turn the curve," but once improvement started, it was exponential. The cycle time measure for "referral to case open" was initially 57 days. Two years later, it was 30 days. The cycle time "referral to deny" began at 97 days, and 2 years later was down to 39 days. Most importantly, the cycle time "referral to first authorization" decreased from an initial 189 days to just 49 days! It was at this time that I shared the outcome data with the team. They were ecstatic! I asked the team to list the problems they believed we had solved through our PIT's efforts. They listed (1) improved staffing, (2) increased staff morale and decreased turnover (all the positions were now filled), (3) better understanding of the job expectations and the rationale behind those expectations, (4) improved teamwork, and (5) more efficient and effective work space. They have maintained enthusiastic support of the PIT, and participation remains high. The team is still highly focused on problem-solving. I have learned that when assuming leadership of a department in which one has no prior experience, a structured team approach to information gathering, assessment of data, identification of problems, and implementation of action plans can be highly effective in the resolution of priority problems.

— Vickie Lemmon

 Would this be a suitable approach for you? Why?

The Solution provides an effective method to handle the situations presented in The Challenge.

The *Chapter Checklist* provides a quick summary of key points in the chapter. To help you keep in mind the broad themes of the chapter, read it immediately *before* you start reading the chapter.

The *Tips* offer guidelines to follow for each chapter before applying the information presented in the chapter.

The *Terms to Know* in every chapter include all the key terms used in that chapter. You might find it helpful to review this list before reading the chapter and to look up in the Glossary any definitions that are unfamiliar.

Chapter 14   Selecting, Developing, and Evaluating Staff   **301**

CHAPTER CHECKLIST

The manager plays a key role in the selection and development of staff. As a role model, the manager is also key in the establishment of the type of work environment that exists. Managers must be supportive and develop their staff to their highest potential. They must have accurate position descriptions and tools for evaluation of employee performance. These are integral to role development and professional socialization. Managers must also use various communication methods to empower their employees. Coaching and implementation of empowerment strategies positively contribute to overall staff performance as well.

- The interviewer should do the following:
  - Prescreen the applicants.
  - Prepare questions in advance.
  - Control the environment.
  - Provide role clarification.
  - Be a good listener.
  - Give honest answers to questions.
  - Provide closure.
  - Inform the applicant when he or she will be notified.
- The applicant should do the following:
  - Be on time and dressed appropriately.
  - Review the organization's mission and goals.
  - Prepare questions in advance.
  - Answer questions honestly and completely.
  - Note appreciation for the interview.
- Development of the staff includes the following:
  - Organized and efficient orientation
  - Plans for education, team building, and professional socialization

  - Active coaching
  - Implementation of empowerment strategies
- Development of accurate position descriptions and tools for evaluation of employees is integral to role development and professional socialization. Nurse managers should use various communication methods, including coaching techniques.
- Role theory describes how individuals perceive their position in an organization.
- Distinction and clarity among the various positions are imperative if partnerships in quality patient care are to exist.
  - The position description serves several purposes:
    - Provides written guidelines that describe roles and responsibilities
    - Reflects the position's overall function and obligations
    - Serves as a contract between manager and employee
    - Reflects current practice guidelines for the position
- Performance appraisals are a method of providing feedback to the employee in relation to individual performance.
  - Types of structured (traditional) performance appraisals include the following:
    - Forced distribution method
    - Graphic rating scales
    - Rating scale
  - Types of flexible (collaborative) performance appraisals include the following:
    - Behaviorally anchored rating scales (BARS)
    - Management by objective (MBO)
    - Peer review

TIPS FOR CONDUCTING AN INTERVIEW

- Prescreen the applicant and schedule a time for the interview.
- Prepare questions in advance. Be concise but thorough.
- Control the environment for noise and interruptions.
- Explain and clarify the role for which the applicant is interviewing.
- Be a good listener.
- Answer questions honestly.

- Inform the applicant when he or she will be informed of the decision.

TERMS TO KNOW

coaching
empowerment
halo or recent behavior bias effect
horn effect
performance appraisal
position description
role ambiguity
role conflict
role theory

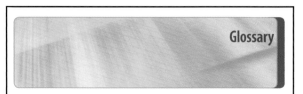

Glossary

Absenteeism The rate at which an individual misses work on an unplanned basis. (Ch. 24)

Accommodation An unassertive, cooperative approach to conflict in which the individual neglects personal needs, goals, and concerns in favor of satisfying those of others. (Ch. 22)

Accountability The expectation of explaining actions and results. (Ch. 23)

Accreditation Process by which an authoritative body determines that an organization meets certain standards to such a degree that the organization is able to meet the standards as a whole and without ongoing monitoring of each aspect of performance. (Ch. 6)

Acknowledgment Recognition that an employee is valued and respected for what he or she has to offer to the workplace, team, or group; acknowledgments may be verbal or written, public or private. (Ch. 17)

Active listening Focusing completely on the speaker and listening without judgment to the essence of the conversation; an active listener should be able to repeat accurately at least 95% of the speaker's intended meaning. (Ch. 17)

Activity or productivity report A report typically including units of service provided, number of beds, number of occupied beds, number of patients typically cared for per day, and average length of stay. (Ch. 13)

Advocate One who proactively speaks for another to ensure certain needs or wishes are met. (Ch. 21)

Agenda A written list of items to be covered in a meeting and the related materials that meeting participants should read beforehand or bring along. Types of agendas include structured

agendas, timed agendas, and action agendas. (Ch. 26)

Allocation of scarce resources Distribution of resources needed for care but which may exceed budget levels. (Ch. 22)

Apparent agency Doctrine whereby a principal becomes accountable for the actions of his or her agent; created when a person holds himself or herself out as acting on behalf of the principal; also known as *apparent authority.* (Ch. 4)

Associate nurse A licensed nurse in the primary care model who provides care to the patient according to the primary nurse's specification when the primary nurse is not working. (Ch. 12)

At-will employee An individual who works without a contract. (Ch. 18)

Autocratic An authoritarian style that places control within one person's position. (Ch. 5)

Autonomy Personal freedom and the right to choose what will happen to one's own person. (Ch. 4)

Average daily census (ADC) Average number of patients cared for per day for a reporting period. (Ch. 13)

Average length of stay The number of patient days in a specific time period divided by the number of discharges in that same time period. (Ch. 13)

Avoiding An unassertive, uncooperative approach to conflict in which the avoider neither pursues his or her own needs, goals, and concerns nor helps others to do so. (Ch. 22)

Bar coding systems/bar code technology Systems that encode data electronically into a format of bars and spaces that represents letters or numbers. (Ch. 10)

(599)

The *Glossary* at the end of the text lists alphabetically all the boldfaced terms from the chapters.

The *Application Activities* are a built-in, perforated tool to help you self-assess and evaluate your learning and understanding of the content in the text.

CHAPTER 16 APPLICATION ACTIVITY

Leading Change

INTRODUCTION

This section contains one application activity that asks students to propose a plan for an actual or hypothetical change in a nursing situation. Guidelines and a sample plan will guide the development of the plan. The best outcome for this activity is for students to implement their plans in actual healthcare organizations. The ultimate outcome is the development of effective change management skills by further enhancing students' conceptual foundations about roles and approaches in leading change.

ACTIVITY 16-1

The use of planned change models for less complex, low-level change can be effective. Most organizational change, however, takes place in groups, units, and departments responsive to influences outside and inside (open system). Thus, managing the influencing factors of a change situation in conjunction with a plan's elements for the change can lead to creative results.

Using the guidelines for planning a change, the change planning worksheet, and the sample of a plan for a hypothetical change, develop a plan for a change. Select a change situation, either an actual or a hypothetical one, and follow the problem-solving format of the planning worksheet to (1) assess the change situation, (2) develop an activity plan for implementation supported by sound change theories and principles, and (3) decide on methods to evaluate the change process and outcomes. The activity plan should reflect several potentially feasible outcome scenarios to work toward and specifically identified resources, timelines, responsible parties, and strategies to achieve each outcome. Discuss your proposed plan with your peers, instructors, and individuals in the change situation.

The following worksheet provides a general framework for planning low-level change. The worksheet headings and sections outline essential points to consider. The guidelines explain the completion of the worksheet section by section.

Guidelines
Section I: Situational Assessment and Analysis

Developing an appropriate plan for a change requires an accurate assessment of the situation needing the change. Effective assessment results in accurate identification of the key elements operating in the situation, not to be confused with symptoms of the need. The elements may be human, technological, system, or other. The need may be a problem needing resolution, a need requiring innovative action, or a measure improving quality.
Part A
Describe the actual situation needing change, naming and briefly describing the who, what, when, where, why, and how elements.

Contents

Part 3: Changing the Status Quo

Part 4: Interpersonal and Personal Skills

Part 1

Core Concepts

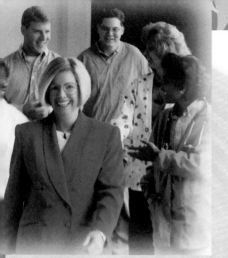

Chapter

1

Managing, Leading, and Following

Michael R. Bleich

Colleen P. Kosiak

*L*eading, managing, and following are integral parts of professional nursing practice. Constructive behaviors associated with these concepts influence patient care and organizational outcomes, regardless of position title. By examining self-motivation and confidence in relation to power, authority, influence, decision-making, conflict, and change, the professional nurse can enhance his/her skill and ability to lead, manage, and follow with meaning and purpose.

Objectives

- Relate leadership and other organizational theories to behaviors that serve as important functions of professional nursing.
- Examine how self-knowledge and emotional intelligence affect an appreciation of power, influence, and authority needed in professional nursing practice.
- Develop strength in those personal attributes needed to effectively lead, manage, and follow.
- Apply effective leading, managing, and following behaviors to change and conflict situations encountered when delivering patient care.

- Demonstrate decision-making when leading, managing, and following in complex clinical settings.

Questions to Consider

- *Do you consider leading, managing, and following behaviors critical to patient, family, peer, and professional perceptions of your capabilities as a professional nurse?*
- *How does effective followership promote successful leadership and management?*
- *What cultural and life experiences influence the lens through which you view power, influence, and authority? What experiences influence how you view leading, managing, and following?*
- *Which experiences influence how you deal with complex decision-making, such as that related to conflict and change management?*
- *How can traditional and emerging leadership, management, and organizational theories guide your professional practice?*

The Challenge

Paula L. Hibbard, BSN, MS
Nurse Manager, Children's Mercy Hospital, Kansas City, Missouri

For a charge nurse in a pediatric hospital, working with the families of patients is integral to achieving patient outcomes. Not only must we provide care and support for our pediatric patients, we must also embrace the child's family and its needs as a unit. As a nurse manager, I take responsibility to support the care-provider staff, who, in turn, diligently address physiologic, emotional, social, and spiritual problems for patients and those in the patients' family networks.

One morning, when getting report from the night charge nurse, a volatile family interaction was brought to my attention regarding patient placement on our unit and subsequent care concerns. This patient was well known to the staff from frequent inpatient and out-patient admissions to the hospital. During report, the information exchanged was not specific: the family was upset when the patient was admitted postoperatively to our unit, and the night surgical resident had listened to these family's concerns.

To investigate, I first spoke with the patient's day shift nurse, who confirmed receiving the same report from the night nurse. Then, when rounding with the surgical team, I communicated to the senior resident and staff the family's frustration regarding the admission and care concerns.

As the team entered the patient's room, the father was visibly upset and defensive. "After surgery last evening our family requested that (our child) be admitted to the unit where he usually stays when he is hospitalized. The staff on that unit knows us well and is knowledgeable about (our child)." The challenge was that our unit staff had expertise in doing the specialized post-surgical assessments and interventions required for this child, yet the patient and family had vested trust and security in the staff on the other unit. Hospital patient placement guidelines had been followed in placing this patient on our unit. The senior resident responded to the father stating that the issues were nursing related and did not involve the surgical team.

 What do you think you would do if you were this nurse?

INTRODUCTION

Too often, nurses who are new to the profession believe that their skill and ability in performing clinical procedures are what make them appear professional to those receiving care, to their peers, or to the public. They may believe that leading and managing is left to those who hold management positions or that being a follower means blindly adhering to the direction of others. Many nurses fail to realize that their professional nursing image and success are equally dependent on effective leading, managing, and following actions. These behaviors are the first lens through which patients, families, co-workers, supervisors and other professionals view them and gain confidence in their abilities. In all clinical settings, it is an expectation that effective leadership, management, and followership will be incorporated into practice to contribute to the healthcare team. Furthermore, nurses must be able to shift easily among these roles within moments when necessary. Examples of these behaviors are presented later in this chapter.

Many organizations face the challenge of making the best use of scarce nursing resources. Professional nurses are expected to hone the skills aligned with leading, managing, and following to meet the organization's mission and goals, including averting medical errors, achieving patient satisfaction, and promoting positive patient outcomes. In addition, organizations expect professional nurses to contain costs when delivering or overseeing patient care, contribute to quality improvement and other change initiatives, and engage in high-level interactions with other healthcare team members to resolve clinical and organizational problems.

In this chapter and in Chapters 2 and 3, various perspectives of the concepts of leading (leadership), managing (management), and following (follower-ship) are presented. There is overlap in these concepts, meaning that a nurse must lead, manage, and follow concurrently! In this chapter, we highlight the distinctiveness of each concept separately for ease of understanding the differences.

In health care, **leadership** can be defined as the use of individual traits and personal power to interact constructively with patients experiencing complex clinical problems for which there are no standardized solutions and to guide interdisciplinary healthcare providers in strategy development to resolve these problems. In partnership, a broad end-point vision or goal is agreed upon. To achieve the goals, steps to implement the strategy are created, with the knowledge that these steps often require adaptation along the way as new knowledge emerges. The nurse leader builds relationships to empower others to set and achieve clinical or organizational goals. Effective leaders communicate direction, use principles to guide the process, and project an air of self-assuredness. These leadership traits evoke security in those associated with the task at hand, which, in turn, fosters reasonable risk-taking (see the Research and Literature Perspectives).

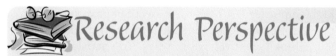

Research Perspective

Upenieks, V. (2003). Nurse leaders' perceptions of what compromises successful leadership in today's acute inpatient environment. *Nursing Administration Quarterly, 27,* 140-152.

Magnet™ hospitals have been recognized for excellence in nursing based on the hospital's unique organizational characteristics. The positive nursing environment of Magnet hospitals is one created by nursing leaders (Lewis & Matthews, 1998). In discussion with nurse leaders Wood Allen (1998) identified five factors that influence leadership development: personal life factors, self-confidence, influence of significant people, progression of experiences and success, and innate leader qualities and tendencies.

Using Kanter's Structural Theory of Organizational Behavior as a conceptual framework, Upenieks (2003) interviewed 16 nurse leaders (nine from nonmagnet hospitals and seven from Magnet institutions) to explore successful nursing leadership in the current healthcare setting. The finding from this study supported Kanter's Theory of Organizational Behavior with nurse leaders, which indicates that access to empowerment structures produced a positive climate. Nurse leader effectiveness was thought to be influenced by (1) nursing administration leadership characteristics of visibility, responsiveness, passion for nursing, and business astuteness; (2) an organizational culture that is supportive and committed to the professional qualities and expertise of nurses; (3) teamwork among nurses and healthcare employees that is collaborative and respectful; and (4) compensation. A majority of those interviewed believed that nurse leaders who have growth opportunities derived from new challenges, information and resource access, and formal and informal power will be successful in attaining professional goals and enhancement.

IMPLICATIONS FOR PRACTICE

Through open communication that increases nurses' access to information and knowledge at the organizational level, nurse leaders are in key positions to provide nurses with opportunities to participate in decision-making at various levels within the organization. They must be innovative and knowledgeable about business practices in today's financially constrained healthcare environment to effectively secure adequate compensation for nurses and the adequate supplies necessary to achieve optimal professional performance.

Literature Perspective

Jooste, K. (2004). Leadership: a new perspective. *Journal of Nursing Management, 12,* 217-223.

In today's fast-paced, challenging, and fluid healthcare environment, nurses are in leadership roles at various levels within organizations. These nurses are impacted by many diverse influences, including professional, political, and economical forces. The role of the nurse leader is changing. The nurse leader of today needs to be a person of vision who creates a learning environment in which nurses are encouraged to manage their own activities.

Jooste has developed an "arch of leadership" (p. 220) that includes the concepts of clarity, commitment, self-image, price, and behavior as tools to identify effective leadership characteristics and aid in recognizing and resolving health-management problems. At the pillars, or ends of the arch, are the concepts of clarity and behavior. The first pillar in the arch, where everything begins, is clarity. The leader should develop a vision and ensure it is communicated to followers. Committed individuals take action and follow through to completion.

At the keystone (center) of the arch is self-image, and that involves inner leadership. Through enhanced self-awareness, understanding one's own assumptions and beliefs, taking action based on values and purpose, individuals can realize their own resources and potential. Price, more than an hourly rate or salary, has to do with how employees are treated by management and administration. How employees perceive their value to management will in turn impact their satisfaction, loyalty, and behavior towards clients. The other pillar in the arch is the concept of behavior. A leader should develop a clear vision of the future and, by increasing followers' involvement in planning and decision-making, instill this vision in them.

There are challenges facing the nurse leader of the future. Leaders will need strong communication and negotiation skills to interact with multidisciplinary groups and informed patients. In this rapidly evolving healthcare environment, nurse leaders need to be aware of past change and anticipate future change to plan strategically and look creatively for ways to manage scarce resources, to retain staff in a time of shortages, and to maximize everyone's abilities.

IMPLICATIONS FOR PRACTICE

Nurse leaders have the opportunity to actively participate in shaping the future of health care and nursing practice using knowledge from the past and present. The future nurse leader will need new leadership skills and styles that are different from those used in the past to be successful in the environment of the future.

Think of leadership as being responsible for a ship sailing into uncharted waters that encounters unplanned and complex obstacles. The leader uses knowledge and skills from previous journeys to develop new strategies and responses to the obstacles, while inspiring the crew to engage fully in critical decision-making and draw on their own experiences, constantly re-evaluating plans to safely reach shore. Leadership should not involve coercion or manipulation of others; the constructive leader informs the followers of the goal or target to be attained so that solutions can be co-created. In the event that leadership is misused, coercive relationships with followers form, often involving unethical decision-making and the withholding of information about the true goal to be achieved. In the scenario just presented, imagine the treacherous results of coercive leadership.

Management refers to persons holding top positions of authority (such as a Nurse Director or Chief Nursing Officer). Management here is defined as the work of any individual who guides others through a series of routines, procedure, or predefined practice guidelines. Management tasks are afforded to any staff member who shares the responsibility for the work of others and who has the accountability to ensure that these practices are carried out. Seeing that actions are carried out in a predetermined time frame (such as those associated with medication administration or other time-sensitive procedures) is a challenging management task! Patient-side nurses are very much managers in the context just described.

Management differs from leadership in that the behaviors and activities required occur in patient situations with less ambiguity; the outcomes are generally known and a sequence of actions to achieve outcomes is prescribed, either in writing or through historical practices that are embedded in the organization's culture. This does not mean that clinical management is simple or does not require professional judgments, because the actions required may involve complex judgments and skills in performing high-risk interventions from which to choose courses of action. The activities to be carried out have a different type of decision structure, but they are just as important.

To summarize, management tasks are used by all nurses to guide and promote interactions with care providers who follow critical paths, algorithms, or clinical protocols to meet patient and family care expectations. In this context, management involves the use of power to expediently guide task attainment known to be necessary for clinical and organizational success (such as in assignment making, medication administration and evaluation, and interdisciplinary discharge planning). In management, a set of best-practice/evidence-based norms is introduced, made known to others, and used to accomplish goals.

Followership is defined as a complementary set of actions taken by individuals that contribute to problem-solving, task attainment, and evaluation using healthy and assertive behaviors to support those who are leading (forging into unknown, complex problem-solving) or managing (adhering to predetermined actions to achieve outcomes). The dynamic interplay between leaders, managers, and followers (often a single individual carrying out one or more of these roles) creates a culture that contributes to patient, family, and healthcare team achievement. Followers promote clinical and organizational outcomes while practicing acquiescence to individuals leading or managing the team over certain tasks, such as direction setting, politicking, pacesetting, or planning. Followership is not a passive process, but rather a set of behaviors that demonstrates collaboration, influence, and action with the leader.

Together, the behaviors that reflect leading, managing, and following enhance each other. All interdisciplinary healthcare providers, including professional nurses, experience situations in which they will lead, manage, and follow. Some positions, such as charge nurse or nurse manager, are formal positions requiring advanced leading and managing behaviors to establish organizational goals and objectives, oversee human resources, provide staff with performance feedback, facilitate change, and manage conflict to meet patient care and organizational requirements. In other positions, the role itself demands shifting between leading, managing, and following, almost on a moment by moment basis. For instance, nurses lead, manage, and follow in daily clinical practice through assignment making, patient and family problem-solving, discharge planning, patient education, and coaching and mentoring staff.

Exercise 1–1

Using the definitions of leadership, management, and followership, imagine that you are faced with a critically ill patient whose family members are spread throughout the country. Some family members are holding vigil at the patient-side, while others are calling the patient care unit incessantly taking time away from other patient care responsibilities. You recognize the family's care and concern, yet you want to move out of a reactive stance to take a proactive position. How would you solve this problem as a leader? A manager? A follower? In which role are you most comfortable? Least comfortable? Which role leads to the best outcome for all parties?

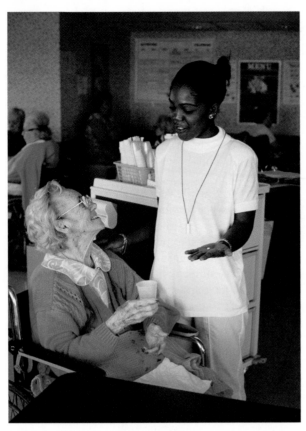

Many nurse leaders are motivated by a strong desire to care for those who cannot care for themselves.

- Having self-awareness (the ability to step outside and see oneself in the context of what is happening while recognizing and owning feelings associated with an event)
- Managing emotions (naming, claiming, and taming feelings such as fear, anxiety, anger, and sadness and taking appropriate actions to progress through feelings in a healthy manner; avoiding passive-aggressive and victim responses)
- Motivating oneself (focusing on a goal, often with delayed gratification, such that emotional self-control is achieved and impulses are stifled)
- Being empathetic (valuing differences in perspective and showing sensitivity to the experiences of others in a way that demonstrates ability to reveal another's perspective on a situation)
- Handling relationships (exhibiting social appropriateness and using social skills to help others manage emotions)

Emotionally intelligent nurses have credibility as leaders, managers, and followers because they possess awareness of patient, family, and organizational needs, have an ability to collaborate, show insight into others, and commit to self-growth. When coupled with performing clinical tasks and critical thinking, the emotionally intelligent nurse demonstrates expanded capabilities. The synergy associated with credibility and capability fuse to become markers of professional nursing. Without self-reflective skills, growth in emotional intelligence is stymied, work becomes routinized, and a nurse can experience a lack of synchrony with others. Box 1-1 is a composite of the attributes that add to the credibility and capability of nurses to lead, manage, and follow.

PERSONAL ATTRIBUTES NEEDED TO LEAD, MANAGE, AND FOLLOW

Leading, managing, and following require different skills from those associated with the technical aspects of nursing. Goleman (1995) and others refer to **emotional intelligence**—that is, possessing social skills, interpersonal competence, psychological maturity, and emotional awareness such that these skills then "help people harmonize" and become "increasingly valued in the workplace" (p. 160). Nurses have countless interactions within the course of a workday. In each interaction, leaders, managers, and followers should use and hone the development of their abilities within five domains associated with being an emotionally intelligent practitioner. The domains address:

Exercise 1-2

Referring back to Exercise 1-1, how would a nurse with highly developed emotional intelligence lead, manage, or follow in reference to problem-solving? Emotional intelligence is developed through insight into one's self, positive "self-talk," journal recording, and other methods that promote awareness of situations, biases, and the like. Develop a personal recipe for enhancing your own emotional intelligence.

BOX 1-1

Attributes of Leaders and Managers

Use focused energy and stamina to accomplish a vision

Use critical-thinking skills in decision-making

Trust personal intuition, then back up intuition with facts

Accept responsibility willingly and follow up on the consequences of actions taken

Identify the needs of others

Deal with people skillfully: coaches, communicates, counsels

Demonstrate ease in standard/boundary setting

Examine multiple options to accomplish the objective at hand flexibly

Are trustworthy and handle information from various sources with respect for the source

Motivate others assertively toward the objective at hand

Demonstrate competence or are capable of rapid learning in the arena where change is desired

THEORY DEVELOPMENT IN LEADING, MANAGING, AND FOLLOWING

Theory has several important functions for the nursing profession. First, theory can help address important questions for which answers are needed. Second, theory (and the expanding array of research methods available to researchers) adds to evidenced-based care and management practices (Goode, 2004). Third, theory directs and sharpens the ability to predict or guide clinical and organizational problem-solving and outcomes. Nurses often have less exposure to organizational theories than clinical theories. Leadership, management, and organizational theories are still evolving as the complexity of healthcare organizations grow and the variables that influence care delivery increase and become more apparent. Unfortunately, a single universal theory to guide all organizational and human interactions does not exist. Theory development plays an important role in health care today, where constant interplay exists among workforce supply, consumer/patient demand, healthcare economics, workforce planning, work environment, research and data support, technology, workforce development, and leadership (Bleich, Hewlett, Santos, Rice, Cox, & Richmeier, 2003).

Theory development associated with leading, managing, and following concepts has been a process of testing, discarding, expanding, creating, and applying. These theories overlap. Terms such

as leadership theory, transformational leadership, servant leadership, management theory, motivational theory, and even attempts at followership theories are inter-related and cannot be categorized in any mutually exclusive manner. Developing theories for leading, managing, and following is a complicated task. Furthermore, the theories that leaders, managers, and followers use are drawn from yet another set of theories, many addressed in this book. These include: change theory, conflict theory, economic theory, clinical theories, individual and group interaction theories, communication theories, and many more.

The development of leadership, motivation, and management theory rapidly evolved at the beginning of the 20th century when people moved in masses to industries that were aimed at mass production. As the population shifted from agricultural communities to urban manufacturing environments, the factors that promoted efficient production were studied. Leadership theory grew by the examination of the influence of charismatic leaders on the workforce, followed by the uncovering of the motivational factors that supported worker job satisfaction and, later, the environmental determinants that contributed to or deterred workers from achieving production quotas (note that the theories developed in manufacturing industries were then applied to other nonmanufacturing settings).

Leadership theory developed as a system of knowledge to extrapolate the traits and behaviors of leaders who were considered to be successful at influencing situations, people, and events to attain organizational goals, especially productivity. Leadership theory was first studied by sociologists and psychologists. It is readily apparent today that leadership is a process of interacting with others, and, therefore, motivational theories naturally overlapped with leadership theory. Motivational theories were attempts to explain how nonmanagement workers sustained behaviors to accomplish goals, or how leaders and corresponding environmental factors influenced worker productivity. Motivational theories were developed primarily by psychologists.

Management theory comprised the body of knowledge that describes how managers should conduct themselves to keep an organization operating effectively. Management theory encompassed variables such as how work is organized, planning is accomplished, change is managed, and production quotas are determined. Because of the diverse nature of activities that contribute to management theory development, representatives from a broad range of disciplines, including managers, psychologists, sociologists, and anthropologists, have contributed to its development.

Again, leadership, motivational, management, and other related organizational theories overlap, although they are often presented as distinctive, depending on the discipline of the theorist. Regardless, each area of theory development continues to evolve, incorporating new knowledge about organizational culture; structure and function; motivation; learning and development; team functioning; and other contemporary factors, such as globalization, diversity, generational differences, and gender equity.

The Theory Boxes in this chapter are organized as an overview to highlight two sets of theoretical work that are commonly referenced: leadership theories (including management and followership concepts) and motivational theories (because of the magnitude of research that explored human behavior and reward structures). Note in the tables that as more disciplines embraced leadership and management theory development that other theories have grown increasingly rich and multidimensional. The complex factors associated with clinical care and organizational functioning explain why no single theory fully addresses the totality of leading, managing, and following.

Theory Box

LEADERSHIP THEORIES

THEORY/CONTRIBUTOR	KEY IDEA	APPLICATION TO PRACTICE
Trait Theories Trait theories were first studied from 1900 to 1950. These theories are sometimes referred to as the Great Man theory, from Aristotle's philosophy extolling the virtue of being "born" with leadership traits. Stogdill (1948) is usually credited as the pioneer in this school of thought.	Leaders have a certain set of physical and emotional characteristics that are crucial for inspiring others toward a common goal. Some theorists believe that traits are innate and cannot be learned; others believe that leadership traits can be developed in each individual.	Self-awareness of traits is useful in self-development (e.g., developing assertiveness) and in seeking employment that matches traits (drive, motivation, integrity, confidence, cognitive ability, and task knowledge).
Style Theories Sometimes referred to as group and exchange theories of leadership, style theories were derived in the mid-1950s because of the limitations of trait theory. The key contributors to this renowned research were Shartle	Style theories focus on what leaders do in relational and contextual terms. The achievement of satisfactory performance measures requires supervisors to pursue effective relationships with their subordinates, while comprehending	To understand "style," it is useful to obtain feedback from followers, superiors, and peers, such as through the Managerial Grid Instrument developed by Blake and Mouton (1985). Employee-

Theory Box—cont'd

LEADERSHIP THEORIES

THEORY/CONTRIBUTOR	KEY IDEA	APPLICATION TO PRACTICE
(1956), Stogdill (1963), and Likert (1961).	the factors in the work environment that influence outcomes.	centered leaders tend to be the leaders most able to achieve effective work environments and productivity.
Situational-Contingency Theories The situational-contingency theorists emerged in the 1960s and early to mid-1970s. These theorists believed that leadership effectiveness depends on the relationship among (1) the leader's task at hand, (2) his or her interpersonal skills, and (3) the favorableness of the work situation. Examples of theory development with this expanded perspective include Fiedler's (1967) Contingency Model, the Vroom and Yetton (1973) Normative Decision-Making Model, and House and Mitchell's (1974) Path-Goal theory.	Three factors are critical: (1) the degree of trust and respect between leaders and followers, (2) the task structure denoting the clarity of goals and the complexity of problems faced, and (3) the position power in terms of where the leader was able to reward followers and exert influence. Consequently, leaders were viewed as able to adapt their style according to the presenting situation. The Vroom-Yetton model was a problem-solving approach to leadership. Path-Goal theory recognized two contingent variables: (1) the personal characteristics of followers and (2) environmental demands. On the basis of these factors, the leader sets forth clear expectations, eliminates obstacles to goal achievements, motivates and rewards staff, and increases opportunities for follower satisfaction based on effective job performance.	The most important implications for leaders are that these theories consider the challenge of a situation and encourage an adaptive leadership style to complement the issue being faced. In other words, nurses must assess each situation and determine appropriate action based on the people involved.
Transformational Theories Transformational theories arose late in the last millennium when globalization and other factors caused organizations to fundamentally reestablish themselves. Many of these attempts were failures, but great attention was given to those leaders who effectively transformed structures, human resources, and profitability balanced with quality. Bass (1990), Bennis and Nanus (1985), and Tichy and Devanna (1986) are commonly associated with the study of transformational theory.	Transformational leadership refers to a process whereby the leader attends to the needs and motives of followers so that the interaction raises each to high levels of motivation and morality. The leader is a role model who inspires followers through displayed optimism, provides intellectual stimulation, and encourages follower creativity.	Transformed organizations are responsive to customer needs, are morally and ethically intact, promote employee development, and encourage self-management. Nurse leaders with transformational characteristics experiment with systems redesign, empower staff, create enthusiasm for practice, and promote scholarship of practice at the patient-side.

Theory Box

MOTIVATIONAL THEORIES

THEORY/CONTRIBUTOR	KEY IDEA	APPLICATION TO PRACTICE
Hierarchy of Needs Maslow is credited with developing a theory of motivation, first published in 1943.	People are motivated by a hierarchy of human needs, beginning with physiologic needs, then progressing to safety, social, esteem, and self-actualizing needs. In this theory, when the need for food, water, air, and other life-sustaining elements is met, the human spirit reaches out to achieve affiliation with others, which promotes the development of self-esteem, competence, achievement, and creativity. Lower-level needs will always drive behavior before higher-level needs will be addressed.	When this theory is applied to staff, leaders must be aware that the need for safety and security will override the opportunity to be creative and inventive, such as in promoting job change.
Two-Factor Theory Herzberg (1991) is credited with developing a two-factor theory of motivation, first published in 1968.	Hygiene factors, such as working conditions, salary, status, and security, motivate workers by meeting safety and security needs and avoiding job dissatisfaction. Motivator factors, such as achievement, recognition, and the satisfaction of the work itself, promote job enrichment by creating job satisfaction.	Organizations need both hygiene and motivator factors to recruit and retain staff. Hygiene factors do not create job satisfaction; they simply must be in place for work to be accomplished. If not, these factors will only serve to dissatisfy staff. Transformational leaders use motivator factors liberally to inspire work performance.
Expectancy Theory Vroom (1964) is credited with developing the expectancy theory of motivation.	Individuals' perceived needs influence their behavior. In the work setting, this motivated behavior is increased if a person perceives a positive relationship between effort and performance. Motivated behavior is further increased if there is a positive relationship between good performance and outcomes or rewards, particularly when these are valued.	Expectancy is the perceived probability of satisfying a particular need based on past experience. Therefore, nurses in leadership roles need to provide specific feedback about positive performance.

Theory Box—cont'd

MOTIVATIONAL THEORIES

THEORY/CONTRIBUTOR	KEY IDEA	APPLICATION TO PRACTICE
OB Modification Luthans (1973) is credited with establishing the foundation for Organizational Behavior Modification (OB Mod), based on Skinner's work on operant conditioning.	OB Mod is an operant approach to organizational behavior. OB Mod Performance Analysis follows a three-step ABC Model: A, antecedent analysis of clear expectations and baseline data collection; B, behavioral analysis and determination; and C, consequence analysis, including reinforcement strategies.	The leader uses positive reinforcement to motivate followers to repeat constructive behaviors in the workplace. Negative events that de-motivate staff are negatively reinforced, and the staff is motivated to avoid certain situations that cause discomfort. Extinction is the purposeful nonreinforcement (ignoring) of negative behaviors. Punishment is used sparingly because the results are unpredictable in supporting the desired behavioral outcome.

THE PROMISE OF COMPLEXITY THEORY

Too often, theories are believed to have been developed in the distant past. However, new theories are being created, tested, and put into practice all the time—a role and function of nurse scientists and others. **Complexity theory** is emerging from the work of physical sciences and, more recently, social sciences. It is addressed here because healthcare organizations and nursing curricula are embracing complexity science as a new way of viewing both clinical and organizational issues that have not responded to traditional science, or top-down hierarchies.

Classic science developed theory on assumptions concerning the examination of the "parts" of the patient and the division of organizational tasks to understand the "whole." Complexity science promotes the idea that the world is full of systems that interact and adapt through relationships. The interactions may appear to be random, rather than controlled, and decisions emerge that make sense through the interactions. Stated another way, professional nurses are being responsive to patient and family dynamics, disease interactions, nonhierarchical communications and decision-making, and the identification of new patterns of human responses through the use of complexity science. Complexity science, therefore, expands the repertoire of nursing interventions beyond cause and effect strategies.

In complexity theory, traditional organizational hierarchy plays a less significant role as the "keeper of high level knowledge." It is replaced with decision-making distributed among the human assets within an organization without regard to hierarchy. Leaders try less to control the future and spend more time influencing, innovating, and responding to the many factors that influence health care, such as those previously described. In complexity science, every voice counts, and every encounter between and among patients and staff adds to effective decision-making.

In reference to leadership, management, and followership, how do these definitions differ using complexity science principles?

Leadership was defined as dealing with the unknown, formulating solutions in reaction to complex presenting circumstances. The definition suggests that responding to and drawing on human resources is important when navigating unknown circumstances, and complexity science supports the idea that overprescribing solutions to complex problems fails to yield the best solution. Leadership, then, does not require hypervigilant control over events, but rather, an engaged interaction with the event and people who are part of it!

The earlier definition of management has less of a role in complexity sciences. The nature of organizations requires that certain processes be put into place and standardized. When problems are of a routine nature, they can often be solved using linear step-by-step prescriptive models. Complexity science does not attempt to replace decisions that can be standardized through cause and effect science, but rather is extended to complement situations in which this approach is not ideal. Nevertheless, pattern analysis, examining relationships, and being open to complexity approaches if causal strategies are not effective are a fit with complexity science.

Followership is a central tenet of complexity sciences. No longer is the follower a passive participant, but rather a central player in the networks that command a full expression of ideas, stories, and lessons learned. As stated earlier, the follower acquiesces to the leader at times. In complexity science, the leader is not hierarchically related to the follower. Rather, each individual brings to the problem-solving network and the particular patient/family encounter the capacity to lead, manage, and follow. It is the flow among and between these roles in which individuals in formal positions foster an environment that empowers, encourages risk-taking, and diminishes fear and organizational silence on matters that are critical to patient and organizational outcomes.

Marion and Uhl-Bien (2001) identify five ways in which complexity science encourages individuals to lead, manage, and follow. Those who use complexity principles:

Develop Networks   A network is any related group with common involvement in an area of focus or concern. Networks are found within organizations, but also beyond organizational boundaries. For example, a nursing program is not considered a part of the hospital or agency setting where clinical experiences take place; however, common interests (supply and preparation of a qualified workforce and demand for clinical services) make this network critically important for both organizations.

Encourage Nonhierarchical, "Bottom-up" Interaction Among Workers   As noted earlier, those who lead, manage, and follow are not considered to be within the traditional hierarchy. Shared governance is an example of decision-making in which all staff at any level in the hierarchy are engaged in shaping policy and practices that affect patient care. In this model, each nurse is a valued human resource.

Become a Leadership "Tag"   The term *tag* references the philosophic, patient-centered, and values-driven characteristics that give an organization its personality, sometimes called "attractors." Although the performance of procedures and functions may be similar in clinical settings, the intangible "caring" attractor can drive organizational performance in a manner that exemplifies caring, while another organization focuses on cost-efficiencies. The term "tag" refers to these distinctions.

Focus on Emergence   The concept of emergence addresses how individuals in positions of responsibility engage with and discover, through active organizational involvement, those networks that are best suited to respond to problems in creative, surprising, and artful ways, those who think "out of the box." Emergence is tied to unleashing constructive energy rather than constraining energy.

Think Systematically   The principles of systems thinking theory have been characterized by Anderson and Johnson (1997) as:

Thinking of the "Big Picture"   The nurse who looks past her/his assignment and comprehends the needs of all units of the hospital, or who can focus on the needs of all the residents in a long-term care facility, or who can think through the complications of emergency department overcrowding in an urban setting is seeing the big picture.

Balancing Short- and Long-Term Objectives   The nurse who recognizes the consequences of actions taken today on the long-term effect of the organization or patient care, such as the decision not to perform cancer treatment, is able to guide thinking about how to balance decision making for quality outcomes.

Recognizing the Dynamic, Complex, and Interdependent Nature of Systems   Everything is simply connected to everything. Patients are connected to families and friends. Together, they are connected to communities and cultures. Communities and cultures make up the fabric of society. The cost of health care is linked to local economies, and local businesses are connected to global industries. Identifying and understanding these relationships helps to solve problems with full recognition that small decisions can have a large impact.

Measurable Versus Nonmeasurable Data Systems thinking triggers a "tendency to 'see' only what we measure. If we focus our measuring on morale, working relationships, and teamwork, we might miss the important signals that only objective statistics can show us. On the other hand, if we stay riveted on 'the numbers,' on how many 'widgets' go out the door, we could overlook an important, escalating conflict between the purchasing and production departments" (Anderson and Johnson, 1997, p. 19).

■ Exercise 1–3

Identify a clinical scenario in which a complex problem needs to be addressed. Who would you include in a network to engage in creative problem-solving? Identify one member of the network, and map the potential connections of that individual that could influence problem resolution. Concentrate on the power of these influencing individuals. The patient/family are part of the network. What role would they play in problem-solving? How would you encourage nonhierarchical interaction among workers? Cite instances (personally or professionally) in which a small change in a system has had a big effect.

TASKS OF LEADING, MANAGING, AND FOLLOWING

When dealing with theory and concepts, it is sometimes easy for developing professionals to lose sight of the practical behaviors that are needed to put these ideas into practice. Gardner (1990) recognized this when he described tasks of leadership in his book *On Leadership* (Box 1-2). The purpose of describing tangible behaviors associated with leading, managing, and following is intended to facilitate an understanding of the distinctions between the tasks and the definitions of leadership, management, and followership presented earlier in the chapter.

Gardner's Tasks of Leadership

Gardner's leadership tasks are presented in Table 1-1 to provide a contrast between clinical positions, leaders who hold management positions, and executive leader positions. Note that each role represents the interests of the organization, although the locus of attention is different.

Envisioning Goals Leading requires envisioning goals, not in isolation but in partnership with others. In the case of patient care, leading is required to help patients envision their life when outcomes are unknown. It might be aimed at helping a patient envision walking again, participating in family events, or changing a lifestyle pattern. In the case of leading peers (not dissimilar to working with patients and family members), leader competence, trustworthiness, self-assuredness, decision-making ability, and prioritization skills are needed to envision crafting solutions to problems. Imagine leading a change to an electronic health record from a traditional paper record: the leader would need the aforementioned abilities to engage with, to convince or persuade staff that this change is

BOX 1-2

Gardner's Tasks of Leadership

1. Envisioning goals
2. Affirming values
3. Motivating
4. Managing
   - Planning and setting priorities
   - Organizing and institution building
   - Keeping the system functioning
   - Setting agendas and making decisions
   - Exercising political judgment
5. Achieving workable unity
6. Developing trust
7. Explaining
8. Serving as symbol
9. Representing the group
10. Renewing

Table 1-1 CONTRASTING LEADING/MANAGING BEHAVIORS OF NURSES IN CLINICAL, MANAGEMENT, AND EXECUTIVE POSITIONS

Gardner's Task	Behaviors		
	Clinical Position	**Management Position**	**Executive Position**
Envisioning goals	Visioning patient outcomes for single patients/families; assisting patients in formulating their vision of future well-being	Visioning patient outcomes for aggregates of patient populations and creating a vision of how systems support patient care objectives; assisting staff in formulating their vision of enhanced clinical and organizational performance	Visioning community health and organizational outcomes for aggregates of patient populations to which the organization can respond
Affirming values	Assisting the patient/family to sort out and articulate personal values in relation to health problems and the effect of these problems on lifestyle adjustments	Assisting the staff in interpreting organizational values and strengthening staff members' personal values to more closely align with those of the organization; interpreting values during organizational change	Assisting other organizational leaders in the expression of community and organizational values; interpreting values to the community and staff
Motivating	Relating to and inspiring patients/families to achieve their vision	Relating to and inspiring staff to achieve the mission of the organization and the vision associated with organizational enhancement	Relating to and inspiring management, staff, and community leaders to achieve desired levels of health and well-being and appropriate use of clinical services
Managing	Assisting the patient/family with planning, priority-setting, and decision-making; making sure that organizational systems work in the patient's behalf	Assisting the staff with planning, priority-setting, and decision-making; making sure that systems work to enhance the staff's ability to meet patient care needs and the objectives of the organization	Assisting other executives and corporate leaders with planning, priority-setting, and decision-making; ensuring that human and material resources are available to meet health needs
Achieving workable unity	Assisting patients/families to achieve optimal functioning to benefit the transition to enhanced health functions	Assisting staff to achieve optimal functioning to benefit transition to enhanced organizational functions	Assisting multidisciplinary leaders to achieve optimal functioning to benefit patient care delivery and collaborative care
Developing trust	Keeping promises to patients and families; being honest in role performance	Sharing organizational information openly; being honest in role performance	Representing nursing and executive views openly and honestly; being honest in role performance

Table 1-1 CONTRASTING LEADING/MANAGING BEHAVIORS OF NURSES IN CLINICAL, MANAGEMENT, AND EXECUTIVE POSITIONS—cont'd

Gardner's Task	Behaviors		
	Clinical Position	Management Position	Executive Position
Explaining	Teaching and interpreting information to promote patient/family functioning and well-being	Teaching and interpreting information to promote organizational functioning and enhanced services	Teaching and interpreting organizational and community-based health information to promote organizational functioning and service development
Serving as symbol	Representing the nursing profession and the values and beliefs of the organization to patients/families and other community groups	Representing the nursing unit service and the values and beliefs of the organization to staff, other departments, professional disciplines, and the community at large	Representing the values and beliefs of the organization and patient care services to internal and external constituents
Representing the group	Representing nursing and the unit in task forces, total quality initiatives, shared governance councils, and other groups	Representing nursing and the organization on assigned boards, councils, committees, and task forces, both internal and external to the organization	Representing the organization and patient care services on assigned boards, councils, committees, and task forces, both internal and external to the organization
Renewing	Providing self-care to enhance the ability to care for staff, patients, families, and the organization served	Providing self-care to enhance the ability to care for staff, patients, families, and the organization served	Providing self-care to enhance the ability to care for patients, families, staff, and the organization served

necessary, and to proceed with setting direction. Envisioning goals is contingent upon trustful relationships, shared information, and agreement on mutual expectations.

Establishing **vision** is an important leadership concept. "Visioning" requires the leader to assess the current reality, determine and specify a desired end-point state, and then strategize to reduce the tension between the two states in a positive manner. If done well, the nurse and the patient, or nurses within an organization, experience creative tension. Creative tension is positive tension that moves the patient toward the desired goal. However, if the nurse fails to engage the patient or fails to recognize the root cause of a clinical problem, then emotional tension (distress) results. Emotional tension drains the energy of those experiencing the change.

Therefore, exceptional visioning skills are an important function of leading. Visioning gives direction to accelerate change.

Affirming Values **Values** are the inner forces that give purpose, direction, and precedence to life priorities. An organization, through its members, has composite values that are expressed through its mission and philosophy. Leaders have values that influence decision-making and priority-setting. People (either patients or peers being influenced by the leader) also have values that undergird their goals and are manifested through behavior. Values are a deep-seated, persuasive force driving how we choose to act and respond to others.

The word "value" conjures up an image of something that has worth; our actions reflect our values. A leader continuously clarifies and acknowledges the values that underlie the need to solve problems or create something new. This is because values are powerful forces that promote acceptance of change and drive achievement toward a goal.

Motivating   When we let our values drive our actions, values become a source of motivation. **Motivation** is tapping into what we value, personally and professionally, and reinforcing these factors to achieve growth and movement toward the vision. Motivators are the reinforcers that keep positive actions alive and tap the inner drive. Motivators fuel the fires that generate the desire to engage in change. Theories of motivation identify and describe the forces that motivate people. Examples of motivation theory are presented in the theory box on Motivation, earlier in this chapter.

Managing   The ability to manage is an important aspect of leading, especially when the leader holds a position of influence in an organization (e.g., a nurse manager). Being an effective manager is not the same as being an effective leader and vice versa. Ideally, those charged with managing are also good leaders and good followers, because there are few organizational positions that require one set of

behaviors over the other. Good leaders need management skills and abilities, and good managers need leading skills and abilities. The tasks of management are discussed later in this chapter.

Achieving Workable Unity   Another leadership challenge is to achieve workable unity between and among the parties being affected by change and to avoid, diminish, or resolve conflict so that vision can be achieved (see Chapters 16 and 22). Conflict-resolution skills are essential for leaders. When a dispute occurs, as a result of conflicting values or interests, following a defined set of principles to guide conflict resolution is a great aid. In their classic work, Ury, Brett, and Goldberg (1988) describe a highly effective approach for restoring unity and movement toward positive change, as shown in Box 1-3.

Developing Trust   A hallmark task of leadership is to behave in a way that is trustworthy. Trust is developed when leaders are clear with others about "where we are headed" and that the way to achieve high levels of performance is through building on strengths rather than entrapment of poor performance. Inherent in this concept is the behavior of truth telling. Although leaders cannot always share

---

BOX 1-3

Principles of Conflict Resolution

1. Put the focus on interests:
   Examine the real issues of all parties.
   Be expedient in responding to the issues.
   Use negotiation procedures and processes such as ethics committees and other neutral sources.
2. Build in "loop-backs" to negotiation:
   If resolution fails, allow for a "cooling off" period before reconvening.
   Review the likely consequences of not proceeding with all parties so that they understand the full consequences of failure to resolve the issue.
3. Build in consultation before and feedback after the negotiations:
   Build consensus and use political skills to facilitate communication before confrontation, if anticipated, occurs.

Work with staff or patients after the conflict to learn from the situation and to prevent a similar conflict in the future.
Provide a forum for open discussion.
4. Provide necessary motivation, skills, and resources:
   Make sure that the parties involved in conflict are motivated to use procedures and resources that have been developed; this requires ease of access and a nonthreatening mechanism.
   Ensure that those working in the dispute have skills in problem-solving and dispute-resolution.
   Provide the necessary resources to those involved to offer support, information, and other technical assistance.

Modified from Ury, W., Brett, J., & Goldberg, S. (1988). *Getting disputes resolved: Designing systems to cut the costs of conflict.* Cambridge, MA: Program of Negatiation at Harvard Law School.

all information, it is unwise to misdirect others in their thinking and actions. Trust, according to Lencioni (2002), is the key component of a team. Without it, the team is dysfunctional. Trustworthiness is reflected in actions and communications.

Explaining Leading and managing require a willingness to communicate and explain—again and again. The art of communication requires the leader to do the following:

1. Know what information needs to be shared.
2. Know the parties who will receive the information. Ask, "What will they 'hear' in the process of the communication?" Information that addresses the listener's self-interest must be presented.
3. Provide the opportunity for dialogue and feedback. Face-to-face communication is preferred because it affords immediate feedback to the leader and offers the opportunity to clarify information. Written feedback, such as through e-mail, is useful to reinforce key messages or to follow-up on inquiries, but too often it is becoming a primary method of communication over other preferred strategies.
4. Know that giving too much information can temporarily paralyze the listener and divert energy away from key responsibilities.
5. Be willing to repeat information in different ways, at different times. The more diverse the group being addressed, the more important it is to avoid complex terms, concepts, or ideas. Information should be kept simple. Remember, a message is heard when a person is ready to hear it, not before.
6. Always explain why something is being asked or is changing. The values behind the change should be reinforced.
7. Acknowledge loss, and provide the opportunity for honest communication about what will be missed, especially if change is involved.
8. Be sensitive to nonverbal communication. It may be necessary in complex situations to have someone reinterpret key points and provide feedback about the clarity of the message after the meeting. Leaders must use every opportunity for explaining as a vehicle to fine-tune communication skills. (See Chapter 17 for more on communication.)

Serving as Symbol Every leader has the opportunity to be an ambassador for those they represent. Nurses may be symbolically present for patients and families, represent their department at an organizational event, or be involved in community public relations events. Serving as a symbol reflects unity and collective identity.

Representing the Group More than being present symbolically, there are many opportunities for leaders to represent the group through active participation. Progressive organizations are creating more opportunities for employee participation, involvement, and innovation (such as organizations seeking **Magnet recognition**). Employees may be invited to participate on human resource committees, safety and security task forces, improvement committees, and other nursing department groups. Nurses offer an important "voice" in each of these leadership opportunities. When decision-making is decentralized, and layers of management are compressed, nurses are given more leadership accountability. Leaders should treat these newfound opportunities with respect and honestly try to represent the group with openness and integrity. Ultimately, leaders must understand the organization's objectives and contribute to its mission and purpose.

Renewing Leaders can generate energy within and among others. A true leader does not expend the group's energy or allow it to lose focus. In organizations and nursing practice, there is a constant need to find a balance between problem-solving (energy-expending) and vision-setting (energy-producing). When changes are made based on vision, they can be made with renewed spirit and purpose, if well led. Taking time in staff meetings to celebrate individual accomplishments or creating a "Hall of Honor" to post photos, letters, and other forms of positive feedback renews the spirit of workers.

Furthermore, leaders must be proponents of self-care—eat a balanced diet, get adequate sleep and exercise, and participate in other wellness-oriented activities—to maintain their perspective and the necessary energy level. Likewise, they must ensure that their constituents are given similar opportunities for physical and mental renewal. Gardner (1990) states that, "The consideration leaders must never forget is that the key for renewal is the release of human energy and talent" (p. 136).

This requires focused energy and personal well-being.

Bleich's Tasks of Management

The ability to manage is very much aligned with how an organization structures its key systems and processes to deliver service. In the legendary *I Love Lucy* television series, the episode in which Lucy and Ethel work in a candy factory serves as a classic example of the role and energy that workers exude to achieve an acceptable work product. Recall the extraordinary effort of wrapping each piece of candy to specification as it passed by on a conveyor belt. The process was designed such that two workers stood side-by-side, each taking an alternating piece of candy and a wrapper, and wrapped the candy according to specifications. Simple and clear. Yet when worker productivity was challenged (poor directions, a nonsupportive supervisor, and limited worker training to the task at hand), the workers "gamed" the system to give the appearance of success! If you recall, the supervisor suggested that "one more mess up" would result in firing. The supervisor—who never truly observed, coached, or gave feedback to her workers—ends up declaring, "Speed it up!" and hilarity ensues as the rate of production approaches near-bedlam, thereby yielding even more errors.

This example highlights the roles of managing and following. Healthcare delivery is composed of processes of care that are far more complex than the candy factory example (observe a dietary tray line sometime, though!), and targeted behaviors are associated with each. A **process of care** specifies the desired sequence of steps that have been designed to achieve clinical standardization. Nurses are challenged to follow a process of care when they give medications, perform clinical procedures, make nursing assessments, conduct patient education, and complete charting responsibilities. Effective managing depends on recognizing that these systems and processes exist, that efficiency and effectiveness is built in (or not built in) to these systems, and that there are prescribed roles for individual workers to comprehend. Data-driven outcome measurements are critical to good management. Likewise, honest feedback, coaching, and mentoring are also key elements. Rewards for individual and team effectiveness reinforce desired behaviors. Box 1-4 lists tasks of management that are essential to effective functioning.

Many healthcare settings have a dire need to reallocate managers' time so that the patient care delivery system can be designed in more effective, efficient, patient-oriented, and staff-friendly ways. Workforce issues are commonly associated with the work environment. Leaders will help guide workplace transformation, but managers must sustain the spirit of clinical system functioning (Bleich & Hewlett, 2004).

Exercise 1–4

Examine one structured process in the delivery of patient care from start to finish (e.g., food ordering, preparation, and delivery). Who is responsible for each step in the process? Who has the responsibility and authority for managing the process? What data are available in the organization to measure how well the process is working?

BOX 1-4

Bleich's Tasks of Management

1. Identify systems and processes for which the manager has responsibility and accountability
2. Verify minimum and optimum standards/specifications for staff to achieve
3. Validate the knowledge, skills, and abilities of available staff; capitalize on strengths; and strengthen areas in need of development
4. Devise and communicate a comprehensive "big picture" plan for the division of work, honoring the complexity and variety of assignments made at an individual level
5. Eliminate barriers/obstacles to work effectiveness
6. Measure the equity of workload, and use data to support judgments about efficiency and effectiveness
7. Offer rewards and recognition to individuals and teams
8. Recommend ways to improve systems and processes
9. Involve others in decision-making when appropriate or relevant

Images associated with followers portray workers who are passive, uninspired, not intellectual, and waiting for direction. In reality, the effective follower is willing to be led, to share time and talents, to create and innovate solutions to problems synergistically, and to take direction from the manager. Simultaneously, followers must perform their assigned structured duties. These duties are not devoid of critical-thinking or decision-making (Box 1-5).

Followers complement leaders and managers with their skills. Followers and leaders fill in the gaps that exist to build on each other's cognitive, technical, interpersonal, and emotional strengths. Followers, showing sensitivity to leaders, offer respite in times of stress. Followers need and respond to feedback from leaders to stay on course. The follower must acquiesce to the skills and abilities of the leader or manager to promote teamwork. This does not mean that the follower does not have the skills and abilities of the leader or manager, as the follower may be thrust into one of those roles when circumstances demand. Box 1-5 lists the tasks of followership.

The relationship between followers and leaders or managers is complex. Burns (2000) states, "It would seem so simple at first glance—that leaders lead and followers follow. When the leader dreams the dream or takes the initiative or issues the call, does the follower even hear the leader?" (p. 11).

There are also times when the leader is the follower and vice versa. In any given work shift, there may be a charge nurse who holds a leading–managing role. During a shift, the charge nurse assesses resources needed, sees the unit as a complete entity, notes where patients may be admitted or discharged, and delegates according to this "big picture" view. Throughout the shift, critical clinical events arise that are better led by one of the senior staff nurses. Ideally, the charge nurse and senior staff nurse shift their relationship so that the functioning of the unit is balanced. Assignments are temporarily adjusted, and talents and skills of individual nurses are deployed to patients and families in need, all with little or no fanfare. But, examine the complexity, respect, and team achievement factors at play as the system adapts.

LEADING, MANAGING, AND FOLLOWING IN A DIVERSE ORGANIZATION

The healthcare industry is spiraling through unparalleled change, often away from the traditional industrial models that have reigned throughout the 20th century. The culture in most healthcare organizations today is more ethnically diverse; has an expansive educational chasm, from non–high

---

BOX 1-5

Bleich's Tasks of Followership

1. Is individually accountable while working within the context of organizational systems and processes; does not change the way work is done for personal gain or short cuts
2. Honors the standards and specifications required to deliver acceptable care/service
3. Offers knowledge, skills, and abilities to accomplish the task at hand
4. Collaborates willingly with leaders and managers; avoids passive-aggressive or nonassertive responses to work assignment
5. Includes data collection as part of daily work activities as a self-guide to efficiency and effectiveness and to contribute to outcome measurement
6. Demonstrates accountability for individual actions within the team effort
7. Takes reasonable risks as an antidote for fearing change or unknown circumstances
8. Gives feedback on the efficiency and effectiveness of systems and processes that affect outcomes of care/service; values well-designed work
9. Gives and receives feedback to other team members, leaders, and managers to enhance a culture of nurturance and support

school graduates to doctoral-prepared clinicians; has multiple generations of workers with varying values and expectations of the workplace; involves the increased use of technology to support all aspects of service functioning; and challenges workers, patients, families, and communities environmentally with medical waste, antibiotic-resistant strains of microorganisms, and other risks.

These and other variables make leading, managing, and following increasingly challenging. A leader must address the needs of the diverse community of those seeking care. Language and cultural barriers create the opportunity for misunderstanding. Those who manage the systems and processes of care may find a temporary workforce, individuals unfamiliar with organizational standards of care and practice, as their primary resource. Followers may have leaders of other generations with values different from their own, and, therefore, the opportunity for conflict is omnipresent.

Developing the leading, managing, and following skills and abilities noted throughout this chapter will sustain professional nurses to adapt to and accept differences as a positive rather than a negative force in daily work life. Building on gender strengths; generational values, gifts, and talents; cultural diversity; varying educational and experiential perspectives; and a mobile and flexible workforce is rewarding. It is also rewarding to be led in different ways, to experience the strength of a good manager, and to achieve positive outcomes as a follower knowing that the team approach generated a successful work experience.

The Solution

Nurses must frequently face situations involving competing priorities. In this case, the priorities involved hospital placement guidelines concerning the specialized skills of the staff in our unit versus the perceived familiarity of the patient and his family by staff in another unit. It is the responsibility of every member of a healthcare team to identify the physical and emotional needs of patients and their families to manage their care effectively. The importance of relationship-based care and the trust of the patient/family with staff are of critical importance. As the nurse manager, I was responsible for providing leadership to the staff by conducting a more in-depth inquiry about what the unknown needs of the patient/family were, and I modeled relationship-building and showed self-confidence in addressing unknown concerns. I did this with confidence in my communication and teamwork skills and my staff's abilities.

As a leader, I did not have a "grand plan" in mind to solve this situation but knew that by involving the father and other members in a network of problem-solvers that a best solution would emerge. As a follower, I used principles from complexity science to co-create with my staff decisions that contributed to a new care plan. After the surgical team left the room, I immediately sat down with the father and let him take the lead in expressing his concerns. I knew he was the best person to inform me how he felt, what he had experienced, and what might be done differently next time.

Using management knowledge, I described the hospital policies regarding placement of patients postoperatively and explained to the father the reason for the admission to the unit. Staff followed risk-management protocols to document the problem and the resolution tactics. All in all, this scenario shows how I moved fluidly from leader, manager, and follower, building relationships that led to a vastly improved outcome for this patient and family.

— Paula L. Hibbard

 Would this approach be suitable for you? Why?

CHAPTER CHECKLIST

This chapter addresses the attributes and tasks of leading, managing, and following and presents the case that professional nurses require the knowledge, skill, and ability to move in and out of these roles with ease, whether in clinical or management positions. Emotional intelligence is defined in terms of self-understanding, and the argument is made that emotional intelligence is as critical to professional practice as are cognitive and technical skills. Healthcare organizations are experiencing major changes and increasing diversity in those being served and those serving; diversity presents new challenges and opportunities for leaders, managers, and followers. Multiple theories are used in today's healthcare system to address emerging organizational and care needs.

- The personal attributes needed for effective leading and managing include the following:
  - Focused energy and stamina to accomplish the vision
  - Ability to make decisions in an intelligent manner
  - Willingness to use intuition, backed up with facts
  - Willingness to accept responsibility and to follow up
  - Sincerity in identifying the needs of others
  - Skill in dealing with people, for example, through coaching, communicating, or counseling
  - Comfortable standard- and boundary-setting
  - Flexibility in examining multiple options to accomplish the objective at hand
  - Trustworthiness and a good "steward of information"
  - Assertiveness in motivating others toward the objective at hand
  - Demonstrable competence and quick learning in the arena where change is desired
- The tasks of leading include the following:
  - Envision goals
  - Affirm values
  - Motivate

- Manage
  - Planning and priority-setting
  - Organizing and institution-building
  - Keeping the system functioning
  - Setting agendas and making decisions
  - Exercising political judgment
- Achieve workable unity
- Develop trust
- Explain
- Serve as symbol
- Represent the group
- Renew
- The tasks for managing include the following:
  - Identify systems and processes
  - Verify minimum and optimum standards/specifications
  - Validate the knowledge, skills, and abilities of available staff
  - Devise and communicate a comprehensive "big picture" plan
  - Eliminate barriers/obstacles to work effectiveness
  - Measure the equity of workload
  - Offer rewards and recognition to individuals and teams
  - Recommend ways to improve systems and processes
  - Involve others in decision-making
- The tasks for following include:
  - Recognize how individual responsibilities fit into organizational systems
  - Honor the standards and specifications
  - Offer knowledge, skills, and abilities
  - Collaborate willingly with leaders and managers
  - Include data collection as part of daily work activities
  - Demonstrate accountability for individual actions
  - Take reasonable risks
  - Give feedback on the efficiency and effectiveness of systems
  - Give and receive feedback to and from other team members, leaders, and managers

TERMS TO KNOW

complexity theory
emotional intelligence
followership
leadership
Magnet recognition
management
management theory
motivation
process of care
values
vision

REFERENCES

Anderson, V., & Johnson, L. (1997). *Systems thinking basics: From concepts to causal loops.* Waltham, MA: Pegasus Communications.

Bass, B. M. (1990). From transactional to transformational leadership: Learning to share the vision. *Organizational Dynamics, 18,* 19-31.

Bennis, W. G., & Nanus, B. (1985). *Leaders: The strategies for taking charge.* New York: Harper & Row.

Blake, R. R., & Mouton, J. S. (1985). *The managerial grid III.* Houston: Gulf Publishing.

Bleich, M., & Hewlett, P. (May 31, 2004). Dissipating the "Perfect Storm"—Responses from nursing and the health care industry to protect the public's health. *Online Journal of Issues in Nursing. 9*(2), Manuscript 4. Retrieved March 25, 2005 from www.nursingworld.org/ojin/topic24/tpc24_4.htm.

Bleich, M., Hewlett, P., Santos, S., Rice, R., Cox, K., & Richmeier, S. (2003). Analysis of the nursing workforce crisis: A call to action. *American Journal of Nursing, 103*(4), 66-73.

Burns, J. M. (2000). Leadership and followership: Complicated relationships. In B. Kellerman & L. R. Matusak (Eds.), *Cutting edge leadership 2000.* College Park: The James Academy of Leadership.

Fiedler, F. A. (1967). *A theory of leadership effectiveness.* New York: McGraw-Hill.

Gardner, J. W. (1990). *On leadership.* New York: Free Press.

Goleman, D. P. (1995). *Working with emotional intelligence.* New York: Bantam Books.

Goode, C. J. (2004, April). *Using evidence to transform your work environment.* Presented at the meeting of Nursing Leadership: Rising on the wings of change, Phoenix, AZ.

Herzberg, F. (1991). One more time: How do you motivate employees? In M. J. Ward & S. A. Price (Eds.), *Issues in nursing administration: Selected readings.* St. Louis: Mosby.

House, R. J., & Mitchell, T. R. (1974, Autumn). Path-goal theory of leadership. *Journal of Contemporary Business, 3,* 81-97.

Jooste, K. (2004). Leadership: a new perspective. *Journal of Nursing Management, 12,* 217-223.

Lencioni, P. M. (2002). *The five dysfunctions of a team: A leadership fable.* San Francisco: Jossey-Bass.

Lewis, C. K., & Matthews, J. H. (1998). Magnet program designates exceptional nursing services. *American Journal of Nursing, 98*(12), 51-52.

Likert, R. (1961). *New patterns of management.* New York: McGraw-Hill.

Luthans, F. (1973). *Organizational behavior.* New York: McGraw-Hill.

Marion, R., & Uhl-Bien, M. (2001). Leadership in complex organizations. *The Leadership Quarterly, 12,* 389-418.

Maslow, A. (1943). A theory of human motivation. *Psychological Review, 50,* 370-396.

Shartle, C. L. (1956). *Executive performance and leadership.* Englewood Cliffs, NJ: Prentice Hall.

Stogdill, R. M. (1948). Personal factors associated with leadership: A survey of the literature. *Journal of Psychology, 25,* 35-71.

Stogdill, R. M. (1963). *Manual for the leader behavior description questionnaire, form XII.* Columbus: The Ohio State University, Bureau of Business Research.

Tichy, N. M., & Devanna, M. A. (1986). *The transformational leader.* New York: John Wiley & Sons.

Upenieks, V. (2003). Nurse leaders' perceptions of what compromises successful leadership in today's acute inpatient environment. *Nursing Administration Quarterly, 27,* 140-152.

Ury, W., Brett, J., & Goldberg, S. (1988). *Getting disputes resolved: Designing systems to cut the costs of conflict.* San Francisco: Jossey-Bass.

Vroom, V. H. (1964). *Work and motivation.* New York: John Wiley & Sons.

Vroom, V. H., & Yetton, P. (1973). *Leadership and decision-making.* Pittsburgh: University of Pittsburgh Press.

Wood Allen, D. (1998). How nurses become leaders: Perceptions and beliefs about leadership development. *Journal of Nursing Administration, 28*(9), 15-20.

Yauk, S., Hopkins, B. A., Phillips, C. D., Terrell, S., Bennion, J., & Riggs, M. (2005). Predicting in-hospital falls: Development of the Scott and White Falls Risk Screener. *Journal of Nursing Care Quality, 20,* 128-133.

SUGGESTED READINGS

Bass, B. M., & Avolio, B. J. (1994). *Improving organizational effectiveness through transformational leadership.* Thousand Oaks, CA: Sage Publications.

Begun, J. W., & White, K. R. (1999). The profession of nursing as a complex adaptive system: Strategies for change. *Research in Sociology of Health Care, 16,* 189-203.

Birute, R., & Lewin, R. *Third possibility leaders: the invisible edge women have in complex organizations.* Retrieved March 25, 2005, from http://plexusinstitute.org/services/stories/show.cfm?id=28.

Boyle, D. K., Bott, M. J., Hansen, H. E., Woods, C. Q., & Taunton, R. L. (1999). Managers' leadership and critical care nurses' intent to stay. *American Journal of Critical Care, 8,* 361-371.

Bridges, W. (1991). *Managing transitions: Making the most of change.* Reading, MA: Addison-Welsey.

Clegg, A. (2000). Leadership: Improving the quality of patient care. *Nursing Standard, 14,* 43-45.

Cohen, A. R., & Bradford, D. L. (1989). *Influence without authority.* New York: John Wiley & Sons.

Covey, S. (1991). *Principle-centered leadership.* New York: Summit.

Gladwell, M. (2000). *The tipping point.* Boston: Little, Brown.

Grossman, R. J. (2000). Emotions at work: Health care organizations are just beginning to recognize the importance of developing a manager's emotional quotient, or interpersonal skills. *Health Forum Journal, 43,* 18-22.

Jaworski, J. (1996). *Synchronicity: The inner path of leadership.* San Francisco: Berrett-Koehler Publishers.

Katzenbach, J. R., & Smith, D. K. (1993). *The wisdom of teams: Creating the high-performance organization.* New York: Harper Business.

Kellerman, B. (1999). *Reinventing leadership: Making the connection between politics and business.* New York: State University of New York Press.

Kinnaman, M., & Bleich, M. (2004). Collaboration: Aligning resources to create and sustain partnerships. *Journal of Professional Nursing, 20,* 310-322.

Lentz, S. (1999). The well-rounded leader: Knowing when to use consensus and when to make a decision is crucial in today's competitive health care market. *Health Forum Journal, 42,* 38-40.

McDaniel, R. R. (1997). Strategic leadership: A view from quantum and chaos theories. *Health Care Management Review, 22,* 21-37.

McNichol, E. (2000). How to be a model leader. Nursing Standard, 14, 24.

Noll, D. C. (1997). Complexity theory 101. *Medical Group Management Journal, 44*(3), 22, 24-26, 76.

Northouse, P. G. (2001). *Leadership theory and practice* (2nd ed.). Thousand Oaks, CA: Sage Publications.

Perra, B. M. (2000). Leadership: The key to quality outcomes. *Nursing Administration Quarterly, 24,* 56-61.

Plsek, P. E., & Wilson, T. (2001). Complexity, leadership, and management in healthcare organizations, *BMJ, 323,* 746-749.

Pugh, D. S., & Hickson, D. J. (1997). *Writers on organizations* (5th ed.). Thousand Oaks, CA: Sage Publications.

Rainey, H. G., & Watson, S. A. (1996). Transformational leadership and middle management: Towards a role for mere mortals. *International Journal of Public Administration, 19,* 764-800.

Trott, M. C., & Windsor, K. (1999). Leadership effectiveness: How do you measure up? *Nursing Economics, 17,* 127-130.

Useem, M. (1998). *The leadership moment.* New York: Three Rivers Press.

Van Wynen, E. A. (1997). Information processing styles: One size doesn't fit all. *Nurse Educator, 22,* 44-50.

Weeks, D. (1994). *The eight essential steps to conflict resolution.* New York: G. Putney Sons.

Zimmerman, B., Lindberg, C., & Plsek, P. (2001). *Edgeware: Insights from complexity science for health care leaders.* Irving, TX: VHA.

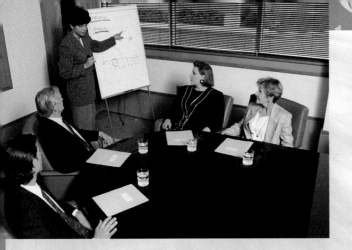

Developing the Role of Leader

Michael L. Evans

This chapter is focused on leadership and its value in advancing the profession of nursing. Leadership development is explained with examples of how to survive and thrive in a leadership position. The differences between the emerging and entrenched workforce generations are explored, and the desired characteristics of a leader for the emerging workforce are described. Leadership in a variety of situations, such as clinical settings, community venues, organizations, and political situations, are described. This chapter provides an introduction to the opportunities, challenges, and satisfaction of leadership.

Objectives

- Analyze the role of leadership in creating a satisfying working environment for nurses.
- Evaluate transactional and transformational leadership techniques for effectiveness and potential for positive outcomes.
- Value the leadership challenges in dealing with generational differences.
- Compare and contrast leadership and management roles and responsibilities.
- Describe leadership development strategies and how they can promote leadership skills acquisition.

- Analyze leadership opportunities and responsibilities in a variety of venues.

- Explore strategies for making the leadership opportunity positive for both the leader and the followers.

Questions to Consider

- Is there one best way to lead?
- Are some people just born to be leaders, or can leadership be taught and learned?
- What are the special leadership challenges of the "20-something" generation?
- How can the leader keep from "burning out"?
- What kinds of opportunities are available for nurses to lead if they are not members of the "management team"?

The Challenge

Rosemary Luquire, PhD, RN, CNAA
Senior Vice President, Patient Care & Chief Quality Officer, St. Luke's Episcopal Health System,
   Houston, Texas

Houston, known as the Bayou City, is accustomed to frequent flooding. Located 60 miles from the Gulf of Mexico, tropical storms and hurricanes are not uncommon for the region. On Tuesday, June 5, 2001, Tropical Storm Allison moved across the city and dropped 2.5 inches of rain, causing some street flooding. St. Luke's Episcopal Hospital, a 948-bed tertiary hospital (26 stories high) in the Texas Medical Center, established an emergency command center in accordance with its emergency preparedness plan. Tropical Storm Allison then moved northward, and the skies cleared. On Friday, June 8, the storm turned and moved back over Houston, creating massive flooding and loss of power throughout the Texas Medical Center. Between 5 PM on June 8 and 5 AM on June 9, 14 inches of rain fell; 36 inches of rain fell within 24 hours in northern Houston. The Bayou City was completely overwhelmed with this "500-year flood" as families fled to their rooftops to be saved by emergency personnel.

On the evening of Friday, June 8, St. Luke's had approximately 600 patients, 110 of whom were critically ill patients; many were on life support devices such as ventilators. I arrived at the hospital before flooding isolated the Texas Medical Center. I was the only senior executive on site. The evening staff was asked to stay and provide patient care, as the storm precluded the arrival of any additional help. In the early morning hours, authorities notified me that the facility would lose all electrical power within an hour. Amid an environment of crisis, isolation, and uncertainty, critical decisions needed to be made quickly. Should patients be evacuated? Who should be evacuated while elevators were still functioning? How could the safety of patients and staff be ensured? When everything is a priority, how do you decide what is truly a priority?

 What do you think you would do if you were this nurse?

WHAT IS A LEADER?

A leader is an individual who works with others to develop a clear vision of the preferred future and to make that vision happen. Oakley and Krug (1994) call that type of **leadership** *enlightened leadership*, or the ability to elicit a vision from people and to inspire and empower those people to do what it takes to bring the vision into reality. Leaders bring out the best in people.

Leadership is a very important concept in life. Great leaders have been responsible for helping society move forward and for articulating and accomplishing one vision after another throughout time. Dr. Martin Luther King, Jr., called his vision a dream, and it was developed because of the input and lived experiences of countless others. Mother Teresa called her vision a calling, and it was developed because of the suffering of others. Steven Spielberg calls his vision a finished motion picture, and it is developed with the collaboration and inspiration of many other people. Florence Nightingale called her vision nursing, and it was developed because people were experiencing a void that was a barrier to their ability to regain or establish health.

Atchison (2004) asserts that leaders have followers. An individual can have an impressive title, but that title does not make that person a leader. No matter what the person with that title does, he or she can never be successful without having the ability to inspire others to follow. "Commitment to follow a leader results when the follower has transcended self-interest. Commitment is the glue that binds the followers to the leader" (Atchison, 2004).

Covey (1992) identifies eight characteristics of effective leaders. Effective leaders are continually engaging themselves in lifelong learning. They are service-oriented and concerned with the common good. They radiate positive energy. For people to be inspired and motivated, they must have a positive leader. Effective leaders believe in other people.

They lead balanced lives and see life as an adventure. Effective leaders are synergistic; that is, they see things as greater than the sum of the parts. Finally, effective leaders engage themselves in self-renewal.

Exercise 2–1

List Covey's eight characteristics of effective leaders on the left side of a piece of paper. Next to each word, list any examples of your activities or attributes that reflect the characteristic. Some areas may be blank; others will be full. Think about what this means for you personally.

Healthcare organizations are complex. In fact, health care is complex. Continual learning is essential to stay abreast of new knowledge, to keep the organization moving forward, and to continue delivering the best possible care. There is an emphasis on organizations becoming learning organizations, providing opportunities and incentives for individuals and groups of individuals to learn continuously over time. A learning organization is one that is continually expanding its capacity to create its future (Senge, 1994). Leaders are responsible for building organizations in which people continually expand their ability to understand complexity and to clarify and improve a shared vision of the future—"that is, they are responsible for learning" (p. 340).

The roles of manager and leader are often considered interchangeable, but they are actually quite different. The manager may also be a leader, but the manager is not required to have leadership skills within the context of moving a group of people toward a vision. The term "manager" is a designated leadership position. Leadership is an abilities role, and it is most effective if the manager is also a leader. **Management** can be taught and learned using traditional teaching techniques. Leadership, however, can also be taught, but is usually a reflection of rich personal experiences.

Management and leadership are both important in the healthcare environment. The problem facing healthcare organizations is that they are overmanaged and underled (Atchison, 1990). Because we can teach new managers, but our leaders are developed over time and through experience, it is important that we value, support, and provide our leaders with the one thing vital for good leadership—good followership. Leadership is a social process involving leaders and followers interacting. Followers need three qualities from their leaders: direction, trust, and hope (Bennis, 1989). The trust is reciprocal. Leaders who trust their followers are, in turn, trusted by them.

The manager is concerned with doing things correctly in the present. The role of manager is very important in work organizations because managers make sure that operations run smoothly and that well-developed formulas are applied to staffing situations, economic decisions, and other daily operations. The manager is not as concerned with developing creative solutions to problems as using strategies to address today's issues. Covey (1992) believes that a well-managed entity may be proceeding correctly but, without leadership, may be proceeding in the wrong direction.

Leadership as an Important Concept for Nurses

Nurses must have leadership to move forward in harmony with changes in society and in health care. Within work organizations, certain nurses are designated as managers. These individuals are important to ensuring that care is delivered in a safe, efficient manner. Nurse leaders are also vital in the workplace to elicit input from others and to formulate a vision for the preferred future.

Moreover, leadership is key for nursing as a profession. The public depends on nurses to advocate for the public's needs and interests. Nurses must step forward into leadership roles in their workplace, in their professional associations, and in legislative and policy-making arenas.

Nurse leadership is vital. Nurses depend on their leaders to set goals for the future and the pace for achieving them. The public depends on nurse leaders to move the consumer advocacy agenda forward.

Leadership as a Primary Determinant of Workplace Satisfaction

Nurse satisfaction within the workplace is an important construct in nursing administration and healthcare administration. Turnover is extremely costly to any work organization in terms of money, expertise, and knowledge, as well as care quality. Thus, being mindful of nurse satisfaction is an economic as well as professional concern.

An amalgamation of several dozen interviews of healthcare workers (including physicians), when asked what followers desire from leaders, produced the following responses in rank order:

1. Respect
2. Control of the decisions that most affect me
3. Rewards and recognition
4. Balance of life—colleagues and family, job and home, work and play
5. Professional development (Atchison, 2004).

The effective leader in healthcare settings works with followers to find a way to create the perception that these important aspects of work life are actualized.

The leader, not the manager, inspires others to work at their highest level. The presence of strong leadership sets the tone for achievement in the work environment. Effective leadership is the basis for an effective workplace, and, therefore, creating leadership succession is an important consideration. This means that in addition to supporting current leaders in their roles, new leaders must be encouraged and developed.

Exercise 2-2

Follower behavior nurtures and supports—or deteriorates—leader behavior. Identify the behavior you exhibited during your most recent clinical experience. What was supportive? What did not support the leader?

THE PRACTICE OF LEADERSHIP

Leadership Approaches

How one approaches leadership depends on experience and expectations. Many leadership theories and styles have been described. Two of the most popular theory-based approaches are transactional leadership and transformational leadership.

Transactional Leadership   A transactional leader is the traditional "boss" image. In a **transactional leadership** environment, employees understand that there is a superior who makes the decisions with little or no input from subordinates. Transactional leadership relies on three methods to move followers: (1) offering rewards to staff or followers for desired work, (2) monitoring work performance and correcting followers when a problem is noted, and (3) waiting until a problem occurs and then dealing with the issue retrospectively (Dunham-Taylor, 2000). Transactional leadership relies on the power of organizational position and formal authority to reward and punish performance. Followers are fairly secure about what will happen next and how to "play the game" to get where they want to be. A transactional leader uses a *quid pro quo* style to accomplish work (e.g., I'll do x in exchange for you doing y). The transactional leader is more likely to opt for status quo and is usually found in stable environments.

Transformational Leadership   A transformational leader is one who seeks and welcomes input from followers as goals are formulated and decisions are made. The **transformational leadership** style is described by Markham (1998) as collaborative, consultative, and consensus-seeking and as ascribing power to interpersonal skills and personal contact. Covey (1992) states, "The goal of transformational leadership is to transform people and organizations in a literal sense, to change them in mind and heart; enlarge vision, insight, and understanding; clarify purposes; make behavior congruent with beliefs, principles, or values; and bring about changes that are permanent, self perpetuating, and momentum-building" (p. 287).

Kouzes and Posner (2002) identify five key practices in transformational leadership: (1) challenging the process, which involves questioning the way things have been done in the past and thinking creatively about new solutions to old problems; (2) inspiring shared vision or bringing everyone together to move toward a goal that all accept as desirable and achievable; (3) enabling others to act, which includes empowering people to believe that their extra effort will have rewards and will make a difference; (4) modeling the way, meaning that the leader must take an active role in the work of change; and (5) encouraging the heart by giving attention to those personal things that are important to people, such as saying "thank you" for a job well done and offering praise after a long day. This type of leader seems particularly suited to the nursing environment. The Research Perspective box suggests that this type of leader increases nurse satisfaction. Transformational leadership is hard work; it takes investment of time and energy to bring out the best in people.

Research Perspective

Dunham-Taylor, J. (2000). Nurse executive transformational leadership found in participative organizations. *Journal of Nursing Administration, 30*(5), 241-250.

Transformational leaders have been found to increase nurse satisfaction in healthcare settings. Transformational leaders empower the workgroup to achieve a vision, whereas the transactional leader monitors work performance and corrects it as needed. In this study, nurse executives ($n = 396$) were asked to describe leadership characteristics, personal power level, and hospital organizational climate. At the same time, three of their staff members ($n = 1115$) were asked to describe their perceptions of the nurse executives' leadership style. Nurse executives who rated themselves as transformational leaders found this claim substantiated by their staff, although the nurse executives tended to rate themselves higher than their staff members. Staff who rated their executive as more of a transformational leader also reported more satisfaction, more effectiveness, and more extra effort put forth in their job. Staff satisfaction decreased as the executive was rated as transactional. Higher transformational scores were seen as the nurse executive possessed higher educational degrees. Furthermore, the larger hospitals tended to be more participative and to attract the transformational nurse executive.

IMPLICATIONS OF PRACTICE

Nurse executives who function in a transformational leadership style tend to have more satisfied employees. The existing cadre of transformational leaders need to serve as mentors and role models to other nurse executives, as well as for young nurses, so that the next generation of nurse executives will assume a transformational leadership style. An empowering, receptive environment is essential to the recruitment and retention of young nurses.

Leadership is the ability to influence people to work toward meeting certain goals. Often this influence requires an ongoing commitment to role-modeling and reinforcing behaviors. The intensity of repeating such influence multiple times can be wearing. In the chaos of health care, nurse leaders face constant change and many challenges. The leader who lasts through these relationships is influential.

Barriers to Leadership

Leadership demands a commitment of effort and time. Many barriers exist to both leading and following. Good leadership and good followership go hand in hand, and both make the mission or the organization stronger. However, there are barriers to leadership.

False Assumptions Some people have false assumptions about leaders and leadership. For example, some believe that position and title are equivalent to leadership. Having the title of Chief Executive Officer or Chief Nursing Officer does not guarantee that a person will be a good leader. Inspired and forward-moving organizations often select these executives specifically because of their ability to forge a vision and lead others toward it. However, a good executive is not necessarily a good leader. Furthermore, assuming a management or administrative role does not automatically confer the title of leader on an individual. Leadership is an earned honor and an action-oriented responsibility.

Others believe that workers who do not hold official management positions cannot be leaders. Some nursing units are managed by the nurse manager but led by the ward secretary or unit clerk. Leaders are those who do the best job of sharing their vision of where the followers want to be and how to get there. Many new nurse managers make the mistake of assuming that along with their new job comes the mantle of leadership. Leadership is an earned right and privilege.

Time Constraints Leadership requires a time commitment; it does not just happen. The leader must fully comprehend the situation at hand, investigate and research options, assume the responsibility to communicate the vision to others, and continually reevaluate the organization or the team to ensure that the vision remains relevant and attainable. All of these activities take time. The 21st century has been described as the period of doing more with less. Everyone is busy. Finding time to lead is, therefore, a barrier for many who have inspirational ideas but lack time to develop the skills needed to lead effectively.

Exercise 2–3

Define a clinical or management issue that sparks your passion. Assume you have 6 weeks to make a difference. Create a plan identifying your leadership tasks, the support required from others, and the time frame to move the issue toward resolution. Think about what your message is and how and when you will deliver it. Think about what you would do if no one was responsive to your issue. Think about why the issue may be important for you but not for others.

LEADERSHIP DEVELOPMENT

Leadership effectiveness depends on mastering the art of persuasion and communication. Success depends on persuading followers to accept a vision by using convincing communication techniques and making it possible for the followers to achieve the shared goals. There are several important leadership tasks that, when used effectively, will help ensure success (Box 2-1). These are discussed in the following sections.

Select a Mentor

A **mentor** is someone who models behavior, offers advice and criticism, and coaches the novice to develop a personal leadership style. A mentor is a confidante and coach as well as a cheerleader and teacher. In other words, a mentor is knowledgeable and skilled. Where do you find a mentor? Usually, a mentor is someone who has experience and some success in the leadership realm of interest, such as in a clinical setting or in an organization. A

BOX 2-1

Leadership Development Tasks

1. Select a mentor.
2. Lead by example.
3. Accept responsibility.
4. Share the rewards.
5. Have a clear vision.
6. Be willing to grow.

respected faculty member; a nurse manager, director, or clinician; or an organizational officer or active member may be a mentor. Mentorship is a two-way street. The mentor must agree to work with the novice leader and must have some interest in the novice's future development. A mentor can be close enough geographically to allow both observation and practice of leadership behaviors, as well as timely feedback. A mentor may also be geographically remote and yet well-connected to the mentee. A mentor should provide advice, feedback, and role-modeling. In addition, the mentor has a right to expect assistance with projects, respect, loyalty, and confidentiality. In a mentoring relationship, aspiring leaders soak up knowledge and experience and should expect to return it by serving as a mentor to a young, aspiring leader in the future.

Lead by Example

An effective leader knows that the most effective and visible way to influence people is to lead by example. Desired behavior can be modeled. For example, if an organization has a vision of becoming a political player in the state or community, the leader should be seen engaging in political activities. If the goal is to have improved relationships between followers, the leader must exhibit respect and patience with followers. A key skill to develop is the ability to understand that the leader serves the followers. The effective leader does not send members to do a job, but rather leads them toward a mutual goal as a team.

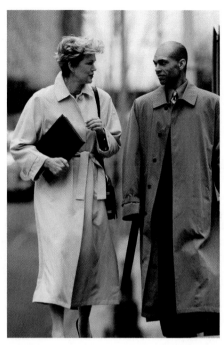

Leading by example helps developing leaders see the mission in action.

Accept Responsibility

Even when the outcome is below expectations, the leader is ultimately responsible for the organization or activity. Effective leaders sometimes react in strange ways when negative outcomes occur. Sometimes these leaders seek to blame others or to make excuses for undesirable or unintended outcomes. Some refuse to accept any responsibility at all. In accepting responsibility, the leader needs to know that there is reward in victory and growth in failure. No one plans to fail, but an effective leader sees failures as opportunities to learn and grow so that previous failures are never repeated. This is called *experience*.

Share the Rewards

An effective leader is as eager to share the glory as to receive it. The more respect and trust are shared with others, the more they are returned to the leader. Followers who believe their major task is to make the leader look good will soon tire of the task. Empowerment, the act of sharing power with others, is a dynamic process. In essence, sharing power has a synergistic effect that increases power overall. Followers who think the leader is working to make them look good will follow eagerly. Followers form a network and a support base for the leader.

Have a Clear Vision

Leaders see beyond where they are and see where they are going. Strong leaders are proactive and futuristic. The effective leader knows why the journey is necessary and takes the time and energy to inspire others to go along. Failing to have a vision is a slow trip to irrelevance (Wieck, 2000). The ability to communicate and promote the vision is a vital part of achieving it. Effective leaders share their vision and empower followers to come along to achieve it. They also share their leadership skills and successes toward achievement of a goal.

Be Willing to Grow

Thinking that growth for the person or organization is automatic is a misconception. Complacency leads to stagnation. Leaders must continually read about new ideas and approaches, experiment with new concepts, capitalize on a changing world, and seek or create continuing education opportunities to enhance their abilities to lead. Growth takes risk, planning, investment, and work. Setting goals that complement the vision will help the aspiring leader know where to invest time and energy to grow into the desired role.

Leadership development is a lifetime endeavor. Effective leaders are constantly striving to improve their leadership skills. The good news is that leadership skills can be learned and improved. A commitment to improvement strengthens the leader's ability to lead effectively and elevates the bar for followers to achieve. As organizations and health care change, the leader is better able to work effectively with an increasingly diverse workforce. The best leaders bring out the best in their followers, as seen in the Literature Perspective.

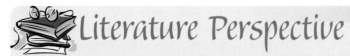

Literature Perspective

Drucker, P. F. (1999). *Management challenges for the 21st century.* New York: HarperBusiness.

Peter F. Drucker has written about leadership and management for more than a half a century. In his recent book about the 21st century, Drucker focuses on the priorities of new millennium workers. Tomorrow's workers will be knowledge workers who require a different kind of leadership style. They expect to be treated as associates rather than as subordinates. After their initial orientation period, the knowledge worker expects to know more about the job than the supervisor. The challenges and issues of leading tomorrow's workforce are already in the arena of ideas; those corporations and leaders who face these challenges today will dominate tomorrow. Those who do not will fall behind and may not survive. Using a team approach will continue to be an effective way to get the work of organizations done, but the new paradigm will be flexibility and change. There is no longer one right way to do things, nor is there one right organization. A primary challenge will be using the best of all leadership and management practices to create an environment that will attract and retain tomorrow's knowledge worker.

IMPLICATIONS OF PRACTICE

Health care has been slower to respond to the changing needs and expectations of the new worker. Dominated by an aging leadership cohort, health care will have to refocus on challenging and appreciating the knowledge worker while creating an environment that allows the knowledge worker to be more marketable and more self-directed. The new workforce wants to be led instead of managed; Drucker's concepts for a new workplace will allow that to happen.

DEVELOPING LEADERS IN THE EMERGING WORKFORCE

Generational differences have always created challenges in the workplace. At the dawn of the 21st century, the workplace found an **emerging workforce** with vastly different goals, priorities, and work preferences than their Baby Boomer parents. Helping each generation understand and tolerate others is often a delicate orchestration of needs and wants, incentives and motives. Transgenerational leadership must focus on building an understanding and acceptance of each other.

The Emerging Workforce: The 1965 to 1985 Generation

Part of this cohort, born between 1965 and 1976, represents the smallest workforce entry pool since 1930, with just 44 million, compared with the 77 million Baby Boomers preceding them and the 70 million Generation Ys following them. They have a mindset and work ethic that Baby Boomers do not understand. Their younger siblings, the Generation Ys, who were born between 1977 and 1985, share many of the same approaches to work but bring their own challenges with no brand loyalty and a blatant disregard for status symbols.

In looking at what these emerging workforce members want in their leaders, a recent study of a national sample of student nurses indicates that they want a leader who is receptive to people, a team player, honest, a good communicator, approachable, knowledgeable, motivating, and competent and has a positive attitude and good people skills (Wieck, Prydun, & Walsh, 2002). Rather than managing details of work, nurse managers have to be able to lead the group through coaching and mentoring.

Successfully leading the emerging workforce means the leader must shape a vision and win the 20-somethings to it. The vision must be one that excites them because fun and balance are an important part of their lives. A vision that is powerful enough can transform the workplace.

The successful leader must mobilize the followers to act. The required actions must provide value to the followers (e.g., learning a new skill or attaining certification or recognition). The younger generations are happy to follow as long as they can retain balance in their lives, have information about and input into the decisions that affect them, and see some benefit in the activity. It is the leader's challenge to provide the type of environment where younger-generation followers want to follow.

The Entrenched Workforce: The 1946 to 1965 Generation

Baby Boomers, born after World War II, see work life very differently compared with the emerging workforce. Boomer workers are much more likely to believe in the power of collective action, based on their successes with social movements in their formative years in the 1960s. They tend to mistrust authority and are very comfortable with the process of getting to a goal. They find the journey of getting to the goal almost as important as reaching the goal. They are tolerant of, even dependent on, meetings and ongoing discussions that the younger generation finds tedious and wasteful.

The preferred leader of the **entrenched workforce** shares some of the characteristics of the younger generation's leader, such as being motivational, honest, approachable, competent, and knowledgeable. However, Baby Boomers also expect their leader to be professional, be supportive, and have high integrity, a concept not even mentioned by the younger generation (Wieck, Prydun, & Walsh, 2002).

Challenges for the entrenched workforce are sharing leadership with the younger generation, empowering them to lead in their own model rather than trying to make them into second-generation Baby Boomers, and retaining the younger leaders in leadership ranks. Many younger employees are opting out of traditional work roles to become entrepreneurs. They take their leadership potential with them where there are few older role models for them to follow. A risk for aging Boomers is that the best and the brightest potential leaders will lose interest in leading and will opt for personal satisfaction and wealth accumulation rather than leadership and service roles.

The challenges of generational acceptance are one of many facing 21st century leaders. Attention to the needs of both the leader and the follower will create an environment where everyone thrives.

■ Exercise 2-4

List the names of the people with whom you work most frequently. Determine to which workforce (emerging or entrenched) each belongs. Describe known benefits of the workplace that support each generation's view. (One list may be longer than the other.) What elements of benefits are present in the personnel policies and workplace practices that benefit each? What elements are absent?

SURVIVING AND THRIVING AS A LEADER

The key to leadership is to believe in the vision and to enjoy the journey. The leader has a responsibility to self and followers to stay healthy and enthusiastic for the mission of the group. Surviving and thriving as a leader is based on the rules in Box 2-2. Each element is discussed in the following sections.

The Leader Must Maintain Balance

Time management is essential for an effective leader. Many new leaders, in their zeal to be accessible to their constituents, lose control of their lives. A good strategy for retaining or regaining control is to get control of communication. Good leaders use the simplest and fastest method of communication that makes them accessible but does not tie them down. The keys to success are setting priorities and keeping in control. Planned telephone time and e-mail are excellent ways to keep control of time. Attending to matters as they come up, handling each question or piece of mail once and only one at a time, and focusing on the task at hand without distractions are just some of the time-management strategies used by effective leaders. Saving time, like wasting time, is a learned habit and can therefore be unlearned or relearned.

BOX 2-2

The Five Rules of Leaders

1. Maintain balance.
2. Generate self-motivation.
3. Build self-confidence.
4. Listen to constituents.
5. Maintain a positive attitude.

The Leader Must Generate Self-Motivation

Leaders who expect their followers to provide them with motivation, to be grateful for the time spent on followers' needs, and to offer frequent and lavish praise are in for a painful awakening. Followers in organizations, work situations, and elected constituencies feel they have earned the right to criticize the leader by being followers. Followers will have an opinion about everything. Sometimes the comments are favorable, and sometimes they are unfavorable. The reason that self-motivation is so essential is because the leader can expect very little external motivation. Most leaders are risk-takers and self-starters who are enthused by and believe in the vision they have created. Enthusiasm leads to an energized base that is a hallmark of a vibrant, healthy organization.

The Leader Must Work at Building Self-Confidence

An effective leader must have self-confidence. This confidence comes from an acceptance of self, despite imperfections. Self-confidence is a self-perpetuating virtue. Effective leaders perform an honest self-appraisal on a regular basis and work to feel good about the job they are doing. A leader who is surrounded by people who enhance the leader's own characteristics makes a formidable leadership team and strengthens self-confidence in the ability to lead.

The more confident a leader feels, the more likely it is that success will follow. Success builds self-confidence. Two important factors are related to developing self-confidence. One is avoiding the tendency to become arrogant. The other is maintaining self-confidence despite setbacks.

The Leader Must Listen to the Constituents

Followers always have something to say. Leaders must listen to their constituents and determine whether action is indicated. Active listening, which in the U.S. culture includes looking the person in the eye and offering questioning probes, shows an interest in what a person is saying. However, listening does not obligate the leader to any course of action. Clear boundaries must be communicated.

A smart leader listens to all sides and makes decisions based on the vision and direction that is best for the group.

The Leader Must Have a Positive Attitude

Positive attitude is vital to leadership success. No one wants to follow a pessimist anywhere. People expect the leader to have the answers, to know where the organization is going, and to take the initiative to get the group to their goal. A positive attitude can be a great ally in sharing and maintaining the vision. Attitude is a choice, not a foregone conclusion. The effective leader uses positive thinking and positive messages to create an environment in which followers believe in the organization, the leader, and themselves. The problems and challenges in health care demand that nurses seek and fill leadership positions in a positive and future-oriented manner.

Exercise 2–5

Using the five rules for leaders, create a personal description of how you maintain balance, generate self-motivation, build self-confidence, listen to constituents, and maintain a positive attitude.

THE NURSE AS LEADER

Leadership Within the Workplace

Staff Nurse as Leader   A common misconception is that leaders within the workplace are the managers. Leaders within the workplace are not necessarily those who are entrusted with the role and title of manager. The workplace manager is one who is a status quo maintainer, that is, the focus is on the day-to-day operations. The manager is concerned about budgets, financial performance, staffing, employee evaluations, and employee education and training. All of these important activities are paramount concerns of the manager of an operational unit in health care. In contrast, the workplace leader is one who has the ability to envision a preferred future for the quality of the working environment. The leader understands that nurse satisfaction is a central construct of many of the most successful nursing-service delivery systems (Evans, 1999).

Workplace leaders lead nurses to satisfaction and have ideas for increasing the level of workplace satisfaction for nurses on the team. Leaders are those who creatively pose solutions to problems and capitalize on opportunities in the workplace. Furthermore, they support staff nurses, who impose numerous ideas about patient safety issues. Nurses who believe that they have good ideas for future improvements should volunteer for opportunities to lead. There might be practice councils, clinical unit standards committees, or legislative committees to pose new solutions. If the hospital or other workplace has no formalized mechanism for nurse input into organizational decision making, staff nurses who are leaders should clarify their vision and work to make it happen.

Developing leadership skills for staff nurses can happen in several ways. Some of these may be employment opportunities (practice councils), others may be professional opportunities (the district nurses association), and still others might be clinical opportunities (heart association). Leadership can be developed, and staff nurse leaders can help establish workplaces that are satisfying and rewarding. Magnet™ facilities, for example, depend on staff nurse leadership to create the intensity of quality work.

Nurse Manager as Leader Management and leadership, although different constructs, can be a strong combination for success. The nurse in the role of manager ensures that the day-to-day elements of the workplace are done correctly. Just as the effective manager pays attention to employee selection, hiring, orientation, continuing employee development, and financial accountability, in the role of leader, the manager raises the level of expectations and helps employees reach their highest level of potential excellence. A primary role of the leader is to inspire (Atchison, 1990).

Developing with staff nurses a shared vision of the preferred future is a goal of the nurse manager in the role of leader. Staff members tend to resist change that is thrust upon them. When nurses are active participants in change, from its inception, they are far more likely to be invested in outcomes.

An essential element of success for the nurse manager as a leader is the inclusion of staff nurses in decision-making. This contribution can enhance their organizational commitment and create a sense of pride in successful outcomes. The nurse manager inspires staff by involving them in changing the workplace to make it more satisfying. In so doing, the nurse manager also develops personal leadership skills.

Nurse Executive as Leader A primary goal of the nurse executive is leadership within the workplace. The nurse executive has an outstanding opportunity to shape the future of professional practice within a working environment by creating opportunities for staff nurses and managers to have optimal input into organizational decision-making related to the future. The nurse executive thus helps create a shared vision of the preferred future.

The concept of empowerment is important to the role of leadership for the nurse executive in a work organization. Empowerment theory suggests that power must be given away or shared with others in the organization. Staff nurses may be encouraged to have input into decisions or they may be given considerable information about how decisions are made. The ability to make or influence changes in the organization is a powerful tool. Nurses must believe that their input and ideas are considered when change occurs. Having input in decisions, having some control over the environment, and receiving feedback about actions taken or not taken all contribute to a feeling of being empowered to have control over one's practice and one's life.

The importance of managers and executives being leaders rather than managers is a recurring theme in nursing literature. The fact is both management and leadership skills in the nurse executive are essential. The ability to balance the day-to-day operating knowledge with the ability to lead a nursing service organization into the future is a winning combination.

Nursing Student as Leader Students have many opportunities to learn and practice leadership skills. The goals for leadership at the student level should be kept within a realistic framework. Allowing the student to practice novice leadership skills within the security of an educational program is a

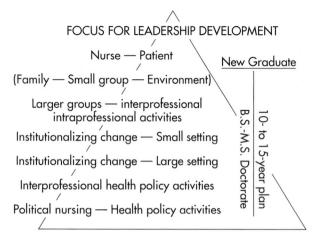

Figure 2-1   A leadership trajectory. (From Fagin, C. [2000]. *Essays on nursing leadership.* New York: Springer.)

reasonable expectation. Novice leadership skills that contribute to future leadership success involve learning how to work in groups, deal with difficult people, resolve conflict, reach consensus on an action, and evaluate actions and outcomes objectively (Figure 2-1). These opportunities create skills that can lead to some expertise that could transfer to initial practice.

Fagin (2000) describes a 10- to 15-year leadership development plan for neophyte nurses that builds on their leadership skills from their beginning nurse-patient experiences. The reality of student development toward true leadership expertise takes place over a long period and should not be expected during the first year or two of nursing school or nursing practice. Nevertheless, every leader started somewhere. Movement toward an increasingly complex leadership experience allows the new nurse to move from leading and planning with an individual to working with groups, such as families or communities. Further leadership development occurs during interactions with larger groups and through instituting changes in research and application of new techniques and moving toward health policy and political activities. With increasing educational achievement and career experience come increasing complexity of leadership capabilities.

Most countries have some type of national student nurses' association, as well as regional, state, and school-based associations. These types of organizations offer an opportunity for student nurses to become involved in service to their future profession. Programs of study in schools of nursing are appropriately heavy on nursing theory and clinical practice. Through involvement in the student association, the nursing student is able to understand the bigger picture of nursing as a profession.

The best way to begin involvement is to become active in the local chapter of the student association. If the student is interested in student association activities, there are opportunities to serve on committees or in elected positions on the board of directors at local, regional, state, and national levels. Examples of leadership development at the national level include serving on liaison committees with nurse leaders; attending leadership development educational programs; attending and leading events at local, state, and national meetings and conventions; and interacting with the leaders of complementary professional nursing organizations.

Organizational Leadership in Organizations

The American Nurses Association and State Affiliates   In the United States, the best and most important step to take in becoming a leader within the nursing profession is to join a professional organization. Many nurses today take part in several organizations. However, membership in the American Nurses Association (ANA) and the state constituent member associations shapes career growth and mobility. Volunteering for local or committee memberships is a valued and useful way to learn and to grow within the association.

After becoming established and known in the local association, running for elected office in the local district association is a way many leaders within professional associations start their leadership careers. It is not unusual to be unsuccessful in the first attempt at running for an elective office in the professional association, but persistence can do two things: It can help with name recognition, and it can let members know that you are serious about being an association leader.

Many of the leaders within the ANA, after having begun their association leadership in the district association, later held office in the state constituent member associations. Volunteering for committee assignments and running for elected office in the state association establish leadership interest within the professional association. Leadership efforts at the national association level are usually more successful after establishing a record of successful leadership in the state constituent member association.

This pathway of professional involvement and leadership, from the student association to the district association to the state association and to the national association, may seem like a linear progression to more global opportunities for leadership in the profession. However, many very successful nursing leaders conceptualize the progression as circular rather than linear. Many well-known leaders who have held high office in the ANA do not then retire from professional involvement, but rather take their experience and expertise to return to offices and committee appointments at the district level and at the state levels or to contribute to other revenues.

Professional Specialty Organizations Professional nursing specialty organizations play an important role in disseminating information to members in such areas as clinical practice (e.g., Oncology Nursing Society), role area (e.g., American Organization of Nurse Executives), and interest groups (e.g., Southern Nursing Research Society). Many of the professional specialty organizations maintain a national or regional presence rather than having state or local chapters. Some of them have local chapters (e.g., Association of periOperative Registered Nurses), especially in the larger, more populated areas across the country. The major impact of the professional specialty organization is sharing and dissemination of information, discussion of mutual clinical or role concerns, and education regarding the latest technical innovations in the field. Leadership opportunities are available to present posters or papers at local, regional, or national conferences, as well as to serve on committees and boards.

Leadership in the Community

Nurses as Community Opinion Leaders Nurses are valued and respected members of their communities. As trusted professionals, nurses have an opportunity to serve as catalysts in leadership opportunities in the community. In partnership with others in the community, nurses can help build a more just, more peaceful, and more healthful society.

Many avenues are available for nurses to serve as community opinion leaders. Attendance at civic gatherings, such as city commission and school board meetings, is an excellent way to be aware of what is happening and to offer input from a nursing perspective. For instance, when the school board begins deliberating whether the budget will accommodate a registered nurse for every school or whether to replace them with a trained clerk who can record vaccinations, a nursing voice in the audience could clarify the importance of school nurses to a school population. Writing letters to the editor of a newspaper and participating in public forums give the nurse an avenue to share expertise and mold community opinion.

Nurses as Community Volunteers Many opportunities exist for volunteer participation in the community. Nurses bring a unique leadership skill set to community activities. The ability to understand complex systems as well as to understand interpersonal dynamics and communication techniques, constitutes knowledge that is valuable in community volunteer opportunities.

Leadership in mobilizing volunteers for health fairs, screening activities, and educational events is a community need that nurses can and do fill. Such activities promote health and advance the health of the community in important ways. Nurses can also lead efforts to engage others in the community in volunteer activities. In addition, nurses can organize individuals in the community to help develop a vision for the future of the community's health, healthcare opportunities, and healthcare delivery.

From the perspective of the nurse as a community leader, there is a unique opportunity to work with schools, city or county governments, and other community entities to formulate a vision for improving the health of the community through disease prevention and health promotion. The nurse can be a catalyst for a community to recognize present problems and to develop a plan to reach a preferred future.

Leadership Through Appointed and Elected Office

Nurses are valuable leaders in elected and appointed offices at the local, state, and national levels. Because of the trustworthiness of nurses in general, nurses should be able to mobilize resources to raise monies, develop support, and get elected to offices. The numbers of nurses in offices at all three levels of government are continually growing. The ANA Political Action Committee (PAC) and the state constituent member association PACs provide assistance to nurses who want to run for office. Nurses who are elected members of governmental bodies are able to exert their leadership to shape the vision of the government to help meet the needs of the citizens.

Local Offices   Leadership opportunities in elected or appointed positions in the local government include school boards, city councils, and community boards dealing with various community initiatives. At the local level, nurses who serve on elected or appointed boards and councils bring a unique perspective, even when the major focus of the entity appears to be totally unrelated to health care. Leadership in this case is casting a vision of a healthy, thriving community.

State Offices   Leadership opportunities at the state level in elected or appointed positions include being elected to state legislatures or appointment to state boards, such as the state board of nursing or the state board of health. The state constituent member association of the ANA often has a role in recommending names of qualified members to be considered for appointment to various boards and committees in the state. Nurses who are members have the highest likelihood of being supported or recommended by the state association or national association.

National Offices   A few nurses have been successful in getting elected to the U.S. Congress as representatives. No nurse has yet been elected U.S. Senator, but many opportunities exist for nurses to be appointed to federal boards and commissions. The ANA and the state constituent member associations often play a role in putting forth nominations of members for appointment to such bodies.

The Challenge of Leading

The nurse is in a trusted role as nurturer and provider of care to the most vulnerable in our society. Nurses who choose leadership roles have many of the needed talents to serve their followers and their profession. Visionary and responsible leadership is vital to the future success of nursing as an art and a science. Professional nursing has been blessed with excellent leaders in the past and will continue to be led by the visionary nurse leaders of tomorrow.

The Solution

The following priorities were set:
- Patient safety
- Occupant safety
- Return to normal function as quickly as possible

Unit nursing staff were instructed to review their emergency preparedness manuals the evening of June 8 and ensure that they had flashlights and water. They were instructed to divide into teams and watch each other's patients, allowing some of the staff to rest. It was clear that the staff needed to pace themselves because it would be hours before additional personnel would arrive. Staff were reassured by frequent rounds made by the supervisors and calls to the units from the Command Center.

As water rushed into the basement of the facility, the departments of pharmacy and radiology moved their supplies higher and dry cereal, bread, and milk were obtained from the cafeteria to sustain patients over the coming hours. The Network Services Department (hospital telephone and page operators) was relocated to higher ground. At 3 AM, as a power shortage became imminent, the decision to triage stable patients who were on life support devices was made. These patients were located on four different floors and were evacuated, starting at the highest floor and working down before elevators lost power. Patients were transferred to an adjacent medical tower building that had an outpatient ambulatory surgery center linked to the hospital via a skybridge. Anesthesiologists, residents, respiratory therapists, and nurses worked collaboratively to triage patients. Some critical care patients were evacuated down stairwells as elevators failed. All critically ill patients who were too unstable to evacuate were placed on ventilators with battery backup. It became apparent that power was needed quickly to maintain ventilator support because batteries would be drained. As soon as roads were passable, external diesel generators were obtained and connected to provide power to ventilators, which then created the need to test for carbon dioxide levels. A human chain was created to deliver medical supplies, water, food, and lights to staff.

Staff were educated to deliver IVs without pumps and take blood pressures the old fashioned way, with a manometer and a flashlight. Food was provided to patients and staff from volunteer agencies such as the Salvation Army. Patient and staff comfort was difficult to maintain in an un–air-conditioned, 26-story tower in the summertime. Patients were triaged for discharge; all admissions were carefully screened by a medical director and nurses because the City of Houston was short 3000 hospital beds for an extended period. Nine days after the flood, all beds and essential services were functioning, and the hospital was open for all admissions.

Nurses often have not learned the necessary skills for triage and disaster response. An understanding of emergency plans and quick critical thinking skills are imperative to surviving a natural disaster.

— Rosemary Luquire

 Would this be a suitable approach for you? Why?

CHAPTER CHECKLIST

The role of the nurse leader is to share a vision and provide the means for followers to reach it. When the group succeeds, the leader succeeds. Members of different generations have different expectations and different needs from those of a leader. Various leadership opportunities are available; it is up to the nurse to take advantage and contribute to the progress of the nursing profession.

- Excellent leadership in any working environment can improve recruitment and retention efforts and result in satisfied employees.
- Two leadership approaches contrast the leader role:
  - Transactional leaders rely on the power of the organizational position to reward or punish performance in order to control employees.
  - Transformational leaders ascribe power to interpersonal skills and personal contact in transforming people to make them want to progress.
- Key elements to becoming an effective leader can be learned and practiced:
  - Select an effective and willing mentor.
  - Lead by example through role modeling.
  - Share the rewards with followers.
  - Have a clear vision that followers can support.
  - Be willing to grow and change to meet current needs.
- The emerging workforce (born 1965 to 1976) want a leader who has good people skills and a nurturing attitude. The entrenched workforce (born 1946 to 1965) wants a leader who is tolerant of the process of change and who exhibits high integrity and professionalism.
- There are many opportunities to lead in nursing. To thrive in a leadership position, the nurse must do the following:
  - Maintain balance.
  - Generate self-motivation.
  - Build self-confidence.
  - Listen to constituents.
  - Have a positive attitude.

TIPS FOR BECOMING A LEADER

If you want to become an effective leader, here are some tips.

- Take advantage of leadership opportunities and practice your leadership skills.
- Expect to stumble occasionally, but learn from your mistakes and continue. Every leader has made mistakes. The truly inspired leaders have learned from them and moved forward.
- Get some help—a caring mentor is the best way to develop leadership ability. The mentor can give you the benefit of experience and will serve as a resource to get feedback on actions and to explore options.
- Take risks. A person does not become a leader by maintaining the status quo. Leaders forge a vision and bring followers forward. However, change involves risks. Do not be fool-hardy, but do not be complacent, either.

TERMS TO KNOW

emerging workforce
entrenched workforce
leadership
management
mentor
transactional leadership
transformational leadership

REFERENCES

Atchison, T. A. (2004). *Followership: A practical guide to aligning leaders and followers.* Chicago: Health Administration Press.

Atchison, T. A. (1990). *Turning health care leadership around.* San Francisco: Jossey-Bass.

Bennis, W. (1989). *On becoming a leader.* Reading, MA: Addison-Wesley.

Covey, S. R. (1992). *Principle-centered leadership.* New York: Simon & Schuster.

Dunham-Taylor, J. (2000). Nurse executive transformational leadership found in participative organizations. *Journal of Nursing Administration, 30*(5), 241-250.

Evans, M. L. (1999). Nursing's role and outcomes in practice and advanced practice. In C. A. Anderson (Ed.), *Nursing student to nursing leader: The critical path to leadership development.* Albany, NY: Delmar.

Fagin, C. (2000). *Essays on nursing leadership.* New York: Springer Publishing.

Kouzes, J., & Posner, B. (2002). *The leadership challenge.* San Francisco: Jossey Bass.

Markham, G. (1998). Gender in leadership. *Nursing Management, 3*(1), 18-19.

Marriner-Tomey, A. (1993). *Transformational leadership in nursing.* St. Louis: Mosby.

Oakley, E., & Krug, D. (1994). *Enlightened leadership.* New York: Simon & Schuster.

Senge, P. M. (1994). *The fifth discipline: The art and practice of the learning organization.* New York: Doubleday.

Tappen, R. M. (2000). *Nursing leadership and management: Concepts and practice* (4th ed.). Philadelphia: FA Davis.

Vance, C. (1999). Mentoring: The nursing leader and mentor's perspective. In C. A. Anderson (Ed.), *Nursing student to nursing leader: The critical path to leadership development.* Albany, NY: Delmar.

Wieck, K. L. (2000). A vision of nursing: The future revisited. *Nursing Outlook, 48*(1), 7-8.

Wieck, K. L., Prydun, M., & Walsh, T. (2002). What Emerging Workforce nurses want in their leaders. *Journal of Nursing Scholarship, 34*(3), 283.

SUGGESTED READINGS

Barger, S. E. (2000). Professional practice: The practice of leadership. *Journal of Professional Nursing, 16*(2), 72.

Bower, F. L. (2000). *Nurses taking the lead: Personal qualities of effective leadership.* St. Louis: Mosby.

Labarre, P. (2000, March). Do you have the will to lead? *FastCompany,* 222-230.

Northouse, P. G. (2001). *Leadership: Theory and practice* (2nd ed.). Thousand Oaks, CA: Sage Publishers.

Shtogren, J. A. (Ed.). (1999). *Skyhooks for leadership.* New York: American Management Association.

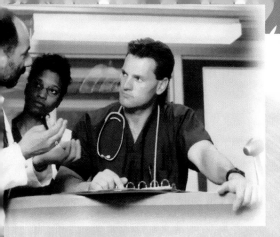

3

Developing the Role of Manager

Ana M. Valadez
Dorothy A. Otto

*T*his chapter identifies key concepts related to the roles of the nurse manager. It describes basic manager functions, illustrates management principles that are inherent in the role of professional practice, and identifies descriptive competencies for the nurse manager. Role-development is crucial to forming the right questions to ask in a management or clinical situation that will help the practitioner identify problems and anticipate needs. This chapter provides an overview for the further development of practical skills.

Objectives

- Analyze roles and functions of a nurse manager.
- Analyze the relationship of the nurse manager with others.
- Analyze management of healthcare settings.
- Evaluate management resource allocation/distribution.
- Evaluate behaviors of professionalism of the nurse manager.

Questions to Consider

- Why do you want to be a nurse manager?
- In what type of practice setting would you like to be a nurse manager?
- How do you manage current resources?
- Do you yearn to have increased involvement in key decisions, changing systems, working with people, or improving patient care?
- How will your clinical expertise be used in the setting?

The Challenge

Joyce Burdett, RN, BSN
Nurse Manager, Covenant Health System, Lubbock, Texas

I know that although the nursing shortage remains a challenge for many of us in management, my biggest challenge is not a shortage of professional staff. In fact, I only have one open position, and, thanks to the staff that do their own recruiting for our unit, we are doing well. My biggest challenge as a nurse manager is how to make the best use of my professional staff skills and not waste them on redundant tasks. Case in point is the lack of the electronic medical record. To give you an example, the professional staff completes an admission packet on every new patient that is 15 pages long, and one of the forms has three subsections. If the nurse truly does a good admission assessment, it will take him/her at least an hour and a half to complete it. As we continue to add more regulatory information, such as HIPPA or Medicare, the admission packet can only increase, rather than decrease, in size.

The nurse managers have been involved in evaluating different electronic record systems, and we thought we had one; however, the system was not large enough to accommodate our expansive health system that has more than one central area of operation. Currently, we think that electronic recording is 3 years down the pike for us.

 What do you think you would do if you were this nurse?

INTRODUCTION

Chapter 1 provided a general overview of leading and managing. In this chapter, we look at management from different perspectives. The underpinnings of role theory began with management theory, a science that has undergone numerous changes in the past century. In the early 1900s, the theory of scientific management was embraced—a theory based on the idea that there is one best way to accomplish a task. Practice in the 1930s through the 1970s was dominated by participative, humanistic leadership theories. Although changes in healthcare delivery no doubt are affecting the roles of nurse managers, the relevance of role theory remains a constant. Conway's (1978) historic definition, "**role theory** represents a collection of concepts and a variety of hypothetical formulations that predict how actors will perform in a given role, or under what circumstances certain types of behaviors can be expected" (p. 17), is still appropriate today.

The evolutionary process of management theories has affected how managers address workers' concerns and needs. The beginning management theories discounted concern for workers' psychological needs and focused on productivity and efficiency. When theories relating to human relations came about, workers' needs and motivations became focal points for the nurse manager. Conversely, situational theories, such as the Path-Goal theory, focused on the environment, clarifying the relationship between the pathway employees take and the outcome or goal they wish to obtain.

What is involved in management? A self-appraisal might lead a potential nurse manager to ask him/herself the following questions: Do I have career goals that include gaining experience and education to become a nurse manager? What specific knowledge, skills, and personal qualities do I need to develop to be most effective in practice? What support systems have I established? If changes need to be made, they must be matched with changes in healthcare agencies and within the larger social system. A nurse manager must recognize the need for growth within, which then translates into improvement of one's practice. A prerequisite for self-actualization is a bond between the nurse and the community, because a nurse manager's patients and staff make up the community. Consider also, what is the **role** of the nurse manager? Practicing nurse managers illustrate role perceptions. Some nurse managers would cite decision-making and problem-solving as major roles, for which maintaining objectivity is sometimes a special challenge.

Others would identify collaboration, especially with other departments, to enhance quality patient outcomes. Truly effective care is the result of efforts by the total healthcare team. Effective collaboration includes honesty, directness, and listening to others' points of view. However, management is more complex than this.

THE MANAGEMENT ROLE

Management is a generic function that includes similar basic tasks in every discipline and in every society. However, before the nurse manager can be effective, he or she must be well-grounded in nursing practice. Drucker (1974), in his classic writings, identified five basic functions of a manager:

- Establishes objectives and goals for each area and communicates them to the persons who are responsible for attaining them
- Organizes and analyzes the activities, decisions, and relations needed and divides them into manageable tasks
- Motivates and communicates with the people responsible for various jobs through teamwork
- Analyzes, appraises, and interprets performance and communicates the meaning of measurement tools and their results to staff and superiors
- Develops people, including self

Table 3-1 shows how these basic management functions apply to the nurse manager.

Managers develop efforts that focus on the individual. Their aim is to enable the person to develop his or her abilities and strengths to the fullest and to achieve excellence. Thus, a manager has a role in helping people develop goals that are realistic. Goals should be set high enough, yet be attainable. Active participation, encouragement, and guidance from the manager and from the organization are needed for the individual's developmental efforts to be fully productive. Nurse managers who are successful in motivating staff are often providing an environment that facilitates accomplishment of goals, resulting in personal satisfactions.

The nurse manager must possess qualities similar to those of a good leader: knowledge, integrity, ambition, judgment, courage, stamina, enthusiasm, communication skills, planning skills, and administrative abilities. The arena of management versus leadership has been addressed by numerous authors, and although there are differences in points of view, there are some similarities between managers and leaders.

Managers address complex issues by planning, budgeting, and setting target goals. They meet their goals by organizing, staffing, controlling, and solving problems. By contrast, **leaders** set a direc-

Table 3-1 BASIC MANAGER FUNCTIONS AND NURSE MANAGER FUNCTIONS

Basic Manager Functions	Nurse Manager Functions
Establishes and communicates goals and objectives	Delineates objectives and goals for assigned area Communicates objectives and goals effectively to staff members who will help attain goals
Organizes, analyzes, and divides work into tasks	Assesses and evaluates activities on assigned area Makes sound decisions about dividing up daily work activities for staff
Motivates and communicates	Stresses the importance of being a good team player Provides positive reinforcement
Analyzes, appraises, and interprets performance and measurements	Completes performance appraisals of individual staff members Communicates results to staff and management
Develops people, including self	Addresses staff development continuously through mentoring and preceptorships Furthers self-development by attending educational programs and seeking specialty certification credentialing

Based on Drucker, P. F. (1974). *Management tasks, responsibilities and practices.* New York: Harper & Row.

Table 3-2 LEADER, MANAGER, AND FOLLOWER TRAITS

Leader Traits	Manager Traits	Follower Traits
Values commitments, relationships with others, and esprit de corps in the organization	Emphasizes organizing, coordinating, and controlling resources (e.g., space, supplies, equipment, people)	Perceives the needs of both the leader and other staff
Provides a vision that can be communicated and has a long-term effect on the organization that moves it in new directions	Attends to short-term objectives/goals	Demonstrates cooperative and collaborative behaviors
Communicates the rationale for changing paths; charts new paths that lead to progress	Maximizes results from existing resources	Exerts the power to communicate through various channels
Endorses and thrives on taking risks that bring about change	Interprets established policy, procedures, and mandates	Remains fully accountable for actions while relinquishing some autonomy and conceding certain authority to the leader
Demonstrates a positive feeling in the workplace and relates the importance of workers	Moves cautiously; dislikes uncertainty	Exhibits willingness to both lead and follow peers, as the situation warrants, allowing for competency-based leadership
	Enforces policy mandates, contracts, etc. (acts as a gatekeeper)	Assumes responsibility to understand what risks are acceptable for the organization and what risks are unacceptable

tion, develop a vision, and communicate the new direction to the staff. Managers address complexity, whereas leaders address change. Another way of looking at management in contrast to leadership and followership is to look at the common traits of each. In Table 3-2, the characteristics of a leader are compared with those of a manager and a follower.

Exercise 3–1

In a small group, discuss how patients pay for services of hospitals, clinics, hospices, or private provider offices. Hypothesize about what portion of those costs represents nursing care. How does a manager contribute to cost-effectiveness?

The literature abounds with complexities that nurse managers face in the everyday roles they encounter when leading their staff. One of those roles is one of creating a positive workplace environment. Manion (2003) conducted a study with 24 healthcare workers to ascertain the joy they experienced in their work. One half of the sample comprised managers, and the age group included Baby Boomers as well as Generation X-ers. Although the participants described many factors in their interviews, three prevailed: (1) work represented progress; (2) the work provided connections with other people; and (3) competence was required. The model of joy that evolved from the interviews demonstrated that the three factors described above all play a part in providing a joyful work environment as long as the internal factors were present within the person. These factors included self-esteem, beliefs, attitudes, values, and competence. The model gives leaders ideas on how they can create a positive work environment. Because more time is spent at work than at home, if joy is present in the person's work environment, life can be more pleasant and satisfying.

The nurse manager is the environmentalist of the unit. In other words, the manager is always assessing the context in which people practice to determine how changes there can affect people's performance. No changes occur within an organization that are not visible in the larger societal context. Thus, we see violence in the workplace today, just as we see it in society as a whole. As a result, the nurse manager's role also requires knowing how to prevent violence, how to diffuse explosive situations, and how to create and enforce a zero-tolerance policy. The nurse manager can explicate that "what happens out there" could, and likely will, happen within an organization's confines. Clearly, one of the roles a manager must fulfill is translating what is happening in a societal sense into the possibilities of the organization. This requires that the nurse manager be involved in strategic planning that can translate to all with whom the manager works.

Quantum theory elucidates the complexity and unpredictability of events. Because nurse managers will continue to practice in an unstable, rapidly changing healthcare environment, quantum theory may be the most significant theory for nurse managers of the 21st century. Porter-O'Grady (2003) speaks to the rules of leadership changing. He addresses the chaos created by a rapidly changing healthcare environment, both from the clinical as well as the structural unit. Porter-O'Grady refers to 10 factors that depict the direction in which health care is moving: (1) Portability of health care leads to shorter recovery periods following less invasive techniques. (2) The more fluid medical care models discharge patients quicker, but the education of nurses still adheres to learning practices that require longer patient stays. (3) The shift from inpatient to speedy outpatient services is increasing. (4) Shorter care stays shift the aftercare from health provider to care-recipient and significant others. (5) Payment models previously never questioned are now subjected to reviews for appropriateness in relation to procedure and fee requested. (6) Healthcare provider shortages are impacting the services given to changing client populations. (7) Work stress and conflict are occurring between the mature worker whose loyalty is institutionally based and the younger worker who values the work, not the institution. (8) Rapidly changing technology demands extreme adaptability from the healthcare provider. (9) Managers have the accountability for temporary workers who give service to an institution yet are employed by an outside company. (10) There is an increased stress on managers who are required to address system problems that take them away from their service unit. All of these factors present a challenging work environment to the manager, who needs different skills to manage clinical work effectively. However, these challenges can be invigorating to talented, creative nurses.

To be successful in day-to-day operations, a manager must be concerned with relationships. Chaleff (1995) developed a model of followership to reorient individuals. "Courageous followership is built on the platform of courageous relationship. The courage to be right, the courage to be wrong, the courage to be different from each other. Each of us sees the world through our own eyes and experiences" (p. 4). Chaleff describes five dimensions of the relationship: the courage to assume responsibility, the courage to serve, the courage to challenge, the courage to participate in transformation, and the courage to leave by separating from a leader or group. Table 3-3 poses the possible corollary role of the manager for supporting this courage development in **followers.**

Table 3-3 THE MANAGER'S COROLLARY TO THE COURAGE OF FOLLOWERS

Dimension of the Relationship	
Follower	Manager
Courage to assume responsibility	Demonstrates trust in individual autonomy
Courage to serve	Advocates for service role
Courage to challenge	Poses dilemmas to encourage behavior
Courage to participate in transformation	Designs opportunities to develop transformational abilities
Courage to leave by separating from a leader or group	Risks separation

Reprinted with permission of the publisher. From Chaleff, I. (1995). *The courageous follower: Standing up to and for our leaders.* San Francisco: Berrett-Koehler Publishers, Inc. All rights reserved. www.bkconnection.com.

CONSUMING RESEARCH

The nurse manager's role calls for a twofold responsibility: that of being a participant in research and that of being an interpreter of research. Nursing literature, especially in nursing administration journals, reflects that nurse managers are contributing to research either by doing unit research or contributing to large-scale agency research projects. Likewise, the nurse manager also interprets published research findings that have implications for the staff or the patients and makes every effort to incorporate the findings into unit activities so that both staff and patients can benefit from evidence-based care. Nurse managers, as first-line managers, are also in the position of identifying best nursing practices that can be researched through collaborative efforts of service and educational institutions.

MENTORING

A manager also should be concerned about preparing successors. Although mentoring individuals for the purpose of attaining greater heights in career development is not a new concept, the use of mentors for women was not addressed until the late 1970s. Cherry and Jacob (2005) include the role of mentoring as another role that nurses in leadership/management positions must embrace. They view mentoring as an interactive, multifaceted role that assists the staff with setting realistic attainable goals. Through mentoring their staff, nurse managers can help boost staff self-confidence, thereby helping them to gain professional satisfaction as they reach their goals. Nurse managers not only give clinical guidance to their staff but also they can be instrumental in assisting them with their present work and their career development.

ORGANIZATIONAL CULTURE

In the ever-changing environment of health care, nurse managers need to know the **organizational culture** of their hospitals and how it supports their unit's mission and goals. Laschinger (2004) reports on a study conducted on a random sample of 500 staff nurses working in the Ontario teaching hospitals. The study looked at the nurses' perception of respect and organizational justice. The instrument used addressed interactional justice (the perceptions of the quality of interactions among persons who are affected by decisions and subsequent outcomes), structural empowerment, respect, work pressures, emotional exhaustion, and work effectiveness. Two hundred and eighty questionnaires were returned, yielding a 52% response rate. The results revealed that the nurses did not perceive their managers as sharing information about eminent changes in their work environment, or showing any compassion for the nurses' response to the changes. The nurses also felt that the managers rarely provided them with rationale for changes in their work environment, showed little concern, and did not deal with them in a truthful way. The study highlighted the importance of a positive organizational environment for nurses to feel respected in their work environment. A consistent factor in the results was the importance of good interpersonal relationships with both managers and colleagues in the organization.

DAY-TO-DAY MANAGEMENT CHALLENGES

The nurse manager who meets the day-to-day management challenges must be able to achieve an acrobatic balance of three sources of demand: upper management requests, consumer demands, and staff needs. The manager has to ensure that the staff has opportunities for providing upper management with input regarding changes that affect them and also has to make unit and staff needs known to upper management. The consumers of health services today are much better educated and accustomed to providing input into decisions that affect them. The nurse manager needs to respect their requests, yet maintain care in the broad context of safety and efficiency. The staff needs recognition and independence when carrying out their roles and responsibilities. The nurse manager needs to have a sense of when to relinquish control, thus allowing decision-making at the point of service. Furthermore, the nurse manager influences staff nurses' satisfaction/dissatisfaction with the work environment, as the Research Perspective shows.

Research Perspective

Johnson, J.E., Buelow, J. (2003, July-August). Providing staff feedback to nurse managers using internal resources. *Journal of Nursing Administration, 33*(7/8), 391-396.

This descriptive study was conducted in an acute-care hospital located in a rural community that competes with large, urban hospitals for nurses. The problem the hospital was facing was RN turnover that had increasingly been climbing since 1999 and was beginning to mimic the problem as seen on the national level. The investigators felt that, although an outside consulting firm was surveying the nurses in relation to employee satisfaction, at least two components of the survey were bothersome: (1) it did not provide a comprehensive view of the nurses work environment and (2) 2 years were too long to wait for another survey and its subsequent results.

The purpose of this project was to provide timely feedback to the nurse managers that they could use to improve their work environment, thus retaining their RN staff. The questionnaire was designed to elicit information concerning organizational and departmental factors that were dissatisfying to the nurses as well as areas of satisfaction that the nurses wished to maintain. Other important components of the study included keeping the questionnaire short, yet informative, and ensuring that the results could be calculated easily. Following an extensive literature review, the survey was designed to fit all in one page, be completed in 10 minutes, and to elicit information in five categories: demographics, unit practices, administrative practices, stress, and additional questions that required short, narrative responses. The overall response rate was 82% (76 of 96 surveys returned); individual department reports were created and given to the nurse managers. The reports included the greatest satisfiers and dissatisfiers, administrative practices that RNs viewed as dissatisfying and areas where RNs reported they almost always felt stressed. By and large, the greatest satisfiers were shift hours and co-workers. Only 5 of the 19 organizational/managerial factors found in the literature were listed as dissatisfiers, and the list included training and education, new nurse orientation, opportunity for advancement, physical work environment, and input into policy and procedure.

IMPLICATIONS FOR PRACTICE

Whereas the identification of RN perceptions is of extreme value to the nurse managers, if left just as reported without further follow-up, more harm than good would be accomplished. Hence, a plan of action was developed that included nurse managers working together to address their own department's practices and stresses. Managers could share with each other their unit satisfiers so that they could be used on other units, thereby canceling out some of the dissatisfiers. Administrators and managers were encouraged to work together and learn from the nurses new satisfiers that would add value to the unit environment and nurse retention. Overall, one overriding positive about this study was that best source for identifying workplace issues remains with the primary providers of care, the RNs.

Nurse managers also must be credible clinicians in the areas they manage. A critical factor in being an excellent nurse manager is understanding how to ensure optimal patient outcomes, involve families or significant others in the plan of care, and allocate resources and technology in a fair and ethical manner. The nurse manager-clinician is confronted with complex and ambiguous patient-care situations. Sometimes, decisions are made to meet one important patient care need at the expense of another. That is an important message to convey to staff.

Exercise 3-2

Select a nurse manager and a staff nurse follower in one of your clinical facilities. Observe them over a certain time (e.g., 2 to 4 hours). Compare the styles they exhibit. Is power shared or centralized? Are interactions positive or negative? What is the nature of their conversations? How does your summation of this observation relate to managerial, leadership, and followership characteristics?

Workplace Violence

Nurse managers continue to be responsible for ensuring the safety of their staff and patients. Workers in high-risk areas, such as the emergency department, require special attention. For the nurse manager, "special attention" translates to his or her staff receiving adequate on-the-job training. Such training may include effective techniques relating to crisis intervention and handling highly agitated people who may be armed. Violence at home can also affect a worker's outlook and productivity. Nurse managers will have to address this problem if it exists on their unit. Because the nurse manager's workforce may include a majority of women, information that addresses violence against women should be readily available. Bradley and Moore (2004) speak to negligent hiring as an emerging trend that makes healthcare agencies liable for workplace violence. Although some healthcare workers may be well-versed (police, security guards) on protective techniques used with violent employees, nurses, who often experience violent assaults, do not have adequate training to protect themselves. Top-level administrators are ultimately responsible for employee violence in their own setting; however, managers who lack training in policy practices have an increased risk for nonadherence to state/federal employee selection requirements.

MANAGING HEALTHCARE SETTINGS

Managing healthcare settings is always challenging for the nurse manager, and the current nursing shortage has made the challenge paramount. Tonges, Baloga-Altieri and Atzori (2004) have reported an interesting approach directed toward addressing the nursing shortage and resource allocations. At the 500-bed Robert Wood Johnson University Hospital in New Jersey, a Nurse Practice Committee (NPC) was formed in 2000 specifically to address a variety of issues relating to the nursing shortage. What is unique about this committee is the membership composition. The committee has equal representation of staff nurses and management staff, a $500,000 budget for a 3-year period, and all members have voting privileges. This type of forum has had good, tangible results, such as

creating several new nurse positions, including a telemetry transport nurse and nurse expeditor, both of which bring about quicker, more efficient care to the patient. The intangible benefits center around improved communication, not only between managers and staff nurses but also among nurses practicing in different service areas throughout the hospital. Although many have said that the nursing shortage may have brought about "the best of times" for nursing, managers will continue to address many healthcare challenges. With inpatient care shifting to outpatient/community-based care, and with the push for health promotion versus a disease-treatment model, the role of the nurse manager may be redefined. One certainty remains: regardless of how manager roles evolve over time, the nurse manager remains "the link" that pulls together and coordinates many patent-care services so that cost-effective, efficient care is available to the consumer of health care, the patient.

The Institute of Medicine (IOM) report, *Keeping Patients Safe* (2004), speaks to the creation of work environments that are more conducive to nurses providing safer patient care. For this to happen, many changes will be required of those in leadership roles, beginning with top-level administration and filtering through the hierarchy to unit managers. Managers need to address the five management practices that have been found to be effective when instituting change and achieving patient safety in high-risk organizations. These practices include: (1) managing the change process actively; (2) balancing the tension between efficiency and reliability; (3) creating a learning environment; (4) creating and sustaining trust; and (5) involving the workers in the work-redesign and the workflow decision-making. This report also addresses and supports the use of evidence-based management, a new concept that is not yet widely known; however, evidence-based practice is supported from systematic research findings, and the same should apply to management practices. Evidence-based management should reflect application of empirical research into everyday managing practices. Another IOM report that is significant for nurse managers is *Crossing the Quality Chasm/A New Health Care System for the 21st Century* (2001). This report proposes six "improvement" aims for today's lower-performing healthcare system. The aims include: *safety* in patient practices that are intended to help rather than hinder the recipient care; providing *effective* patient services grounded on scientific knowledge and eliminating services that are of no benefit to the patient; ascribing to *patient-centered* care that considers the patient's needs and wants and ensures that patient values guide clinical decisions; giving care that is *timely* and that reduces the negative delay effects to both the recipient and provider of care; addressing *efficiency,* thereby avoiding not only waste of supplies/equipment but also energy; and giving *equitable* care that does not vary in quality because of gender, ethnicity, or socioeconomic status.

High technology will continue to modify nurse managers' roles. For example, because of the ability to perform more complex surgery through surgicenters, nurse managers will find themselves practicing with short-term or ambulatory-care admissions. A key to successful management is interdependence. A critical component of interdependence is collaboration, which uses the different strengths of each person. Collaboration requires one to be flexible and broadminded and to have a strong self-concept. Sullivan and Decker (2001) addressed the concept of collaboration from the perspective of conflict management. When collaboration is used to solve a conflict, the energies of all parties are focused on solving the problem versus defeating the opposing party.

The staff often looks to the nurse manager to lead them in addressing workplace issues with higher levels of administration. To do this, the nurse manager must possess two sets of skills: (1) the ability to address power sources in one's work environment and define power-based strategies, such as in organizing a following of other nurse managers with similar concerns, and (2) the ability to effectively place pressure on the power holders so that needed changes can occur. Employees' "buy in" to a change sometimes needs to be thought out carefully.

The staff also looks to the nurse manager to lead them in ethical, value-based management. The manager's commitment to the mission, vision, and purpose must be demonstrated in everyday behavior, not merely recited on special occasions. This ongoing commitment lends stability in a time of constant change. In other words, although the approach to an issue may change, the core values remain, and the nurse manager is the one who must lead the group in the changed behavior to reflect the mission, vision, and purpose. Without this evidence that is almost palpable, staff nurses may be skeptical about the manager's commitment to the organization and to them. This contemporary commitment reflects an understanding of the core values and a relationship with the world as it is today. The nurse manager then must translate this commitment to the staff so that they know they are valued in accomplishing the work of the unit that furthers the mission of the organization. One way of demonstrating that employees are valued is by recognizing staff through various means. Employees who have gone beyond the scope of their job to meet the needs of the patient, department, or institution deserve recognition. An award may reflect the institution's philosophy, beliefs, and mission, as exemplified in one institution's "Quality Credo"—communication, competent performance, personal leadership, respect, and teamwork.

Exercise 3–3

The Vice-President for Patient Care Services for the local health department has just undergone a tremendous challenge because of a natural disaster of flooding in the vicinity. Many staff members, despite their own family needs, assisted flood victims with their needs, which ranged from crisis care to adequate follow-up of chronic disorders. The Vice-President for Patient Services wants to establish a recognition program for the staff who gave endless hours to their community. How would you approach establishing this recognition program? What resources would you need, and where would you go to seek the needed resources?

MANAGING RESOURCES

Each of these concepts inherent in managing resources is addressed in depth elsewhere in this book, but the key point is that the manager must manage each and integrate each with the others. The practice settings of tomorrow will no doubt continue to include in-hospital care; however, numerous innovative practice models operating from a community-based framework also may be found. Predictors of effective outcomes to ensure quality patient care include rationed and multi-tiered distribution of healthcare services, such as health maintenance organizations (HMOs), preferred provider organizations (PPOs), or independent private payment plans; very precise outcome-oriented quality-assurance measures, such as critical pathways; and concerted efforts to control spiraling health costs by increasing productivity and efficiency of healthcare providers. Other practice models, differentiated practice, shared governance, and restructured work environments make use of all levels of healthcare personnel.

The manager is responsible for managing all resources designated to the unit of care. This includes all personnel, professional and nonprofessional, under the manager's span of control. The wise manager quickly determines that a unit must function economically and, in so doing, realizes that there are many opportunities to reshape how nursing is delivered. Budget and personnel have always been considered critical resources. However, as technology improves, informatics must be integrated with budget and personnel as a critical resource element. Basing practice on research findings (evidence-based care), networking through the Internet with other nurse managers, sharing concerns and difficulties, and being willing to step outside of tradition can assist future managers in decisions about resource utilization.

MANAGED CARE

Managed care, a healthcare delivery option introduced in the 1980s, has clearly affected the role and responsibilities of all nurses (Sportsman & Valadez, 2001). This is especially true of nurses working in managerial positions. The goal of managed care is to provide needed services efficiently and at an appropriate cost. In essence, this goal requires nurse managers to know and incorporate business principles into patient-care practices. Nurse managers who know business principles become conduits for ensuring safe, effective, affordable care.

CASE MANAGEMENT

Case management, a method used to provide care for many years in outpatient service areas, is now, because of managed care, an option of care in acute care settings (Sullivan & Decker, 2001). The key to effective case management is coordination of care, with identified time frames for accomplishing appropriate care outcomes. The nurse manager is often the overseer of the case managers, and in some settings, the nurse manager is the immediate

supervisor of the case managers. Case management involves components of case selection, multidisciplinary assessment, collective planning, coordination of events, negotiation, and evaluation and documentation of the outcomes of patient status in measures of cost and quality. Case managers are employed in acute care settings, rehabilitation facilities, subacute facilities, community-based programs, home care, and insurance companies. These managers must possess a broad range of personal, interpersonal, and management skills.

INFORMATICS

Informatics is in a stage of constant change, and it highlights two roles that have prevailed for nurse managers: educator and research translator. Both of these roles have become easier to accomplish because informatics, through the electronic medical record, has given quick and ready access to current and retrospective clinical patient data. The accessibility and use of the Internet facilitates the education of staff, patients, and their families. Nurse managers have taken advantage of informatics to gain quick access to patient classification systems that denote acuity of care and access to personnel hours that relate directly to patient acuity. A manager must ensure that the staff's data input is accurate and must also demonstrate leadership in synthesizing how the data are used to deliver care. In addition, managers must be early adapters of the technology to demonstrate its value in performance.

BUDGETS

Budgetary allocations, whether they are related to the number of dollars available to manage a unit or in full-time equivalent employee formulas, may be the direct responsibility of nurse managers. For highly centralized organizations, only the administrative group at the executive level decides on the budgetary allocations. As healthcare organizations adopt "flat" organizational structures and decentralize responsibilities to the patient care areas, nurse managers allocate fiscal resources for their designated unit. In the decentralized organizational model, nurse managers must have the business and financial skills to be able to prepare and justify a

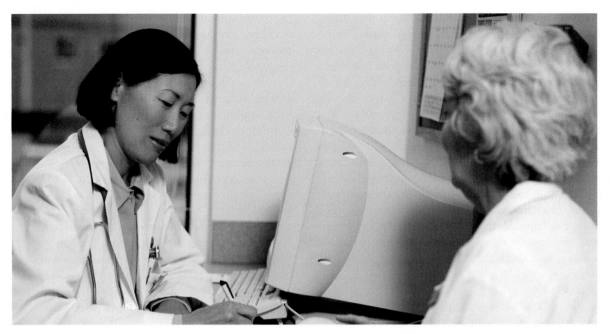

Patient care is shifting from in-hospital settings to outpatient and community settings.

detailed budget that reflects the short- and long-term needs of the unit.

Perhaps the most important aspect of a budget is the provision for a mechanism that allows some self-control, such as decision-making at the point of service (POS), which does not require previous hierarchical approval and a rationale for budgetary spending.

Exercise 3–4

Visit a city health department or an adult daycare facility. What type of information system is used? Are both paper (hard copy) and computer sources used? What can you assume about the budget, based on the physical appearance of the setting? Does any equipment appear dated? How do the employees (and perhaps volunteers) function? Do they seem motivated? Ask two or three to tell you, in a sentence or two, the purpose (vision and mission) of the organization. Can you readily identify the nurse manager? What does the manager do to manage the three critical resources of personnel, finances, and technologic access?

QUALITY INDICATORS

The nurse manager is consistently concerned with the quality of care that is being delivered on his or her unit. The **quality indicators** developed by the American Nurses Association (ANA), such as The National Database of Nursing Quality Indicators (NDNQI) (http://nursingworld.org/readroom/fssafe99.htm), are good resources for the nurse manager. The NDNQI measures are specifically concerned with patient safety and aspects of quality of care that may be affected by changes in the delivery of care. The quality indicators address staff mix and nursing hours for acute-care settings as well as other care components. The NDNQI project is designed to assist healthcare organizations in identifying links between nursing care and patient outcomes.

PROFESSIONALISM

Nurse managers must set examples of professionalism, which include academic preparation, roles and function, and increasing autonomy. The ANA's classic "Nursing's Social Policy Statement" (2003) provides significant ideals for all nurses, specifically autonomy, self-regulation, and accountability. Nurses are guided by a humanistic philosophy that includes the highest regard for self-determination, independence, and choice in decision-making, whether for staff or for patients. The policy statement can be used by the nurse manager as a framework for a broader understanding of nursing's connection with society and nursing's accountability to those who receive nursing care that facilitates "health and healing" in a caring relationship. For example, a nurse manager's professional philosophy should include the patient's rights. These rights have traditionally identified such basic elements as human dignity, integrity, honesty, confidentiality, privacy, and informed consent. Additional basic rights now include self-determination through advance directives (living wills, directives to physicians and family or surrogates, medical power of attorney) and the right to healthcare accessibility.

Exercise 3–5

Mr. Jones, a patient who had foot surgery 3 days ago, has asked Donna D., a young nurse on a surgical orthopedic unit, several times during her 12-hour day shift for some medication for pain. Donna D.'s assessment of Mr. Jones leads her to believe that he is not having that much pain. Although the patient does have an oral medication order for pain, Donna D. independently decides to administer a placebo by subcutaneous injection and documents her medication intervention. Mr. Jones does not receive any relief from this subcutaneous medication. When the 12-hour night nurse relieves Donna D., Donna D. gives the nurse a report of her intervention concerning Mr. Jones' pain. The following morning, the night nurse reports Donna D.'s medication intervention to you, the nurse manager. You will have to address Donna's behavior. What will you do? What resources will you use to handle Donna D.'s behavior? How will you demonstrate professionalism?

Professionalism is all-encompassing; the way a manager interacts with personnel, other disciplines, patients, and families reflects a professional philosophy. Professional nurses are ethically and legally accountable for the standards of practice and nursing actions delegated to others. Conveying high standards, holding others accountable, and shaping the future of nursing for a group of healthcare providers are inherent behaviors in the role of a manager.

The **Nursing Licensure Compact** is another aspect of professionalism that is being legislated by several states. This legislation allows a nurse to have a single licensure that is recognized by the "compact" states, thus facilitating mobility across states. Although the compact promotes better compliance with rules and regulatory processes of boards of nursing, nurse managers will probably assume additional responsibility to ensure that a nurse practicing in a "compact" state maintains a home state license in only one state at a time and that the nurse meets the requirement for licensure in the designated home state (http://www.ncsbn.org/nlc/rnlpvncompact_mutual_recognition_state.asp, February, 2005).

The nurse manager is the closest link to the direct care staff. That individual sets the tone, creates the environment, and manages within the context while providing professional role-modeling to develop future managers and leaders. That person influences staff in their decisions to stay or leave. The nurse manager is critical to the success of any healthcare endeavor.

The Solution

Of course, the ideal would be to eliminate our time-consuming task of documenting immediately by putting an electronic record system in place, but I know that is not an option. Two serendipitous happenings will help us to deal with the immediate problem. One of my staff nurses, who is very frustrated with the redundant documentation, took it upon herself to evaluate the admission packet, and guess what she discovered? There are at least four places where pain, height, and weight must be documented. Other patient assessment needs, such as skin, are documented three times. I am taking advantage of our Magnet™ status preparation and using the profes-

sional staff council meeting to bring up the problem. My unit staff nurse representative will take the evaluation of the admission packet and present it to the council to get their input as to what can be done to save precious nurse time while we wait for the electronic record to become a reality. My hunch is that the council will work at reducing some of the documentation redundancy, because they will have to address it in the Magnet proposal.

— Joyce Burdett

 Would this be a suitable approach for you? Why?

CHAPTER CHECKLIST

The role of the nurse manager is multifaceted and complex. Integrating clinical concerns with management functions, synthesizing leadership abilities with management requirements, and addressing human concerns while maintaining efficiency are the challenges facing a manager. Thus, the nurse manager's role is to ensure effective operation of a defined unit of service and to contribute to the overall mission of the organization and quality of care by working through others.

- There are five basic functions of a manager:
  - Establishing and communicating goals and objectives
  - Organizing and analyzing activities and decisions and dividing them into tasks
  - Motivating and communicating with others
  - Analyzing, appraising, and interpreting performance
  - Developing people
- A nurse manger is responsible for the following:
  - Relationships with those above themselves, peers, and staff for whom they are accountable
  - Professionalism
  - Management of resources

TIPS FOR IMPLEMENTING THE ROLE OF NURSE MANAGER

Aspects of the role of the nurse manager include being a leader as well as a follower. To implement the role, the nurse manager must profess to the following:

- Management philosophy that values people
- Commitment to patient-focused quality-care outcomes that address customer satisfaction
- Desire to learn healthcare changes and their effect on his or her role and functions

TERMS TO KNOW

case management
follower
leader
managed care
manager
Nursing Licensure Compact
organizational culture
quality indicators
quantum theory
role
role theory

REFERENCES

American Nurses Association (ANA). (2003). *Nursing's social policy statement* (NP-107). Washington, DC: American Nurses Publishing.

Bradley, D. B., & Moore, H. L. (2004). Preventing workplace violence from negligent hiring in health care. *Journal of Nursing Administration, 34*(3), 157-161.

Chaleff, I. (1995). *The courageous follower: Standing up to and for our leaders.* San Francisco: Berrett-Koehler.

Cherry, B., & Jacob, S. R. (2005). *Contemporary nursing, issues, trends and management.* St. Louis: Elsevier-Mosby.

Conway, M. E. (1978). Theoretical approaches to the study of roles. Cited in Hardy, M. E. & Conway, M. E. (1978). *Role theory: Perspectives for health professionals.* New York: Appleton-Century-Crofts.

Drucker, P. F. (1974). *Management tasks, responsibilities and practices.* New York: Harper & Row.

Institute of Medicine (IOM). (2004). *Keeping patients safe: Transforming the work environment of nurses.* Washington, DC: The National Academy Press.

Institute of Medicine (IOM). (2001). *Crossing the Quality Chasm: A New Health System for the 21st Century.* Washington, DC: The National Academy Press.

Johnson, J. E., & Buelow, J. (2003, July-August). Providing staff feedback to nurse managers using internal resources. *Journal of Nursing Administration, 33*(7/8), 391-396.

Laschinger, H. K. P. (2004). Hospital nurses' perception of respect and organizational justice. *Journal of Nursing Administration, 34*(7/8), 354-363.

Manion, J. (2003, December). Joy at work. *Journal of Nursing Administration, 33*(12), 652-659.

National Council of State Boards of Nursing. Nurse Licensure Compact Implementation. Retrieved August 30, 2005 from http://www.ncsbn.org/nlc/rnlpvncompact_mutual_recognition_state.asp.

The National Database of Nursing Quality Indicators (NDNQI). Retrieved August 30, 2005 from http://nursingworld.org/quality.

Porter-O'Grady, T. (2003, February). A different age for leadership, part 1. *Journal of Nursing Administration, 33*(2), 105-110.

Sportsman, S., & Valadez, A. M. (2001). Managed care and the law. Chapter 14. Cited in O'Keefe, M. E. *Nursing practice and the law: Avoiding malpractice and other legal risks*. Philadelphia: F.A. Davis.

Sullivan, E. J., & Decker, P. J. (2001). *Effective leadership and management in nursing* (5th ed.). Upper Saddle River, NJ: Prentice Hall.

Tonges, M. C., Baloga-Altieri, B., & Atzori, M. (2004). Amplifying nursing's voice through a staff-management partnership. *Journal of Nursing Administration, 34*(3), 134-139.

SUGGESTED READINGS

Cameron, K. S., & Quinn, R. E. (1994). *PRISM5: Changing organizational culture: A competing values workbook*. Ann Arbor, MI: University of Michigan. Cited in Jones, K. R., & Redman, R. W. (2000, December). Organizational culture and work redesign: Experiences in three organizations. *Journal of Nursing Administration, 30*(12), 604-610.

Cathcart, D., Jeska, S., & Karmas, J. (2004). Span of control matters. *Journal of Nursing Administration, 34*(9), 395-399.

Duchscher, J. E., & Cowin, L. (2004). Multigenerational nurses in the workplace. *Journal of Nursing Administration, 34*(11), 493-501.

Ferguson, L. M., & Day, R. A. (2004). Supporting new nurses in evidence-based practice. *Journal of Nursing Administration, 34*(11), 490-492.

Greenberg, J., & Baron, R. A. (2000). *Behavior in organizations* (7th ed.). Upper Saddle River, NJ: Prentice Hall.

Hardy, M. E., & Conway, M. E. (1988). *Role theory: Perspectives for health professionals* (2nd ed.). Norwalk, CT: Appleton & Lange.

Lang, T. A., Hodge, M., & Olson, V. (2004). Nurse-patient ratios: A systematic review on the effects of nurse staffing on patient, nurse employee, and hospital outcomes. *Journal of Nursing Administration, 34*(7/8), 326-337.

Lavoit-Tremblay, M. (2004). Creating a healthy workplace: A participatory organizational intervention. *Journal of Nursing Administration, 34*(10), 469-474.

Lunney, M., Delaney, C., & Duffy, M. (2005). Advocating for standardized nursing languages in electronic health records. *Journal of Nursing Administration, 35*(1), 1-3.

Sams, L., Penn, B. K., & Facteau, L. (2004). The challenge of using evidence-based practice. *Journal of Nursing Administration, 34*(9), 407-414.

Tiedeman, M. E., & Lookinland, S. (2004). Traditional models of care delivery: What have we learned? *Journal of Nursing Administration, 34*(6), 291-297.

Vestal, K. (2004, December). Making time for leadership. *Nurse Leader: From Management to Leadership, 2*(6), 8-9.

Wolf, G., Bradle, J. & Nelson, G. (2005). Bridging the strategic leadership gap: A model program for transformational change. *Journal of Nursing Administration, 35*(2), 54-60.

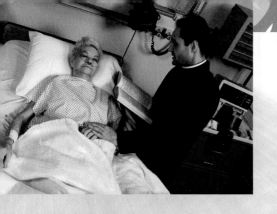

Legal and Ethical Issues

Ginny Wacker Guido

T his chapter highlights and explains key legal and ethical issues as they pertain to managing and
leading. Negligence and malpractice, informed consent, types of liability, selected federal and state
employment laws, ethical theories, and ethical principles are discussed. This chapter provides specific guidelines for preventing legal liability and guides the reader in applying ethical decision-making models in everyday clinical practice settings.

Objectives

- Examine nurse practice acts, including
  the legal difference between licensed
  registered nurses and licensed practical
  (vocational) nurses that a manager
  must know.
- Apply various legal principles,
  including negligence and malpractice,
  privacy, confidentiality, reporting
  statutes, and doctrines that minimize
  one's liability, in leading and managing
  roles in professional nursing.
- Evaluate informed-consent issues,
  including patient rights in research and
  medical literacy from a nurse
  manager's perspective.
- Analyze ethical principles, including
  autonomy, beneficence,
  nonmaleficence, veracity, justice,
  paternalism, fidelity, and respect for
  others.
- Apply the Code of Ethics for Nurses
  from the manager's perspective.
- Apply managers' rights and
  responsibilities from a legal and an

ethical perspective to selected
examples.
- Examine legal implications of resource
  availability versus service demand
  from a manager's perspective.
- Analyze key aspects of employment
  law, and give examples of how these
  laws benefit professional nursing
  practice.

- Apply five guidelines that a nurse
  manager or leader can implement to
  encourage a professional, satisfying
  work setting.
- Analyze decision-making when legal
  and ethical situations overlap, using
  the Theresa M. Schiavo case as the
  framework for this analysis.

Questions to Consider

- *What are the most common potential legal liabilities for
  nurse managers? Can these potential legal liabilities be
  avoided or minimized?*
- *What is the role of the nurse manager in incorporating
  ethical principles into ongoing relationships with staff and
  patients?*
- *What federal employment laws affect nurse managers'
  work settings?*
- *What is the role of the nurse manager in determining which
  course of action to implement when a legal or ethical
  dilemma arises?*

The Challenge

Nancy Joyner BA, MS, RN, CHPN
Resource Nurse Palliative Care, Altru Health System, Grand Forks, North Dakota

One of the most important tenants of the philosophy of hospice is to neither prolong life nor hasten death. An issue that hospice nurses often confront concerns the nutrition and hydration support for patients in the terminal stages of their illnesses. Questions that arise include whether the patient should have artificial hydration or nutrition to provide comfort in light of the fact that such additional hydration may cause more distress and an exacerbation of the primary disease state. For example, giving intravenous fluids may cause congestive heart failure or pulmonary edema to develop, thus hastening death.

A recent case example illustrates this concern. An elderly patient had deteriorated to the extent that she was able to use only mouth swabs soaked in water for her primary hydration. Family members were concerned that she was not eating and was not able to swallow fluids, and, therefore, she was not receiving the hydration that she needed to sustain life. They equated this lack of hydration with the belief that the patient was starving to death. Family members approached the hospice nurse to begin intravenous fluids. The hospice nurse spent some time with the family, explaining that the additional fluids would cause congestive heart failure to develop, ultimately hastening death and diminishing the comfort level of their loved one. The family members rejected this concept and insisted that the physician be contacted for an order to begin intravenous fluids. The physician supported the family, stating that the hospice needed to "treat the family and not only the patient," and he ordered a bolus of intravenous fluids. The patient died shortly afterward, leaving the family members relieved that they had done something to assist the patient and the hospice nurse knowing that the primary tenant of hospice had been violated.

 What do you think you would do if you were this nurse?

INTRODUCTION

The role of professional nursing continues to expand and incorporate increasing higher levels of expertise, specialization, autonomy, and accountability from both legal and ethical perspectives. This expansion has forced new concerns among nurse managers and leaders and a heightened awareness of the interaction of legal and ethical principles. Areas of concern include professional nursing practice, legal issues, ethical principles, labor-management interactions, and employment. Each of these areas is individually addressed in this chapter.

PROFESSIONAL NURSING PRACTICE

Nurse Practice Acts

The scope of nursing practice, those actions and duties that are allowable by a profession, is defined and guided individually by each state in the nurse practice act and by **common law.** Common law is "derived from principles rather than rules and regulations and consists of broad and comprehensive principles based on justice, reason, and common sense" (*Bishop v. United States*, 1971, p. 418). Common-law principles govern most interactions affecting nursing; they are based on a traditional justice perspective rather than a caring relationship. The state **nurse practice act** is the single most important piece of legislation for nursing because it affects all facets of nursing practice. Furthermore, the act is the law within the state, and state boards of nursing cannot grant exceptions, waive the act's provisions, or expand practice outside the act's specific provisions.

Nurse practice acts and common law define three categories of nurses: licensed practical or vocational nurses (LPNs and LVNs, respectively); licensed registered nurses (RNs); and advanced practice nurses. The nurse practice acts, along with common law, set educational and examination requirements, provide for licensing by individuals who have met these requirements, and define the functions of each category of nurse, both in general and in specific terminology. The nurse practice act must be read to ascertain what actions are allowable for the three categories of nurses. Some states have separate acts for licensed RNs and LPNs/LVNs. If two acts exist, they must be reviewed at the same time to ensure that all allowable actions are included in one of the two acts and that there is no overlap between the acts. Additionally, state acts are not consistent in defining or delineating advanced nursing roles.

Each practice act also establishes a state board of nursing. The main purposes of state boards of nursing are twofold. One purpose is to ensure enforcement of the act, serving to regulate those who come under its provisions and prevent those not addressed within the act from practicing nursing. The second purpose is to protect the public, ensuring that those who present themselves as nurses are licensed to practice within the state. The National Council of State Boards of Nursing (NCSBN) serves as a central clearinghouse, further ensuring that individual state actions against a nurse's license are recorded and enforced in all states in which the individual nurse holds licensure.

These various boards of nursing develop and implement rules and regulations regarding the discipline of nursing and must be read in conjunction with the nurse practice act. Often any changes within the state's definition of nursing practice occur through modifications in the rules and regulations, rather than in the act itself. This mandates that nurses and their nurse managers periodically review both the state act and the board of nursing rules and regulations.

Because each state has its own nurse practice act and state courts hold jurisdiction on the common law of the state, all nurses are well advised to know and understand the provisions of the state's nurse practice act. This is especially true in the areas of diagnosis and treatment; states vary greatly on whether nurses can diagnose and treat or merely assess and evaluate. An acceptable action in one state may be the practice of medicine in a bordering state.

With the advent of multistate licensure, the need to know and understand provisions of state nurse practice acts has become even more critical. Multistate licensure permits an RN the right to be licensed in one state and to legally practice in states belonging to the compact without obtaining additional state licenses. For the purposes of the law, the state nurse practice act that regulates the practice of the RN is the state in which the patient or client resides, not the state in which the nurse holds his or her license. Many of the nurses practicing under multistate licensure are working with patients in a variety of states through telenursing, which involves the use of telecommunications technology, such as telephone triage and advice. Others work for agencies or clinics that serve patients across state borders.

All nurses must know applicable state **law** and use the nurse practice act for guidance and appropriate action. Nurse managers have this same basic responsibility to apply legal principles in their practice. However, they are also responsible for monitoring the practice of employees under their supervision and for ensuring that personnel maintain current and valid licensure. Unless nurse managers remain current with the nurse practice act in their state or with nurse practice acts in all states in which they supervise employees, there is constant potential for liability.

Exercise 4–1

Read your state's nurse practice act, which includes rules and regulations that the state board of nursing has promulgated for the profession. You may need to read two acts if RNs and LPNs/LVNs come under different licensing boards. Does your state address advanced practice? How do the definitions of nursing vary for RNs, LPNs/LVNs, and advanced practice nurses? Describe why it is vital that the nurse manager understands these distinctions.

Negligence and Malpractice

Nurse managers frequently serve as mentors and consultants for nurses whom they supervise. It is imperative that nurse managers have a full appreciation for this area of the law as negligence/malpractice continue to be the major causes of action brought against nursing staff members. Managers cannot guide and counsel their employees unless they are fully knowledgeable about this area of the law.

Negligence denotes conduct that is lacking in care and typically concerns nonprofessionals. Many experts equate negligence with carelessness, a deviation from the **standard of care** that a reasonable person would deliver. **Malpractice**, sometimes referred to as *professional negligence,* concerns professional actions and is the failure of a person with professional education and skills to act in a reasonable and prudent manner. Issues of malpractice have become increasingly important to the nurse as the authority, accountability, and autonomy of nurses have increased. The same types of actions may be the basis for either negligence or malpractice; *Pender v. Natchitoches Parish Hospital* (2003) specifically noted that for malpractice there must be a dereliction of a professional skill. Usually, six elements must be presented in a successful malpractice suit. All of these factors must be shown before the court will find **liability** against the nurse or institution. Table 4-1 outlines these elements.

Negligence and malpractice have two commonalities. Both concern actions that are a result of omission (the failure to do something that the reasonable, prudent person or nurse would have done) and commission (acting in a way that causes injury to the patient). Both also concern nonintentional actions; injury results, but the individual who caused the harm never intended to hurt the patient. Remember: the most important point in determining whether an action was truly malpractice or negligence is the nonintentional action on the part of the nurse.

Elements of Malpractice

Duty Owed the Patient   The first element is duty owed the patient, which involves both the existence of the duty and the nature of the duty. That a nurse owes a duty of care to a patient is seldom hard to establish. Often, this is established merely by showing the valid employment of the nurse within the institution. The more difficult part is the nature of the duty, which involves standards of care that represent the minimum requirements for acceptable practice. Standards of care are established by reviewing the institution's policy and procedure manual, the individual's job description, and the practitioner's education and skills, as well as pertinent standards established by professional organizations, journal articles, and standing orders and protocols. Several sources may be used to determine the applicable standard of care. The American Nurses Association (ANA), as well as a cadre of specialty organizations, publishes standards for nursing practice.

The overall framework of these standards is the nursing process. In 1988, the ANA first published Standards for Nurse Administrators, a series of nine standards incorporating responsibilities of nurse administrators across all practice settings. Accreditation standards, especially those published yearly by the Joint Commission on Accreditation of Healthcare Organizations (JCAHO), also assist in establishing the acceptable standard of care for healthcare facilities. In addition, many states have healthcare standards that affect individual institutions and their employees.

Nurse managers are directly responsible for ensuring that standards of care, as written in the hospital policy and procedure manuals, is current and that all nursing staff follow these standards of care. Should a standard of care be revised or changed, nurse managers must ensure that all staff members who are expected to implement this altered standard are apprised of the revised standard. If the new standard entails new skills, man-

Table 4-1	ELEMENTS OF MALPRACTICE
Elements	**Examples**
Duty owed the patient	Failure to monitor a patient's response to treatment
Breach of the duty owed	Failure to communicate change in patient status to the primary healthcare provider
Foreseeability	Failure to ensure minimum standards are met
Causation	Failure to provide adequate patient education
Injury	Fractured hip and head concussion after a patient fall
Damages	Additional hospitalization time; future medical and nursing care needs and costs

agers must ensure that staff members are educated before they implement the new standard. For example, if the institution alters a policy regarding nurses removing invasive lines, the nurse manager must first ensure that all nurses who will be performing this skill understand how to perform the skill safely, possible complications that could occur, and the most appropriate interventions to take should those complications occur.

Breach of the Duty of Care Owed the Patient   The second element required in a malpractice case is proven breach of the duty of care owed the patient. Once the standard of care is established, the breach or falling below the standard of care is easy to show. However, the standard of care may differ depending on whether the injured party is trying to establish the standard of care or whether the hospital's attorney is establishing an acceptable standard of care for the given circumstances. The injured party will attempt to show that the acceptable standard of care is a much higher standard of care than that shown by the defendant hospital and staff. **Expert witnesses** give testimony in court to determine the applicable and acceptable standard of care on a case-by-case basis and to assist the judge and jury in understanding nursing standards of care.

A case example, *Sabol v. Richmond Heights General Hospital* (1996), shows this distinction. A patient was admitted to a general acute care hospital for treatment after attempting to commit suicide by drug overdose. While in the acute care facility, the patient became increasingly paranoid and delusional. A nurse sat with the patient and tried to calm him. Restraints were not applied because the staff feared this would compound the situation by raising his level of paranoia and agitation. The patient got out of bed, knocked down the nurse who was in his room, fought his way past two nurses in the hallway, ran off the unit, and jumped from a third-story window, fracturing his arm and sustaining other relatively minor injuries.

Expert witnesses for the patient introduced standards of care pertinent to psychiatric patients, specifically those hospitalized in psychiatric facilities or in acute care hospitals with separate psychiatric units. The court ruled that the nurses in this general acute care situation were not professionally negligent in this patient's care. The court stated that the nurses' actions were consistent with basic professional standards of practice for medical-surgical nurses in an acute care hospital. They did not have, nor were they expected to have, specialized psychiatric nursing training and would not be judged as if they did.

Foreseeability   The third element needed for a successful malpractice case, **foreseeability,** involves the concept that certain events may reasonably be expected to cause specific results. The nurse must have prior knowledge or information that failure to meet a standard of care may result in harm. The challenge is to show what was foreseeable given the facts of the case at the time of the occurrence, not when the case finally comes to court. Some of the more common areas concerning forseeability concern medication errors, patient falls, and failure to adhere to physician orders. For example, in *Sisters of St. Joseph of Texas, Inc. v. Cheek* (2001), a postoperative patient was allowed to remain immobile, despite written orders for early ambulation. The patient subsequently died from a pulmonary embolus.

Causation   The fourth element of a malpractice suit is causation, which means that the nurse's actions or lack of actions directly caused the patient's harm; the patient did not merely experience some type of harm. There must be a direct relationship between the failure to meet the standard of care and the patient's injury. Note that it

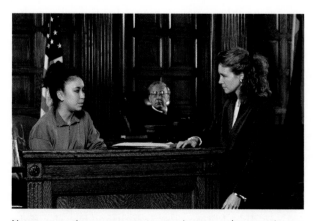

Nurses sometimes serve as expert witnesses whose testimony helps the judge and jury understand the applicable standards of nursing care.

is not sufficient that the standard of care has been breached, but that the breach of the standard of care must be the direct cause-and-effect factor for the injury. For example, in *Burns v. UHS of New Orleans, Inc.* (2003), the nursing staff was not liable for alleged injuries caused by a saline lock, despite the fact that the patient was inadvertently discharged with the saline lock in place. Once notified of the omission, the nursing staff appropriately informed the patient that he should return to have the saline lock removed by professional staff rather then removing the saline lock himself.

Injury   The resultant injury, the fifth malpractice element, must be physical, not merely psychological or transient. In other words, there must be some physical harm incurred by the patient before malpractice will be found against the healthcare provider. Although there are some specific exceptions to the requirement that a physical injury must result, they are extremely limited and usually involve very specific relationships, such as the parent–child relationship. Pain and suffering are allowed when they accompany actual physical injuries.

Damages   Finally, the injured party must be able to prove damages, the sixth element of malpractice. Damages are vital because malpractice is nonintentional. Thus, the patient must show financial harm before the courts will allow a finding of liability against the defendant nurse and/or hospital.

A nurse manager must know the applicable standards of care and ensure that all employees of the institution meet or exceed them. The standards must be reviewed periodically to ensure that the staff members remain current and attuned to advances in technology and newer ways of performing tasks. If standards of care appear outdated or absent, the appropriate committee within the institution is notified so that timely revisions can be made. Finally, the nurse manager must ensure that all employees meet the standards of care. This may be done by (1) performing or reviewing all performance evaluations for evidence that standards of care are met, (2) reviewing patient charts randomly for standards of care documentation, and (3) inquiring of employees what constitutes standards of care and appropriate references for standards of care within the institution.

Exercise 4–2

Read a policy and procedure manual at a community nursing service with which you are familiar. Are any policies outdated? Find out who is in charge of revising and writing policies and procedures for the agency. Take an outdated policy and revise it, or think of an issue that you determine should be included in the policy and procedure manual and write such a policy. Does your rewritten or new policy define standards of care? Where would you find criteria for ensuring that your policy and procedures fit a national standard? As the nurse manager within the healthcare setting, how would you go about ensuring that staff members whom you supervise follow the standards of care as outlined in the policy and procedure manual? How would you inform/teach the staff about the new policy?

LIABILITY: PERSONAL, VICARIOUS, AND CORPORATE

Personal liability defines each person's responsibility and accountability for individual actions or omissions. Even if others can be shown to be **liable** for a patient injury, each individual retains personal accountability for his or her actions. The law sometimes allows other parties to be liable for certain causes of negligence. Known as **vicarious liability,** or substituted liability, the doctrine of **respondeat superior** (let the master answer) makes employers accountable for the negligence of their employees. The rationale underlying the doctrine is that the employee would not have been in a position to have caused the wrongdoing unless hired by the employer, and the injured party will be allowed to suffer a double wrong merely because most employees are unable to pay damages for their wrongdoings. Nurse managers can best avoid these issues by ensuring that the staff they supervise know and follow hospital policy and procedure and deliver competent nursing care.

Nurses often believe that the doctrine of vicarious liability shields them from personal liability; the institution may be sued, but not the individual nurse or nurses. However, patients injured because of substandard care have the right to sue both the institution and the nurse. This includes potentially suing the nurse's nurse manager if he or she knowingly allowed substandard care to be given to a patient. In addition, the institution has the right under **indemnification** to counter-sue the nurse for damages paid to an injured patient. The principle of indemnification is applicable when the employer is held liable based solely on the actions of the staff member's negligence and the employer pays monetary damages because of the employee's negligent actions.

Corporate liability is a newer trend in the law and essentially holds that the institution has the responsibility and accountability for maintaining an environment that ensures quality healthcare delivery for consumers. Corporate liability issues include negligent hiring and firing issues, failure to maintain safety in the physical environment, and lack of a qualified, competent, and adequate staff. In *Wellstar Health Systems, Inc. v. Green* (2002), a hospital was held liable to an injured patient for the negligent credentialing of a nurse practitioner.

Nurse managers play a key role in assisting the institution to avoid corporate liability. For example, the nurse manager is normally delegated the duty to ensure that staff members remain competent and qualified, that personnel within their supervision have current licensure, and that incompetent, illegal, or unethical practices are reported to the proper persons or agencies. Nurse managers also play a pivotal role in whether a nurse remains employed on the unit or is discharged or reassigned.

CAUSES OF MALPRACTICE FOR NURSE MANAGERS

Nurse managers are charged with maintaining a standard of competent nursing care within the institution. Several potential sources of liability for malpractice among nurse managers may be identified; guidelines to prevent or avoid these pitfalls should be developed.

Assignment, Delegation, and Supervision

The field of nursing management involves supervision of various personnel who directly provide nursing care to patients. Supervision is defined as the active process of directing, guiding, and influencing the outcome of an individual's performance of an activity. The nurse manager retains personal liability for the reasonable exercise of assignment,

delegation, and supervision activities. The failure to assign, delegate, and supervise within acceptable standards of professional nursing practice may constitute malpractice. In addition, in a newer trend in the law, failure to delegate and supervise within acceptable standards may extend to direct corporate liability for the institution.

Delegation, used throughout all of nursing history, has evolved into a complex, work-enhancing strategy that has the potential for varying levels of legal liability. Prior to the early 1970s, nurses used delegation to direct the multiple tasks performed by the various levels of staff members in a team-nursing model. Subsequently, the concept of primary nursing and assignment became the desirable nursing model in acute care settings, with the focus on an all-professional staff, requiring little delegation but considerable assignment of duties. By the mid-1990s, a nursing shortage had again shifted the nursing model to a multilevel staff, with the return of the need for delegation.

It is necessary for the nurse manager to know certain definitions regarding this area of the law. *Delegation* involves at least two people, a delegator and a delegatee, with the transfer of authority to perform some type of task or work. A working definition could be that delegation is the transfer of responsibility for the performance of an activity from one individual to another, with the delegator retaining accountability for the outcome. In other words, delegation involves the transfer of responsibility for the performance of tasks and skills without the transfer of accountability for the ultimate outcome. Examples include the registered nurse (RN), who delegates patients' personal care tasks to certified nursing aides who work in a long-term care setting. In delegating these tasks, the RN retains the ultimate accountability and responsibility for ensuring that the delegated tasks are completed in a competent manner.

Typically, delegation involves the tasks and procedures that are given to unlicensed assistive personnel, such as certified nurse's aides, orderlies, assistants, attendants, and technicians. However, delegation can also occur with licensed to licensed staff members. For example, if one RN has the accountability for an outcome and asks another RN to perform a specific component of the overall function, that is delegation. This is typically the type of delegation that occurs between professional staff members when one member leaves the unit/ work area for a meal break.

Delegation is complex, because it involves relationships and communication (Anthony, Standing, & Hertz, 2000). Multiple players, usually with varying degrees of education and experience and different scopes of practice, are involved in the process. Understanding these variances and communicating effectively to the delegatee involves an understanding of competencies and the ability to communicate with all levels of staff personnel.

Assignment is the transfer of both the accountability and the responsibility from one person to another. This is typically what happens between professional staff members. The nurse manager assigns patient care responsibilities to other professional nurses working in the same unit of the institution or community healthcare setting. The level of accountability for the nurse manager who assigns as opposed to delegates is fairly obvious, although there can be some accountability in both instances. The degree of knowledge concerning the skills and competencies of those one supervises is of paramount importance. The doctrine of respondeat superior has been extended to include "knew or should have known" as a legal standard in both assigning and delegating tasks to the individuals one supervises. If it can be shown that the nurse manager assigned/delegated tasks appropriately and had no reason to believe that the nurse to whom tasks were assigned/delegated was not competent to perform the task, the nurse manager potentially has no personal liability or minimal personal liability. The converse is also true; if it can be shown that the nurse manager was aware of incompetence in a given employee or that the assigned/delegated task was outside the employee's capabilities, the nurse manager becomes substantially liable for the subsequent injury to a patient.

Nurse managers have a duty to ensure that the staff members under their supervision are practicing in a competent manner. The nurse manager must be aware of the staff's knowledge, skills, and competencies and should know whether they are maintaining their competencies. Knowingly allowing a staff member to function below the acceptable standard of care subjects both the nurse manager and the institution to potential liability. For example, in *Fairfax Nursing Home, Inc. v. Department of Health and Human Services* (2003), a nursing home was held liable for inadequate

practices and procedures in monitoring ventilator-dependent patients. In that case, a professional staff member delegated the task of suctioning a ventilator-dependent patient to a nurse's aide. After suctioning the patient, the aide failed to ensure that the ventilator was reconnected to the patient's tracheostomy, and the patient subsequently died. The professional nurse was also found to be liable for her failure to ensure that the task had been correctly performed.

Some nurse practice acts also legislate fines and discipline for the nurse manager who assigns/delegates tasks or patient care loads that make a nursing assignment unsafe. Means of ensuring continuing competency are expected and may include continuing education programs and assignment of a staff member to work with a second staff member to improve technical skills.

Duty to Orient, Educate, and Evaluate

Most healthcare institutions have continuing education departments to orient nurses who are new to the institution and to supply in-service education addressing new equipment, procedures, and interventions to existing employees. Nurse managers also have a duty to orient, educate, and evaluate. Nurse managers and their representatives are responsible for the daily evaluation of whether nurses are performing competent care. The key to meeting this requirement is reasonableness and is determined by courts on a case-to-case basis. Nurse managers should ensure that they promptly respond to all allegations, whether by patients or staff, of incompetent or questionable nursing care. Nurse managers should thoroughly investigate allegations, recommend options for correcting the situation, and follow up on recommended options and suggestions.

In *Bunn-Penn v. Southern Regional Medical Corporation* (1997), a male emergency center technician was accused of sexually assaulting a female patient. Before this incident, nurses had complained to the nurse manager that the male technician seemed too eager to assist female patients and that he stayed too long with female patients while they were undressing. The nurse manager spoke to the technician about these concerns. The nurse manager gave him detailed instructions regarding how he was to conduct himself in the future. She then monitored his activities carefully and noted no further evidence of inappropriate behavior. In finding that there was no liability on the part of the hospital, the court was positive in its praise of the nurse manager, noting that she had fulfilled her duty by counseling and monitoring the employee and in acting promptly when the issues were first presented to her. The court also noted that the nurse manager had monitored this employee for an 18-month period and had filed favorable periodic reviews in his personnel folder.

Exercise 4–3

You are the nurse manager of a busy operating room in a large metropolitan hospital, serving both adult and pediatric clients. A case is scheduled involving a child who will have a hip arthroplasty. The surgical technician usually scheduled to the pediatric cases is unavailable to assist with this case, so you schedule a surgical technician who has assisted with multiple hip arthroplasties, but never one performed on a younger child. After the procedure, the child has permanent damage to his sciatic nerve and his parents file a lawsuit against the surgical technician, you as the nurse manager, and the hospital. How will the court react to such a case? What would their findings likely be in such an instance and why?

Failure to Warn

A newer area of potential liability for nurse managers is **failure to warn** potential employers of staff incompetencies or impairment. Information about suspected addictions, violent behavior, and incompetency is of vital importance to subsequent employers. If the institution has sufficient information and suspicion to warrant the discharge of an employee or force a resignation, subsequent employers should be advised of those issues. Additionally, the state board of nursing or agency that oversees disciplinary actions of professional and nonprofessional nursing staff should also be notified whenever there is cause to dismiss an employee for incompetency or impairment, unless the employee voluntarily enters a peer-assistance program.

One means of supplying this information is through the use of *qualified privilege* to certain communications. In general, qualified privilege concerns communications made in good faith between persons or entities with a need to know. Most states now recognize this privilege and allow previous employers to give factual, objective information to subsequent employers. Note, however, that the previous employee must have listed the nurse manager or institution as a reference before this privilege arises.

Staffing Issues

Three issues arise under the general term *staffing*. These include: maintaining adequate numbers of staff members in a time of advancing patient acuity and limited resources; floating staff from one unit to another; and using temporary or "agency" staff to augment hospital staffing. Each area is addressed separately.

Accreditation standards, specifically those of JCAHO and the Community Health Accreditation Program (CHAP), as well as other state and federal standards, mandate that healthcare institutions provide adequate staffing with qualified personnel. This applies not only to the number of staff but also to the legal status of the staff. For instance, some areas of an institution, such as critical care areas, postanesthesia care areas, and emergency centers, must have greater percentages of RNs than LPNs/LVNs. Other areas, such as the general nursing areas and some long-term-care areas, may have equal or lower percentages of RNs to LPNs/LVNs or nursing assistants. Whether understaffing exists in a given situation depends on the number of patients, care acuity scores, and number and classification of staff. Courts determine whether understaffing existed on an individual case basis.

California was the first state to adopt legislation that mandates fixed nurse-to-patient ratios. Although Governor Schwarzenegger has attempted to delay the enactment of this legislation, the Third District Court of Appeals, in March of 2005, refused to postpone the amended 1:5 nurse-to-patient ratio (Dauner, 2005). Fifteen other states are also working on enacting such legislation. California law, which requires set nurse-to-patient ratios for all areas of acute-care nursing, became effective January 1, 2004 (California Launches Experiment, 2003). A separate lawsuit filed by the California Hospital industry requesting that the ratios not be enforced at all times has also been met with defeat. The judge in that case upheld the current law, noting that the interpretation that the new ratios not be enforced at all times made the nurse-patient ratios meaningless (Court Rejects Hospital Suit, 2004).

Although the institution is ultimately responsible for staffing issues, nurse managers may also incur liability because they directly oversee numbers of personnel assigned to a given unit. Courts have looked to the constant exercise of professional judgment, rather then reliance on concrete nurse-patient ratios, in cases involving staffing issues. Thus, nurse managers should exercise sound judgment to ensure patient safety and quality care rather than relying on exact nurse-to-patient ratios. For liability to incur against the nurse manager, it must be shown that a resultant patient injury was directly due to staffing issues and not to the incompetent or inappropriate actions of an individual staff member. To prevent nurse manager liability, he or she must show that sufficient numbers of competent staff were available to meet nursing needs.

Harrell v. Louis Smith Memorial Hospital (1990) was the precedent case concerning adequate staffing. The case centered on a lawsuit for negligence to provide adequate staffing and concerned the ability of an emergency department staff to adequately diagnose and intervene appropriately with a patient who had experienced a myocardial infarction. The court concluded that the hospital was required to provide staff competent to exercise a reasonable degree of care and skill when delivering health care to patients. Their degree of expertise, not staffing ratios, led to the ultimate death of the patient.

Exercise 4-4

Judy Jones, RN, has worked in the emergency department for several years. She is currently advanced cardiac life support (ACLS) certified, as are the other emergency care nurses. The hospital policy requires ACLS certification for employment in critical care areas. One of the areas covered in attaining this certification is that the individual is taught to intubate a patient. A new hospital policy expressly forbids the intubation of patients by nurses; only physicians may intubate patients. A crisis occurred in the emergency center one evening, and Judy Jones competently intubated a patient in full cardiac arrest. What would you do about this issue?

Guidelines for nurse managers in short-staffing issues include alerting hospital administrators and upper-level managers of concerns. First, however, the nurse manager must do whatever is under his or her control to alleviate the circumstances, such as approving overtime for adequate coverage, reassigning personnel among those areas he or she supervises, and restricting new admissions to the area. Second, nurse managers have a legal duty to notify the chief operating officer, either directly or indirectly, when understaffing endangers patient welfare. One way of notifying the chief operating officer is through formal nursing channels, for example, by notifying the nurse manager's direct supervisor. Upper management must then decide how to alleviate the short staffing, either on a short-term or on a long-term basis. Appropriate measures could be closing a unit or units, restricting elective surgeries, hiring new staff members, or temporarily reassigning personnel from other departments. Once the nurse manager can show that he or she acted appropriately, used sound judgment given the circumstances, and alerted his or her supervisors of the serious nature of the situation, the institution and not the nurse manager becomes potentially liable for staffing issues.

Some institutions have resorted to the use of mandatory overtime as a means of alleviating nursing shortages. Although few states have enacted legislation regarding this issue, mandatory overtime has become a major issue in nursing today. In a time when there is an aggressive national movement to reduce adverse patient outcomes, fatigued nurses and other healthcare providers are routinely requested to work additional hours. This demand for additional work coverage confronts ethical nursing practice standards that mandate that nurses not engage in any practice that can compromise patient outcomes. These issues are well addressed in the American Nurses Association's *Code of Ethics for Nurses* (2001), provisions 3 and 4.

Floating staff from unit to unit is the second issue that concerns overall staffing. Institutions have a duty to ensure that all areas of the institution are staffed adequately. Units temporarily overstaffed because of low patient census or a lower patient acuity ratio usually float staff to units that are less well staffed. Although floating nurses to areas with which they have less familiarity and expertise can increase potential liability for the nurse manager, leaving another area understaffed can also increase potential liability.

Before floating staff from one area to another, the nurse manager should consider staff expertise, patient-care delivery systems, and patient-care requirements. Nurses should be floated to units as comparable to their own unit as possible. This requires the nurse manager to match the nurse's home unit and float unit as much as is possible or to consider negotiating with another nurse manager to cross-float a nurse. For example, a manager might float a critical care nurse to an intermediate care unit and float an intermediate care unit nurse to a general unit. Or the nurse manager might consider floating the general unit nurse to the postpartum unit and floating a postpartum nurse to labor and delivery. Open communications regarding staff limitations and concerns, as well as creative solutions for staffing, can alleviate some of the potential liability involved and create better morale among the floating nurses. A positive option is to cross-train nurses within the institution so that nurses are familiar with two or three areas and can competently float to areas in which they have been cross-trained.

An older but still relevant legal case shows that employees also have some responsibility in the area of cross-training. In *David W. Francis v. Memorial General Hospital* (1986), an intensive care nurse refused to float to an orthopedic unit because he felt that he was unqualified to act as a charge nurse on that unit. The hospital offered to orient him, but he declined and was subsequently terminated. The court sided with the employer, noting that the employee's unwillingness to be oriented or to even try working with hospital administration undermined his case.

The use of temporary or "agency" personnel has created increased liability concerns among nurse managers. Until recently, most jurisdictions held that such personnel were considered **independent contractors** and thus the institution was not liable for their actions, although their primary employment agency did retain potential liability. Today, courts have begun to hold the institution liable under the principle of **apparent agency**. *Apparent authority* or *apparent agency* refers to the doctrine whereby a principal becomes accountable for the actions of his or her agent. Apparent agency is created when a person (agent) holds himself or herself out as acting in behalf of the principal; in the instance of the agency nurse, the patient is unable to ascertain whether the nurse works directly for the hospital (has a valid employment contract) or is working for a different employer. At law, lack of actual authority is no defense. This principle applies when it can be shown that a reasonable patient believed that the healthcare worker was an employee of the institution. If it appears to the reasonable patient that this worker is an employee of the institution, the law will con-

sider the worker an employee for the purposes of corporate and vicarious liability.

At least one case, however, seems to uphold the idea that temporary nurses are independent contractors in cases of liability. In *Hansen v. Caring Professionals, Inc.* (1997), the Appellate Court in Illinois held that a temporary nurse was an independent contractor and not an employee of the temporary nursing agency. The court cited the nurse's filing of a Form 1099 (rather than a W-2 form), the payment of her own employment taxes, and the payment of her own workers' compensation coverage as proof of her independent employment status. However, the hospital did have potential liability because it controlled which patients would be assigned to the agency nurse and directly supervised the agency nurse's clinical performance. Classification may be unimportant; what is important is that the hospital, and thus the nurse manager, may be sued for incompetent care when an agency nurse gives less than competent nursing care.

These trends in the law make it imperative that the nurse manager considers the temporary worker's skills, competencies, and knowledge when delegating tasks and supervising the worker's actions. If there is reason to suspect that the temporary worker is incompetent, the nurse manager must convey this fact to the agency. The nurse manager must also either send the temporary worker home or reassign the worker to other duties and areas. The same screening procedures should be performed with temporary workers as are used with new institution employees.

Additional areas that nurse managers should stress when using agency or temporary personnel include ensuring that the temporary staff member is given a brief but thorough orientation to institution policies and procedures, is made aware of resource materials within the institution, and is made aware of documentation procedures. It is also advisable for nurse managers to assign a resource person to the temporary staff member. This resource person serves in the role of mentor for the agency nurse and serves to prevent potential problems that could arise merely because the agency staff member does not know the institution routine or is unaware of where to turn for assistance. This resource person also serves as a mentor for critical decision-making for the agency nurse.

PROTECTIVE AND REPORTING LAWS

Protective and reporting laws ensure the safety or rights of specific classes of individuals. Most states have reporting laws for suspected child and older adult abuse and laws for reporting certain categories of diseases and injuries. Examples of reporting laws include reporting cases of sexually transmitted diseases, abuse of residents in nursing and convalescent homes, and suspected child abuse. Nurse managers are often the individuals who are responsible for ensuring that the correct information is reported to the correct agencies, thus avoiding potential liability against the institution.

Many states now also have mandatory reporting of incompetent practice, especially through nurse practice acts, medical practice acts, and the National Practitioner Data Bank. In addition, the National Council of State Boards of Nursing has developed an Electronic License Verification System (ELVIS) that monitors nurses' licensure status in all states and U.S. territories for discipline issues, competency ratings, and renewals. Reporting incompetent practice often is restricted to issues of chemical abuse, and special provisions prevail if the affected nurse voluntarily undergoes drug diversion or chemical-dependency rehabilitation. Mandatory reporting of incompetent practitioners is a complex process, involving both legal and ethical concerns. Nurse managers must know what the law requires, when reporting is mandated, to whom the report must be sent, and what the individual institution expects of its nurse managers. When in doubt, the nurse manager should seek clarification from the state board of nursing and hospital administration.

INFORMED CONSENT

Informed consent becomes an important concept for nurse managers in three very different instances. First, staff nurses may approach the nurse manager with questions about informed consent; thus, the nurse manager becomes a consultant for the staff nurse. Secondly, and more often, the nurse manager is queried about patients' rights in research studies that are being conducted in the institution. Third, the issue of medical literacy has implications for the provision of valid informed consent by an ever-growing number of patients.

Remember: informed consent is the authorization by the patient or the patient's legal representative to do something to the patient; it is based on legal capacity, voluntary action, and comprehension. Legal capacity is usually the first requirement and is determined by age and competency. All states have a legal age for adult status defined by **statute;** generally, this age is 18. Competency involves the ability to understand the consequences of actions or the ability to handle personal affairs. State statutes mandate who can serve as the representative for a minor or incompetent adult. The following types of minors may be able to give valid informed consent: **emancipated minors,** minors seeking treatment for substance abuse or communicable diseases, and pregnant minors.

Voluntary action, the second requirement, means that the patient was not coerced by fraud, duress, or deceit into allowing the procedure or treatment. Comprehension is the third requirement, and the most difficult to ascertain. The law states that the patient must be given sufficient information, in terms he or she can reasonably be expected to comprehend, to make an informed choice. Inherent in the doctrine of informed consent is the right of the patient to informed refusal. Patients must clearly understand the possible consequences of their refusal. In recent years, most states have enacted statutes to ensure that the competent adult has the right to refuse care and that the healthcare provider is protected should the adult validly refuse care. This refusal of care is most frequently seen in end-of-life decisions. Box 4-1 lists the information needed for obtaining informed consent.

Nurses often ask about issues concerning informed consent that concern the actual signing of the informed consent document, not the teaching and information that make up informed consent. Many nurses serve as witnesses to the signing of the informed consent document; in this capacity, they are attesting only to the voluntary nature of the patient's signature. There is no duty on the part of the nurse to insist that the patient repeat what has been said or what he or she remembers. Should the patient ask questions that alert the nurse to the inadequacy of true comprehension on the patient's part or express uncertainty while signing the document, the nurse has an obligation to inform the primary healthcare provider and appropriate

BOX 4-1

Information Required for Informed Consent

- An explanation of the treatment/procedure to be performed and the expected results of the treatment/procedure
- Description of the risks involved
- Benefits that are likely to result because of the treatment/procedure
- Options to this course of action, including absence of treatment
- Name of the person(s) performing the treatment/procedure
- Statement that the patient may withdraw his/her consent at any time

persons that informed consent has not been obtained.

The second issue concerns the patient who is part of a research study. Federal laws regulate this area as patients are generally considered to come under the heading of vulnerable populations. Whenever research is involved, be it a drug study or a new procedure, the investigators must disclose the research to the subject or the subject's representative and obtain informed consent. Federal guidelines have been developed that specify the procedures used to review research and the disclosures that must be made to ensure that valid informed consent is obtained.

The federal government mandates the basic elements of information that must be included to meet the standards of informed consent. These basic elements include the following:

1. A statement that the study involves research, an explanation of the purposes of the research and the expected duration of the subject's participation, a description of the procedures to be followed, and identification of any procedures that are experimental.
2. A description of any reasonably foreseeable risks or discomforts to the subject.
3. A description of any benefits to the subjects or others that may reasonably be expected from the research.

4. A disclosure of appropriate alternative procedures or courses of treatment, if any, that may be advantageous to the subject.
5. A statement describing the extent, if any, to which confidentiality of records identifying the subject will be maintained.
6. For research involving more than minimal research, an explanation as to any compensation and an explanation as to whether any medical treatments are available if injury occurs and, if so, what they consist of or where further information may be obtained.
7. An explanation of whom to contact for answers to pertinent questions about the research and research subjects' rights and whom to contact in the event of a research-related injury to the subject.
8. A statement that participation is voluntary, refusal to participate will involve no benefits to which the subject is otherwise entitled, and the subject may discontinue participation at any time without penalty or loss of benefits to which the subject is otherwise entitled (45 CFR, Section 46.116, 1991).

The information given must be in a language that is understandable by the subject or the subject's legal representative. No exculpatory wording may be included—for example, a statement that the researcher incurs no liability for the outcome to the subject. Subjects should also be advised of the following:

1. Any additional costs that they might incur because of the research.
2. Potential for any foreseeable risks.
3. Rights to withdraw at will, with no questions asked or additional incentives given.
4. Consequences, if any, of withdrawal before the study is completed.
5. A statement that any significant new findings will be disclosed.
6. The number of proposed subjects for the study.

Excluded from these strict requirements were studies that use existing data, documents, records, or pathological and diagnostic specimens, if these sources are publicly available or the information is recorded so that the subjects cannot be identified (45 CFR, Section 46.101[b], 1991). Other studies that involve only minimal risks to subjects, such as moderate exercise by healthy adults, may be expedited through the review process (45 CFR, Section 46.110, 1991). Nurse managers need to know the staff understands any research protocol with which their patients are involved.

The advent of the Health Insurance Portability and Accountability Act of 1996 ([HIPAA], Public Law 104-191) has affected how medical record information can now be utilized in research studies. No separate patient permission to use medical-record information is required if de-identified information is used. De-identified information is health information that cannot be linked to an individual; most of the 18 demographic items constituting the protected health information (PHI) must be removed before researchers are permitted to use patient records without obtaining individual patient permission to use/disclose their PHI. The de-identified data set that is permissible for usage may contain the following demographic factors: gender and age of individuals and a three-digit ZIP code. Note that if individuals are 90 years of age or older, they are all listed as 90 years of age.

To prevent the onerous task of requiring patients who have been discharged from healthcare settings to sign such permission forms, researchers are allowed to submit a request for a waiver. The waiver is a request to forego the authorization requirements based on two conditions: (1) the use and/or disclosure of PHI involves minimal risk to the subject's privacy, and (2) the research cannot be done practically without this waiver. Additional information about HIPAA and confidentiality are covered later in the chapter.

Concerns over the past abuses that have occurred in the area of research with children has led to the adoption of federal guidelines specifically designed to protect children when they are enrolled as research subjects. Before proceeding under these specific guidelines, state and local laws must be reviewed for laws regulating research on human subjects. In 1998, Subpart D: Additional Protections for Children Involved as Subjects in Research was added to the code (45 CFR 46.401 et seq.). These sections were added to give further protection to children when they are subjects of research studies and to encourage researchers to involve children, where appropriate, in research.

A final issue with informed consent about which nurse managers should be cognizant con-

cerns **medical literacy** or the inability of a growing number of individuals to understand medical terms and instructions. Comprehending medical jargon is difficult for well-educated Americans; it is virtually impossible for approximately 90 million Americans who have "limited health literacy" (Medical Illiteracy, 2004, paragraph 3). Comprehending medical instructions and terms may be impossible for individuals whose first language is not English, who are unable to read at greater than a second grade level, or who have vision or cognitive problems caused by aging. These individuals have difficulty following instructions that are printed on medication labels (both prescription and over-the-counter), interpreting hospital consent forms, and even understanding diagnoses, treatment options, and discharge instructions.

Nurse managers play a significant role in addressing this growing problem. The first issue to address is awareness of the problem, as many patients and their family members hide the fact that they cannot read or do not understand what healthcare providers are attempting to convey. A second issue involves ensuring that the information and words nurses use to communicate with patients are at a level that the person can comprehend. One means of assisting staff nurses to ensure that patients do understand patient discharge information and medication instructions is to request continuing education classes that address this specific issue. Another means may be by role-modeling methods that staff nurses can use to ensure that patients are fully aware of the instructions they have been given.

Exercise 4–5

A patient is admitted to your surgical center for minor surgery that involves a breast biopsy under local anesthesia. The surgeon has previously informed the patient of the surgery risks, options, desired outcomes, and possible complications. A staff member gives the surgery permit form to the patient for her signature. She readily states that she knows about the surgery and has no additional questions. She signs the form with no hesitation. Her husband, who is visiting with her, states he is worried because she will be awake during the procedure, and he is afraid that something may be said to alarm her. The staff member comes to you for advice. How would you, as the nurse manager, handle this issue? Do you alert the surgeon that informed consent has not been obtained? Do you request that the surgeon revisit the patient and reinstruct her about the surgery?

PRIVACY AND CONFIDENTIALITY

Privacy is the patient's right to protection against unreasonable and unwarranted interference with the patient's solitude. This right extends to protection of the person's reputation as well as protection of one's right to be left alone. Within a medical context, the law recognizes the patient's right to protection against (1) appropriation of the patient's name or picture for the institution's sole advantage, (2) intrusion by the institution on the patient's seclusion or affairs, (3) publication of facts that place the patient in a false light, and (4) public disclosure of private facts about the patient by the hospital or staff. **Confidentiality** is the right to privacy of the medical record.

Institutions can reduce potential liability in this area by allowing access to patient data, either written or oral, only to those with a "need to know." Persons with a need to know include physicians and nurses caring for the patient, technicians, unit clerks, therapists, social service workers, and patient advocates. Usually, this need to know extends to the house staff and consultants. Others wishing to access patient data must first ask the patient for permission to review a record. Administration of the institution can access the patient record for statistical analysis, staffing, and quality-of-care review.

The nurse manager is cautioned to ensure that staff members both understand and abide by rules regarding patient privacy and confidentiality. "Interesting" patients should not be discussed with others, and all information concerning patients should be given only in private and secluded areas. All nurses may need to review the current means of giving reports to oncoming shifts and policies about telephone information. Many institutions have now added, to the nursing care plan, a place to list persons to whom the patient has allowed information to be given. If the caller identifies himself or herself as one of those listed persons, the nurse can give patient information without violating the patient's privacy rights. Patients are becoming more knowledgeable about their rights in these areas, and some have been willing to take offending staff members to court over such issues.

The patient's right of access to his or her medical record is another confidentiality issue. Although the patient has a right of access, individual states mandate when this right applies. Most states give the right of access only after the medical record is completed; thus, the patient has the right to review the record after discharge. Some states do give the right of access while the patient is hospitalized, and therefore, individual state law governs individual nurses' actions. When supervising a patient's review of his or her record, the nurse manager or representative should explain only the entries that the patient questions or about which the patient requests further clarification. The nurse makes a note in the record after the session indicating that the patient has viewed the record and what questions were answered.

Patients also have a right to copies of the record, at their expense. The medical record belongs to the institution as a business record, and patients never have the right to retain the original record. This is also true in instances in which a subpoena is obtained to secure an individual's medical record for court purposes. A hospital representative will verify that the copy is a "true and valid" copy of the original record.

An issue that is closely related to the medical record is that of incident reports or unusual occurrence reports. These reports are mandated by JCAHO and serve to alert the institution to risk management and quality assurance issues within the setting. As such, incident reports are considered internal documents and thus not discoverable (open for review) by the injured party or attorneys representing the injured party. In most jurisdictions where this question has arisen, however, the courts have held that the incident report was discoverable and thus open to review by both sides of the suit.

It is therefore prudent for nurse managers to complete and to have staff members complete incident reports as though they will be open records. It is advisable to omit any language of guilt, such as, "The patient would not have fallen if Jane Jones, RN, had ensured the side rails were in their up and locked position." This document should contain only pertinent observations and all care given the patient, such as radiograph films that were obtained for a potential broken bone, medication that was given, and consultants who were called to examine the patient. It is also advisable not to note the occurrence of the incident report in the official record because that incorporates the incident report "by reference," and there is no way to keep the report from being seen by the injured party or attorneys for the injured party.

A newer concept concerning the right to confidentiality concerns HIPAA Public Law 104-191. Signed into law by then President Clinton in August 1996, this act mandated the development of a centralized electronic database containing all health records for every patient in the United States as well as provisions for confidentiality as part of the medical record. The Secretary of the U.S. Department of Health and Human Services has promulgated comprehensive standards facilitating the transmission of medical data, administrative records, and financial records. PHI, which includes some 18 individual identifiers, is at the crux of the confidentiality aspect of the law. The privacy standards limit how these PHI may be used or shared, mandates safeguards for protecting the health information, and shifts the control of health information from providers to the patient by giving patients significant rights. Healthcare facilities must provide patients with a documented Notice of Privacy Rights, explaining how their PHI will be used or shared with other entities. This document also alerts patients to the process for complaints if they determine that their information rights have been violated.

Nurse managers have the responsibility to ensure that those they supervise uphold these patient rights as dictated by HIPAA and to take corrective actions should these rights not be upheld. A thorough understanding of the provisions of the act is the starting point to ensure that patient confidentiality rights are maintained. To maintain one's currency in this area of the law, nurse managers should continue to seek additional education about the evolving aspects of this law.

POLICIES AND PROCEDURES

Risk management is a process that identifies, analyzes, and treats potential hazards within a given setting. The object of risk management is to identify potential hazards and eliminate them before anyone is harmed or disabled. Risk management activities include writing policies and procedures. Written policies and procedures are a requirement of JCAHO. These documents set standards of care for the institution and direct practice. They must be clearly stated, well delineated, and based on current practice. Nurse managers should review the policies and procedures frequently for compliance and timeliness. If policies are absent or outdated, the nurse manager must request the appropriate person or committee to either initiate or update the policy.

■ *Exercise 4-6*

You are assigned some risk management activities in the nursing facility where you work. In investigating incident reports that were filed by your staff, you discover that this is the third patient this week who has fallen while attempting to get out of bed and sit in a chair. How would you handle this issue? Decide how you would start a more complete investigation of this issue. For example, is it a facility-wide issue or one that is confined to one unit? Does it affect all shifts or only one? What safety issues are you going to discuss with your staff, and how are you going to discuss these issues? Do these falls involve the same staff member? Design a unit in-service class for the staff concerning incident reports and patient safety.

EMPLOYMENT LAWS

The federal and individual state governments have enacted laws regulating employment. To be effective and legally correct, nurse managers must be familiar with these laws and how individual laws affect the institution and labor relations. Many nurse managers have come to fear the legal system because of personal experience or the experiences of colleagues, but much of this concern may be directly attributable to uncertainty with the law or partial knowledge of the law. By understanding and correctly following federal employment laws, nurse managers may actually decrease their potential liability by complying with both federal and state laws. Table 4-2 gives an overview of key federal employment laws.

Equal Employment Opportunity Laws

Several federal laws have been enacted to expand equal employment opportunities by prohibiting discrimination based on gender, age, race, religion, handicap, pregnancy, and national origin. The Equal Employment Opportunity Commission (EEOC) enforces these laws. All states have also enacted statutes that address employment opportunities, and the nurse manager should consider both when hiring and assigning nursing employees.

Table 4-2 SELECTED FEDERAL LABOR LEGISLATION

Year	Legislation	Primary Purpose of the Legislation
1935	Wagner Act; National Labor Act	Unions, National Labor Relations Board established
1947	Taft-Hartley Act	Equal balance of power between unions and management
1948	1962 Executive Order 10988	Public employees could join unions
1963	Equal Pay Act	Became illegal to pay lower wages based on gender
1964	Civil Rights Act	Protected against discrimination based on race, color, creed, national origin, etc.
1967	Age Discrimination	Act protected against discrimination based on age
1970	Occupational Safety and Health Act	Ensured healthy and safe working conditions
1974	Wagner Amendments	Allowed nonprofit organizations to unionize
1990	Americans with Disabilities Act	Barred discrimination against workers with disabilities
1991	Civil Rights Act	Addressed sexual harassment in the workplace
1993	Family and Medical Leave Act	Allowed work leaves based on family and medical needs
1999	Ergonomics Program Standard	Addressed the issue of work-related musculoskeletal disorders
2000	Ergonomics Program Standard Repealed	

The most significant legislation affecting equal employment opportunities today is the amended 1964 Civil Rights Act (1978). Section 703(a) of Title VII makes it illegal for an employer "to refuse to hire, discharge an individual, or otherwise to discriminate against an individual, with respect to his compensation, terms, conditions, or privileges of employment because of the individual's race, color, religion, sex, or national origin." The Equal Opportunities Act of 1972 also amended title VII, so that it applies to private institutions with 15 or more employees, state and local governments, **labor unions,** and employment agencies.

The Civil Rights Act was signed into law in 1991. This act further broadened the issue of sexual harassment in the workplace and supersedes many of the sections of Title VII. Sections of the new legislation define sexual harassment, its elements, and the employer's responsibilities regarding harassment in the workplace, especially prevention and corrective action. The Civil Rights Act is enforced by the EEOC-created in the 1964 act; its powers were broadened in the 1972 Equal Employment Opportunity Act. The primary activity of the EEOC is processing complaints of employment discrimination. There are three phases: investigation, conciliation, and litigation. Investigation focuses on determining whether the employer has violated provisions of Title VII. If the EEOC finds "probable cause," an attempt is made to reach an agreement or conciliation between the EEOC, the complainant, and the employer. If conciliation fails, the EEOC may file suit against the employer in federal court or issue to the complainant the right to sue for discrimination under its auspices, including those relating to staffing practices and sexual harassment in the workplace. The EEOC defines sexual harassment broadly, and this has generally been upheld in the courts. Nurse managers must realize that it is the duty of employers (management) to prevent employees from sexually harassing other employees. The EEOC issues policies and practices for employers to implement, both to sensitize employees to this problem and to prevent its occurrence; nurse managers should be aware of these policies and practices and seek guidance in implementing them if sexual harassment occurs in their units.

Employers may seek exceptions to Title VII on a number of premises. For example, employment decisions made on the basis of national origin, religion, and gender (never race or color) are lawful if such decisions are necessary for the normal operation of the business, although the courts have viewed this exception very narrowly. Promotions and layoffs based on bona fide seniority or merit systems are permissible (*Herrero v. St. Louis University Hospital*, 1997), as are exceptions based on business necessity.

Age Discrimination in Employment Act of 1967

The Age Discrimination in Employment Act of 1967 made discrimination against older men and women by employers, unions, and employment agencies illegal. A 1986 amendment to the law prohibits discrimination against persons older than 40 years. The practical outcome of this act has been that mandatory retirement is no longer allowed in the American workplace.

As with Title VII, there are some exceptions to this act. Reasonable factors other than age may be used when terminations become necessary; such reasonable factors may include a performance evaluation system or certain limited occupational qualifications—for example, the tedious physical demands of a specific job.

Americans with Disabilities Act of 1990

The Americans with Disabilities Act (ADA) of 1990 provides protection to persons with disabilities and is the most significant civil rights legislation since the Civil Rights Act of 1964. The purpose of the ADA is to provide a clear and comprehensive national mandate for the elimination of discrimination against individuals with disabilities and to provide clear, strong, consistent, enforceable standards addressing discrimination in the workplace. The ADA is closely related to the Civil Rights Act and incorporates the antidiscrimination principles established in Section 504 of the Rehabilitation Act of 1973.

The act has five titles; Table 4-3 shows the pertinent issues of each title. The ADA has jurisdiction over employers, private and public; employment agencies; labor organizations; and joint labor-management committees. It defines disability broadly. With respect to an individual, a disability is (1) a physical or mental impairment that substantially limits one or more of the major life activities of such individual, (2) a record of such impairment, or (3) regarded as having such an impairment (ADA, 1990). The overall effect of the legislation is that persons with disabilities will not be excluded from job opportunities or adversely affected in any aspect of employment unless they are not qualified or are otherwise unable to perform the job. The ADA thus protects qualified individuals with disabilities in regard to job application procedures, hiring, compensation, advancement, and all other employment matters.

The number of lawsuits filed under the ADA since its enactment has been extensive. Recent cases have assisted in defining disability eligibility. The following findings have been decided in court regarding disabilities: (1) A nurse with a lifting disability is not qualified for protection under the ADA (*Thompson v. Holy Family Hospital*, 1997),

Table 4-3	AMERICANS WITH DISABILITIES ACT OF 1990
Title	**Provisions**
I	Employment: defines the purpose of the act and who is qualified under the act as having a disability
II	Public services: concerns services, programs, and activities of public entities as well as public transportation
III	Public accommodations and services operated by private entities: prohibits discrimination against persons with disabilities in areas of public accommodations, commercial facilities, and public transportation services
IV	Telecommunications: intended to make telephone services accessible to individuals with hearing or speech impairments
V	Miscellaneous provisions: certain insurance matters; incorporation of this act with other federal and state laws

From Americans with Disabilities Act of 1990.

(2) erratic behavior does not give notice to the employer that the individual has a mental impairment (*Webb v. Mercy Hospital,* 1996), (3) depression and anxiety are not disabling conditions (*Cody v. Cigna Healthcare of St. Louis, Inc.,* 1998), (4) a nurse taking medications for depression is not disabled (*Wilking v. County of Ramsey,* 1997), (5) migraine headaches and latex allergies are not disabilities (*Howard v. North Mississippi Medical Center,* 1996), and (6) pregnancy is not a disability (*Jessie v. Carter Health Care Center, Inc.,* 1996).

The ADA requires an employer or potential employer to make reasonable accommodations to employ persons with a disability. The law does not mandate that individuals with disabilities be hired before fully qualified persons who do not have a disability; it does mandate that those with disabilities not be disqualified merely because of an easily accommodated disability.

This last point was well illustrated by the court in *Zamudio v. Patia* (1997). The court stated that the employer would be required to inform Ms. Zamudio when a position became available for which the reasonable accommodation she required could be met. She would be allowed to apply, but "as a disabled employee seeking reasonable accommodation she did not have to be given preference over other employees without disabilities who might have better qualifications or more seniority" (*Zamudio v. Patia,* 1997, at 808).

Moreover, the court will not impose job restructuring on an employer if the person needing accommodation qualifies for other jobs not requiring such accommodation. In *Mauro v. Borgess Medical Center* (1995), the court refused to impose accommodation on the employer hospital merely because the affected employee desired to stay within a certain unit of the institution. In this case, an operating surgical technician who tested positive for HIV was offered an equivalent position by the hospital in an area where there would be no patient contact. He refused the transfer, desiring accommodation within the operating arena, and was denied such accommodation by the Michigan court.

The act also provides for essential job functions. These are defined by the ADA as those functions that the person must be able to perform to be qualified for employment positions. Courts have assisted in determining these essential job functions. For example, in *Jones v. Kerrville State Hospital* (1998), the court found that an essential job function for a psychiatric nurse is the ability to restrain patients. In *Laurin v. Providence Hospital and Massachusetts Nurses Association* (1998), the ability to work rotating shifts was held to be an essential job function.

The act also specifically excludes the following from the definition of *disability:* homosexuality and bisexuality, sexual behavioral disorders, gambling addiction, kleptomania, pyromania, and current use of illegal drugs (ADA, 1990). Moreover, employers may hold alcoholic persons to the same job qualifications and job performance standards as other employees, even if the unsatisfactory behavior or performance is related to the alcoholism (ADA, 1990). As with other federal employment laws, the nurse manager should have a thorough understanding of the law as it applies to the institution and his or her specific job description and should know whom to contact within the institution structure for clarification as needed.

Affirmative Action

The policy of affirmative action (AA) differs from the policy of equal employment opportunity (EEO). AA policy enhances employment opportunities of protected groups of people; EEO policy is concerned with implementing employment practices that do not discriminate against or impair the employment opportunities of protected groups. Thus, AA can be seen in conjunction with several federal employment laws; for example, in conjunction with the Vietnam Era Veterans' Re-adjustment Act of 1974, AA requires that employers with government contracts take steps to enhance the employment opportunities of veterans with disabilities and other veterans of the Vietnam era.

Equal Pay Act of 1963

The Equal Pay Act makes it illegal to pay lower wages to employees of one gender when the jobs (1) require equal skill in experience, training, education, and ability; (2) require equal effort in mental or physical exertion; (3) are of equal responsibility and accountability; and (4) are performed under similar working conditions. Courts have held that unequal pay may be legal if it is based on seniority, merit, incentive systems, or a factor other than gender. The main cases filed under this law in the area of nursing have been by nonprofessionals.

Occupational Safety and Health Act

The Occupational Safety and Health Administration (OSHA) Act of 1970 was enacted to ensure that healthful and safe working conditions would exist in the workplace. Among other provisions, the law requires isolation procedures, placarding areas containing ionizing radiation, proper grounding of electrical equipment, protective storage of flammable and combustible liquids, and the gloving of all personnel when handling bodily fluids. The statute provides that if no federal standard has been established, state statutes prevail. Nurse managers should know the relevant OSHA laws for the institution and his or her specific area. Frequent review of new additions to the law must also be undertaken, especially in this era of AIDS and infectious diseases, and care must be taken to ensure that necessary gloves and equipment, as specified, are available on each unit.

A newer area in the OSHA standards, the Ergonomics Program Standard, was issued on November 14, 2000, and became effective on January 16, 2001. This standard was created to address the issue of work-related musculoskeletal disorders (MSDs) that result when there is a physical mismatch between the physical capacity of the worker and the physical demands of the workplace. Approximately 1.8 million workers in the United States report work-related MSDs, including carpal tunnel syndrome, tendonitis, and back injuries; 600,000 workers report loss of time from work for these work-related injuries (U.S. Department of Labor, 2001). **Ergonomics,** the science of fitting the job to the worker, is seen as one solution to this issue.

The standard required that the employer provide the following basic information to all employees: (1) common MSDs and their signs and symptoms, (2) the importance of reporting MSDs as soon as possible, (3) how to report MSDs in the workplace, (4) risk factors and job and work activities associated with MSD hazards, and (5) a brief description of OSHA's ergonomics standard. The six elements of the complete ergonomics program include (1) management leadership and employee training, (2) hazard information and reporting, (3) job hazard analysis and control, (4) employee training, (5) MSD management, and (6) program evaluation. The first two elements are required for all jobs that carry a potential risk for MSDs, even if no MSD has been reported, and were to be fully implemented by October 14, 2001 (OSHA Regulations, 1999).

Projected to cost employers $4.5 billion annually, the standard was repealed by the U.S. Senate and House of Representatives on March 6 and 7, 2001. President George W. Bush signed the joint resolution of Congress on March 20, 2001, stating that "Joint Resolution 6 . . . repeals an unduly burdensome and over broad regulation dealing with ergonomics. . . . There needs to be a balance between and an understanding of the costs and benefits associated with Federal regulations. In this instance, though, in exchange for uncertain benefits, the ergonomics rule would have cost both large and small employers billions of dollars and presented employers with overwhelming compliance challenges." He further pledged to "pursue a comprehensive approach to ergonomics that addresses the concerns surrounding the ergonomics rule repealed today" (Bush, 2001, paragraphs 2 and 3).

Family and Medical Leave Act of 1993

The Family and Medical Leave Act of 1993 was passed because of the large numbers of single-parent and two-parent households in which the single parent or both parents are employed full-time, placing job security and parenting at odds. The law also supports the growing demands that aging parents are placing on their working children. The act was written in an attempt to balance the demands of the workplace with the demands of the family, allowing employed individuals to take leaves for medical reasons, including the birth or adoption of children and the care of a spouse, child, or parent who has serious health problems.

Essentially, the act provides job security for unpaid leave while the employee is caring for a new infant or other family healthcare needs. The act is gender-neutral and allows both men and women the same leave provisions.

To be eligible under the act, the employee must have worked for at least 12 months and worked at least 1250 hours during the preceding 12-month period. The employee may take up to 12 weeks of unpaid leave. The act allows the employer to require the employee to use all or part of any paid vacation, personal leave, or sick leave as part of the 12-week family leave. Employees must give the employer 30 days notice, or such notice as is practical in emergency cases, before using the medical leave.

Employment-at-Will and Wrongful Discharge

Historically, the employment relationship has been considered a "free will" relationship. Employees were free to take or not take a job at will, and employers were free to hire, retain, or discharge employees for any reason. Many laws, some federal but predominantly state, have been slowly eroding this at-will employment relationship. Evolving case law provides at least three exceptions to the broad doctrine of employment-at-will.

The first exception is a public policy exception. This exception involves cases in which an employee is discharged in direct conflict with established public policy. Some examples include discharging an employee for serving on a jury, reporting employers' illegal actions (better known as "whistleblowing"), and filing a workers' compensation claim.

Several recent court cases attest to the number of terminations in healthcare settings that serve as retaliation for the employer. More commonly known as "whistleblowing" cases, the healthcare provider in these cases is terminated for one of three distinct reasons: (1) speaking out against unsafe practices, (2) reporting violations of federal laws, or (3) filing lawsuits against employers. Essentially, the Whistleblower Law states that no employer can discharge, threaten, or discriminate against an employee regarding compensation, terms, conditions, location, or privileges of employment because the employee in good faith reported or caused to be reported, verbally or in writing, what the employee had a reasonable cause to believe was a violation of a law, rule, or regulation of state or federal law. For example, in *Roulston v. Tendercare (Michigan), Inc.* (2000), a social services director was dismissed after she confronted the director of nursing for what the social services director called *patient abuse*. The social services director had reported instances of patient abuse to the state Department of Consumer and Industry Services and the Health Care Fraud Unit of the state attorney general's office. The nursing director first attempted to debate the definition of patient abuse, then told the social services director that she had better start thinking like everyone else who worked at the nursing home. The court was satisfied that the social services director's lawsuit against the nursing home for retaliation was appropriate.

In *Fleming v. Correctional Healthcare Solutions, Inc.* (2000), a nurse in a correctional facility was dismissed for reporting financial mismanagement. The nurse was terminated for insubordination, and she sued her former employer for retaliation under the New Jersey whistleblower act. The court upheld her right to sue for wrongful dismissal. Similarly, the court in *UTMB v. Hohman* (1999) allowed a nurse to bring suit for wrongful dismissal when she was discharged for reporting a physician's alleged abuses.

The court in *Taylor v. Memorial Health Systems, Inc.* (2000) enumerated the conditions that must be present to file a valid employer retaliation lawsuit. (1) The whistleblower must disclose or threaten to disclose an allegation in writing and under oath to the state department of professional regulation. (2) The allegation must have been about an activity, policy, or practice of the employer that is or was a violation of a state or federal law, rule, or regulation. (3) The employee must have given the employer written notification and reasonable time to correct the problem. (4) The employee must have suffered retaliation in the form of some actual harm (*Taylor v. Memorial Health Systems, Inc.*, 2000, p. 755). Although states may vary slightly on these elements, this court essentially outlines the elements to consider when contemplating a whistleblower lawsuit.

The second exception to wrongful discharge involves situations in which there is an implied contract. The courts have generally treated employee handbooks, company policies, and oral statements made at the time of employment as "framing the employment relationship" (*Watkins v. Unemployment Compensation Board of Review*, 1997). For example, in *Trombley v. Southwestern Vermont Medical Center* (1999), the court found that the employee handbook outlined the procedure for progressive discipline, mandating that such procedure be followed before a nurse could be terminated for incompetent nursing care.

The third exception to wrongful discharge is a "good faith and fair dealing" exception. The purpose of this exception is to prevent unfair or malicious terminations, and the courts use the exception sparingly. Although this exception is rarely seen in nursing, it remains a valid exception to wrongful discharge of an employee. An older, but still relevant case illustrates its use. In *Fortune v. National Cash Register Company* (1977), an employee was discharged just before a final contract was signed between his employer and another company for which the employee would have received a large commission. The court held that he was discharged in bad faith, solely to prevent payment of his commission by National Cash Register.

Nurse managers are urged to know their respective state laws concerning this growing area of the law, particularly in conjunction with whistleblower laws. Managers should review institution documents, especially employee handbooks and recruiting brochures, for unwanted statements implying job security or other unintentional promises. Managers are also cautioned not to say anything during the preemployment negotiations and interviews that might be construed as implying job security or other unintentional promises to the potential employee. To prevent successful suits for retaliation by whistleblowers, nurse managers should carefully monitor the treatment of an employee after a complaint is filed and ensure that performance evaluations are performed and placed in the appropriate files. The nurse manager should also take steps to correct the whistleblower's complaint or refer the complaint to upper management so that it can effectively be addressed.

Exercise 4-7

Mary Sanchez is the nurse manager for a busy home healthcare agency. She overhears staff members discussing the quality of nursing care that they are forced to deliver to patients because of the number of patients served by the home healthcare agency and limited number of staff. The nurses are especially critical of the number of vacancies for RNs. She fears that the staff may file a formal complaint with the state. What should she do to prevent the filing of such a complaint? If a complaint is filed, what advice would you give Mary Sanchez?

Collective Bargaining

Collective bargaining, also called *labor relations,* is the joining together of employees for the purpose of increasing their ability to influence the employer and improve working conditions. Usually, the employer is referred to as management, and the employees, even professionals, are labor. Those persons involved in the hiring, firing, scheduling, disciplining, or evaluating of employees are considered management and may not be included in a collective bargaining unit. Those in management could form their own group but are not protected under these laws. Nurse managers may or may not be part of management; if they have hiring and firing authority, they are part of management.

Collective bargaining is defined and protected by the National Labor Relations Act and its amendments; the National Labor Relations Board (NLRB) oversees the act and those who come under its auspices. The NLRB ensures that employees are able to choose freely whether they want to be represented by a particular bargaining unit, and it serves to prevent or remedy any violation of the labor laws. Chapter 18 provides a further analysis of this concept.

PROFESSIONAL NURSING PRACTICE: ETHICS

Ethics is an area of professional practice in which nurse managers should have a solid foundation, as this is an area that is becoming increasingly more prominent in clinical practice settings, yet it remains an area in which many nurses feel the most inadequate. This is partially due to the fact that ethics is much more nebulous than are laws and regulations. In ethics, there are no right and wrong answers, just better or worse answers, and nurses seek mentorship and counseling from nurse managers when they encounter difficult situations. Thus, nurse managers must have a deep understanding of ethical principles and their application.

Ethics may be distinguished from the law because ethics is internal to an individual, looks to the ultimate "good" of an individual rather than society as a whole, and concerns the "why" of one's actions. The law, comprising rules and regulations pertinent to society as a whole, is external to oneself and concerns one's actions and conduct. Ethics concerns the individual within society, whereas law concerns society as a whole. Law can be enforced through the courts and statutes, whereas ethics are enforced via **ethics committees** and professional codes.

Today, ethics and legal issues often become entwined, and it is difficult to separate ethics from legal concerns. Legal principles and doctrines assist the nurse manager in decision-making; ethical theories and principles are often involved in those decisions. Thus, the nurse manager must be cognizant of both laws and ethics in everyday management concerns.

Ethical theories and principles are important because they form the essential base of knowledge from which to proceed, rather than giving easy, straightforward answers. Without ethical theories and principles, decisions revolve on personal emotions and values.

Ethical Principles

Although ethical theories are frequently used in nursing to apply to patient care decisions, these same ethical principles are paramount in the effective nurse manager's work. Ethical principles that the nurse manager should consider when making decisions include the eight items listed in Box 4-2. Each of these principles can be used alone, although it is much more common to see more than one ethical principle affecting a nurse's clinical practice. The principle of **autonomy** addresses personal freedom and the right to choose what will happen to one's own person. The legal doctrine of informed consent is a direct reflection of this principle. The principle underlies the concept of progressive discipline because the employee has the option to meet delineated expectations or take full accountability for his or her actions. This principle also underlies the nurse manager's clinical practice because autonomy is reflected in individual decision-making about patient care issues and in-group decision-making about unit operations decisions.

The principle of **beneficence** states that the actions one takes should promote good. This principle is used when nurse managers accentuate the employee's positive attributes and qualities rather than focusing on the employee's failures and shortcomings. Nurse managers also use this principle when they encourage staff members to excel to their fullest potential and when the nurse manager encourages staff members to seek more challenging and satisfying clinical experiences.

The corollary of beneficence, the principle of **nonmaleficence,** states that one should do no harm. For a nurse manager following this principle, performance evaluation should emphasize the employee's good qualities and give positive direction for growth. Destroying the employee's self-esteem and self-worth would be considered doing harm under this principle.

Veracity concerns telling the truth and incorporates the concept that individuals should always tell the truth. The principle also compels that the truth be told completely. Nurse managers use this principle when they give all the facts of a situation truthfully and then assist employees to make decisions. For example, with low patient censuses, employees must be told all the options and then be allowed to make their own decisions about floating to other units, taking vacation time, or taking a day without pay if the institution has such a policy.

Justice is the principle of treating all persons equally and fairly. This principle usually arises in times of short supplies or when there is competition for resources or benefits. This principle is used by nurse managers when they decide which staff members will have holiday and vacation time or paid attendance at national or local conferences. The staff member's overall performance should be considered, rather than who is next on the list to attend a conference or to be allowed time off. Justice is also encountered when deciding who should be floated to another unit/service within the institution or which staff member should be moved to a straight day position rather than remaining on a rotating schedule.

The principle of **paternalism** allows one person to make decisions for another and often is seen as a negative or undesirable principle. Paternalism, however, may be used to assist persons to make decisions when they do not have sufficient data or expertise. Paternalism becomes undesirable when the entire decision is taken from the employee. Nurse managers use this principle in a positive manner by assisting employees in deciding major career moves and plans, helping the staff member to more fully understand all aspects of a possible career change.

Fidelity means keeping one's promises or commitments. Nurse managers abide by this principle

---

BOX 4-2

Ethical Principles

Autonomy	Justice
Beneficence	Paternalism
Nonmaleficence	Fidelity
Veracity	Respect for others

when they follow through on any promises they have previously made to employees, such as a promised leave, a certain shift to be worked, or a promotion to preceptor within the unit.

Many think the principle of **respect for others** is the highest principle and incorporates all other principles. Respect for others acknowledges the right of individuals to make decisions and to live by these decisions. Respect for others also transcends cultural differences, gender issues, and racial concerns. Nurse managers positively reinforce this principle daily in their actions with employees, patients, and peers because they serve as role models for staff members and others in the institution. Nurses also reinforce these principles when they incorporate role-modeling theory in interactions with staff members. See the Theory Box.

Exercise 4-8

The community has been suffering from a severe nursing shortage made worse by a particularly virulent flu that has affected many of the staff members. Upper management is aware of the severity of the shortage and has decreased bed census by 20%; only emergency surgery is being performed until the crisis abates. You are considering reassigning a portion of your critical care staff, including dialysis and emergency care nurses, to the general medical and surgical floors because the crisis is most severe on the general units. None of the staff has been cross-trained specifically to the general units. From an ethical standpoint,

how would you begin to achieve this task? How would you select which nurses to reassign and which nurses to retain in the unit? Would you involve the nurses themselves in the decision-making process? Why or why not?

Codes of Ethics

Ethical codes have been developed to serve as a public expression of the profession's agreement with the society in which it functions by publishing a statement of the obligations and duties a profession has to persons it serves. A written and published code provides non-negotiable standards to both the public it serves and the members who come under its auspices. Professional nursing organizations publish a variety of codes for ethical conduct ranging from an *International Council of Nurses Code of Ethics for Nurses* (International Council of Nurses, 2000) to a variety of codes for nurses in specific countries. The ANA *Code of Ethics for Nurses* (2001) and the *Code of Ethics for Registered Nurses* (Canadian Nurses Association, 2002) are examples of country-specific codes.

The *Code of Ethics for Nurses* (ANA, 2001) should be the starting point for any nurse faced with an ethical issue. The first American nursing code was adopted in 1950, and it focused on the character of the nurse and the virtues that were essential to the profession. In 1968, the focus

Theory Box

MODELING AND ROLE-MODELING THEORY

THEORY/CONTRIBUTOR	KEY IDEA	APPLICATION TO PRACTICE
Modeling and Role-Modeling Theory (based on Maslow's hierarchical ordering of needs)	The theory uses Maslow's hierarchical ordering of needs as the driver for human behavior, allowing the nurse to use these perceived needs to plan and implement interventions. The aim of these interventions involve five common goals: building trust; promoting positive orientation; promoting perceived control; promoting strengths; and setting health-directed mutual goals.	Implementing this model as the basis for leadership decisions may assist in retaining nurses in the profession by developing the interpersonal and interactive relationships needed to create an environment where staff members can express their concerns, desires, needs, and questions.

Arruda, E. (2004). Better retention through nursing theory. *Nursing Management, 36*(4), 16-18.

shifted to a duty-based ethical focus, and the current *Code of Ethics for Nurses* (2001) has blended these duty-based ethics with a historical focus on character and virtue. The *Code of Ethics for Nurses* (2001) has been simplified and updated so that nurses can readily understand and apply its provisions. This nine-point code guides nurses in understanding the extent of their commitment to the patient, themselves, other nurses, and the nursing profession. The code begins with addressing respect for others, as the first provision of the code refers to the "inherent dignity, worth, and uniqueness of every individual" (ANA, 2001, provision 1). Further provisions in the code assist nurses in understanding that patients, whether as individuals, or as members of families, groups, or communities, are their first obligation, and that nurses must not only ensure quality care but also protect the safety of these patients. Nurses and their nurse managers should ensure that the provisions of the code are incorporated into nursing care delivery in all clinical settings.

Ethical Decision-Making Framework

Ethical decision-making involves reflection on the following: who should make the choice; possible options or courses of action; available options; consequences, both good and bad, of all possible options; rules, obligations, and values that should direct choices; and desired goals or outcomes. When making decisions, nurses need to combine all of these elements using an orderly, systematic, and objective method; ethical decision-making models assist in accomplishing this goal.

Ethical decision-making is always a process. To facilitate this process, the nurse manager must use all available resources, including the institutional ethics committee, and communicate with and support all those involved in the process. Some decisions are easier to reach and support. It is important to allow sufficient time for the process so that a supportable option can be reached. The Research Perspective box shows how the ethical principles of nurse managers and staff nurses differ, yet both are vital to quality patient outcomes.

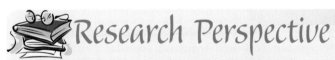

Research Perspective

Kellen, J. C., Oberle, K., Girard, F. & Falkenberg, L. (2004). Exploring ethical perspectives of nurses and nurse managers. *Canadian Journal of Nursing Leadership, 17*(1), 78-87.

The need for this study arose because the nursing shortage reached crisis proportions. Staff nurses must believe that their nurse managers are supportive and hold the same basic nursing values and principles that the staff nurses hold, yet there appears to be a movement by nurse managers from these basic nursing values to a more corporate ethical view. The main question explored in the study was whether "nurse managers are expected to subscribe to a corporate ethic versus a nursing ethic in making decisions and whether these approaches are fundamentally different" (p. 78). The authors reasoned that if the ethics of clinical decision-making differed between the two groups of nurses, problems could arise in the delivery of competent patient-care delivery.

Although the exact methodology was somewhat uncertain, the authors concluded that there were some differences in how the two groups perceived values, particularly in the areas of beneficence and justice. Staff nurses perceived that their nursing care was more aligned with beneficence (the duty to do good) for the individual patient, whereas nurse managers were more concerned with distributive justice (equality and fairness) at the system level. Nurse managers have as their goal the greater good for all persons, as opposed to the individual within the system. Decisions are made by nurse managers about program cuts in consideration of the overall goal of doing good, whereas staff nurses' decisions are about prioritizing care and limiting choice. Ultimately, both groups use fundamental ethical principles; the difference is in the emphasis and level of application (individual versus the overall system).

Continued

The authors concluded that, although the Canadian healthcare system focuses on providing services limiting healthcare costs, the same challenges face both nurse managers and staff nurses: the primacy of individual patient care within the system-wide issues of resource allocation. Nurses at all levels strive to ensure the provision of quality nursing care within fiscal boundaries. Professional values and ethical principles guide them in their decision-making. The nurses at the staff level must observe the impact of decisions made by nurse managers, and these staff nurses must be willing to challenge decisions that place patients at risk. Similarly, nurse managers play a pivotal role in ensuring that the organization continues to enable basic nursing values to be realized. They are thus required to challenge the overall system to ensure that these basic values are not lost.

IMPLICATIONS FOR PRACTICE

First, nurse managers and staff nurses must come to the realization that they hold differing perspectives, yet both groups strive to ensure the best possible nursing care to the patients they serve. One way to begin to assist staff nurses is in involving the staff nurse in decision-making activities. Nurse managers should also ensure that the decision-making process is more transparent, so that staff nurses can better appreciate the constraints under which nurse managers function. Nurse managers must also begin to demonstrate respect for the staff nurse's voice. Second, staff nurses must begin to understand the broader perspectives of the nurse manager's decisions. Although staff nurses have a right to be heard, they also have an obligation to consider all ethical dimensions of decisions that are made, including the need to ensure appropriate allocation of resources.

Exercise 4-9

Joe Rodriquez, age 19, presents to the hospital emergency department with a diagnosis of West Nile Virus. He has a fever of 102° F, chills, and a generalized aching in all his muscles. He reports that he was recently hiking in a wooded portion of the state and was bitten repeatedly by mosquitoes, despite the fact that he used an insect repellant. He and his parents are informed about this condition, including the need for immediate hospitalization and the treatment plan. Joe refuses to be hospitalized, stating that he will follow all medical recommendations at home. He asks to be assigned a home healthcare nurse to assist with his medical treatment. His parents are totally torn between honoring their son's wishes and forcing the admission of their son so that he can receive the needed medical and nursing care.

You are the nurse manager for the emergency department, and staff members approach you about this patient. How would you begin to resolve this dilemma? What type of direction would you give staff members to allow them to come to a satisfactory conclusion?

Ethics Committees

With the increasing numbers of ethical dilemmas in patient situations and administrative decisions, healthcare providers are using hospital ethics committees for guidance. Such committees can provide both long-term and short-term assistance. Ethics committees can provide structure and guidelines for potential problems, serve as open forums for discussion, and function as true patient advocates by placing the patient at the core of the committee discussions.

To form such a committee, the involved individuals should begin as a bioethical study group so that all potential members can explore ethical principles and theories. The composition of the committee should include nurses, physicians, clergy, clinical social workers, nutritional experts, pharmacists, administrative personnel, and legal experts. Once the committee has become active, individual patients or patients' families and additional representatives of members of the healthcare delivery team may be invited to committee deliberations.

Ethics committees traditionally follow one of three distinct structures, although some institutional committees blend the three structures. The autonomy model facilitates decision-making for competent patients. The patient-benefit model uses substituted judgment (what the patient would want for himself or herself if capable of making these issues known) and facilitates decision-making for the incompetent patient. The social justice model considers broad social issues and is accountable to the overall institution.

In most settings, the ethics committee already exists because there are complex issues dividing healthcare workers. In many centers, ethical rounds, conducted weekly or monthly, allow staff members who may later become involved in ethical decision-making to begin reviewing all the issues and to become more comfortable with ethical issues and their resolution.

Blending Ethical and Legal Issues

Blending legal demands with ethics is a challenge for nursing, and no case better portrays this type of difficult decision-making than does the recent case of Theresa M. Schiavo. Ms. Schiavo suffered a cardiac arrest in February, 1990; it is estimated that she was without oxygen for approximately 11 minutes, which is 5 to 7 minutes longer than most medical experts believe is possible without suffering severe and permanent brain damage. She was resuscitated and, at the insistence of her husband, was intubated, placed on a ventilator, and eventually received a tracheotomy. The cause of her cardiac arrest was determined to be a severe electrolyte imbalance caused by an eating disorder. In the 6 years preceding the cardiac event, Ms. Schiavo had lost approximately 140 pounds, going from 250 to 110 pounds.

During the first 2 months after her cardiac arrest, Ms. Schiavo was in a coma. She then regained some wakefulness and was eventually diagnosed as being in persistent vegetative state (PVS). She was successfully weaned from the ventilator and was able to swallow her saliva, both reflexive behaviors. However, she was not able to eat food or drink liquids, which is characteristic of PSV. A permanent feeding tube was placed so that she could receive nutrition and hydration.

Throughout the early years of her PSV, there was no challenge to the diagnosis or to the appointment of her husband as her legal guardian. Four years after her cardiac arrest, a successful lawsuit was filed against a fertility physician who failed to detect her electrolyte imbalance. A judgment of $300,000 went to her husband for loss of companionship and $700,000 was placed in a court-managed trust fund to maintain and provide care for Ms. Schiavo.

Sometime after this successful lawsuit, the close family relationship that Ms. Schiavo's husband and her parents had began to erode, and the public first became aware of Ms. Schiavo's plight. As her court-appointed guardian noted:

> Thereafter, what is for millions of Americans a profoundly private matter catapulted a close, loving family into an internationally watched blood feud. The end product was a most public death for a very private individual. . . . Theresa was by all accounts a very shy, fun loving, and sweet woman who loved her husband and her parents very much. The family breach and public circus would have been anathema to her. (Wolfson, 2005, p. 17)

The court battles regarding the removal or retention of her feeding tube began. There was adequate medical and legal evidence to show that Ms. Schiavo had been correctly diagnosed and that she would not have wanted to be kept alive by artificial means. Laws in the state of Florida, where Ms. Schiavo was a patient, allowed the removal of tubal nutrition and hydration in patients with PVS. The feeding tube was removed and later reinstated following a court order.

In October, 2003, there was a second removal of the feeding tube after a higher court overturned the lower court decision that had caused the feeding tube to be reinserted. With this second removal, the Florida legislature passed what has become to be known as Terri's Law. This law gave the Florida governor the right to demand the feeding tube be reinserted and also appoint a special guardian to review the entire case. The special guardian at litem was appointed in October, 2003. Terri's Law was later declared unconstitutional by the Florida Supreme Court and the U.S. Supreme Court refused to overrule their decision. In early 2005, during the last week's of Ms. Schiavo's life, the U.S. Congress attempted to move the issue to the federal rather than Florida state court system. This fiasco ended with the federal district court in Florida and the 11th Circuit Court of Appeals ruling that there was insufficient evidence to create a new trial, and the U.S. Supreme Court refused to review the findings of these two lower courts (Wolfson, 2005). Ms. Schiavo died on March 31, 2005; she was 41 years of age.

Whichever side of the case one supported, the plight of Terri Schiavo created numerous ethical concerns for the nurses caring for her and for the nurse managers in the clinical setting. Issues that created these conflicts ranged from working with feuding family members, to multiple media personnel attempting to cover the story, to constant editorial and new stories invading the privacy of this individual, to masses of people lined at the borders of the hospice center insisting that she be fed, to individual emotions about the correctness of either keeping or removing the feeding tube. One thing, however, is clear. The nurse managers and nurses caring for the patient had a legal obligation to either remove or reinsert the feeding tube based on the prevailing court decision or legislative act. Their individual reflections about the correctness or justice of such court decrees were secondary to the prevailing court orders.

Nurse managers should ensure that nurses whose ethical values differ from court orders are given: opportunities to voice their concerns and feelings, mechanisms for requesting reassignment, and time for quiet reflection. Although there can be no deviance from one's legal obligation, the nurse manager must ensure that the emotional and psychological well-being of those he or she supervises are also recognized. Merely acknowledging that such discord can occur and allowing positive means to express this concern may be the best solution in handling these difficult legal and ethical patient situations.

Future Ethical Concerns for Nurses

Issues of concern in the near future involve autonomy and independent practice among nurses, quality of care in home and community settings, and development of nurses as leaders in the healthcare delivery field. Issues that continue to permeate ethical concerns for nurses include the patient's right to refuse health care; issues surrounding death and dying, including the issues of hydration and nutrition for patients in persistent vegetative states; nurses' ability to be patient advocates in today's healthcare structure; and the ability to perform competent, quality nursing care in a system that continuously rewards cost-saving measures rather than quality healthcare delivery and that employs increasingly fewer professional nurses. Nursing must begin to address potential issues in a timely manner, particularly as the nursing shortage continues to escalate, because these issues will become more prominent in the future. As with ethical dilemmas in patient care, the more expertise and time one has to resolve issues, usually, the better the outcome.

Nurses need to begin now to look at the issues, professional values, and expectations they face and decide the issues for which they will fight and those that are acceptable as they are. Once these issues are identified, strategies for promoting quality nursing care can be delineated.

The Solution

Several members of the hospice staff met with the ethics committee. They had requested a meeting to assist them in deciding how to best assist patients and families before a second such incident occurred and also to resolve their own feelings about the situation. Actually, after following the Terri Schiavo case in Florida, the nurses were concerned that an issue concerning hydration and nutrition in a patient in a persistent vegetative state could arise and wondered if their current level of patient education was adequate for such issues. They were also concerned that some of the nursing staff might not be fully aware of current legislative and religious positions regarding nutrition and hydration following the Schiavo case.

Following the meeting with the ethics committee, the hospice nurses worked with legal counsel and patient educators in developing guidelines for educating patients, family members, hospice staff, and physicians involved in hospice care. They also developed teaching brochures and pamphlets, written at a fifth-to-sixth grade level, using language that patients and family members could easily understand, and these materials are now used to educate and support family members.

Future plans involve having some of these brochures translated into Spanish, as this area of the country is beginning to see more Hispanic patients.

Since this incident, the hospice staff members have been much more proactive rather than reactive. Educational materials are discussed, questions are answered, and the family is informed that an ethics committee meeting may be convened if they desire such a meeting. Additionally, the nurses have a roster of religious staff who could assist patients and their family members in these decisions. Staff members continue to reassure family members that the primary concern is the comfort and welfare of the patient. Since this approach has been used, there have been no repeats of such instances. Rather, family members know that we are trying to do the very best for the patient and respect the dying process by not prolonging life unnecessarily nor hastening death, but allowing each person to die with dignity.

— Nancy Joyner

 Would this be a suitable approach for you? Why?

CHAPTER CHECKLIST

This chapter addresses the issues of legal and ethical interactions with regard to nurse managers. Legislative and legal controls have been established to clarify the boundaries of professional practice and to protect consumers. Thus, there are some definite answers and guidelines to assist practitioners from the legal and legislative areas. These controls are constantly evolving, and the nurse manager must continually be aware of these changes as they affect the scope of the practice. Ethics has no such answers. Nor are there rules and guidelines that cover all aspects of human life. Nurse managers must explore value systems and become expert in using ethical models, incorporating both ethical theories and principles. The use of a systematic, humanistic approach reduces bias, facilitates decision-making, and allows the best working conditions possible from an ethical standpoint.

- Understanding and using legal and ethical principles are key strategies to be integrated into the role of an effective nurse manager.
- Nurse practice acts define the scope of acceptable practice for licensed registered nurses and licensed practical (vocational) nurses.
- Legal principles, if effectively integrated into all aspects of nursing management, minimize one's potential legal liability.
  - Malpractice is the failure of a person with professional education and skills to act in a reasonable and prudent manner.
  - Causes of malpractice for nurse managers include the following:
    - Issues of assignment, delegation, and supervision
    - Not discharging the duty to orient, educate, and evaluate
    - Failure to warn
    - Staffing issues
  - Liability may be classified as personal, vicarious, corporate, or strict product liability.

- Protective and reporting laws ensure the safety or rights of specific groups of people.
- Informed consent issues that nurse managers most often address concern the witnessing of the documents, research issues, and medical literacy.
- Privacy and confidentiality rights protect the patient from unreasonable and unwanted interference and secure the privacy of the patient's medical record.
- Federal and state governments have enacted a number of employment laws that nurses must understand and follow when dealing with managerial issues. These include the following:
  - Equal Pay Act of 1963
  - Civil Rights Act
  - Age Discrimination Act of 1967
  - Americans with Disabilities Act of 1990
  - Affirmative Action
  - Equal Employment Opportunity Laws
  - Occupational Safety and Health Act
  - Employment-at-Will and Wrongful Discharge
  - Family and Medical Leave Act of 1993
  - Collective Bargaining
- Ethical theories and principles relate to moral actions and value systems and apply to both patient and management situations.
  - Ethical theories justify existing moral principles and are considered universally applicable.
  - Ethical principles that nurse managers use include the following:
    - Autonomy
    - Beneficence
    - Nonmaleficence
    - Veracity
    - Justice
    - Paternalism
    - Fidelity
    - Respect for others
  - Codes of ethics assist nurses in applying ethical principles to professional nursing practice.
  - Ethics committees aid in assisting nurses to implement solutions in everyday clinical practice.

TIPS ON LEGAL AND ETHICAL ISSUES

- Before applying the information presented in the chapter, the following five tips are offered:
  - Read the state nurse practice act carefully to fully comprehend the allowable scope of practice within the given state.
    - Nurse practice acts are the most important legislative actions affecting the practice of nursing.
  - Consult with risk management, the institutional attorney, or the legal department for a fuller understanding of how federal employment laws pertain to the individual nurse manager.
    - Legal issues concern what one did or did not do, not why one acted as she or he did.
    - Legal issues concern societal norms and expectations, rather than the individual within society.
    - HIPAA may prove to be the most important legislation in preserving the privacy rights of patients within the healthcare system.
    - Ethics concern one's motives, attitudes, values, and culture rather than one's actions.
    - Ethics concerns the individual within society rather than society at large.
    - Legal mandates as dictated by court decisions and legislative actions take precedent over ethical issues.
  - Cultivate a group of professional consultants, either within the institution or outside the institution, who can assist with legal-ethical questions. Professional consultants may have great insight into issues as they arise and can assist in preventing problems in the future.
  - Discover who serves on the institutional ethics committee, and develop friendships with selected members. Attend the meetings to see how ethical issues are addressed in the institution. Become an active part of the ethical rounds if they exist in the institution.
  - Think before you act. Remember that it is always easier to hesitate, even briefly, so that the better approach can be implemented than to try to retract or amend something already done or already verbalized.

TERMS TO KNOW

apparent agency
autonomy
beneficence
collective bargaining
common law
confidentiality
corporate liability
emancipated minor
ergonomics
ethics
ethics committee
expert witness
failure to warn
fidelity
foreseeability
indemnification
independent contractor
informed consent
justice
labor union
law
liability
liable
malpractice
negligence
nonmaleficence
nurse practice act
paternalism
personal liability
privacy
respect for others
respondeat superior
standard of care
statute
veracity
vicarious liability

REFERENCES

American Nurses Association (ANA). (2001). *Code of ethics for nurses with interpretive statements.* Washington, DC: Author.

American Nurses Association (ANA). (1988). *Standards for nurse administrators.* Kansas City, MO: Author.

Americans with Disabilities Act of 1990, 42 U.S.C. § 12101 *et seq.* (1990).

Anthony, M. K., Standing, T., & Hertz, J. E. (2000). Factors influencing outcomes after delegation to unlicensed assistive personnel. *Journal of Nursing Administration, 30*(10), 474-481.

Arruda, E. H. (2004). Better retention through nursing theory. *Nursing Management, 36*(4), 16-18.

Bishop v. United States, 334 F. Supp. 415 (D.C. Tex., 1971).

Bunn-Penn v. Southern Regional Medical Corporation, 488 S.E. 2d. 747 (Ga. App., 1997).

Burns v. UHS of New Orleans, Inc., 2003 WL 549037 (La. App., February 19, 2003).

Bush, G. W. (2001). *Ergonomics.* Retrieved March 27, 2001. http://osha-slc.gov/ergonomics-standard.

California launches experiment in enforcing nurse-to-patient ratios. (2003, December 21). Retrieved from http://news.ncmonline.com/news/view_article.html.

Canadian Nurses Association. (2002). *Code of ethics for registered nurses.* Ottawa, ON: Author.

Civil Rights Act of 1964, § 703 et seq. (1978).

Cody v. Cigna Healthcare of St. Louis, Inc., 139 F.3d 595 (8th Cir., 1998).

Court rejects hospital situ to reverse safe staffing law. (2004, May 26). Retrieved from http://www.calnurse.org/can/press/52604.html.

Dauner, D. (2005). California hospitals express disappointment over denial of stay in nurse ratio case. Retrieved from www.calhealth.org.

David W. Francis v. Memorial General Hospital, 726 P.2d 852 (New Mexico, 1986).

Fairfax Nursing Home, Inc. v. Department of Health and Human Services, 123 S. Ct. 901, 71 USLW 3471, 2003 WL 98478 (United States, January 13, 2003).

Fleming v. Correctional Healthcare Solutions, Inc., 751 A.2d 1035 (N.J., 2000).

Fortune v. National Cash Register Company, 272 Mass. 96, 264 N.E.2d 1251 (1977).

45 CFR, Sec. 46.111, 46.101(b), 46.110, and 46.116 (1991).

45 CFR, Sec. 46.401 et seq. (1998).

Hansen v. Caring Professionals, Inc., 676 N.E.2d 1349 (Ill. App., 1997).

Harrell v. Louis Smith Memorial Hospital, 397 S.E. 2d 746 (Georgia, 1990).

Health Insurance Portability and Accountability Act of 1996. Public Law 104-191.

Herrero v. St. Louis University Hospital, 109 F.3d 481 (8th Cir., 1997).

Howard v. North Mississippi Medical Center, 939 F. Supp. 505 (N.D. Miss., 1996).

International Council of Nurses. (2000). *The International Council of Nurses code of ethics for nurses.* Geneva, Switzerland: Author.

Jessie v. Carter Health Care Center, Inc., 926 F. Supp. 613 (E.D. Ky., 1996).

Jones v. Kerrville State Hospital, 142 Fed.3d 263 (5th Cir., 1998).

Kellen, J. C., Oberle, K., Girard F., & Falkenberg, L. (2004). Exploring ethical perspectives of nurses and nurse managers. *Canadian Journal of Nursing Leadership, 17*(1), 78-87.

Laurin v. Providence Hospital and Massachusetts Nurses Association, 150 F.3d 52 (1st Cir., 1998).

Mauro v. Borgess Medical Center, 4:94 CV 05 (Michigan, 1995).

Medical illiteracy putting Americans at risk. (2004). Retrieved from http://www.hollandsentinel.com/stories/040904/new_040904006.shtml.

OSHA Regulations (1999). Standards. 29 CFR Standard. 1910.900.

Pender v. Natchitoches Parish Hospital, 2003 WL 21017235 (La. App., May 7, 2003).

Roulston v. Tendercare (Michigan), Inc., 608 N.W.2d 525 (Mich. App., 2000).

Sabol v. Richmond Heights General Hospital, 676 N. E.2d 958 (Ohio App. 1996).

Sisters of St. Joseph of Texas, Inc. v. Cheek, 61 S. W. 3d 32 (Tex. App., 2001).

Taylor v. Memorial Health Systems, Inc., 770 So.2d 752 (Fla. App., 2000).

Thompson v. Holy Family Hospital, 122 F.3d 537 (9th Cir., 1997).

Trombley v. Southwestern Vermont Medical Center, 738 A.2d 103 (Vt., 1999).

U.S. Department of Labor, Occupational Safety and Health Administration. (2001). *Ergonomics.* Retrieved March 27, 2001. http://www.inventoryops.com/ergonomics.htm.

UTMB v. Hohman, 6 S. W.3d 767 (Tex. App., 1999).

Watkins v. Unemployment Compensation Board of Review, 689 A.2d 1019 (Pa. Commonwealth, 1997).

Webb v. Mercy Hospital, 102 F.3d 958 (8th Cir., 1996).

Wellstar Health System, Inc. v. Green, 2002 WL 31324127 (Ga. App., October 18, 2002).

Wilking v. County of Ramsey, 983 F. Supp. 848 (D. Kan., 1997).

Wolfson, J. (2005). Erring on the Side of Theresa Schiavo: Reflections of the Special Guardian ad Litem. *The Hastings Center Report, 35*(3), 16-19.

Zamudio v. Patia, 956 F. Supp. 803 (N.D. Ill., 1997).

SUGGESTED READINGS

Andrews, D. R. (2004). Fostering ethical competency: An ongoing staff development process that encourages Professional growth and staff satisfaction. *Journal of*

Continuing Education in Nursing, 35(1), 27-33, 44-45.

Cohen, S. (2004). The new manager's guide to surviving and thriving. *Nursing Management, 36*(4), 20-21.

Doane, G., Pauly, B., Brown, H., & McPherson, G. (2004). Exploring the heart of ethical nursing practice: Implications for ethics education. *Nursing Ethics, 11*(3), 240-253.

Dresser, R. (2005). Schiavo's legacy: The need for an objective standard. *The Hasting Center Report, 35*(3), 20-22.

Drew, S. (2004). Ethical decision-making in practice: A triage decision. *Nursing Outlook, 27*(1), 18-20.

Mathes, M. (2004). Ethics, law, and policy: Ethical decision making and nursing. *Medical-Surgical Nursing, 13*(6), 429-431.

Numerof, R. E., Abrams, M., & Ott, B. (2004). Building a nursing leadership infrastructure. *Nurse Leader, 2*(1), 33-37.

O'Connor, M. (2004). Succession planning: A key strategy in nursing leadership education. *Nurse Leader, 2*(5), 24-25.

Pozgar, G. (2004). *Legal aspects of health care administration* (9th ed.). Boston, MA: Jones and Bartlett, Publishers.

Tappen, R. M. (2004). *Essentials of nursing leadership and management* (3rd ed.). Philadelphia, PA: F. A. Davis Company.

Woods, M. (2005). Nursing ethics education: Are we really delivering the good(s)? *Nursing Ethics, 12*(1), 5-18.

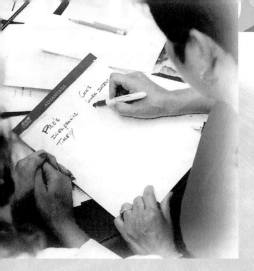

Chapter 5

Making Decisions and Solving Problems

Rose Aguilar Welch

*T*his chapter describes the key concepts related to problem-solving and decision-making. The relationship between these essential skills and critical-thinking is also examined. The primary steps of the problem-solving and decision-making processes, as well as analytical tools used for these processes, are explored. Moreover, strategies for individual or group problem-solving and decision-making are presented.

Objectives

- Use a decision-making format to list options to solve a problem, identify the pros and cons of each option, rank the options, and select the best option.
- Evaluate the effect of faulty information-gathering on a decision-making experience.

- Analyze the decision-making style of a nurse leader/manager.
- Investigate resources on the Internet that focus on critical-thinking,

problem-solving, and decision-making.

Questions to Consider

- *Why are problem-solving and decision-making skills important for professional nursing practice?*
- *How can you enhance your skills in problem-solving and decision-making?*
- *What is the relationship between critical-thinking ability and skill in problem-solving and decision-making?*

The Challenge

Vickie Lemmon, RN, MSN
Director of Clinical Strategies and Operations, Wellpoint, Inc., Ventura, California

Healthcare managers today are faced with numerous and complex issues that pertain to providing quality services for patients within a resource-scarce environment. Stress levels among staff can escalate when problems are not resolved, leading to a decrease in morale, productivity, and quality service. This was the situation I encountered in my previous job as Administrator for California Children Services (CCS). When I began my tenure as the new CCS Administrator, staff expressed frustration and dissatisfaction with staffing, workload, and team communications. This was evidenced by high staff turnover, lack of teamwork, customer complaints, unmet deadlines for referral and enrollment cycle times, and poor documentation. The team was in crisis, characterized by in-fighting, blaming, lack of respectful communication, and lack of commitment to program goals and objectives. I had not worked as a case manager in this program. It was hard for me to determine how to address the problems the staff presented to me. I wanted to be fair, yet felt that I did not have enough information to make immediate changes. My challenge was to lead this team to greater compliance with state-mandated performance measures.

What do you think you would do if you were this nurse?

INTRODUCTION

Problem-solving and decision-making are vital abilities for nursing practice. Not only are these processes involved in managing and delivering care but also they are essential for engaging in planned change. Myriad technologic, social, political, and economic changes have had a dramatic effect on health care and nursing. Increased patient acuity, shorter hospital stays, shortage of healthcare providers, increased technology, and the continuing shift from inpatient to ambulatory and home health care are some of the changes that require nurses to make rational and valid decisions that achieve results. Moreover, increased diversity in employment settings and types of healthcare providers demands efficient and effective decision-making and problem-solving. In addition to the focus on achieving people-oriented and cost-effective results, more emphasis is now placed on involving patients in decision-making and problem-solving and using multidisciplinary teams.

Professional nursing organizations have affirmed that competency in decision-making and problem-solving is essential to nursing practice. The reader can review select position and policy statements by referring to the Internet resources in Table 5-1 (or conduct a search using the organization's name).

Nurses must possess the basic knowledge and skills required for effective problem-solving and decision-making. These competencies are especially important for nurses with leadership and management responsibilities.

Definitions

Problem-solving and *decision-making* are not synonymous terms. However, the processes for engaging in both behaviors are similar. Both skills require **critical-thinking,** which is a high-level cognitive process, and both can be improved with practice.

Decision-making is a purposeful and goal-directed effort that uses a systematic process to choose among options. Not all decision-making begins with a problem situation. Instead, the hallmark of decision-making is the identification and selection of options or alternatives. For example, the nurse manager of a home healthcare agency is strategizing ways to empower the nursing staff. The options under consideration include having the staff create the schedule, having them perform self-evaluations, or having them provide more input in the formulation of agency policy.

Table 5-1 PROFESSIONAL NURSING ORGANIZATIONS

Organization	URL
American Nurses Association	www.nursingworld.org Click "Nursing Issues/Programs" Select "ANA Position Statements" Click on "Ethics and human rights." Select "Nursing and the Patient Self Determination Act."
Canadian Nurses Association	www.cna-nurses.ca Click on "Position Statements." Click on "Research" Click on "Evidence-based Decision Making and Nursing Practice."

Problem-solving, which includes a decision-making step, is focused on trying to solve an immediate problem, which can be viewed as a gap between "what is" and "what should be." This is what Rooney and Hopen (2004b) refer to as a "deviation," where performance is not equal to expectations. They also categorize problems as situations that require intervention due to perceptions of "future threat," as well as situations that are amenable to improvement.

As previously mentioned, effective problem-solving and decision-making are predicated on an individual's ability to think critically. Although critical-thinking has been defined in numerous ways, the National Council for Excellence in Critical Thinking Instruction defines it as the "intellectually disciplined process of actively and skillfully conceptualizing, applying, analyzing, synthesizing, or evaluating information gathered from, or generated by, observation, experience, reflection, reasoning or communication, as a guide to belief and action" (Paul, 1995, p. 110). Critical-thinking is not an isolated process. It is manifested whenever a nurse asks "why," "what," or "how." A nurse who questions why a patient is restless is thinking critically. Compare the analytical abilities between a nurse who assumes a patient is restless because of anxiety related to an upcoming procedure and a nurse who asks if there could be another explanation and proceeds to investigate possible causes. In another example, a novice home health nurse learns that an elderly patient on multiple medications has not been taking the medications as prescribed. The nurse reports back to the supervisor that the patient is "non-compliant."

The supervisor will assume that this nurse is not demonstrating critical-thinking skills. The supervisor's task then is to help the nurse think through the other factors. Critical-thinking is manifested when nurses employ the skills of interpretation, analysis, evaluation, inference, explanation, and self-regulation (Facione & Facione, 1996). It is important for managers to assess their staff members' ability to think critically and enhance their knowledge and skills through staff-development programs, coaching, and role-modeling. Establishing a positive and motivating work environment can enhance attitudes and the disposition to think critically.

Creativity is essential for the generation of options or solutions. Creative individuals can conceptualize new and innovative approaches to a problem or issue by being more flexible and independent in their thinking. It just takes one person to plant a seed for new ideas to generate. This is made clear in Ralph Waldo Emerson's quote, "The creation of a thousand forests is in one acorn."

The model depicted in Figure 5-1 demonstrates the relationship among related concepts such as professional judgment, decision-making, problem-solving, creativity, and critical-thinking. Sound clinical judgment requires critical or reflective thinking. Critical-thinking is the concept that interweaves and links the others. An individual, through the application of critical-thinking skills, engages in problem-solving and decision-making in an environment that can promote or inhibit these skills. It is the manager's task to model these skills and promote them in others.

DECISION-MAKING

The phases of the decision-making process include defining objectives, generating options, identifying advantages and disadvantages of each option, ranking the options, selecting the option most likely to achieve the predefined objectives, implementing the option, and evaluating the result. Box 5-1 contains a form that can be used to complete these steps.

A poor-quality decision is likely if the objectives are not clearly identified or if they are inconsistent with the values of the individual or organization. Lewis Carroll illustrates the essential step of defining the goal, purpose, or objectives in the following excerpt from *Alice's Adventures in Wonderland*.

> One day Alice came to a fork in the road and saw a Cheshire Cat in a tree. "Which road do I take?" she asked. His response was a question: "Where do you want to go?" "I don't know," Alice answered. "Then," said the cat, "it doesn't matter."

Decision Models

The decision model that a nurse uses depends on the circumstances. Is the situation routine and predictable or complex and uncertain? Is the goal of

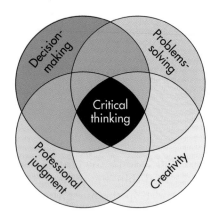

Figure 5-1 Problem-solving and decision-making model. (Modified from Sullivan, E. J., & Decker, P. J. [1992]. *Effective management in nursing.* Menlo Park, CA: Addison-Wesley.)

BOX 5-1

Decision-Making Format

Objective: _____

Desired outcome: _____

Options: _____

_____

_____

Analysis of options:

Option	Advantages	Disadvantages

Rank priority of options (1 being most preferred): _____

_____

Select the best option (implementation plan): _____

_____

Evaluation plan: _____

_____

Theory Box

DECISION MODEL THEORIES

THEORY/CONTRIBUTOR	KEY IDEA	APPLICATION TO PRACTICE
Normative or prescriptive	Used when information is objective, routine decisions are involved, or the problem is structured. Options are known and predictable.	Situations that fall under this category can be handled using agency policy, standard procedures, or analytical tools.
Descriptive or behavioral	Used when information is subjective, nonroutine, and unstructured. Uncertainty exists because options or outcomes are either unknown or unpredictable.	Situations that fall under this category are best handled by gathering more data, using past experience, using creative approaches, or following a group process.
Satisficing	Decision-maker selects the solution that minimally meets the objective or standard for a decision. It is the more conservative method compared to an optimized approach.	This process is the most expedient and may be the most appropriate when time is an issue.
Optimizing	Decision-maker selects the solution that maximally meets the objective or standard for a decision. Usually, this process involves accessing the pros and cons of each known option and listing benefits and costs associated with each option. The goal is to select the most ideal solution.	This process is more likely to result in a better decision, but it takes longer.

Lancaster, J., & Lancaster, W. (1982). *Concepts for advanced nursing practice: The nurse as a change agent.* St. Louis: Mosby; and Sullivan, E. J., & Decker, P. J. (1992). *Effective management in nursing.* Menlo Park, CA: Addison-Wesley.

the decision to make a decision conservatively that is just "good enough" (satisficing) or one that is optimal? Examples of decision models or theories are presented in the Theory Box.

The following scenario illustrates decision theories. Staff nurses on a medical-surgical unit have complained that they cannot obtain access to the computer stations to do their charting in a timely manner. A **satisficing decision** might involve the expedient option of going back to paper and pencil documentation on nursing forms. However, an **optimizing decision** might involve creating a multidisciplinary task force to analyze the problem and propose optional solutions.

Decision-Making Styles

The decision-making style of a nurse manager is similar to the leadership style that the manager is likely to use. A manager who leans toward an auto-cratic style may choose to make decisions independent of the input or participation of others. This has been referred to as the "decide and announce" approach, an authoritative style. On the other hand, a manager who uses a **democratic** or **participative** approach to management involves the appropriate personnel in the decision-making process. Kerfoot (2003) proposes that when organizations fail to use the knowledge of people within the organization (unit or department), the organization will appear "stupid." Through participatory management, organizations can "raise their collective IQ" by taking advantage of individuals who can help the organization achieve desired outcomes. It is imperative for managers to involve nursing personnel in making decisions that affect patient care. One mechanism for doing so is by seeking nursing representation on various committees or task forces. Participative management has been shown to increase work performance and productivity, decrease employee turnover, and enhance employee satisfaction.

Any decision style can be used appropriately or inappropriately. Like the tenets of situational leadership theory, the situation and circumstances should dictate which decision-making style is most appropriate.

The autocratic method results in more rapid decision-making and is appropriate in crisis situations or when groups are likely to accept this type of decision style. However, followers are generally more supportive of consultative and group approaches. Although these approaches take more time, they are more appropriate when conflict is likely to occur, when the problem is unstructured, or when the manager does not have the knowledge or skills to solve the problem. Box 5-2 summarizes the key advantages and disadvantages of decision-making (leadership styles).

Exercise 5–1

Interview colleagues about their most preferred decision-making style. What barriers or obstacles to effective decision-making have your colleagues encountered? What strategies are used to increase the effectiveness of the decisions made? Based on your interview, is the style effective? Why or why not?

Factors Affecting Decision-Making

Numerous factors affect individuals and groups in the decision-making process. The perception of the situation can be influenced by internal and external factors. Internal factors include variables such as the decision-maker's physical and emotional state, personal philosophy, biases, values, interests, experience, knowledge, and attitudes. External factors include environmental conditions, time, and resources. Decision-making options are externally limited when time is short or when the environment is characterized by a "we've always done it this way" attitude.

Values affect all aspects of decision-making, from the statement of the problem/issue through the evaluation. Values, determined by one's cultural, social, and philosophical background, provide the foundation for one's ethical stance. Dr. Michael McDonald, Director of the Centre for Applied Ethics at the University of British Columbia, provides a "Framework for Ethical Decision-Making" (http://www.ethics.ubc.ca/people/mcdonald/decisions.html). The steps for engaging in ethical decision-making are similar to the steps described earlier; however, alternatives or options identified in the decision-making process are evaluated with the use of ethical resources. Resources that can facilitate ethical decision-making include institutional policy; principles such as autonomy, nonmaleficence, beneficence, veracity, paternalism, respect, justice, and fidelity; personal judgment; trusted co-workers; institutional ethics committees; and legal precedent. McDonald poses several questions when considering decision options. One of the most powerful is to "ask yourself what would a virtuous person—one with integrity and experience—do in these circumstances?" (2001, p. 4).

BOX 5-2

Key Advantages and Disadvantages of Decision-Making Styles

DECISION-MAKING STYLES (LEADERSHIP STYLES)	ADVANTAGES	DISADVANTAGES
Autocratic/Authoritarian	Rapid decision-making is necessary—e.g., crisis or emergency High productivity is required	Encourages dependency May result in higher turnover, less motivation, less creativity, increased dissatisfaction
Democratic/Participative	Can result in greater morale, motivation, and creativity.	Takes longer, and may decrease efficiency
Laissez-Faire (hands-off)	Works when staff members can work independently and are committed to the job and organization	Group may flounder if no one emerges to give the group direction

Certain personality factors, such as self-esteem and self-confidence, affect whether one is willing to take risks in solving problems or making decisions. Ask yourself, "Do I prefer to let others make the decisions? Am I more comfortable in the role of 'follower' than leader? If so, why?" Characteristics of an effective decision-maker include courage, a willingness to take risks, self-awareness, energy, creativity, sensitivity, and flexibility. As Mark Twain would say, "Courage is resistance to fear, mastery of fear, not absence of fear."

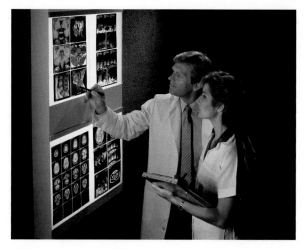

To be part of the solution, followers must be a part of the problem-solving process.

Exercise 5-2

Identify a current or past situation that involved resource allocation, end-of-life issues, conflict among healthcare providers or patient/family/significant others, or some other ethical dilemma. Describe how the internal and external factors previously described influenced the decision options, the option selected, and the outcome.

Group Decision-Making

There are two primary criteria for effective decision-making. First, the decision must be of a high quality; that is, it achieves the predefined goals, objectives, and outcomes. Second, those who are responsible for its implementation must accept the decision. Variables that influence the quality of decisions include the following:

- Was the information used factual, complete, and relevant to the situation?
- What were the behavioral characteristics of the decision-makers?
- Were they able to process the data?
- Is the decision defensible in that the solution generated can be justified?
- Did the benefits of the decision outweigh the risks that were involved?
- How well did the decision solve the problem or meet the identified need/outcome?

Higher-quality decisions are more likely to result if groups are involved in the problem-solving and decision-making process. "Team problem solving is a critical component in any organization's continuous improvement toolkit" (Rooney & Hopen, 2004a, p. 20). When individuals are allowed input into the process, they tend to function more productively, and the quality of the decision is generally superior. Taking ownership of the process and outcome provides a smoother transition. Multidisciplinary teams should be used in the decision-making process, especially if the issue, options, or outcome involve other disciplines.

Research findings suggest that groups are more likely to be effective if members are actively involved, the group is cohesive, communication is encouraged, and members demonstrate some understanding of the group process. In deciding to use the group process for decision-making, it is important to consider group size and composition. If the group is too small, there will be a limited number of options generated and fewer points of view expressed. Conversely, if the group is too large, it may lack structure, and consensus becomes more difficult. Homogeneous groups may be more compatible; however, heterogeneous groups may be more successful in problem-solving. Research has demonstrated that the most productive groups are those that are moderately cohesive. In other words, divergent thinking is useful to create the best decision.

For groups to be able to work effectively, the group facilitator or leader should carefully select members on the basis of their knowledge and skills in decision-making and problem-solving. However, Rooney and Hopen (2004b) assert that group composition should not be based solely on the knowledge that members bring to the table, but teams should include members who already enjoy a positive working relationship. Individuals who are aggressive, are authoritarian, or manifest self-oriented behaviors tend to decrease the effectiveness of groups.

Furthermore, the leader should provide a non-threatening and positive environment in which group members are encouraged to participate actively. Using tact and diplomacy, the facilitator can control aggressive individuals who tend to monopolize the discussion and can encourage more passive individuals to contribute by asking direct, open-ended questions. Providing positive feedback, such as "You raised a good point"; protecting members and their suggestions from attack; and keeping the group focused on the task are strategies that create an environment conducive to problem-solving.

Advantages of Group Decision-Making

The advantages of group decision-making are numerous. The adage "two heads are better than one" illustrates that when individuals with different knowledge, skills, and resources collaborate to solve a problem or make a decision, the likelihood of a quality outcome is increased. More ideas can be generated by groups than by individuals functioning alone. In addition, when followers are directly involved in this process, they are more apt to accept the decision, because they have an increased sense of ownership or commitment to the decision. Implementing solutions becomes easier when individuals have been actively involved in the decision-making process. Involvement can be enhanced by making information readily available to the appropriate personnel, requesting input, establishing committees and task forces with broad representation, and using group decision-making techniques.

The group leader must establish with the participants what decision rule will be followed. Will the group strive to achieve consensus, or will the majority rule? In determining which decision rule to use, the group leader should consider the necessity for quality and acceptance of the decision. Achieving both a high-quality and an acceptable decision is possible, but it requires more involvement and approval from individuals affected by the decision.

Groups will be more committed to an idea if it is derived by consensus rather than as an outcome of individual decision-making or majority rule.

Consensus requires that all participants agree to go along with the solution. Although achieving consensus requires considerable time, it results in both high-quality and high-acceptance decisions and reduces the risk of sabotage.

Majority rule can be used to compromise when 100% agreement cannot be achieved. This method saves time, but the solution may only partially achieve the goals of quality and acceptance. In addition, majority rule carries certain risks. First, if the informal group leaders happen to fall in the minority opinion, they may not support the decision of the majority. Certain members may go so far as to build coalitions to gain support for their position and block the majority choice. After all, the majority may represent only 51% of the group. In addition, group members may support the position of the formal leader, although they do not agree with the decision, because they fear reprisal or they wish to obtain the leader's approval. In general, as the importance of the decision increases, so does the percentage of group members required to approve it.

To secure the support of the group, the leader should maintain open communication with those affected by the decision and be honest about the advantages and disadvantages of the decision. The leader should also demonstrate how the advantages outweigh the disadvantages, suggest ways the unwanted outcomes can be minimized, and be available to assist when necessary.

Disadvantages of Group Decision-Making

Although group problem-solving and decision-making have distinct advantages, involving groups also carries certain disadvantages and may not be appropriate in all situations. As previously stated, group decision-making requires more time. In some situations, this may not be appropriate, especially in a crisis situation requiring prompt decisions.

Another disadvantage of group decision-making relates to unequal power among group members. Dominant personality types may influence the more passive or powerless group members to conform to their points of view. Furthermore, individuals may expend considerable time and energy defending their positions, resulting in the primary objective of the group effort being lost.

Kritek (2002) points out that inequality among individuals results in an "uneven table," setting the stage for dominant behavior. In her book *Negotiating at an Uneven Table: Developing Moral Courage in Resolving our Conflicts*, Kritek identifies 10 "constructive ways of being at an uneven table." These strategies are explored in Chapter 22.

Groups may be more concerned with maintaining group harmony than engaging in active discussion on the issue and generating creative ideas to address it. Group members who manifest a "groupthink" mentality are so concerned with avoiding conflict and supporting their leader and other members that important issues or concerns are not raised. Failure to bring up options, explore conflict, or challenge the status quo results in ineffective group functioning and decision outcomes.

Strategies

Strategies exist to minimize the problems encountered with group problem-solving and decision-making. These strategies include decision-making techniques, such as brainstorming, nominal group techniques, focus groups, and the Delphi technique.

Brainstorming can be an effective method for generating a large volume of creative options. Often, the premature critiquing of ideas stifles creativity and idea generation. When members use inflammatory statements, euphemistically referred to as *killer phrases,* the usual response is for members to stop contributing. Killer phrases include statements such as "It will never work," "Administration won't go for it," "What a dumb idea," "It's not in the budget," "If it ain't broke, don't fix it," or "We tried that before."

The hallmark of brainstorming, a right-brain activity, is to list all ideas as stated without critique or discussion. The group leader or facilitator should encourage people to tag onto or spin off ideas from those already suggested. One idea may be piggybacked on others. Ideas should not be judged, nor should the relative merits or disadvantages of the ideas be discussed at this time. The goal is to generate ideas, no matter how seemingly unrealistic or absurd. It is important for the group leader or facilitator to cut off criticism and be alert for nonverbal behaviors signaling disapproval. Because the emphasis is on the volume of ideas generated, not

necessarily the quality, solutions may be superficial and fail to solve the problem. Group brainstorming also takes longer, and the logistics of getting people together may pose a problem. If the facilitator allows the group to establish the rules for discussion, the aspects that stymie an open discussion often are eliminated by the group's norms or rules of participation.

The nominal group technique, a method designed by Delbecq and Gustafson in the 1970s, allows group members the opportunity to provide input into the decision-making process. Although the group is physically present, participants are asked not to talk to each other as they write down their ideas to solve a predefined problem or issue. After a period of silent generation of ideas, generally no more than 10 minutes, each member is asked to share an idea, which is displayed on a chalkboard or flip chart. Comments and elaboration are not allowed during this phase. Each member takes a turn sharing an idea until all ideas are presented, after which discussion is allowed. Members may "pass" if they have exhausted their list of ideas. During the next step, ideas are clarified, and the merits of each idea are discussed. In the third and final step, each member privately assigns a priority rank to each option. The solution chosen is the option that receives the highest ranking by the majority of participants. The advantage of this technique is that it allows equal participation among members and minimizes the influence of dominant personalities. The disadvantages of this method are that it is time-consuming and requires advance preparation. In addition, it requires that the group physically come together.

The purpose of focus groups is to explore issues and generate information. They can be used to identify problems or to evaluate the effects of an intervention. The groups meet face-to-face to engage in the discussion of issues. Under the direction of a group leader who functions as a facilitator or moderator, the participants are able to validate or disagree with ideas expressed. Because the interaction is face-to-face, potential disadvantages include the logistics of getting people together, time, and issues revolving around group dynamics already mentioned. Nevertheless, if managed effectively, the experience can yield a treasure trove of information. The Research Perspective provides an example of how researchers utilized focus groups.

Research Perspective

Aroskar, M. A., Moldow, G., & Good, C. M. (2004). Nurse's voices: Policy, practice and ethics. *Nursing Ethics, 11*(3). Retrieved April 24, 2005 from the Proquest database.

Using focus groups, researchers sought to identify nurse's ethical concerns due to governmental and institutional policies related to nursing practice and patient care. Four focus groups were conducted with practicing registered nurses (*n* = 36), 33 of which provided or managed direct patient care in a variety of settings. A moderator used a moderator guide developed by a nurse ethicist, nurse social worker, and health policy expert.

During the 2-hour discussions, nurses identified policies that impacted their care of patients, which included ethical implications. Researchers reviewed transcripts to conduct content analysis, and identified major themes. These included the effects of policies focused on cost containment on the nurse's ability to provide quality patient care; the effects of policy, such as nurse-patient ratio and the increased use of unlicensed assistive personnel, on the quality of patient care; effects on patient-education and referral; and the effects on nurses and the profession.

Although the use of focus groups was helpful to provide participants the opportunity to voice their concerns regarding the effects of governmental and institutional policy on patient care, the researchers acknowledged the lack of "younger" nurses and new graduates in the groups, the lack of male nurses in the sample, and the lack of nurses other than those who worked in urban areas.

IMPLICATIONS FOR PRACTICE

Focus groups are a powerful means to gather information. They can be used to gather information to properly identify a problem or collect data to evaluate an intervention. Nurse leaders should be cognizant of the importance of adequately preparing for focus groups, such as identification of the purpose of the focus groups, selection of the participants and moderator or facilitator, and guidelines for conducting the sessions.

Another group decision-making strategy is the Delphi technique. It involves systematically collecting and summarizing opinions and judgments from respondents, such as expert panels, on a particular issue through interviews, surveys, or questionnaires. Opinions of the respondents are repeatedly fed back to them with a request to provide more refined opinions and rationales on the issue or matter under consideration. Between rounds, the results are tabulated and analyzed so that the findings can be reported to the participants. This allows the participants to reconsider their responses. The goal is to achieve a consensus.

There are different variations on the Delphi technique. Nevertheless, the procedure generally calls for anonymous feedback, multiple rounds, and statistical analyses. One advantage of this technique is the ability to involve a large number of respondents, because the participants do not need to assemble together. Indeed, participants may be located throughout the country or world. Also, the questionnaire or survey requires little time commitment on the part of the participant. This technique may actually save time because it eliminates the "off-the-subject" digressions typically encountered in face-to-face meetings. In addition, the Delphi technique avoids the negative or unproductive verbal and nonverbal interactions that can occur when groups work together. Although the Delphi technique has its advantages, using the Delphi technique may result in a lower sense of accomplishment and involvement because the participants are detached from the overall process and do not communicate with each other.

Decision-Making Tools

Several decision-making tools exist to aid a nurse manager in planning a decision-making process or selecting the best decision among the available options. The most common quantitative tools include decision grids and payoff tables. These tools are most appropriately used when information is available and options are known. Nurses in any position can use these tools to help make career decisions.

Decision grids facilitate the visualization of the options under consideration and allow comparison of options using common criteria. Criteria, which are determined by the decision-makers, may include time required, ethical or legal considerations, equipment needs, and cost (Figure 5-2). The relative advantages and disadvantages of the different options should be listed for each option.

Payoff tables require the manager to establish the cost-versus-benefit relationships and the probabilities of certain outcomes using current information and historical data. To illustrate, the manager of a hospital education department is evaluating whether it is better to retain the services of an outside consultant to coordinate an advanced cardiac life support course in the hospital or pay the per-person fees to send the staff elsewhere. The type of information this manager might compile includes a breakdown of the costs for both options, equipment needs, benefits of each option, the number of nurses needing the course, future training needs, and the feasibility of training hospital staff to conduct the course. Examples of these and other analytic tools can be reviewed at http://www.mindtools.com. This commercial website provides links to software and other resources. Click on the links to "decision-making" and/or "problem-solving."

Exercise 5-3

Design a decision grid for a current situation you are experiencing. Identify the components you need to explore in the decision-making process, such as cost, time, resources, advantages, and disadvantages, for the various options you are considering.

PROBLEM-SOLVING

Problem-solving includes the decision-making processes. However, in this case, the trigger for action is the existence of a "problem" or issue. Before attempting to solve a problem, a nurse must ask certain key questions:

1. Is it important?
2. Do I want to do something about it? (e.g., Do I "own" the problem?)
3. Am I qualified to handle it?
4. Do I have the authority to do anything?
5. Do I have the knowledge, interest, time, and resources to deal with it?
6. Can I delegate it to someone else?
7. What benefits will be derived from solving it?

If the answer to questions 1 through 5 is "no," why waste time, resources, and personal energy? At this juncture a conscious decision is made to ignore the problem, refer or delegate it to others, or consult or collaborate with others to solve it. On the other hand, if the answers are "yes," the nurse chooses to accept the problem and thus assume responsibility for it. Once engaged in solving a problem, others

Options under Consideration	Time	Cost	Legal/Ethical Considerations	Equipment Needed

Figure 5-2   Decision grid.

generally assume that you are qualified and have the authority to create the solution.

After identifying the problem, nurse managers must decide whether it is significant enough to require intervention and whether it is even within their control to do anything about it. Sometimes new managers believe they need to "solve" every problem brought to their attention. There are situations, such as some interpersonal conflicts, that are best resolved by the individuals who own the problem. Known as *purposeful inaction*, a "do nothing" approach might be indicated when other persons should resolve problems or if the problem is beyond the manager's control. Consider the following scenario:

> Mary complains to the nurse manager that Sam, a fellow nurse, was rude and abrupt with her during a hallway interchange. How should the nurse manager handle Mary's complaint? Should the manager discuss the problem with Sam? Should Mary be present during the discussion? What are the possible risks or benefits of such an approach? Alternatively, should the manager assist Mary in developing her communication skills so that Mary can address the problem herself?

Exercise 5–4

Using the decision-making format presented in Box 5-1, list other options for this scenario and the advantages and disadvantages of each approach. Rank the options in order of most desirable to least desirable, and select the best option. Determine how you would implement and evaluate the chosen option.

Some decisions are "givens" because they are based on firmly established criteria in the institution, which may be based on the traditions, values, doctrines, culture, or policy of the organization. Every manager has to live with mandates from persons higher in the organizational structure. Although managers may not have the authority to

control certain situations, they may be able to influence the outcome. For example, because of losses in revenue, administration has decided to eliminate the clinical educator positions in a home health agency and place the responsibility for clinical education with the senior home health nurses. It is beyond the manager's control to reverse this decision. Nevertheless, the manager can explore the nurses' fear and concerns regarding this change and facilitate the transition by preparing them for the new role.

In these examples, it is a misnomer to refer to the approach as *do nothing*, because there is deliberate action on the part of the manager. This approach should not be confused with the laissez-faire (hands off) approach taken by a manager who chooses to do nothing when intervention is indicated.

Problem-Solving Process

Several models or approaches to problem-solving exist. The traditional process for problem-solving is illustrated in Figure 5-3. This figure gives the appearance of a sequential and linear process. However, the problem-solving process is a dynamic one. Although individuals can certainly follow the problem-solving steps, a team approach is more likely to succeed.

Define the Problem, Issue, or Situation   "The main principles for diagnosing a problem are know the facts, separate the facts from interpretation, be objective and descriptive, and determine the scope of the problem. Nurses also need to determine how to establish priorities for solving problems. For example, do you tend to work on problems that are encountered first, that appear to be the easiest, that take the shortest amount of time to solve, or that may have the greatest urgency?

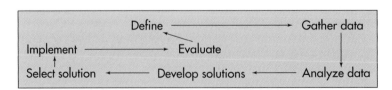

Figure 5-3   The problem-solving process.

The most common cause for failure to resolve problems is the improper identification of the problem/issue; therefore, problem recognition and identification are considered the most vital steps. The quality of the outcome depends on accurate identification of the problem. The problem is likely to recur if the true underlying causes are not targeted. Problem identification is influenced by the information available; by the values, attitudes, and experiences of those involved; and by time. Sufficient time should be allowed for the collection and organization of data. All too often, an inadequate amount of time is allocated for this essential step, resulting in unsatisfactory outcomes.

Kritek (2002) asserts there are two primary phases in solving a problem: identifying/understanding the problem and identifying/selecting the best solution to resolve it. However, she believes that a common error is to skip step number one and proceed directly to step number two. As a result, too few options may be determined, or solutions may be implemented for an unrelated problem. Why does this happen? Kritek holds that the likely explanation is that people may avoid the step that requires the problem to be named and understood because it can reveal negative aspects about themselves that they may not want to address. However, Yoder-Wise (2004) encourages us to look at our strengths, not just the problems. This may help minimize the inevitable distress that emerges when engaging in the problem-solving process. She reminds us we should ask questions such as, "What is good?" "What isn't a problem?" and "What are our strengths?" (p. 147).

It is important to differentiate between the actual problem and the symptoms of a problem. Consider the problem of an inadequately stocked emergency cart from which emergency medications are often missing and equipment fails to function properly. Individuals charged with resolving this problem may discover that this is symptomatic of the underlying problem, perhaps inadequate staffing or staffing mix. Based on the proper identification of the problem in this scenario, a possible solution might be to assign the task of checking and stocking the emergency cart to the unlicensed personnel in the unit.

In work settings, problems often fall under certain categories that have been described as the four M's: manpower, methods, machines, and materials. A fishbone diagram, also known as a *cause-and-effect diagram,* is a useful model for categorizing the possible causes of a problem. The diagram graphically displays, in increasing detail, all of the possible causes related to a problem to try to discover its root causes. This tool encourages problem solvers to focus on the content of the problem and not be sidetracked by personal interests, issues, or agendas of team members. It also collects a snapshot of the collective knowledge of the team and helps build consensus around the problem. The "effect" is generally the problem statement, such as decreased morale, and is placed at the right end of the figure (the "head" of the fish). The major categories of causes are the main bones, and these are supported by smaller bones, which represent issues that contribute to the main causes. Refer to the chapter's Solution for an example of a fishbone diagram.

Exercise 5–5

Using a fishbone diagram, identify all the factors (causes) that are at the root of a problem you are currently facing in the workplace. After you have listed as many issues as possible, share the diagram with a work colleague. Are there other issues you did not consider? Where do most of the factors influencing the problem fit: manpower, methods, machines, or materials?

Gather Data After the general nature of the problem is identified, individuals can focus on gathering and analyzing data to resolve the issue. Assessment, through the collection of data and information, is done continuously throughout this dynamic process. The data gathered consist of objective (facts) and subjective (feelings) information. Information gathered should be valid, accurate, relevant to the issue, and timely. Moreover, individuals involved in the process must have access to information and adequate resources to make cogent decisions. Generally, decisions based on "intuition" only should be avoided. Nursing lore places value on actions based on intangible and invisible "gut feeling" responses. However, in the era of evidence-based practice, reliance on intuition alone can cause problems.

Analyze Data Data are analyzed to further refine the problem statement and identify possible solutions or options. It is important to differentiate a problem from the symptoms of a problem. For example, a nurse manager is dismayed by the latest continuous quality improvement (CQI) report indicating nurses are not documenting patient-teaching. Is this evidence that patient-teaching is not being done? Is lack of documentation the actual problem? Perhaps it is a symptom of the actual problem. On further analysis, the manager may discover that the new computerized documentation system is not user-friendly. By distinguishing the problem from the symptoms of the problem, a more appropriate solution can be identified and implemented.

Develop Solutions   The goal of generating options is to identify as many choices as possible. Occasionally, rigid "black and white" thinking hampers the quality of outcomes. A nurse who is unhappy with his or her work situation and can think of only two options—stay or quit—is displaying this type of thinking.

Being flexible, open-minded, and creative, attributes of a critical-thinker, is critical to being able to consider a range of possible options. Everyone has preconceived notions and ideas when confronted with certain situations. Although putting these notions on hold and considering other ideas is beneficial, it is difficult to do. However, asking questions such as the following can allow a person to consider other viewpoints:

- Am I jumping to conclusions?
- If I were [insert name of role model], how would I approach it?
- How are my beliefs and values affecting my decision?

Select a Solution   The decision-maker should then objectively weigh each option according to its possible risks and consequences, as well as positive outcomes that may be derived. Criteria for evaluation might include variables such as cost, effectiveness, time, and legal or ethical considerations. The options should be ranked in the order in which they are likely to result in the desired goals or objectives.

The solution selected should be the one that is most feasible and satisfactory and has the fewest undesirable consequences. Nurses must consider whether they are picking the solution because it is the best solution or because it is the most expedient. Being able to make cogent decisions based on thorough assessment of a situation is an important yardstick of a nurse's effectiveness.

Implement the Solution   The implementation phase should include a contingency plan to deal with negative consequences, should they arise. In essence, the decision-maker should be prepared to institute "plan B" as necessary.

Evaluate the Result   Considerable time and energy are usually spent on identifying the problem or issue, generating possible solutions, selecting the best solution, and implementing the solution. However, not enough time is typically allocated for evaluation and follow-up. It is important to establish early in the process how evaluation and monitoring will take place, who will be responsible for it, when it will take place, and what the desired outcome is. Be prepared to make mistakes and take responsibility for them. The key is to learn from mistakes and use the experiences to help guide future actions, or, as Henry Ford said, "Failure is only the opportunity to begin again more intelligently."

Individuals and groups may not adopt a structured problem-solving approach because it takes too much time, the process may be boring, people are too busy to get involved, and participants may perceive there is little or no recognition for their participation. Leaders should be cognizant of these potential barriers to prevent or minimize them.

Regardless of the model or approach taken, using a systematic approach helps address issues in an organized and focused manner. All nurses, whether they are managers, leaders, or followers, need adequate problem-solving and decision-making skills to be effective in their roles.

The Solution

In a previous job, I had used multidisciplinary process improvement teams (PITs), which consisted of key stakeholders, to initiate process improvement. I chose to give this concept a try in this setting. Our team consisted of the Public Health Nurse (PHN) case managers, the CCS case workers, the billing and claims staff, the CCS Medical Director, clerical and support staff, and myself. I believed that a group approach to these problems would yield the most information and gain the greatest support for any changes that would be made. The team met weekly for an hour. We began by identifying our customers and key stakeholders and their expectations. This was extensive and took a few months to complete. Key stakeholders included the clients (children) and their parents, the providers (physicians and hospitals), pharmacies, vendors, schools, other insurance plans, the tax payers (in the form of the State and County), our own team members, and other agencies. The expectations for each stakeholder were listed, discussed for clarity, and recorded. During this exercise, the team learned a great deal about each person's job duties (there were a few surprises) and about the effect each person's job had on other team members' ability to do their job. As the team began understanding each person's job and issues, they focused less on blaming and more on how to change our processes.

Next, the team brainstormed (divergent thinking) a list of issues. The numerous issues were then grouped according to similarity, and duplicates were eliminated. Multivoting was then used to determine the three highest-priority issues. Our number one problem related to cycle time. When a client is referred to CCS, determination of eligibility, opening (or denying) the case, and authorizing care are key cycles. Patient care is often coordinated based on the client's eligibility, and delays in service can result when the process is not completed in a timely manner. The reasons for our failure to meet these deadlines seemed overwhelming and confusing. We needed a method to find the root-causes to improve our performance. We chose to use a fishbone diagram, also known as a cause-and-effect diagram (Figure 5-4). Our problem was "New referrals are not completed within 45 days." We categorized our known barriers on the four "bones" of the fish, manpower, methods, machines, and materials. Once we had identified the factors contributing to our problem, we prioritized them and generated action plans for each major factor. These action plans were extensive and involved implementing training and education programs, re-designing work space for greater efficiency, purchasing more equipment, revising job descriptions, increasing provider outreach activities, and more. Performance data did not improve during the initial year of our PIT, and I chose not to share it with staff to avoid demoralizing them. My management team and I were taking a leap of faith that our process would eventually result in the desired outcome of meeting the performance metrics.

It took 18 months for CCS to "turn the curve," but once improvement started, it was exponential. The cycle time measure for "referral to case open" was initially 57 days. Two years later, it was 30 days. The cycle time "referral to deny" began at 97 days, and 2 years later was down to 39 days. Most importantly, the cycle time "referral to first authorization" decreased from an initial 189 days to just 49 days! It was at this time that I shared the outcome data with the team. They were ecstatic! I asked the team to list the problems they believed we had solved through our PIT's efforts. They listed (1) improved staffing, (2) increased staff morale and decreased turnover (all the positions were now filled), (3) better understanding of the job expectations and the rationale behind those expectations, (4) improved teamwork, and (5) more efficient and effective work space. They have maintained enthusiastic support of the PIT, and participation remains high. The team is still highly focused on problem-solving. I have learned that when assuming leadership of a department in which one has no prior experience, a structured team approach to information gathering, assessment of data, identification of problems, and implementation of action plans can be highly effective in the resolution of priority problems.

— Vickie Lemmon

 Would this be a suitable approach for you? Why?

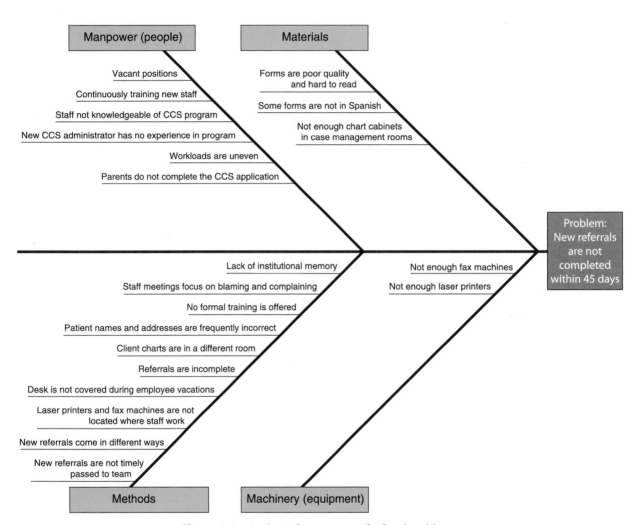

Figure 5-4   Analysis of root causes of referral problems.

CHAPTER CHECKLIST

The ability to make good decisions and encourage effective decision-making in others is a hallmark of nursing leadership and management. A nurse manager or leader is in a good position to facilitate effective decision-making by individuals and groups. This requires good communication skills, conflict resolution and mediation skills, knowledge of the vagaries of group dynamics, and the ability to foster an environment conducive to effective problem-solving, decision-making, and creative thinking.

- The main steps of the traditional problem-solving process are as follows:
  - Define the problem, issue, or situation.
  - Gather data.
  - Analyze data.
  - Develop solutions and options.
  - Select a solution with a desired outcome.
  - Implement the solution.
  - Evaluate the result.
- A decision-making format involves the following:
  - Listing options
  - Identifying the pros and cons of each option
  - Ranking the options in order of preference
  - Selecting the best option
- If you want to make sound decisions or solve problems effectively, information gathered must be as follows:
  - Accurate
  - Relevant
  - Valid
  - Timely
- The situation and circumstances should dictate the leadership style used by managers to solve problems and make decisions. Analytical tools are helpful in planning and illustrating decision-making activities.

TIPS FOR DECISION-MAKING AND PROBLEM-SOLVING

- Seek additional information from other sources, even if it does not support the preferred action.
- Learn how other people approach problem situations.
- Talk to colleagues and superiors who you believe are effective problem-solvers and decision-makers. Observe these positive role models in action.
- Research journal articles and relevant sections of textbooks to increase your knowledge base.
- Risk using new approaches to problem resolution through experimentation, and calculate the risk to self and others.

TERMS TO KNOW

autocratic
creativity
critical-thinking
decision-making
democratic
optimizing decision
participative
problem-solving
satisficing decision

REFERENCES

Aroskar, M. A., Moldow, G. & Good, C. M. (2004). Nurse's voices: Policy, practice and ethics. *Nursing Ethics, 11*(3). Retrieved April 24, 2005, from the Proquest database.

Facione, N. C. & Facione, P. A. (1996). Externalizing the critical thinking in clinical judgment. *Nursing Outlook, 44*, 129-136.

Kerfoot, K. (2003). Organizational intelligence/organizational stupidity: The leader's challenge. *Nursing Economics, 21*(2), 91. Retrieved April 24, 2005, from the Proquest database.

Kritek, P. (2002). *Negotiating at an uneven table: Developing moral courage in resolving our conflicts.* San Francisco: John Wiley & Sons.

Lancaster, J., & Lancaster, W. (1982). *Concepts for advanced nursing practice: The nurse as a change agent.* St. Louis: Mosby.

McDonald, M. (2001). A framework for ethical decision-making. Retrieved April 2, 2001, from http://www.ethics.ubc.ca/mcdonald/deicisions.html.

Paul, R. W. (1995). *Critical thinking: How to prepare students for a rapidly changing world.* Santa Rose, CA: Foundations for Critical Thinking.

Rooney, J. J. & Hopen, D. (2004a). Part I: Problem solving should be like treasure hunting. The *Journal for Quality and Participation, 27*(3), 20. Retrieved April 7, 2005, from the Proquest database.

Rooney, J. J. & Hopen, D. (2004b). Part II: What's in? What's out: Defining your problem. The *Journal for Quality and Participation, 27*(4), 34. Retrieved April 24, 2005, from the Proquest database.

Sullivan, E. J., & Decker, P. J. (1992). *Effective management in nursing.* Menlo Park, CA: Addison-Wesley.

Yoder-Wise, P. (2004). The problem with problem-based learning. *The Journal of Continuing Education in Nursing, 35*(4), 147. Retrieved April 1, 2005, from the Proquest database.

INTERNET RESOURCES

California Academic Press: www.calpress.com

Center for Critical Thinking and Foundation for Critical Thinking at Sonoma State University: www.criticalthinking.org

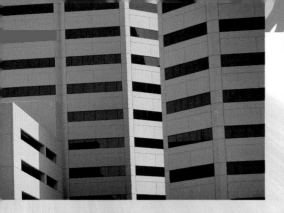

6

Healthcare Organizations

Mary E. Mancini

*T*his chapter presents an overview of existing and emerging healthcare organizations, their characteristics, and their designs. Economic, social, and demographic factors that influence organizational
development are discussed. A major emphasis is placed on management and leadership responses that professional nurses must consider in planning the delivery of nursing care in the changing environment. Leaders,
managers, followers, and nursing students engaged in active practice must be aware of the changing dynamics if they are to be effective healthcare professionals and advocate for patients, families, and community.

Objectives

- Identify and compare characteristics that are used to differentiate healthcare organizations.
- Classify healthcare organizations by major types.
- Analyze economic, social, and demographic forces that drive the development of healthcare organizations.

- Explain the implications of healthcare organizational evolution for nursing leadership and management roles.

Questions to Consider

- *What are the changes that have taken place in healthcare organizations in your geographic region in the past 5 years?*
- *What changes have taken place in specific characteristics of ownership, service orientation, teaching status, and financing of healthcare organizations in your community?*
- *What economic, social, and demographic factors are forces driving the development of healthcare organizations in your community?*
- *What leadership and management functions are nurses performing as healthcare organizations in your geographic region evolve?*

The Challenge

Beth A. Smith, RN, MSN, MBA
Director, Case Management, W.A. Foote Memorial Hospital, Jackson, Mississippi

Our hospital system is faced with the challenge of caring for a large number of uninsured patients who do not receive basic health care. When they do seek health care, it is often because they have an advanced disease process that consequently requires high-cost treatment and support. One such patient was a 42-year-old, uninsured, self-employed seasonal worker with no current income, assets, or support systems. He underwent a partial laryn-gectomy for his throat cancer. When he was ready to be discharged, he still required tube feedings, a tracheostomy with humidified air, intravenous antibiotics, and speech therapy. I needed to balance virtually nonexistent resources with great needs.

 What do you think you would you do if you were this nurse?

INTRODUCTION

Organizations are collections of individuals brought together in a defined environment to achieve a set of predetermined objectives. Economic, social, and demographic factors affect the purpose and structuring of the system, which in turn interact with the mission, philosophy, and structure of healthcare organizations.

Healthcare organizations provide two general types of services: illness care (restorative) and wellness care (preventive). Illness care services help the sick and injured. Wellness care services promote better health as well as illness and accident prevention. In the past, most organizations (e.g., hospitals, clinics, public health departments, community-based organizations, and physicians' offices) focused their attention on illness services. Recent economic, social, and demographic changes have placed emphasis on the development of organizations that focus on the full spectrum of health, especially wellness and prevention, to meet consumers' needs in more effective ways. Emphasis is being placed on the role of the nurse as both a designer of these restructured organizations and a healthcare leader and manager within the organizations. For example, the manner in which chronic and acute illnesses are managed are dramatically different from such a decade ago. Nurses take a much more active and independent role in providing these services. Similarly, as population numbers increase and the demand for nurses exceeds the supply, we can anticipate more changes in how nurses function within the healthcare system.

An increased focus on continuous performance improvement and benchmarking demands that organizations constantly consider their own practices and make appropriate changes, including those related to the organization's culture and the role of nurses within the organization.

Nurses practice in many different types of healthcare organizations. Nursing roles develop in response to the same social, cultural, economic, legislative, and demographic factors that shape the organizations in which they work. As the largest group of healthcare professionals providing direct and indirect care services to consumers, nurses have an obligation to be involved in the development of healthcare, social, and economic policies that shape healthcare organizations.

CHARACTERISTICS AND TYPES OF ORGANIZATIONS

Responding to the rapidly changing nature of the economic, social, and demographic environment at the national, state, and local level, the United States healthcare system is in a continual state of flux as are the organizations within this system. Organizations either anticipate or respond to these environmental changes.

Institutional Providers

Acute-care hospitals, long-term care facilities, and rehabilitation facilities have traditionally been classified as institutional providers. Major characteristics that differentiate institutional providers as well as other healthcare organizations are (1) types of services provided, (2) length of direct care services provided, (3) ownership, (4) teaching status, and (5) accreditation status.

Types of Services Provided The types of services offered is a characteristic used to differentiate institutional providers. Services can be classified as either general or special care. Facilities that provide specialty care offer a limited scope of services, such as those targeted to specific disease entities or patient populations. Examples of special care facilities include those providing psychiatric care, burn care, children's care, women's and infants' care, or oncology care. Alternatively, facilities, such as general hospitals, provide a wide range of services to multiple segments of the population.

Length of Direct Care Services Provided Another characteristic that is used to differentiate healthcare organizations is the duration of the care provided. According to the American Hospital Associations (AHA, 2004), most hospitals are acute-care facilities giving short-term, episodic care. The AHA defined an acute-care hospital as a facility in which the average length of stay is less than 30 days. Chronic care or long-term facilities provide services for patients who require care for extended periods in excess of 30 days. In acute-care institutions, patients are discharged as soon as their conditions are stabilized. An example of a long-term facility is a geriatric organization that provides care services from onset of impairment until death. Many institutions have components of both short-term and long-term services. They may provide acute care, home care, hospice care, ambulatory clinic care, day surgery, and an increasing number of other services, such as day care for dependent children and adults or focused services, such as Meals-on-Wheels. The term *healthcare network* refers to interconnected units that either are owned by the institution or have cooperative agreements with other institutions to provide a full spectrum of wellness and illness services. The spectrum of care services provided are typically described as **primary care** (first-access care), **secondary care** (disease-restorative care), and **tertiary care** (rehabilitative or long-term care). Table 6-1 describes the continuum of care and the units of healthcare organizations that provide services in the three phases of the continuum.

■ *Exercise 6–1*

Using the local telephone directory, determine the types and numbers of primary care, secondary care, and tertiary care services available. Table 6-2 provides an example of a format for collecting data.

Table 6-1 CONTINUUM OF HEALTHCARE ORGANIZATIONS

Type of Care	Purpose	Organization or Unit Providing Services
Primary	Entry into system Health maintenance Long-term care Chronic care Treatment of temporary nonincapacitating malfunction	Ambulatory care centers Physicians' offices Preferred provider organizations Nursing centers Independent provider organizations Health maintenance organizations School health clinics
Secondary	Prevention of disease complications	Home health care Ambulatory care centers Nursing centers
Tertiary	Rehabilitation Long-term care	Home health care Long-term care facilities Rehabilitation centers Skilled nursing facilities Assisted living programs/retirement centers

Table 6-2 CHARACTERISTICS AND TYPES OF HEALTHCARE ORGANIZATIONS

Healthcare Organization	Characteristics					
	Type	Services	Own	Fin	Tchg	Multi
Veterans Administration	Institution	General	Federal	NP	Y	Y
Academic Medical Center	Institution	General	Private	NP	Y	Y
Community General	Institution	General	Private	NP	N	Y
Public Hospital	Institution	General	County	NP	Y	N
Shriners Burn Hospitals	Institution	Specialty	Private	NP	N	N
Prepaid Health Plan	HMO	General	Private	NP-P	N	N
Public Health Department	Community	General	State	NP	N	N
Women's and Infants' Project	Community	Specialty	State	NP	N	N
Geriatric Corporation	Institution	Long term	Private	NP	N	Y
Visiting Nurses Association	Community	Specialty	Private	NP	N	N

Fin, Financing; *HMO*, health maintenance organization; *Multi*, multiunit; *N*, no; *NP*, non-profit; *Own*, ownership; *P*, profit; *Tchg*, teaching status; *Y*, yes.

Ownership   Ownership is another characteristic used to classify healthcare organizations. Ownership establishes the organization's legal, business, and mission-related imperative. Healthcare organizations have three basic ownership forms: public, private non-profit, and for-profit. **Public institutions** provide health services to individuals under the support and/or direction of local, state, or federal government. These organizations must answer directly to the sponsoring government agency or boards and are indirectly responsible to elected officials and taxpayers who support them. Examples of these service recipients at the federal level are veterans, members of the military, American Indian, and prisoner healthcare organizations. State-supported organizations may be health service teaching facilities, chronic care facilities, and prisoner facilities. Locally supported facilities include county- and city-supported facilities. Table 6-2 shows how several common healthcare organizations are classified. **Private non-profit (or not-for-profit) organizations**—often referred to as *voluntary agencies*—are controlled by voluntary boards or trustees and provide care to a mix of paying and charity patients. In these organizations, excess revenue over expenses is redirected into the organization for maintenance and growth rather than returned as dividends to stockholders. These organizations are required to serve people regard-less of their ability to pay. Non-profit organizations located in impoverished urban and rural areas are often economically disadvantaged by the amounts of uncompensated care that they provide. Some states, such as New York, have created charity pools to which all non-profit organizations in the state are required to contribute to offset financial problems of the disadvantaged institutions. Historically, non-profit organizations have been exempt from paying taxes as they commit to providing an important community service. The owners of such organizations include churches, communities, industries, and special interest groups such as the Shriners. It is important for nurses to understand the impact of ownership on how organizations are structured, the services they provide and the patients they serve.

For-profit organizations are also referred to as *proprietary organizations*. Investor-owned hospitals operate with the specific intent of earning a profit by providing healthcare services to individuals who can afford to pay for these services. Organizations such as private or public insurers who provide healthcare insurance coverage are known as **third-party payers**. Owners may be individuals, partnerships, corporations, or multisystems. Many for-profit organizations, like the not-for-profit ones, receive supplementary funds through private and public sources to provide special services and research. This funding allows them to provide financial assistance to patients who can afford ordinary care but are not in a position to finance catastrophic occurrences such as vital organ failure, birth of premature or sick infants, or transplant operations.

Multi-hospital systems, which are defined as two or more institutional providers having common owners, represent a significant development that has taken place in the past two decades. Investor-owned, multi-hospital systems are becoming increasingly popular. Nursing homes, home care, psychiatric services, and health maintenance organizations (HMOs) are commonly units in such systems.

Ownership can impact efficiency. Although hospital ownership is defined legally, there are significant differences within the three sectors related to teaching status, location, bed size, and corporate affiliation. For-profit hospitals, which represent 14% of the beds in short-term, acute-care hospitals, are typically nonteaching, suburban facilities with small-to-medium bed capacity and the ability to access group purchasing cooperatives that lower non-salary expenses. For-profit hospitals tend to have higher hospital charges and lower wage and salary costs that most likely represent an aggressive approach to maximizing return on investment.

Ownership results in differential treatment relative to regulatory requirements. Public and non-profit hospitals are tax exempt and have a concomitant responsibility to provide mandated community service such as delivering care to the poor and indigent. Thus, one can expect operational differences between and among the three ownership sectors. Ownership impacts the organization's level of effort in regard to the provision of uncompensated care. Those organizations with taxing authority or direct support from local or state government have a clear mandate to care for indigent patients and receive at least some level of dedicated funds to do so. For-profit hospitals offer fewer unprofitable services and actively seek to avoid providing uncompensated care and are required to pay taxes that can have an impact on their bottom line. To keep their nonprofit status, these facilities must make a good-faith effort to provide community service and charity care. Unfortunately, the literature provides conflicting and inconclusive evidence in regard to the impact of ownership on hospital financial performance.

Teaching Status Teaching status is a characteristic that can differentiate healthcare organizations. The term **teaching institution** is applied to academic health centers—those directly affiliated with a school of medicine and at least one other health profession school—and affiliated teaching hospitals—those that provide only the clinical portion of a medical school teaching program. Studies have shown that although care is usually more costly at teaching hospitals than at nonteaching hospitals, teaching hospitals generally offer better care because of their access to state-of-the-art technology and researchers. The higher costs of teaching hospitals have been attributed to the unique missions these institutions tend to pursue, including graduate medical education, biomedical research and the maintenance of stand-by capacity for highly specialized patient care. In a study of 3552 hospitals, Koenig and colleagues (2003) estimated these mission-related components account for 27.6% of costs per case in teaching hospitals.

Traditionally, teaching hospitals have received government reimbursement to cover these additional costs. There are, however, intrinsic costs of providing a medical training program that are not fully reimbursed by the government. Maintaining a teaching program places a financial burden on hospitals relative to the direct cost of the program and the indirect cost of the inefficiencies surrounding the training process. These inefficiencies include (1) salaries of physicians who supervise students' care delivery and participate in educational programs such as teaching rounds and seminars; (2) duplicated tests or procedures; and (3) delays in processing patients related to the teaching process. Currently, these expenses are reimbursed based on a formula that takes into consideration the cost of caring for the low-income and uninsured patients who populate most academic teaching programs. Revisions in this reimbursement are occurring as states reduce subsidies for the education of physicians. Hospitals make strategic decisions about their level of participation in physician training. Because of the additional costs, few for-profit hospitals sponsor teaching programs. Teaching hospitals are usually located close to their affiliated medical school. They tend to be larger and located in more urban and economically depressed inner-city areas than their non-teaching counterparts. Teaching hospitals, therefore, tend to exhibit weaker economic performance compared with non-teaching hospitals.

> **Exercise 6-2**
> Return to the data you started in the first exercise, and add financial and teaching status information.

Accreditation Status   Whether or not a healthcare organization has been accredited by an external body as having the structure and process necessary to provide high quality care is another characteristic that can be used to distinguish one organization from another. Private organizations play significant roles in establishing standards and ensuring care delivery compliance with standards by accrediting healthcare organizations. Examples of these organizations are the Joint Commission on Accreditation of Healthcare Organizations (JCAHO), and The National Committee for Quality Assurance (NCQA). More information on accrediting organizations is provided later in this chapter.

Consolidated Systems and Networks

Healthcare organizations are being organized into **consolidated systems** through both the formation of for-profit or not-for-profit multi-hospital systems and the development of **networks** of independently owned and operated healthcare organizations.

Consolidated Systems   Consolidated systems tend to be organized along five levels. The first level includes the large national hospital companies, most of which are investor owned. The second level involves large voluntary affiliated systems, which provide members with access to capital, political power, management expertise, joint venture opportunities, and links to health insurance services or, as in Canada, to a national healthcare coverage program. The third level involves regional hospital systems that cover a defined geographic area, such as an area of a state. The fourth level involves metropolitan-based systems. The fifth level is composed of the special interest groups that own and operate units organized along religious lines, teaching interests, or related special interests that drive their activities. This level often crosses over the regional, metropolitan, and national levels already described. Through the creation of multiunit systems, an organization has greater marketing, policy, and contracting potentials.

Networks   Healthcare markets with 100,000 or more residents are generally served by one to three health networks. The networks usually follow one of three organizational models: public utilities, for-profit businesses, or loose alliances. Public utility models are organized and governed just like today's public utilities, for example, the county water department. Their aim is serving large regional populations. In most markets, two or three competing markets have emerged that require significant capital, causing many traditional not-for-profit providers to shift to for-profit status. Loose alliances take the shape of loosely connected "virtual" networks that emulate integrated health systems through contracts and linked computer systems.

Ambulatory-Based Organizations

Many health services are provided on an ambulatory basis. The organizational setting for much of this care has been the group practice or private physician's office. A growing form of group practice is prepaid group practice plans, referred to as managed care systems, which combine care delivery and financing and provide comprehensive services for a fixed prepaid fee. A goal of these services is to reduce the cost of expensive acute hospital care by focusing on out-of-hospital preventive care and illness follow-up care. Group practice plans take various forms. One form has a centralized administration that directs and pays salaries for physician practice (e.g., HMOs).

The HMO is a configuration of healthcare agencies that provide basic and supplemental health maintenance and treatment services to voluntary enrollees who prepay a fixed periodic fee without regard to the amount of services used. To be federally qualified, an HMO company must offer inpatient and outpatient services, treatment and referral for drug and alcohol problems, laboratory and radiology services, preventive dental services for children younger than 12 years, and preventive healthcare services in addition to physician services.

Independent practice associations (IPAs) (or professional associations [PAs]) are a form of group practice in which physicians in private offices are paid on a **fee-for-service** basis by a prepaid plan to deliver care to enrolled members. Preferred provider organizations (PPOs) operate similarly to IPAs; contracts are developed with private practice physicians, but fees are discounted from their usual and customary charges. In return, physicians are guaranteed prompt payment.

Nurse practitioners' leadership in managing patients in these group practices has contributed greatly to their success. Examples of this can be found by reviewing literature related to nurses' activities at Kaiser Permanente HMO and the Harvard Community Health Plan.

Numerous freestanding ambulatory centers are developing. These organizations include surgicenters, urgent care centers, primary care centers, and imaging centers.

Exercise 6–3

Again return to the data started in the first exercise and add information about the status of the multiunit systems that are in place.

Other Organizations

Although hospitals, nursing homes, health departments, visiting nurse services, and private physicians' offices have made up the traditional primary service delivery organizations, it is important to recognize the increasing role being played by other organizations that may be freestanding or units of hospitals or other community organizations. These include community service organizations, subacute facilities, and a proliferating number of home health agencies, long-term care facilities, and hospices. Additionally, nurse-owned/nurse-organized services and self-help voluntary organizations contribute to the overall service provision. This rapid growth was spurred by the implementation of the prospective payment system, which resulted in early discharge of many patients from acute-care facilities. These patients require highly technical continuing nursing care to maintain a stable status. The focus of these organizations is on the care of individuals and their family and significant others, rather than a focus on the community as a whole. Many of these organizations are functioning as PPOs, and this is expected to be a continuing pattern in the future.

Community Services Community services, including public health departments, are focused on the treatment of the community rather than that of the individual. The historical focus of these organizations has been on control of infectious agents and provision of preventive services under the auspices of public health departments. Local, state, and federal governments allocate funds to health departments to provide a variety of necessary services. These funds provide personal health services that include maternal and child care, care for communicable diseases such as AIDS and tuberculosis, services for children with birth defects, mental health care, and investigation of epidemiology and treatment of bioterrorism threats and attacks such as anthrax. Monies are also allocated for environmental services, such as ensuring that food services meet established standards, and for health resources, such as control of reproduction, promotion of safer sex, and breast cancer screening programs. Local health departments have been provided some autonomy in determining how to use funds that are not assigned to categorical programs.

School health programs whose funds are also allocated to them by local, state, and federal governments traditionally have been organized to control infectious disease outbreaks; to detect and refer problems that interfere with learning; to treat on-site injuries and illnesses; and to provide basic health education programs. Increasingly, schools are being seen as primary care sites for children.

Visiting nurse associations, which are voluntary organizations, have provided a large amount of the follow-up care for patients after hospitalization and for newborns and their mothers. Some are organized by cities, and others serve entire regions. Some operate for profit; others do not.

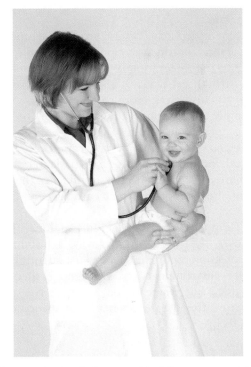

Visiting nurse associations provide follow-up care at home for many. (Copyright 2005 by JupiterImages Corporation.)

Subacute Facilities As hospitals began to discharge patients earlier in their recuperation, the subacute facility emerged as a healthcare organization. Initially, many of these facilities were old-style nursing homes refurbished with the high-tech equipment necessary to deal with patients who have just come out of surgery or who are still acutely ill and have complex medical needs. Today, many are newly built centers or new businesses that have taken over hospitals that were shut down in the merger mania of recent years.

Home Health Organizations Home health organizations have numerous configurations; they may be freestanding or owned by a hospital and may be for-profit or not-for-profit organizations. Professional nurses with expert skills in assessing patients' self-care competencies and in building structures to overcome patients' and families' social and emotional deficits in providing sick and palliative care are needed to meet home care needs. Home care agencies staffed appropriately with adequate numbers of professional nurses have the potential to keep elderly persons, those with disabilities, and persons with chronic illnesses comfortable and safe at home. An increasing number of restrictions on home care by managed care companies are threatening the adequate performance of this function.

Home care is the fastest growing segment in health care. The organizational design will likely change to the integration of a functional and divisional structure because the home health service industry is becoming more complex and is changing rapidly. For example, reimbursement for home care is primarily an arrangement of contract pricing and capitation. The integration of clinical, financial, human resources, and patient outcome information are factors that will influence the organizational design of the home care agency.

Long-Term Care and Residential Facilities Long-term care (LTC) facilities provide rehabilitation and professional nursing services. Residential facilities are environments in which no skilled care is provided but where residents who have special needs are offered safe, sheltered environments in which to live.

Hospice Hospices can be located on inpatient nursing units, such as the kind commonly found in Canada, the United Kingdom, and Australia, or in the home or residential centers in the community. The concept of hospice or palliative care was launched at St. Christopher Hospice in London. Hospices focus on confirming rather than denying the reality of death and thus provide care that ensures dignity and comfort.

Nurse-Owned and Nurse-Organized Services Nursing centers, which are nurse-owned and nurse-operated places where care is provided by nurses, are another form of community-based organization. Many nursing centers are administered by schools of nursing and serve as a base for faculty practice and research and clinical experience for students. Others are owned and operated by groups of nurses. These centers have a variety of missions. Some focus on care for specific populations, such as the homeless, or on care for people with AIDS. Others have taken responsibility for university health services. Some have assumed responsibility for school health programs in the community, and others operate employee wellness programs, hospices, and home care services. Some are freestanding, and others are units of hospitals. Church-affiliated organizations, sometimes operating as parish or shul (a service of synagogues) nursing facilities, are also examples of nurse-based organizations.

Self-Help Voluntary Organizations Other organizations are the self-help/self-care organizations. These organizations also come in various forms. They are often composed of and directed by peers who are consumers of healthcare services. Their purpose is most often to enable patients to provide support to each other and raise community consciousness about the nature of a specific physical or emotional disease. AIDS support groups and Alcoholics Anonymous are two examples. Community geriatric organizations, frequently sponsored by healthcare organizations and offering multiple services for promoting wellness and rehabilitation, are increasing rapidly.

Supportive and Ancillary Organizations

Organizations involved in the direct provision of health care are supported by a number of other organizations whose operations have a significant effect on provider organizations, as well as on the overall performance of the health system. These organizations include regulatory organizations, accrediting bodies, third-party financing organizations, pharmaceutical and medical equipment supply corporations, and various professional, educational, and training organizations.

Exercise 6–4

Identify supportive and ancillary organizations operating in your community. Can you determine whether nurses are playing leadership or staff roles in those organizations and what functions are incorporated into existing nursing roles?

Regulatory Organizations Regulatory organizations set standards for the operation of healthcare organizations, ensure compliance with federal and state regulations developed by governmental administrative agencies, and investigate and make judgments regarding complaints brought by consumers of the services and the public. They approve organizations for licensure as providers of health care. Healthcare organizations are regulated by a number of different federal, state and local agencies to protect the health and safety of the patients and communities they serve. A number of different regulatory agencies monitor functions in healthcare organizations. These include the Centers for Medicare and Medicaid Services, the U.S. Food and Drug Administration, the Occupational Health and Safety Administration, the Equal Employment Opportunity Commission, and state licensing boards for various health professions. Regardless of the type of organization in which they work, nurses are often involved in these processes. Therefore, all nurses need to be familiar with the regulations that impact their organization.

Established in 1965, Medicare is the country's largest health insurance program, providing healthcare funding for more than 40 million individuals. This makes the federal government the primary payer of healthcare costs in the United States. The Medicare program is not limited to individuals aged 65 or older. Persons with certain permanent illnesses, such as end-stage renal disease, also receive Medicare health benefits. Because of the size of the Medicare market, the federal government serves as the leading regulator of healthcare services in this country.

The Centers for Medicare and Medicaid Services (CMS) administer the Medicare and Medicaid programs. Participation in these programs is regulated by a complex set of rules outlined in a lengthy set of guidelines—The Conditions of Participation (CoP). These guidelines are established to improve quality and protect the health and safety of Medicare and Medicaid beneficiaries by specifying the requirements that organizations must meet to be eligible to receive Medicare and Medicaid reimbursement.

To be in compliance with the CoP, hospitals must meet the requirements of the Quality Assessment and Performance Improvement Program. The program is designed to ensure that hospitals systematically examine the quality of care provided and that they use the data obtained to develop and implement projects that improve quality, enhance patient safety, and reduce medical errors. Through its Quality Improvement Organization program (formally called Peer Review), CMS provides a financial incentive for hospitals to report quality data that will be used by patients to help them make decisions about hospital care and the establishment of minimum quality standards for healthcare facilities.

Nurses are actively involved in CMS quality improvement processes. The level of their participation may be as participants in facility-based quality or utilization management activities or they may be involved as case managers. Nurse case managers can serve in a number of different roles, but they frequently serve as the organization's interface with the physician. In this role, these case managers routinely monitor for appropriate physician documentation of medical necessity and other required CoP elements. In the ambulatory or acute-care setting, the case managers typically work with physician advisors to ensure that care follows the recognized standards and facilitates patient flow to the appropriate setting for care.

Nurses also play key roles in developing, implementing, and evaluating the review processes of these regulatory agencies. Nursing leaders have active roles in establishing standards and ensuring that organizations comply with standards in their roles as members of healthcare organizations providing both direct and indirect services to patients and as members of, or advisors to, regulatory agencies.

Accrediting Bodies Accreditation refers to the approval, recognition, or certification by an official review board that an organization has met certain promulgated standards. CMS is responsible for the enforcement of its standards through its certification activities. For a healthcare organization to participate in and receive payment from either Medicare or Medicaid, the organization must be certified as being in compliance with the CoP. One manner that an organization can be recognized as complying with the CoP is through a survey process conducted by a state agency on behalf of CMS. Alternatively, an organization can be surveyed and accredited by a national accrediting body holding **"deeming authority"** for CMS. To obtain deeming authority, an accreditation organization must undergo a comprehensive evaluation by CMS to ensure that the standards of the accrediting organization are at least as rigorous as CMS standards. Healthcare organizations accredited by an organization with CMS deeming authority are therefore "deemed" as meeting Medicare and Medicaid certification requirements. A number of states accept national accreditation by an approved accrediting agency in lieu of other types of regulatory activity. For these reasons, healthcare organizations often seek accreditation by an accrediting body with deeming authority rather than through a multiple survey process conducted by state agencies and CMS.

Healthcare organizations commonly seek accreditation by either The American Osteopathic Association (AOA) or The Joint Commission on Accreditation of Healthcare Organizations (JCAHO). Both of these organizations have been granted "deeming" authority by CMS. The AOA is a professional association specifically for osteopathic healthcare organizations. They accredit osteopathic acute-care hospitals, mental health facilities, substance abuse centers, and physical rehabilitation centers. The Joint Commission is an independent, not-for-profit organization that currently accredits more than 15,000 healthcare organizations in the United States and internationally. The explicit mission of the Joint Commission is to continuously improve the safety and quality of care provided to the public through the provision of health care accreditation and related services that support improvement of performance in healthcare organizations. The Joint Commission accredits approximately 80% of acute-care hospitals in the United States as well as numerous ambulatory surgicenters, clinical laboratories, critical access hospitals, HMOs, preferred provider organizations

(PPOs), home healthcare agencies, hospices, and acute-care hospitals.

Third-Party Financing Organizations   Organizations that provide financing for health care comprise another subset of supportive and ancillary organizations. As noted earlier, the government, through the Centers for Medicare and Medicaid Services, finances a large portion of the population and represents the largest third-party organization involved in healthcare provision. Private health insurance carriers, who account for most of the remaining financing, are composed of not-for-profit and for-profit components. Blue Cross/Blue Shield is an example of a not-for-profit insurance company. The Blues, as they are often called, have led the move of insurers from fee-for-service insurance to managed care. This has been both a cost-reduction mechanism and a marketing response to the managed care concept introduced by HMOs and the arrangements discussed previously in relation to physician practice agreements. Commercial insurance companies represent the private sector.

Third-party financing organizations have a major effect on the actual delivery of health care. They do so by identifying those procedures, tests, services, or drugs that will be covered under their healthcare insurance programs. In addition, they indirectly impact the configuration of the healthcare delivery system through the use of their significant political influence. As the cost of health care increases and the number of medically uninsured and underinsured grows, pressure increases for significant changes in healthcare reimbursement. Reconfiguration of the current system is certain to bring with it restructuring of the organizations responsible for delivery of healthcare services. An understanding of the interrelated changes in healthcare organizations can be gained by examining the results of the 1982 enactment by Congress of the Tax Equity and Fiscal Reimbursement Act (TEFRA), which introduced the prospective payment system for Medicare reimbursement.

Pharmaceutical and Medical Equipment Supply Corporations   About one tenth of all healthcare expenditures is allocated to drugs and medical equipment, and this is increasing. When other healthcare supply organizations, such as healthcare information system corporations, are considered, the estimated percentage may rapidly escalate toward the one-quarter mark. Nurses, as primary users of these products, play a significant role in healthcare organizations in setting standards for safe and efficient products that meet both consumers' and organizations' needs in a cost-effective manner. Supply organizations often seek nurses as customers and as participants in market surveys for the design of new products, services, and marketing techniques. Nurses are employed by these organizations as designers of new products, marketing representatives, and members of the sales and research staffs. Examples of the roles nurses play can be seen by studying organizations that employ nurses to design new products and market them through production and distribution of a newsletter and ongoing continuing-education presentations.

Professional, Educational, and Training Organizations Professional organizations have as their primary goal the protection and enhancement of the interests of the service delivery organizations and their disciplines. Because of their direct impact on the healthcare delivery system as well as their tremendous political influence, professional healthcare organizations must be considered in any discussion of health care in this country. Professional organizations operate at the local, state, and national levels and perform a number of functions, including protection and support through political lobbying; education; and the development and maintenance of standards for caregivers, resources, environment, and care. Examples of these are the American Nurses Association, the American Medical Association, American Pharmacists Association, and the American Hospital Association. In addition to the professional organizations, labor organizations representing healthcare organization employees play an increasing role in healthcare organization development. Educational and training organizations, such as the American Heart Association, contribute to the development of healthcare organizations through the creation and dissemination of practice standards.

Organizational Relationships

Organizational relationships are complex. Additionally, as in business, some organizations have experienced (or will) acquisitions or mergers.

Integration As the healthcare industry faces continuing and increasing pressure to be both efficient and effective, healthcare organizations are entering into a number of different organizational relationships. Organizations can come together to form affiliations, consortiums, and consolidations that result in multi-hospital systems and/or multi-organizational arrangements. When organizations that provide similar services come together, the arrangement is referred to as **horizontal integration**. An example of horizontal integration is a group of acute-care facilities that come together to provide coverage for an expanded region. When organizations align to provide a full array or continuum of services, the arrangement is referred to as **vertical integration**. Organizations brought together in a vertical integration might include an acute-care facility, a rehabilitation facility, a home care agency, an ambulatory clinic, and a hospice. Benefits attributed to vertical integration include enhanced coordination of services, efficiency, and customer services.

Acquisitions and Mergers The economic forces of capitated payments and **managed care** are causing healthcare organizations to reorganize, restructure, and reengineer to decrease waste and economic inefficiency. Many organizations are forming multi-institutional alliances that integrate healthcare systems under a common organizational infrastructure. These alliances are accomplished through acquisitions or mergers. Acquisitions involve one organization directly buying another. Mergers involve combining two or more organizations and their assets to form a new entity. Mergers can also happen within organizations as departments or patient care units come together. People, structure, culture, and political issues or organizational change can be very traumatic and lead to dysfunctional outcomes if they are not managed (Armstrong-Stassen & Cameron, 2003).

FORCES THAT INFLUENCE HEALTHCARE ORGANIZATIONS

Economic, social, and demographic factors provide the input for future development and act as major forces driving the evolution of healthcare organizations.

Economic Factors

During the past two decades, decisions surrounding the financing of health care have shaped the supply, configuration, and distribution of healthcare organizations and substantially changed the provision of health care in the United States. Although the overall number of hospitals has decreased, the demand for health services has grown (American Hospital Association, 2004). This increase has been particularly notable in the ranks of the needy and uninsured. According to the Kaiser Commission (2003), nearly two thirds of non-elderly Americans receive health insurance coverage through their employers, and Medicare covers almost all the elderly at some level. Still, millions of individuals lack health insurance either because their employers do not offer it, or they simply cannot afford to pay for it. In October 2003, the Census Bureau reported the number of uninsured jumped in 2002 by 2.4 million, the largest increase in a decade, to 43.6 million or 15.2% of the population.

An increase in the number of persons without health insurance has a significant impact on the communities in which they live and the healthcare organizations where they seek care. In its 2003 report, "A Shared Destiny; Effects of Uninsurance on Individuals, Families, and Communities," the Institute of Medicine notes that the presence of a large number of uninsured people in a community could affect the availability of medical care for everyone. The uninsured strain the resources of hospitals and divert tax dollars away from other necessary public health programs. The financial strain impacts the financial performance of local governments and healthcare providers alike. The report goes on to say that it is misguided, even dangerous, to assume that lack of health insurance only harms those who are uninsured. It hurts everyone when immunizations are missed and infectious diseases flourish or when chronic care is missed and an acute exacerbation occurs. In a study by Castel et al. (2003), analysis of state level data from 1994 to 1999 found higher uninsurance rates to be a significant predictor of the level of uncompensated care incurred by hospitals. In 2001, hospitals in the United States provided $21.6 billion of uncompensated care, threatening the economic viability of many of these organizations. The radical restructuring of the healthcare system that is required to reduce the continuing

escalation of economic resources into the system and to make health care accessible to all citizens will necessitate ongoing changes in healthcare organizations.

In addition to struggling to respond to the increasing numbers of uninsured patients and the concomitant increase in the amounts of uncompensated care, healthcare organizations are being confronted daily with the financial pressures associated with rapidly escalating drug costs, expensive new technology, and spiraling personnel costs associated with healthcare labor shortages (Kaiser Commission, 2003, 2004). The Centers for Medicare and Medicaid Services reported that in 2003, overall health spending rose 7.7%, with healthcare spending reaching 15.3% of the Gross Domestic Product (CMS, 2005). With costs escalating for legitimate reasons, one could reasonably expect that reimbursement would be increasing as well. This is, unfortunately, not the case.

Contemporaneous with cost inflation, payments by all payer groups are being reduced. The Kaiser Commission (2003) reports that both state and local governments are facing increasing financial pressure from the growing numbers of uninsured persons who are seeking health care at public expense as a result of losing their healthcare coverage due to unemployment. Beyond the higher cost associated with the increased enrollment due to layoffs, as the economy contracts, state and local government face declining revenues that result in fewer resources to pay for the expanding programs. With the majority of state budgets in financial crisis, the common response has been massive state reductions, including major cutbacks in Medicaid eligibility levels, covered services, and payments to physicians and hospitals.

Compounding the impact of the direct reduction in governmental payments and subsidies on healthcare organizations is the expansion of managed care as a healthcare insurance product. During the past decade, the U.S. healthcare system has become increasingly competitive. As managed care plans compete for business primarily on their rate structures, these plans emphasize controlling patient access to care and lowering payments to providers. As payments to hospitals are reduced, access to care for the uninsured is eroded because these hospitals have less financial capacity to provide charity care.

The complexity of controlling costs is currently and will remain a major issue driving development of the healthcare system. Perhaps the most immediate change will be in the increasing direct involvement of employers as healthcare costs rise and as financing-mandated employee benefit programs remains a major concern for corporations. This involvement is currently taking the form of evaluating and restructuring employee use of health care and designing benefits packages to control costs. Another form of control of healthcare organization services is the development of local coalitions consisting of community health providers, consumers, and corporations acting to unify business initiatives in healthcare cost containment and to provide consumers with input into health planning and policy development. Wellness programs designed to modify consumers' use of and demand for services such as health-promotion campaigns, ergonomic programs to reduce work-related injuries such as carpal tunnel syndrome, and fitness and exercise programs are other industrial corporate initiatives being introduced to reduce costs. Again, nurses are assuming key roles in managed care and in organizing and directing wellness programs.

Nurses have a major role to play in demonstrating that access to care and quality management are essential components of cost control. With the increasing involvement of industry, business management techniques will assume greater emphasis in healthcare organizations. Leadership will need to be taken by nurses to redesign roles and restructure healthcare organizations. Nurse leaders and managers will need to go beyond obtaining education in business techniques to gaining skill in adapting that knowledge to meet the specific needs of delivery of cost-effective, quality care.

Social Factors

Increasing consumer attention to disease prevention and promotion of healthful lifestyles is redefining relationships of healthcare organizations and their patients. Patients are becoming increasingly active in care planning, implementation, and evaluations and are seeking increased participation with their providers. Demands will be made of healthcare organizations for more personal, responsive, and coordinated care. As such, development of strategies that allow patients to become empowered controllers of their own health status is essential. Responsive structural changes in service delivery

will be needed to maintain congruence with new missions and philosophies developed in response to cultural demands and social changes. Continuous evaluation will be needed to assess cost and quality outcomes related to these changes. Maintaining focus on the quality of care provided as well as access to care will be required so that bottom-line costs do not overshadow quality care provisions. Nursing's history of work with the development of patient-centered interactive strategies places nurses in a position to assume leadership roles in this area of organizational development.

Demographic Factors

Geographic dispersion, regional access to care, incomes of the population, aging of the population, and immigration trends are among the demographic factors influencing the design of healthcare organizations. Changing economic and demographic characteristics of many communities are resulting in a larger number of uninsured and underinsured individuals. Geographic isolation often limits access to necessary health services and impedes recruitment of healthcare personnel. Community-based rural health networks that provide primary care links to urban health centers for teaching, consultation, personnel sharing, and the provision of high-tech services are one solution for meeting needs in rural areas. Federal and state funding, which includes incentives for healthcare personnel to work in rural areas, is another approach. Strategic planning by nursing is critical to address community needs.

A major influence exerted on healthcare organizations comes from the aging of the population. By the year 2025, more than 18% of the population is expected to be older than 65 years of age. The numbers of "the old-old," those older than 80, are increasing dramatically. Although this segment of the population does not necessarily have dependency needs, a need exists for more long-term beds, supportive housing, and community programs. To meet these emerging needs of elderly persons, new healthcare organizations will continue to evolve, be evaluated, and be restructured based on findings. New roles for nurses as leaders and managers of elderly care are evolving, such as the roles being played by advanced nurse practitioners in directing the care of patients who have become members of geriatric care organizations, such as retirement centers.

Another significant effect on the system will come from the increasing number of individuals and families who are unable to afford care to meet even their most basic needs. These individuals may be truly indigent or may be the working poor who are but one paycheck or illness from being hungry or homeless. Without a broad array of basic healthcare services affordable and available to these individuals, failure to treat a minor problem, such as high blood pressure, can result in a high-cost illness such as a cerebrovascular accident. This lack of healthcare provision is compounded by the number of people excluded from coverage due to preexisting health conditions, job loss, or immigration status.

A THEORETICAL PERSPECTIVE

Systems Theory

Systems theory attempts to explain productivity in terms of a unifying whole as opposed to a series of unrelated parts (Thompson, 1967). Systems can be either closed—self-contained—or open—interacting with both internal and external forces. In systems theory, a system is described as being comprised of four elements: structure, technology, people, and their environment. Systems theorists focus on the interplay among these elements in a framework of inputs—resources such as people, money, or materials; throughputs—the processes that produce a product from the inputs; and outputs—the product of inputs and throughput.

The theoretical concepts of systems theory have been applied to nursing and to organizations. Systems theory presents an explanation of organizational evolution that is similar to biological evolution. Systems theory produces a model that explains the process of healthcare organization evolution (Figure 6-1). The survival of the organization, as portrayed throughout this chapter, is dependent on its evolutionary response to changing environmental forces; it is seen as an open system. The response to environmental changes brings about internal changes, which produce changes that alter environmental conditions. The changes in the environment, in turn, act to bring about changes in the internal operating conditions of the organization.

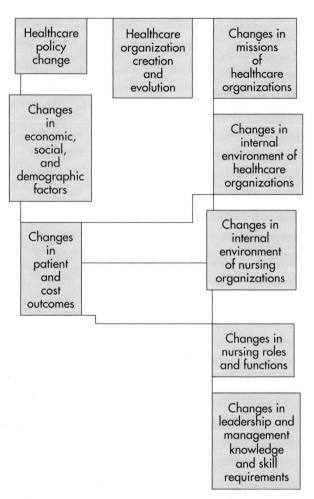

Figure 6-1   Healthcare organizations as open systems.

A very simplified example of this can be seen by again studying the implementation of the prospective payment system that was caused by the economic driving force of escalating healthcare costs in the 1990s. Ambulatory surgery, same-day admissions, and hospital- and community-based home care organizations are some of the internal healthcare organization changes that resulted from an environmentally driven policy change—the cap that was placed on reimbursing expenses incurred by hospitalized patients. These internal organizational developments placed pressure on the external environment to create mechanisms to respond to increasing percentages of the population with self-care deficits who were returning to the community.

This open systems approach to organizational development and effectiveness emphasizes a continual process of adaptation of healthcare organizations to external driving forces and a response to the adaptations by the external environment, which generates continuing inputs for further healthcare organization development. This open system is in contrast to a closed system approach that views a system as being sufficient unto itself and thus is untouched by that which happens around it. (The effects of external forces on internal structures of healthcare organizations are discussed in Chapter 7.)

Chaos Theory

Unfortunately, health care as an industry is not always as predictable and orderly as systems theorists would have us believe. In contrast with the somewhat orderly universe described in systems theory, whereas an organization can be viewed in terms of a linear, cause-and-effect model, chaos theory sees the universe as filled with unpredictable and random events (Hawking, 1987). According to the proponents of chaos theory, organizations must be self-organizing and adapt readily to change in order to survive. Organizations, therefore, must accept that change is inevitable and unrelenting. When one embraces the tenets of chaos theory, one gives up on any attempt to create a permanent organizational structure. Using creativity and flexibility, successful managers will be those who can tolerate ambiguity, take risks, and experiment with new ideas that respond to each day's unique situation or environment. They will not rest upon a successful transition or organizational model because they know the environment within which it flourished is fleeting. The successful nurse leaders will be those individuals who are committed to life-long learning and problem-solving. The Theory Box notes key elements of systems and chaos theories.

Exercise 6-5

Think about the economic, social, and demographic changes you can identify in your community. How will they influence healthcare organizations and the provision of health care in your community? How can systems theory and chaos theory help provide a context for discussing these trends?

NURSING ROLE AND FUNCTION CHANGES

Leadership and management roles for nurses are proliferating in healthcare organizations that are developing or evolving in response to environmental driving forces. The proportion of nursing jobs in the community is increasing. Nurses need new knowledge and skills to coordinate the care of patients or communities with the many other disciplines and organizational units that are providing the continuum of care. Our society needs nurses who can engage in the political process of policy development, coordinate care across disciplines and settings, use conflict management techniques to create win-win situations for patients and providers in resolving the healthcare system's delivery problems, and use business savvy to market and prepare financial and organizational plans for the delivery of cost-effective care. The Research Perspective box suggests how nurse leaders can have an impact and mitigate the negative effects of organizational restructuring.

Theory Box

Systems Theory	Definition: A system comprises four elements (structure, technology, people, and environment) forming a unified whole.
	Viewed as inputs, throughputs, and outputs
	Closed systems—self contained
	Open systems—interacting with internal and external forces
Chaos Theory	Definition: The universe is chaotic and requires organizations to be self-organizing and adaptive to survive.
	Viewed as unpredictable and random events
	Constant change results in little long-term stability

Research Perspective

Cummings, G., Hayduk, L. & Estabrooks, C. (2005) Mitigating the impact of hospital restructuring on nurses: The responsibility of emotionally intelligent leadership. *Nursing Research, 54*(1), 2-12.

Faced with significant changes in patient demands and financial reimbursement strategies, in order to remain viable hospitals responded with major reorganization efforts. These efforts often resulted in the reduction of nursing personnel. Nurses who continued to work in the reorganized environment reported decreased job satisfaction, significant negative physical and emotional sequelae, and decreased opportunities to provide quality patient care. The purpose of this study was twofold. First, the authors sought to develop a theoretical model that explained the impact of hospital restructuring on nurses. The second purpose was to determine the extent that emotionally intelligent leadership (as measured by an inventory of thirteen leadership competencies) could mitigate the impact of hospital restructuring on nursing staff.

The authors used a survey methodology and reported on the responses from 6536 nurses practicing in Alberta, Canada. Analysis of the data indicated that nurses who work for leaders who demonstrate a resonant leadership style— one that reflects the art of hearing their workers' feelings and responding empathically—reported less emotional exhaustion, fewer psychosomatic syndromes, better emotional health, more satisfaction with supervision and their job, and fewer unmet patient care needs.

IMPLICATIONS FOR PRACTICE

These findings provide nursing leadership with specific interventions and learned behaviors that can provide opportunities to enhance their effectiveness. The authors put forth the suggestion that by investing energy into relationships with their nurses, they can positively impact not only the health and welfare of the staff but also ultimately improve patient care outcomes.

Whether influenced by systems or chaos theory, today's healthcare organizations are in a dynamic state. Nurses must be continuously alert to assessing both the internal and external environment for forces that act as inputs to changes needed in their healthcare organization and for the effects of changes that are made. Awareness of the changing status of healthcare organizations and the ability to play a leading role in creating and evaluating adaptation in response to changing forces will be a central function of nurse leaders and managers in healthcare organizations. Nurses need to develop a foundation of leadership and management knowledge that they can build on through a planned program of continuing education. Even in tumultuous times within the healthcare industry, nursing leaders have demonstrated their ability to strengthen the quality of both their organizations and the practice of nursing. As healthcare organizations continue to transform, tomorrow's nurses—whether leaders, managers, or followers—need to carry these lessons forward.

The Solution

I contacted the hospital case manager, who arranged for this patient to have access to special programs in the hospital to fund the medications and support the case management expenses. We arranged for the patient to be seen by a state agency that provides emergency funds for utilities and phone service and assisted him with a Medicaid application with a request for a retroactive initiation date. Finally, we contacted Hospice and the American Cancer Society to support the tube-feeding expenses and worked with other agencies to delay billings until Medicaid was available. Clearly, today's nurse manager has to be connected with the extended resources in the community to ensure care for patients who require assistance.

— Beth A. Smith

 Would this be a suitable approach for you? Why?

CHAPTER CHECKLIST

Knowledge of types of healthcare organizations and characteristics used to differentiate healthcare organizations provides a foundation for examining the operation of the healthcare system. Understanding the economic, social, and demographic forces driving changes in healthcare organizations identifies needs that organizations must be designed to fit. Recognizing that alterations in the environment and in healthcare organizations are mutually interactive is necessary to determine the effects of change and the steps that need to be taken in response to the constant changes. Changes in nursing roles as well as in the settings in which services are provided requires that nurses expand their knowledge and skills. These changes are part of a continual evolution that demands a foundation in leadership and management knowledge that serves as a basis for future development.

- ■ Key characteristics that differentiate types of healthcare organizations are:
  - Clinical services provided
  - Length of services provided
  - Ownership
  - Teaching status
  - Geographic location
  - Accreditation status
- ■ Major types of healthcare organizations are as follows:
  - Institutional providers
  - Acute-care facilities
  - Long-term facilities
  - Rehabilitation facilities

- Consolidated systems and networks
- Ambulatory-based organizations
- Other organizations
  - Community services
  - Subacute facilities
  - Home-health organizations
  - Long-term care and residential facilities
  - Hospice
  - Nurse-owned/nurse-organized services
  - Self-help voluntary organizations
- Supportive and ancillary
  - Regulatory organizations
  - Accrediting bodies
  - Third-party payers (insurers)
  - Pharmaceutical and medical equipment supply corporations
  - Professional, educational and training organizations
- ■ Economic forces driving the development of healthcare organizations are numerous and are continually evolving, escalating the percentage of the Gross National Product comprised of healthcare costs.
  - An increasing number of uninsured patients threatens the health of the community.
  - Decreasing reimbursement threatens the economic viability of healthcare organizations.
  - Social forces driving development of healthcare organizations include the following:
    - A focus of society that is changing from illness to health (wellness)
    - An increasing demand by individuals that they participate in designing their own customized care plans

Continued

- Demographic forces driving development of health-care organizations include the following:
  - The increasing percentage of society that is composed of elderly individuals
  - An increasing percentage of poor people who do not have the financial resources to have access to care
  - The inability of communities to provide ready and economical access to needed health services
- Implications of healthcare organization evolution for leadership and management role functions of professional nurses include the following:
  - An increased ability to attune to the altered environmental driving forces that predict and direct necessary changes in healthcare organizations
  - An increased ability to attune to the healthcare organization's internal environment to predict and direct changes required in both the internal and external environment

- Knowledge and skill both in influencing the development of and in developing healthcare policy at the federal, state, local, and organizational levels
- Knowledge and skill in coordinating and collaborating with peers and other disciplines providing services within a point of service and in networks created by the interconnection of many points of service
- Skill in using business knowledge in planning and evaluating delivery of health care in healthcare organizations that must market cost and outcome effectiveness to survive
- Knowledge and skill in planning and directing group work, which promotes optimal health statuses with minimal use of personnel and material resources

TIPS ON HEALTHCARE ORGANIZATIONS

- Knowledge of economic, social, and demographic changes is essential to redesigning healthcare organizations to meet society's needs.
- Increasing consolidation of healthcare services that provide all levels of care necessitates the development of communication systems that provide information on patients receiving services at the various points of care in the network.
- Diversified positions will be available for professional nurses in the various organizations that are developing to enhance the provision of care.
- New configurations of healthcare delivery will demand that professional nurses continually develop new knowledge in leadership and management.

TERMS TO KNOW

accreditation
consolidated systems
deeming authority
fee-for-service
for-profit organization
horizontal integration
managed care
networks
primary care
private non-profit (or not-for-profit) organization
public institution
secondary care
teaching institution
tertiary care
third-party payers
vertical integration

REFERENCES

American Hospital Association. (2004). *American Hospital Association/Health Forum Annual Survey Data Report.* Chicago: American Hospital Association.

Armstrong-Stassen, M., & Cameron, S. J. (2003) Dimensions of control and nurses reactions to hospital amalgamation. *International Journal of Sociology and Social Policy, 23*(8-9), 104-128.

Cady, R. F. (2003). DHHS's Final Rule on the Quality Assessment and Performance Improvement Program. *JONA's Healthcare Law, Ethics, and Regulation.* June 2003. *5*(2), 29-31.

Castel, L. D., Timbie, J. W., Sendersky, V., Curtis, L. H., Feather, K. A. & Schulman, K. A. (2003). Toward estimating the impact of changes in immigrants' insurance eligibility on hospital expenditures for uncompensated care. *Health Service Research, 3*(1), 1.

Centers For Medicare and Medicaid Services. (2005). Highlights—National Health Expenditures, 2003. www.cms.hhs.gov/statistics/nhe/historical/highlights

Coakley, E., & Scoble, K. B. (2003). A reflective model for organizational assessment and interventions. *Journal of Nursing Administration, 33*(12), 660-669.

Cummings, G., Hayduk, L., & Estabrooks, C. (2005). Mitigating the impact of hospital restructuring on nurses: The responsibility of emotionally intelligent leadership. *Nursing Research, 54*(1), 2-12.

Hawking, S. (1987). *A brief history of time.* Bantom Press, London.

Institute of Medicine. (2003). *A shared destiny: Effects of uninsurance on individuals, families, and communities.* Washington, DC: National Academies Press.

Kaiser Commission on Medicaid and the Uninsured. (2003). *The uninsured in America: A chartbook.* 5th edition. Washington, DC: Henry J. Kaiser Family Foundation.

Kaiser Commission on Medicaid and the Uninsured. (2004). *Health care coverage in America.* Washington, DC: Henry J. Kaiser Family Foundation.

Koenig, L., Dobson, A., Ho, S., Siegel, J. M., Blimenthal, D., & Weissman, J. S. (2003). Estimating the mission-related costs of teaching hospitals. *Health Affair, 22*(6), 112-122.

Thompson, J. D. (1967). *Organization in action.* New York: McGraw-Hill.

Dubbs, N. L. Bazzoli, G. J, Shortell, S. M. & Kralovec, P. D. (2004). Reexamining organizational configurations: An update, validation, and expansion of the taxonomy of health networks and systems. *Health Services Research, 39*(1), 207-220.

Etheridge, P. (1997). The Carondelet experience. *Nursing Management, 28*(3), 26-28.

Hess, R. (2004). From bedside to boardroom—nursing shared governance. *Online Journal of Issues in Nursing, 9*(1).

Kast, F. E., & Rosenweiz, J. E. (1991). General systems theory: Applications for organizations and management. In M. J. Ward & S. A. Price (Eds.), *Issues in nursing administration: Selected readings* (pp. 60-73). St. Louis: Mosby.

Levit, K., Smith C., Cowan C., Lazenby H., Sensenig A., & Catlin A. (2003). Trends in U.S. health care spending, 2001. *Health Affairs, 22*(1), 154-164.

Porter-O'Grady, T. (1996). The seven basic rules for successful redesign. *Journal of Nursing Administration, 26*(1), 46-55.

United States Government Accountability Office. (2004). CMS needs additional authority to adequately oversee patient safety in hospitals. *GAO-04-850, a report to congressional requesters.* www.gao.gov/cgi-bin/getrpt?GAO-04-850.

Upenieks, V. V. (2003). The interrelationship of organizational characteristics of Magnet hospitals, nursing leadership, and nursing job satisfaction. *Health Care Management, 22*(2), 83-98.

SUGGESTED READINGS

Bernstein, S. J. (2004). VA health services research: Lessons for the world's health care organizations. *American Journal of Managed Care, 10* (11; pt 2), 825-827.

INTERNET RESOURCES

Centers for Medicare and Medicaid Services: www.cms.gov

Community Health Assessment Program: www.chapinc.org

Government Accountability Office: www.gao.gov

Indian Health Services: www.ihs.gov

Joint Commission on Accreditation of Healthcare Organizations: www.jcaho.org

Kaiser Family Foundation—Kaiser Commission on Medicaid and the Uninsured: www.kkf.org

National Committee on Quality Assurance: www.ncqa.org

Veterans Health Benefits: www.va.gov/health_benefits

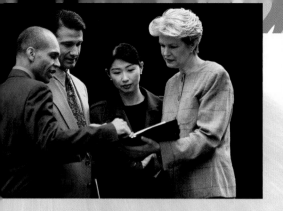

Chapter

7

Understanding and Designing Organizational Structures

Mary E. Mancini

This chapter explains key concepts related to organizational structures and provides information on designing effective structures. This information can be used to help new managers function in an organization and to design structures that support work processes. An underlying theme is designing organizational structures that will respond to changes taking place in the current healthcare environment.

Objectives

- Analyze the relationships among mission, vision, and philosophy statements and organizational structure.
- Analyze factors that influence the design of an organizational structure.
- Relate types of organizational structures with three distinguishing characteristics of each.
- Evaluate the forces that are necessitating reengineering of organizational systems.

Questions to Consider

- What is the nursing organization's reason for being?
- What are the beliefs and values regarding patients, patient care, and the employees?
- What characteristics of the nursing organization's structure would best serve patients' and employees' needs and support work processes? At what level are decisions about each made?
- What would a futuristic organizational chart look like? What management strategies would be prevalent in this organization?

The Challenge

Rebecca M. Patton, RN, MSN, CNOR
Director of Nursing , University Hospitals Health System, Richmond Heights Hospital,
  Cleveland, Ohio

This is a newly acquired hospital in my health system. The hospital went through three different owners during the past 5 years. As a result, there were at least three sets of operating policies directing care. When I was appointed Director of Nursing, there was an organizational plan in place, but several of the head nurse positions and supervisor positions were vacant.

The standard of care, as a result, was driven by three different sets of policies, and sometimes there was no nursing administrator available to clarify which practice to follow or even to be aware of the fact that there was a major clinical conflict.

What do you think you would do if you were this nurse?

INTRODUCTION

Professional nurses work mostly in organizations. Learning to determine how an organization accomplishes its work, how to operate productively within an organization, and how to influence organizational processes is essential to a successful professional nursing practice. An organization's mission, vision, and philosophy form the foundation for its structure and performance as well as the development of the professional practice models it uses (Ingersoll, Witzel, & Smith, 2005; Laschinger & Finegan, 2005). *Organization* as it is used here refers to the structure that is designed to support organizational processes. An organization's **mission,** or reason for the organization's existence, influences the design of the structure, for example, to meet the healthcare needs of a designated population, to provide supportive and stabilizing care to an acute care population, or to prepare patients for a peaceful death. The **vision** is the articulated goal to which the organization aspires. A vision statement conveys an inspirational view of how the organization wishes to be described at some future time. It suggests how far to strive in all endeavors. Another key factor influencing structure is the organization's **philosophy.** A philosophy expresses the values and beliefs that members of the organization hold about the nature of their work, about the people to whom they provide service, and about themselves and others providing the services. Figure 7-1 reflects how these elements interrelate.

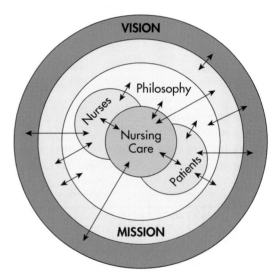

Figure 7-1 The interrelationship of mission, vision, and philosophy.

Exercise 7–1

Consider how you might use the information in the Introduction (1) to analyze an organization that you are considering joining to determine whether it fits your professional development plans, (2) to assess the functioning of an organization that you are already a member of, or (3) to make a plan to reengineer the structure or philosophy to better accomplish the mission of an organization you are considering joining or are already a member of. Use Figure 7-1 as a test for interrelatedness.

MISSION

The mission statement defines the organization's reason or purpose for being. The mission statement identifies the organization's customers and the types of services offered, such as education, supportive nursing care, rehabilitation, acute care, and home care. It enacts the vision statement.

The mission statement sets the stage by defining the services to be offered, which, in turn, identify the kinds of technologies and human resources to be employed. The mission statement of healthcare systems typically refers to the larger community they serve as well as the specific patient populations to whom they provide care. Hospitals' missions are primarily treatment-oriented; the missions of ambulatory care group practices combine treatment, prevention, and diagnosis-oriented services; long-term care facilities' missions are primarily maintenance and social support–oriented; and the missions of nursing centers are oriented toward promoting optimal health status for a defined group of people. The definition of services to be provided and its implications for technologies and human resources greatly influence the design of the **organizational structure**, the arrangement of the work group.

Nursing, as a profession providing a service within a healthcare agency, formulates its own mission statement that describes its contributions to achieve the agency's mission. One of the purposes of the nursing profession is to provide nursing care to clients. The statement should define nursing based on theories that form the basis for the model of nursing to be used in guiding the process of nursing care delivery. Nursing's mission statement tells why nursing exists within the context of the organization. It is written so that others within the organization can know and understand nursing's role in achieving the agency's mission. The mission should be the guiding framework for decision-making. It should be known and understood by other healthcare professionals, by clients and their families, and by the community. It indicates the relationships among nursing and patients, agency personnel, the community, and health and illness. This statement provides direction for the evolving statement of philosophy and the organizational structure. It should be reviewed for accuracy and updated routinely by professional nurses providing care. Units that provide specific services such as intensive care, cardiac services, or maternity services also formulate mission statements that detail their specific contributions to the overall mission.

VISION

Vision statements are future-oriented, purposeful statements designed to identify the desired future of an organization. They serve to unify all subsequent statements toward the view of the future and to convey the core message of the mission statement. Typically, vision statements are brief, consisting of only one or two phrases or sentences. A vision statement appropriate to the patient care unit described in Box 7-1, for example, might be as follows: To be the premier neurosurgical nursing unit in the state.

PHILOSOPHY

The philosophy is a written statement that articulates the values and beliefs held about the nature of the work required to accomplish the mission and the nature and rights of both the people being served and those providing the service. It states the nurse managers' and practitioners' vision of what they believe nursing management and practice are and sets the stage for developing goals to make that vision a reality. It states the beliefs of nurse managers and staff as to how the mission or purpose will be achieved. For example, the mission statement may incorporate the provision of individualized care as an organizational purpose. The philosophy statement would then support this purpose through an expression of a belief in the responsibility of nursing staff to act as patient advocates and to provide quality care according to the wishes of the patient, family, and significant others.

Philosophies are evolutionary in that they are shaped both by the social environment and by the stage of development of professionals delivering the service. The nursing staff reflects the values of the times. The values acquired through education are reflected in the nursing philosophy. Technology developments can also help shape philosophy. For example, information systems can provide people with data that allow them greater control over their work; workers are consequently able to make more decisions and take more autonomous action.

BOX 7-1

Mission and Philosophy for a Neurosurgical Unit

Mission Statement

This unit's purpose is to provide high-quality nursing care for neurosurgical patients during the acute phase of their illness that facilitates their progression to the rehabilitation phase. We strive to cultivate a multidisciplinary approach to the care of the neurosurgical patient and provide multiple educational opportunities for the professional development of neurosurgical nurses.

Philosophy

The philosophy is based on Roy's Adaptation Model and on the American Association of Neurosurgical Nursing Conceptual framework.

Patients

We believe

- It is the right of the patients to make informed choices concerning their treatment.
- Patients have a right to high-quality nursing care and opportunities for improving their quality of life, regardless of the potential outcomes of their illness.
- The patient/family/significant other has a right to exercise personal options to participate in care to the extent of individual abilities and needs.

Nursing

We believe

- Neuroscience nursing is a unique area of nursing practice because neurosurgical interventions and/or neurological dysfunction affect all levels of human existence.
- The goal of the neuroscience nurse is to engage in a therapeutic relationship with his or her patients to facilitate adaptation to changes in physiological, self-concept, role performance, and interdependent modes.
- The ultimate goal for the neuroscience nurse is to foster internal and external unity of patients to achieve optimal health potentials.

Nurse

We believe

- The nurse is the integral element who coordinates nursing care for the neurosurgical patient using valuable input from all members of the patient care team.
- The nurse has an obligation to assume accountability for maintaining excellence in practice.
- The nurse has three basic rights: human rights, legal rights, and professional rights.
- The nurse has a right to autonomy in providing nursing care based on sound nursing judgment.

Nursing Practice

We believe

- Nursing practice must support and be supported by activities in practice, education, research, and management.
- Insofar as possible, patients must be assigned one nurse who is responsible and accountable for their care throughout their stay on the neurosurgical unit.
- The primary nurse is responsible for consulting and collaborating with other healthcare professionals in planning and delivering patient care.
- The contributions of all members of the nursing team are valuable, and an environment must be created that allows each member to participate fully in the delivery of care in accord with his or her abilities and qualifications.
- The nursing process is the vehicle used by nurses to operationalize nursing practice.
- Data generated in nursing practices must be continually and consistently collected and analyzed for the purpose of managing the quality of nursing practice.

Courtesy Upstate Medical University, University Hospital, Syracuse, NY (W. Painter, J. Van Nest-Kinne).

Philosophies require updating to reflect the extension of rights brought about by such changes. Box 7-1 shows an example of a philosophy developed for a neurosurgical unit with the leadership of a nurse manager and clinical instructor.

Exercise 7–2

Obtain a copy of the philosophy of a nursing department and identify behaviors that you observe on a unit of the department that relate or do not relate to the beliefs and values expressed in the document.

ORGANIZATIONAL CULTURE

An organization's mission, vision, and philosophy both shape and reflect organizational culture. **Organizational culture** is the reflection of the norms or traditions of the organization and is exemplified by behaviors that illustrate values and beliefs. Examples include rituals and customary forms of practice, such as celebrations of promotions, publications, degree attainment, professional performance, weddings, and retirements. Other examples of norms that reflect organizational culture are the characteristics of the people who are recognized as heroes by the organization and the behaviors—either positive or negative—that are accepted or tolerated within the organization.

In organizations, culture is demonstrated in two ways that can be either mutually reinforcing or conflict-producing. Organizational culture is typically expressed in a formal manner via written mission, vision, and philosophy statements; job descriptions; and policies and procedures. Beyond formal documents and verbal descriptions given by administrators and managers, organizational culture is also represented in the day-to-day experience of staff and patients. To many, it is the lived experience that reflects the true organizational culture. Do the decisions that are made within the organization consistently demonstrate that the organization values its patients and keeps their needs at the forefront? Are the employees treated with trust and respect or are the words used in recruitment ads simply empty promises with little evidence to back them up? When there is a lack of congruity between the expressed organizational culture and the experienced culture, confusion, frustration, and poor morale often result.

Organizational culture can be effective and promote success and positive outcomes or it can be ineffective and result in disharmony, dissatisfaction, and poor outcomes for patients, staff, and the organization. A number of workplace variables are impacted by organizational culture (Martin, Gustin, Uddin, & Risner, 2004). When seeking employment or advancement, nurses need to assess the organization's culture and develop a clear understanding of existing expectations as well as the formal and informal communication patterns. Various techniques and tools are available to assist the nurse in performing a cultural assessment of an organization (Forsythe, 2005). With a solid understanding of organizational culture, nurses will be better able to be effective change agents and help transform the organizations in which they work.

FACTORS INFLUENCING ORGANIZATIONAL DEVELOPMENT

To be most effective, organizational structures must reflect the organization's mission, vision, philosophy, goals, and objectives. Organizational structure defines how work is organized, where decisions are made, and the authority and responsibility of workers. It provides a map for communication and outlines decision-making paths. As organizations change through acquisitions and mergers, it is essential that structure changes to accomplish revised missions.

Probably the best theory to explain today's nursing organizational development is the chaos (complexity, nonlinear, quantum) theory. (See Chapter 6 and the Index.) In essence, chaos theory suggests that lives—and organizations—are really web-like. Pulling on one small segment rearranges the web; a new pattern emerges; yet, the whole remains. This theory, applied to nursing organizations, suggests that differences logically exist between and among various organizations and that the constant environmental forces continue to affect the structure, its functioning, and the services.

The issues in healthcare delivery, with their concomitant changes, such as reimbursement regulation and the development of networks for delivery of health care, have profound effects on organizational structure designs. Consumerism, the consumer demand that care be customized to meet individual needs, necessitates that decision-making be done where the care is delivered. Change is ongoing as efforts are made to reduce cost and improve outcomes of health care. Increased consumer knowledge and greater responsibility for selecting healthcare providers and options have resulted in consumers who demand customized care. Competition for clients is another factor influencing structure design. These three factors—consumerism, change, and competition—necessitate reengineering healthcare structures. Whereas **redesign** is a technique to analyze tasks to improve efficiency, and **restructuring** is a technique to enhance organizational productivity, **reengineering** involves a total overhaul of an organizational structure. It is a radical reorganization of the totality of an organization's structure and work processes. In reengineering, fundamentally new organizational expectations and relationships are created. An example of where reengineering is required is technological change, particularly in information services, that provides a means of customizing care. Its potential for making all information concerning a client immediately accessible to direct caregivers has the potential for a profound positive impact on healthcare decision-making.

Regardless of the level of changes made within an organization—redesign, restructuring, or reengineering—the impact is felt by staff and patients alike. Some of the changes result in improvements, whereas others may not; some of the impacts are expected, whereas others are not. It is critical, therefore, that nurse managers as well as staff nurses are vigilant for both anticipated and unanticipated results of these changes. Nurses need to position themselves to participate in change discussions and evaluations. Ultimately, it is their day-to-day work with their patients that is affected by the decisions made in response to a rapidly changing environment (Burke, 2003, 2004). The Literature Perspective describes the effects of hospital restructuring on nurses who remain employed after layoffs.

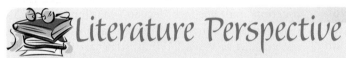 Literature Perspective

Cummings, G. & Estabrooks, C. A. (2003). The effects of hospital restructuring that included layoffs on individual nurses who remained employed: A systematic review of impact. *International Journal of Sociology and Social Policy, 23*(8/9) 8-39.

Healthcare organizations in the United States and Canada—acute care hospitals in particular—have experienced unprecedented changes. The authors categorize these changes into three waves of restructuring. In the mid-1980s, the first wave of restructuring occurred motivated primarily by a desire to maximize the use of registered nurses' time and effort. The results of these efforts include primary nursing and shared governance models. The second wave of restructuring occurred in the 1990s and focused on responding to consumer demands for patient-centered care with emphasis on eliminating inefficiencies, enhancing patient satisfaction, and promoting collaboration amongst caregivers and patients. Ultimately, the goal was to decrease costs and improve quality. Although motives may have been noble, the results were generally mixed. Responding to fiscal challenges and political demands, the third wave of restructuring began in the late 1990s. Widespread reductions in programs as well as in nursing positions were hallmarks of this wave of hospital restructuring.

To better understand the phenomena, the authors undertook a review of the literature on the effects of hospital restructuring that resulted in nursing layoffs. Specifically, they sought to determine the effects on individual hospital nurses. In their review, the authors found significant decreases in job satisfaction, professional efficacy, ability to provide quality care, and physical and emotional health. In addition, they found increases in turnover and disruption of team relationships.

IMPLICATIONS FOR PRACTICE

Survivors of organizational restructuring do not survive unscathed. The effects were greatest for nurses with fewer years of experience and nurses who had experienced multiple restructuring attempts.

During times of restructuring, nurses at all levels must be aware of these potential negative effects and actively develop plans to mitigate them. Research is necessary to identify effective strategies to support nurses and protect patients from the unintended consequences of the identified effects of restructuring.

Exercise 7-3

Arrange to interview a nurse employed in a healthcare agency or use your own experience to identify examples of changes taking place that necessitate reengineering. These may include changes associated with implementation of new reimbursement strategies, development of policies to carry out legislative regulations related to patient confidentiality, or development of chest pain centers for marketing. Identify examples of how previous systems of communication and decision-making were either adequate or inadequate to cope with these changes.

CHARACTERISTICS OF ORGANIZATIONAL STRUCTURES

The characteristics of different types of organizational structures and the theories on which designs are based provide a catalog of options to consider in designing structures that fit specific situations. Knowledge of these characteristics and theories also assists managers in understanding the structures in which they currently function.

An organization is a group of people working together to achieve a purpose. Since time began, people have organized themselves into groups to achieve a common purpose. Organizational theory is based largely on the systematic investigation of the effectiveness of specific organizational designs in achieving their purpose. Organizational theory development is a process of creating knowledge to understand the effect of identified factors, such as (1) organizational culture; (2) organizational technology, which is defined as all the work being carried out; and (3) organizational structure or organizational development. A purpose of such work is to determine how organizational effectiveness might be predicted or controlled through the design of the organizational structure.

Organizational designs are often classified by their characteristics of complexity, formalization, and centralization. Figure 7-2 illustrates specialization, centralization, authority, and responsibility. *Complexity* concerns the division of labor in an organization, the specialization of that labor, the number of hierarchical levels, and the geographic dispersion of organizational units. *Division of labor* and *specialization* refer to the separation of processes into tasks that are performed by designated people. The horizontal dimension of an **organizational chart,** the graphic representation of work units and reporting relationships, relates to the division and specialization of labor functions attended by specialists. **Hierarchy** connotes lines of authority and responsibility. **Chain of command** is a term used to refer to the hierarchy and is depicted in vertical dimensions of organizational charts. Hierarchy vests authority in positions on an ascending line away from where work is performed and allows control of work. Staff members are often placed on a bottom level of the organization, and those in authority, who provide control, are placed in higher levels.

Geographic dispersion refers to the physical location of units. Units of work may be in one building; in several buildings in one location; spread throughout a city; or in different counties, states, or countries. The more dispersed an organization is, the greater are the demands for creative designs that place decision-making related to client care close to the patient and, consequently, far from corporate headquarters. A similar type of complexity exists in organizations that deliver care at multiple sites in the community, such as school health programs in which care delivery sites are located in schools that usually are at great distances from the corporate office that has overall responsibility for the school health program.

Formalization is the degree to which an organization has rules, stated in terms of policies that define a member's function. The amount of formalization varies among institutions. It is often inversely related to the degree of specialization and the number of professionals within the organization.

Exercise 7-4

Review a copy of a nursing department's organizational chart and identify the divisions of labor, the hierarchy of authority, and the degree of formalization.

Centralization refers to the location where a decision is made. Decisions are made at the top of a centralized organization. In a decentralized organization, decisions are made at or close to the patient-care level. Highly centralized organizations delegate *responsibility*—the obligation to perform the task—without the *authority*—the right to act—necessary to carry out the responsibility. For example, some hospitals have delegated—transferred responsibility and authority to act—admission decisions to the charge nurse (decentralized), whereas others require the nurse supervisor or

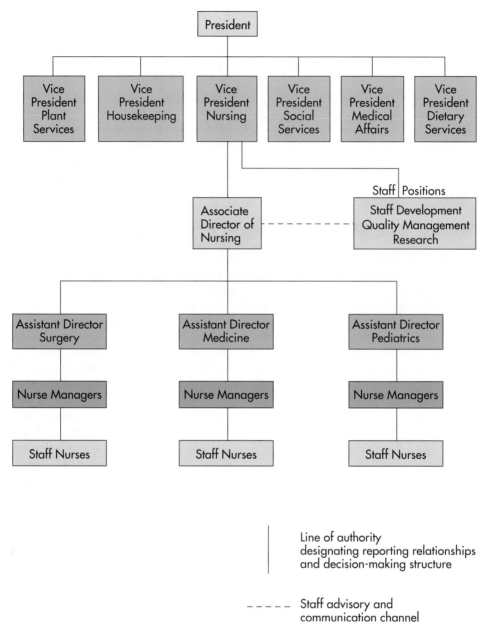

Figure 7-2   A bureaucratic organizational chart depicting specialization of labor, centralization, hierarchical authority, and line and staff responsibilities.

chief nurse executive to make such decisions (centralization).

Exercise 7-5
Review nursing policies in a city health department, a school health office, a home health agency, and a hospital. Are there common policies? Does one of the organizations have more detailed policies than others? Is this formalization consistent with the structural complexity?

BUREAUCRACY

Many organizational theories in use today find their basis in the works of early 21st century theorists Max Weber, a German sociologist who developed the basic tenets of bureaucracy (Weber, 1947), and Henri Fayol, a French industrialist who crafted 14 principles of management (Fayol, 1949). Initially, **bureaucracy** referred to the centralization of authority in administrative bureaus or government departments. The term has come to refer to an inflexible approach to decision-making or an agency encumbered by "red-tape" that adds little value to organizational processes.

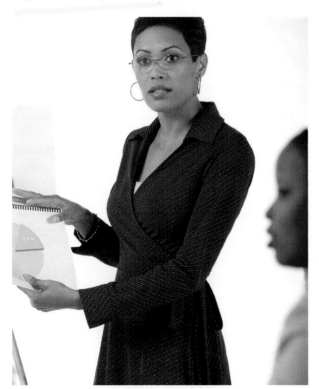

Irrespective of the organizational approach, the chief nurse executive has the authority for nursing services.

Bureaucracy is an administrative concept imbedded in how organizations are structured. It arose at a time of societal development when services were in short supply, workers' and clients' knowledge bases were limited, and technologies for sharing information were undeveloped. Characteristics of bureaucracy arose out of a need to control workers and were centered on the division of processes into discrete tasks. Weber proposed that organizations could only achieve high levels of productivity and efficiency by adherence to what he called "bureaucracy." Weber believed that bureaucracy, based on the sociological concept of rationalization of collective activities, provided the idealized organizational structure. Bureaucratic structures are formal and have a centralized and hierarchical command structure (chain of command). In bureaucratic structures, there is a clear division of labor and well-articulated and commonly accepted expectations for performance. Rules, standards, and protocols ensure uniform actions and limit individualization of services and variance in workers' performance. In bureaucratic organizations, as shown in Figure 7-2, communication and decisions flow from top to bottom. Although it enhances consistency, bureaucracy, by nature, limits employees' autonomy.

In developing his 14 principles of management, Fayol outlined structures and processes that guide how work is accomplished within an organization. Consistent with theories of bureaucracy, his principles of management include division of labor or specialization, clear lines of authority, appropriate levels of discipline, unity of direction, equitable treatment of staff, the fostering of individual initiative, and the promotion of a sense of team work and group pride.

Exercise 7-6
Develop a list of decisions that you as a staff nurse would like to make to optimize care for your patients. Determine where those decisions are made in a nursing organization with which you are familiar. Consider issues such as (1) deciding on visiting schedules that meet your own, your clients', and their significant others' needs and (2) determining a personal work schedule that meets your personal needs and your clients' needs. An example of the latter is talking to the children of a confused elderly client during the evening because they work during the day shift, when you are on duty.

At the time that bureaucracies were developed, these characteristics promoted efficiency and production. As the knowledge base of the general population and employees grew and technologies developed, the bureaucratic structure no longer fit the evolving situation. Increasingly, employees and consumers functioning in bureaucratic situations complain of red tape, procedural delays, and general frustration.

The characteristics of bureaucracy can be present in varying degrees. An organization can demonstrate bureaucratic characteristics in some areas and not in others. For example, nursing staff in intensive care units may be granted autonomy in making and carrying out direct client care decisions, but they may be granted no voice in determining work schedules or financial reimbursement systems for hours worked. One method to determine the extent to which bureaucratic tendencies exist in organizations is to assess the organizational characteristics of labor specialization (the degree to which client care is divided into highly specialized tasks), centralization (the level of the organization on which decisions regarding carrying out work and remuneration for work are made), and formalization (the percentage of actions required to deliver patient care that is governed by written policy and procedures).

Exercise 7-7

Analyze the decisions identified in Exercise 7-6 from a manager's perspective. Is that perspective similar to or different from the original perspective you identified?

Weber and Fayol described decision-making and authority in terms of line and staff functions. **Line functions** are those that involve direct responsibility for accomplishing the objectives of a nursing department, service, or unit. Line positions may include registered nurses, licensed practical/vocational nurses, and unlicensed assistive (or nursing) personnel who have the responsibility for carrying out all aspects of direct care. **Staff functions** are those that assist those in line positions in accomplishing the primary objectives. In this context, the term "staff positions" should not be confused with specific jobs that include "staff" in their names such as "staff nurse" or "staff physician." Staff positions include individuals such as staff development personnel, researchers, and special clinical consultants who are responsible for supporting line positions through activities of consultation, education, role modeling, and knowledge development,

with limited or no direct authority for decision-making. Line personnel have authority for decision-making, whereas personnel in staff positions provide support, advice, and counsel. Organizational charts usually indicate line positions through the use of solid lines and staff positions through broken lines (reminder: in this context, the term "staff position" does not reference staff nurses). Line structures have a vertical line, designating reporting and decision-making responsibility. The vertical line connects all positions to a centralized authority (see Figure 7-2).

To make line and staff functions effective, decision-making authority is clearly spelled out in position descriptions. Effectiveness is further ensured by delineating competencies required for the responsibilities, providing methods for determining whether personnel possess these competencies, and providing means of maintaining and developing the competencies.

Exercise 7-8

Organizational structures vary in the extent to which they have bureaucratic characteristics. Using observations from your current situations, place a check mark (√) in the "Present" column beside the bureaucratic characteristics that you believe apply to the agency. What does this analysis indicate about the bureaucratic tendency of the agency? Do the environment and technologies fit the identified bureaucratic tendency? (Consider the state of development of information systems, method of care delivery, clients' characteristics, workers' characteristics, regulatory status, and competition.)

CHARACTERISTIC	PRESENT
Hierarchy of authority	———
Division of labor	———
Written procedures for work	———
Limited authority for workers	———
Emphasis on written communication related to work performance and workers' behaviors	———
Impersonality of personal contact	———

TYPES OF ORGANIZATIONAL STRUCTURES

In healthcare organizations, there are several common types of organizational structures: functional, service line, matrix, or flat. Nursing orga-

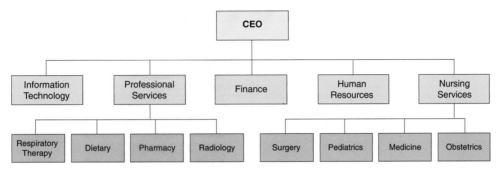

Figure 7-3 Functional structure

nizations often combine characteristics forming a structure that is a hybrid. Shared governance is a term often used to describe the flat types of structures currently being designed to meet the changing needs of nursing organizations.

Functional Structures

Functional structures arrange departments and services according to specialty. This approach to organizational structure is common in healthcare organizations. Departments providing similar functions report to a common manager or executive (Figure 7-3). For example, a healthcare organization with a functional structure would have vice presidents for each major function: nursing, finance, human resources, and information technology.

This organizational structure tends to support professional expertise and encourage advancement. It may, however, result in discontinuity of patient care services. Delays in decision-making can occur if a silo-mentality develops within groups. That is, issues that require communication across functional groups typically must be raised to a senior management level before a decision can be made.

Service-Line Structures

In **service-line structures** (sometimes called product lines), the functions necessary to produce a specific service or product are brought together into an integrated organizational unit under the control of a single manager or executive (Figure 7-4). For example, a cardiology service line at an acute care hospital might include all professional, technical, and support personnel providing services to the cardiac patient population. The manager or executive in this service line would be responsible for the chest pain evaluation center situated within the emergency department, the coronary care unit, the cardiovascular surgery intensive care unit, the telemetry unit, the cardiac catheterization lab, and the cardiac rehabilitation center. In addition to managing the budget and the facilities for these areas, the manager typically would be responsible for coordinating services for the physicians and other providers who admit and care for these patients.

The benefits of a service-line approach to organizational structure include coordination of services, expedited decision-making process, and clarity of purpose. The limitations of this model can include increased expense associated with duplication of services, loss of professional or technical affiliation, and lack of standardization.

Matrix Structures

Matrix structures are complex and designed to reflect both function and service in an integrated organizational structure. In a matrix organization, the manager of a unit responsible for a service reports to both a functional manager and a service or product line manager. For example, a director of pediatric nursing could report to both a vice president for pediatric services (the service line manager) and a vice president of nursing (the functional manager) (Figure 7-5).

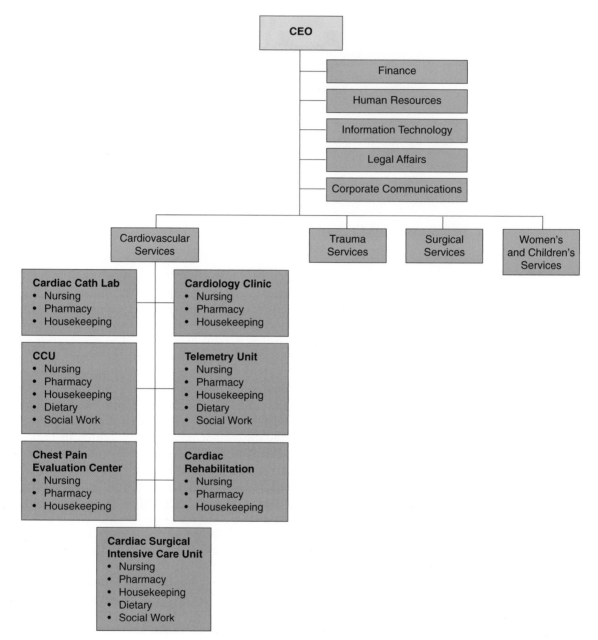

Figure 7-4   Service line structure

Matrix structures can be effective in the current healthcare environment. The matrix design enables timely response to the forces in the external environment that demand continual programming, and it facilitates internal efficiency and effectiveness through the promotion of cooperation among disciplines.

A matrix structure combines both a bureaucratic structure and a flat structure; teams are used to carry out specific programs or projects. A matrix

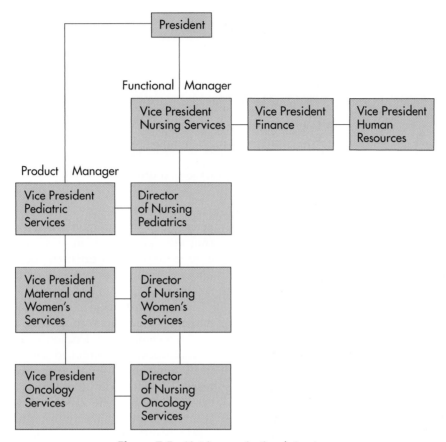

Figure 7-5 Matrix organizational structure

structure superimposes a horizontal program management over the traditional vertical hierarchy. Personnel from various functional departments are assigned to a specific program or project and become responsible to two supervisors—their functional department head and a program manager. This creates an interdisciplinary team.

A line manager and a project manager must function collaboratively in a matrix organization. For example, in nursing, there may be a chief nursing executive, a nurse manager, and staff nurses in the line of authority to accomplish nursing care. In the matrix structure, some of the nurse's time is allocated to project or committee work. Nursing care is delivered in a teamwork setting or within a collaborative model. The nurse is responsible to a nurse manager for nursing care and to a program or project manager when working within the matrix overlay. Well-developed collaboration and coordination skills are essential to effective functioning in a matrix structure. The nature of a matrix

organization with its complex interrelationships requires workers with knowledge and skill in interpersonal relationships and teamwork.

One example of the matrix structure is the patient-focused care delivery model that is being implemented in some facilities. Another example is the program focused on specialty services such as geriatric services, women's services, and cardiovascular services. A matrix model can be designed to cover both a patient-focused care delivery model and a specialty service. Other examples are special healthcare facility programs such as discharge planning, total quality management, and cardiopulmonary resuscitation.

Flat Structures

The primary organizational characteristic of a flat structure is the delegation of decision-making to the professionals doing the work. The term **flat** signifies the removal of hierarchical layers, thereby granting authority to act, and placing authority at

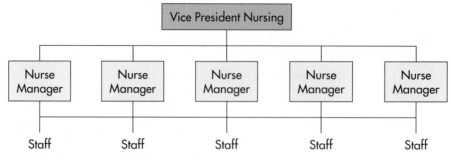

Figure 7-6   Flat organizational structure.

the action level (Figure 7-6). Decisions regarding work methods, nursing care of individual patients, and conditions under which employees work are made where the work is carried out. In a flat organizational structure, decentralized decision-making replaces the centralized decision-making typical of functional structures. Providing staff with authority to make decisions at the place of interaction with clients is the hallmark of a flat organizational structure. Magnet™ hospitals have recognized the benefits of decentralized decision-making and its impact on both nursing satisfaction and patient outcomes (Havens & Johnston, 2004; Manojlovich, 2005).

Flat organizational structures are less formalized than hierarchical organizations. A decrease in strict adherence to rules and policies allows individualized decisions that fit specific situations and meet the needs created by the increasing demands associated with consumerism, change, and competition. Work supported by the Institute for Healthcare Improvement (http://www.ihi.org/IHI/), as an example, capitalizes on decisions being made at the unit level. The focus of this work is to improve patient safety. Therefore, nurses on a clinical unit can make changes in real time rather than use the traditional organizational hierarchy that includes committees and administrative channels.

Decentralized structures are not without their challenges, however. These include the potential for inconsistent decision-making, loss of growth opportunities, and the need to educate managers to communicate effectively and demonstrate creativity in working within these nontraditional structures (McMurray & Williams, 2004).

The degree of flattening varies from organization to organization. Organizations that are decentralizing often retain some bureaucratic char-

acteristics. They may at the same time have units that are operating as matrix structures. **Hybrid** is a term applied to organizational structures that operate with characteristics of different types of structures.

As organizational structures change, some managers are hesitant to relinquish their traditional role in a centralized decision-making process. This reluctance, when combined with recognition of the need to move to a more facilitative role, is partially responsible for the development of hybrid structures. Managers are unsure of what needs to be controlled, how much control is needed, and which mechanisms can replace control. Fear of chaos without control predominates. Education that prepares managers to use leadership techniques that empower nursing staff to take responsibility for their work is one method of minimizing managers' fears. These fears stem from loss of centralized control, as authority with its concomitant responsibilities moves to the place of interaction. The evolutionary development of shared-governance structures in nursing departments demonstrates a type of flat structure being used to replace hierarchical control.

Shared Governance

Shared governance goes beyond participatory management through the creation of organizational structures that allow nursing staff more autonomy to govern their practice (Batson, 2004). Accountability forms the foundation for designing professional governance models. To be accountable, authority to make decisions concerning all aspects of responsibilities is essential. This need for authority and accountability is particularly important for nurses who treat the wide range of human responses to wellness states and illness. Organizations where professional autonomy is encouraged have demonstrated higher levels of staff satisfaction, enhanced productivity, and improved retention (Manojlovich, 2005; Martin et al, 2004).

A major cause of nurses' dissatisfaction with their work revolves around the absence of professional autonomy and accountability. The early Magnet hospital study (McClure, Poulin, Sovie, & Wandelt, 1983), which identified characteristics of hospitals successful in recruiting and retaining nurses, found that nursing departments with structures that provided nurses the opportunity to be accountable for their own practice were the major contributing characteristic to success. Studies of Magnet hospitals demonstrate that governance structures provide nurses with accountability that will be effective in recruiting and retaining nursing staff while also meeting consumers' demands and remaining competitive. These findings continue to be validated and expanded upon (Aiken, Havens, & Sloane, 2000; Kramer & Schmalenberg, 2004; Taylor, 2005). Magnet characteristics are now accepted as impacting not only the quality of the work environment but also the quality of patient care. The Research Perspective box presents a study on the link between workplace empowerment and Magnet hospitals.

Shared or self-governance structures, sometimes referred to as *professional practice models*, go beyond decentralizing and diminishing hierarchies. In an organization that embraces shared governance, the structure's foundation is the professional workplace rather than the organizational hierarchy. Shared governance vests the necessary levels of authority and accountability for all aspects of the nursing practice in the nurses responsible for the delivery of care. The management and administrative level serves to coordinate and facilitate the work of the practicing nurses. Mechanisms are designed outside of the traditional hierarchy to provide for the functional areas needed to support professional practice. These functions include areas such as quality management, competency definition and evaluation, and continuing education. Changing nurses' positions from dependent employees to independent, accountable professionals is a prerequisite for the radical redesign of healthcare organizations that is required to create value for

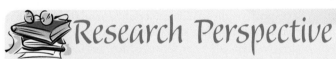

Research Perspective

Spence-Laschinger, H. K., Almost, J., & Tuer-Hodes, D. (2003). Workplace empowerment and Magnet hospital characteristics: Making the link. *Journal of Nursing Administration, 33*(7/8), 410-422.

Built upon Kanter's empowerment theory, this study tested a theoretical model that linked Magnet hospital characteristics, nurses' perception of their level of empowerment in the work environment, and job satisfaction. The model was tested using secondary data analysis from studies in three different work settings in Ontario, Canada. Two of the studies involved staff nurses, and one involved acute care nurse practitioners. Analysis of the three studies all support the hypothesized positive relationship between structural empowerment factors and the Magnet hospital characteristics of autonomy, positive physician-nurse relationships, and control over professional practice. Working in an environment that supports empowered nurses described in terms of the core Magnet characteristics was significantly predictive of the nurses' job satisfaction.

IMPLICATIONS FOR PRACTICE

This study supports the belief that organizational efforts to create a professional work environment and empower nurses will result in positive patient and organizational outcomes. Nurse administrators can use the results from this study to guide their work redesign efforts as they seek to create organizations that provide the highest quality of care by the recruitment and retention of professional nurses into an empowered work environment.

BOX 7-2

Shared-Governance Structure Evolution

Phase One

Representative staff nurses are members of clinical forums, which have authority for designated practice issues and some authority for determining roles, functions, and processes. Managers are members of the management forums, which are responsible for the facilitation of practice through resource management and location. Recommendations for action go to the executive committee, which has administrative and staff membership that may or may not be in equal proportion. The nurse executive retains decision-making authority.

Phase Two

Representative staff nurses belong to nursing committees that are designated for specific management and/or

clinical functions. These committees are chaired by staff nurses or administrators appointed by the vice president of nursing. The nursing committee chairs and nurse administrators make up the nursing cabinet, which makes the final decision on recommendations from the committees.

Phase Three

Representative staff nurses belong to councils with authority for specific functions. Council chairs make up the management committee charged with making all final operational organizational decisions.

---

clients. It requires administrators, managers, and staff to abandon traditional notions regarding the division of labor in healthcare organizations. Structures of shared governance organizations vary. Box 7-2 shows three governance structures in progressive stages of evolution. As shown, evolution is moving structure beyond committees imposed on hierarchical structures to governance structures at the unit level.

Shared governance structures require new behaviors of all staff, not just new assignments of accountability. The areas of interpersonal relationship development, conflict resolution, and personal acceptance of responsibility for action are of particular importance (Burnhope & Edmonstone, 2003). Education, experience in group work, and conflict management are essential for successful transitions.

ANALYZING ORGANIZATIONS

When an organization is analyzed, it is important to scrutinize the various systems that exist to accomplish the work of the enterprise. This includes delineating the processes or procedures that have been developed to coordinate the work to be done. To conceptualize how the organization functions, it is imperative to know the recruitment proce-

dures, the method of selecting individuals for positions, the reporting relationships, the information network, and the governance structure for nurses. A positive organization reflects a fit of the mission, vision, and philosophy with the structure and practices. Understanding the criteria for Magnet facilities (American Nurses Credentialing Center, 2004), irrespective of structure, could form the basis for evaluating nursing services.

EMERGING FLUID RELATIONSHIPS

As the continuum of care moves health services outside of institutional parameters, different skill sets, relationships, and behavioral patterns will be required. Organizations are beginning to lose their traditional boundaries. Old boundaries of hierarchy, function, and geography are disappearing. Vertical integration aligns dissimilar but related entities such as hospital, home care agency, rehabilitation center, long-term care facility, insurance provider, and medical office/clinic. New technologies, fast-changing markets, and global competition are revolutionizing relationships in health care, and the roles that people play and the tasks that they perform have become blurred and ambiguous.

In the future, nurses will no longer practice in geographically limited settings, but rather in systems of care that have extended boundaries. Reframing or changing current organizations will require significant effort focused on a four-dimensional process (human, structural, political, and symbolic). In future organizations, healthcare delivery businesses will be knowledge-based organizations largely comprising specialists who direct their performance through organized feedback from colleagues, customers, and headquarters (Vander Woude & Letcher, 2005). Nurses need to be able to participate as active members of a living-learning organization. Nurses, whether leaders,

managers, or staff, must have the ability to work with other members of the organization and with society at large to design organizational models for care delivery that meet patient/customer needs and priorities. It is essential to take a new look at the nature of the work of nursing and propose innovative models for nursing practice that take into account emerging labor-saving assistive technologies and rapidly changing healthcare needs. Employee participation and learning environments go hand in hand, and work redesign needs to be regarded as a continuous process. It is essential that nurses value their own and others' autonomy to deal successfully in these new structures.

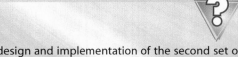

The Solution

Immediately, I established what the management structure would be. For example, I changed the scope of responsibility for the individual managers. I then actively recruited for those positions and put in place specific retention strategies to ensure that those who were already a part of the team were engaged in the new direction. I also created a staff development position to fulfill my strategy of clinical management.

After I created the management team, I created core competencies for the clinical staff. Obviously, staff representatives participated in the establishment and design of the initial set of competencies. Now we are working

on the design and implementation of the second set of competencies that are more unit-specific. It really is exciting to see how the nurses here have focused their energy in meeting this challenge. I am very fortunate, also, that the staff development educator has had experience in a university, and, therefore, she has connections for recruitment, and she is acutely aware of standards and consistency.

— Rebecca M. Patton

 Would this approach be suitable for you? Why?

CHAPTER CHECKLIST

The mission, vision, and philosophy of the organization determine how nursing care is delivered in a healthcare organization. Changes occurring in the organization's mission affect both the culture of the workplace and the philosophies regarding the work required to accomplish the mission. Actualizing new missions and philosophies requires reengineered organizational structures that places decision-making authority and responsibility where care is delivered. Decision-making responsibility requires staff to understand the organization's mission and to participate in the development of mission and philosophy statements.

■ Five factors influencing design of an organization structure are:
  • The types of service performed or the product produced
  • The characteristics of the employees performing the service or producing the product
  • The beliefs and values held by the people responsible for delivering the service concerning the work, the people receiving the services, and the employees
  • The technologies used to perform the service and produce the product
  • The needs, desires, and characteristics of the consumers using the product or service

Continued

- Reengineering, the complete overhaul of an organization's structures, is driven by forces of the following:
  - Change
  - Consumerism
  - Competition
- Bureaucratic structures are characterized by the following:
  - A high degree of formalization
  - Centralization of decision-making at the top of the organization
  - A hierarchy of authority
  - Structures can be organized along the following lines:
    - Functional
    - Service
    - Matrix
    - Flat
- Functional structures are characterized by the following:
  - Departments and services organized according to specialty
  - Discontinuity of patient services due to silomentality, even when structure supports professional expertise and encourages advancement
- Service structures are characterized by the following:
  - Functions necessary to provide a specific service brought together under a single line of authority
- Matrix structures are characterized by the following:
  - Dual authority for product and function
  - Mechanisms such as committees to coordinate actions of product and function managers
  - Success that is dependent on recognition and appreciation of each others' missions and philoso-phies and commitment to the organization's mission and philosophy
- Flat organizations are characterized by the following:
  - Decision-making concerning work performed, decentralized to the level where the work is done
  - Authority, accountability, and autonomy, as well as responsibility, provided to staff performing care
  - Low level of formalization in relation to rules, with processes tailored to meet individual consumer's needs
- Mission, vision, and philosophy determine the characteristics of the organizational structure by doing the following:
  - Describing the consumers and services as a pre-scription for the technologies and human resources needed to accomplish the defined purpose (mission)
  - Creating an ultimate state of existence (vision)
  - Citing values and beliefs that shape and are shaped by the nature of the work and the rights and responsibilities of workers and consumers (philosophy)
  - Designing characteristics that support the service implementation to fulfill the mission and philosophy (structure)
- Shared governance is characterized by the following:
  - The creation of organizational structures that allow nursing staff more autonomy to govern their practice
  - Recruitment and retention of nursing staff while meeting patient needs in an effective and efficient manner

TIPS ON UNDERSTANDING ORGANIZATIONAL STRUCTURES

- The mission of the organization and the mission for the specific unit in which a professional nurse is employed or is seeking employment provide knowledge concerning the major focus for the work to be accomplished.
- Understanding the philosophy of the organization and/or unit where work occurs provides knowledge of the behaviors that are valued in the delivery of client care and in interactions with persons employed by the organization.
- Organizational structures describe channels of communication and decision-making.
- Matrix organizations usually have two persons responsible for the work, and, therefore, it is important to know to whom you are responsible for what.
- For a shared-governance structure to function effectively, mechanisms must be put in place to promote decision-making about client care by the professionals providing the care.
- Professional nurses in staff or followership positions need to understand the mission, vision, philosophy, and organizational structure to maximize their contributions to patient care.

TERMS TO KNOW

bureaucracy
chain of command
flat organization
functional structure
hierarchy
hybrid
line function
matrix structure
mission
organizational chart
organizational culture
organizational structure
philosophy
redesign
reengineering
restructuring
service line
shared governance
staff function
structure
vision

REFERENCES

Aiken, L. H., Havens, D. S., & Sloane, D. M. (2000). The Magnet Nursing Services Recognition Program: A comparison of two groups of Magnet hospitals. *American Journal of Nursing, 100*(3), 26-36.

American Nurses Credentialing Center. (2004). *Health care organization instructions and application process manual.* Washington, DC: Author.

Batson, V. (2004). Shared governance in an integrated health care system. *AORN Online, 80*(3), 493-514.

Burke, R. J. (2003). Hospital restructuring stressors: Support and nursing staff perceptions of unit functioning. *Health Care Manager, 22*(3), 241-248.

Burke, R. J. (2004). Implementation of hospital restructuring and nursing staff perceptions of hospital functioning. *Journal of Health Organizations and Management, 18*(4), 279-289.

Burnhope, C., & Edmonstone, J. (2003). "Feel the fear and do it anyway": the hard business of developing shared governance. *Journal of Nursing Management, 11,* 147-157.

Cummings, G., & Estabrooks, C. C. (2003). The effects of hospital restructuring that include layoffs on individual nurses who remain employed. *International Journal of Sociology and Social Policy, 23*(4), 8-39.

Forsythe, L. L. (2005). Using an organizational culture analysis to design interventions for change. *AORN Journal, 816*(6), 1288-1302.

Fayol, H. (1949). *General and industrial management.* London: Pitman.

Havens, D. S., & Johnston, M. A. (2004). Achieving Magnet hospital recognition: Chief nurse executives and Magnet coordinators tell their stories. *Journal of Nursing Administration, 34*(12), 579-588.

Ingersoll, G. L., Witzel, A. A., & Smith, T. C. (2005). Using organizational mission, vision, and values to guide professional practice development and measurement of nurse performance. *Journal of Nursing Administration, 35*(2), 89-93.

Kramer, M. & Schmalenberg, C. (2004). Essentials of a Magnetic work environment. *Nursing, 34*(6), 50-54.

Laschinger, H. K. S., & Finegan, J. (2005). Using empowerment to build trust and respect in the workplace: A strategy for addressing the nursing shortage. *Nursing Economics, 23*(1), 6-13.

Manojlovich, M. (2005). Predictors of professional nursing practice behaviors in hospital settings. *Nursing Research, 54*(1), 41-47.

Martin, P. A., Gustin, T. J., Uddin, D. E., & Risner, P. (2004). Organizational dimensions of hospital nursing practice: Longitudinal results. *Journal of Nursing Administration, 34*(12), 554-561.

McClure, M. L., Poulin, M. A., Sovie, M. D., & Wandelt, M. A. (1983). *Magnet hospitals, attrition and retention of professional nurses*. Kansas City, MO: American Nurses Association.

McMurray, A. J., & Williams, L. (2004). Factors impacting on nurse managers' ability to be innovative in a decentralized management structure. *Journal of Nursing Management, 12*(5), 348-353.

Spence-Laschinger, H. K., Almost, J., & Tuer-Hodes, D. (2003). Workplace empowerment and Magnet hospital characteristics: Making the link. *Journal of Nursing Administration, 33*(7/8), 410-422.

Taylor, N. T. (2005). The magnetic pull. *Nursing Management, 36*(1), 36-43.

Vander Woude, D. L., & Letcher, D. C. (2005). Becoming a living-learning organization. *Nursing Science Quarterly, 18*(1), 24-30.

Weber, M. (1947). *The theory of social and economic organization*. Parsons, NY: Free Press.

SUGGESTED READINGS

Adams, A., & Bond, S. (2003). Staffing in acute hospital wards: Part 1. The relationship between the number of nurses and ward organizational environment. *Journal of Nursing Management, 11*(5), 287-292.

Aiken, L. H., Clarke, S. P., & Sloane, D. M. (2000). Hospital restructuring: Does it adversely affect care and outcomes? *Journal of Nursing Administration, 30*(10), 457-465.

Aiken, L. H., & Patrician, P. A. (2000). Measuring organizational traits of hospitals: The revised nursing work index. *Nursing Research, 49*(3), 146-153.

Batson, V. (2004). Shared governance in an integrated health care network. *AORN Journal, 80*(3), 493-514.

Carkhuff, M. W. (2004). Advanced organizers: A framework to implement learning readiness in support of broad-scale change. *Journal of Continuing Education in Nursing, 35*(5), 216-221.

Castledine, G. (2004). How to run an efficient and safe nurse-led service. *British Journal of Nursing, 13*(18), 115.

Guinane, C. S., & Davis, N. H. (2004). The science of Six Sigma in hospitals. *The American Heart Hospital Journal, 2*(1), 42-48.

Hess, R. G. (2004). From bedside to boardroom—nursing shared governance. *Online Journal of Issues in Nursing, 9*(1), Manuscript 1.

Kennedy, S. H. (1996). Effects of shared governance on perceptions of work and work environment. *Nursing Economics, 14*(2), 111-116.

Martin, P. A. (2004). Organizational dimensions of hospital nursing practice. *Journal of Nursing Administration, 34*(12), 554-561.

McHugh, N. (2004). Improving staff member satisfaction and productivity through technology. *AORN Journal, 80*(3), 523-526.

Porter-O'Grady, T. (1996). The seven basic rules for redesign. *Journal of Nursing Administration, 26*(1), 46-53.

Poteet, G., & Hill, A. (1988). Identifying the components of a nursing service philosophy. *Journal of Nursing Administration, 18*(10), 29-35.

Schryer, N. (2004). Implementing organizational redesign to support practice: The Tulane model. *Journal of Nursing Administration, 34*(9), 400-406.

Trossman, S. (2004). A magnetic force: ANCC program gains recognition in ensuring excellence in nursing service. *American Journal of Nursing, 104*(12), 68-69.

Upennieks, V. V. (2003). The interrelationship of organizational characteristics of Magnet hospitals, nursing leadership and nursing job satisfaction. *Health Care Manager, 22*(2), 83-98.

Vogeler, S. (2004). The heart of efficiency. *Health Management Technology, 25*(12), 20-25. www.nursingworld.org/ancc/magnet

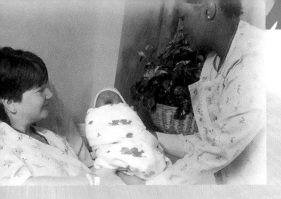

Chapter

8

Cultural Diversity in Health Care

Dorothy A. Otto
Ana M. Valadez

*T*his chapter focuses on the importance of cultural considerations for patients and staff. Although it does not address comprehensive details about any specific culture, it does provide guidelines for actively incorporating cultural aspects into the roles of leading and managing. It presents concepts and principles of transculturalism, describes techniques for managing a culturally diverse workforce, emphasizes the importance of respecting different lifestyles, and discusses the effects of diversity on staff performance. Scenarios and exercises to promote an appreciation of cultural richness are also included.

Objectives

- Evaluate the use of concepts and principles of culture, cultural diversity, and cultural sensitivity in leading and managing situations.
- Analyze differences between cross-cultural, transcultural, multicultural, and intracultural concepts and cultural marginality.
- Describe common characteristics of any culture.
- Illustrate the richness of cultures as they relate to staff and patients through storytelling.

- Evaluate individual and societal factors involved with cultural diversity.
- Compare values and beliefs about illness that affect management of

nursing care interventions involving patients from specific cultures.
- Use tools to address staff and patient cultural diversity.

Questions to Consider

- *Why is it necessary to understand values, beliefs, and rituals held by culturally diverse staff and patients?*
- *What implications would "cultural sensitivity" have for you as a nurse leader or manager?*
- *In what ways do health-related or personal problems vary with the culture of patients and staff?*
- *What specific tools could you use to incorporate cultural diversity into your practice setting?*

The Challenge

Sally C. Fernandez, RN, MSN, ANP
Nurse Manager, Emergency Center, University of Texas M.D. Anderson Cancer Center,
   Houston, Texas

I work with a large staff of females and males from several cultures and they have different perspectives about their assignments. Hispanics, Asians, Asian Indians, and Nigerians provide a challenge for me. If I try to address a work issue, such as assignments, some become defensive. Some males feel that they are superior to me. It might be because I am female. In contrast, I have noticed that some Asians are more submissive and do better with female-to-female interactions. We frequently have a high patient census in the emergency department. There are times when either the charge nurse or I tell staff members to complete a task more quickly within their assignment, due to the number of patients waiting to be seen in the emergency department. This does not set well with some staff, who tend to become defensive. For example, a male staff member of one culture felt he was being "overpowered" by the charge nurse from another culture.

 What do you think you would do if you were this nurse manager?

INTRODUCTION

Nurse leaders and managers are concerned with cultural diversity from two perspectives: the care of a diverse patient population and positive work experiences in a culturally diverse workforce. In its report to the Secretary of Health & Human Resources and Congress, the National Advisory Council on Nurse Education and Practice (NACNEP, 2000) addressed the need for a culturally diverse workforce to meet the healthcare needs of our nation. The Council defined that a national action-oriented agenda is needed to address the under-representation of racial-ethnic minorities in the workforce. To this end, the NACNEP solicited, through the Division of Nursing, an Expert Workgroup on Diversity to advise them on the development of the National Agenda. The workgroup based their recommendations on four overarching goals. The four goals addressed are (1) enhancing efforts to increase the recruitment, retention, and subsequent graduation of minority nurses; (2) promoting leadership development for minority nurses; (3) developing a practice environment that promotes diversity; and (4) promoting the preparation of all nurses so that culturally competent care can be provided. The more recent Sullivan Commission (2005) was equally concerned with diversity of all healthcare professions.

The American Nurses Association (ANA) has a long and vital history supporting ethics, human rights, and numerous efforts to eliminate discriminatory practices against nurses as well as patients. ANA position statements that will be published in 2006 pending review include: *Cultural Diversity in Nursing Practice* (October 22, 1991) and *Discrimination and Racism in Health Care* (March 26, 1998) (ANA NursingWorld, 2005). The ANA *Code of Ethics for Nurses with Interpretative Statements*, Provision 8 states: "The nurse collaborates with other health professionals and the public in promoting community, national, and international efforts to meet health needs" (2001, p. 23). This provision helps the nurse recognize that health care must be provided to culturally diverse populations in the United States and in all continents of the world. Although a nurse may have the inclination to impose his or her own cultural values on others, avoiding this imposition affirms the respect and sensitivity for the values and healthcare practices associated with different cultures. For example, participating in a medical mission trip to provide primary care and treatment with "American drugs" to Indian family members in the mountainous villages of Honduras where natural sources are used to treat injuries, illnesses, and diseases is an imposition of healthcare views. To be more culturally appropriate, the mission team might focus on health assessments in relationship to cultural mores and needs of these indigent people.

Global occurrences offer frequent opportunities for nursing's growing interconnectedness with other countries. The globalization reinforces the significance of international values, standards, and competencies. The International Council of Nurses' (ICN, 2003) *Framework of Competencies for the Generalist Nurse* helps clarify the role of nurses and provides guidelines related to nursing's role and scope of practice in a healthcare delivery system. The framework requires interpretation by each country to allow for flexibility for competencies that are deemed essential and adequately comprehensive to the country's health needs and priorities (Hancock, 2004).

American health care has consistently focused on individuals and their health problems, yet we have failed some people as a group in recognizing their cultural differences, beliefs, symbolisms, and interpretations of illness. Commonly, these patients for whom healthcare practitioners provide care are newcomers to health care in the United States. Similarly, new staff are neither acculturated nor assimilated into the cultural values of the dominant **culture.** The knowledge base necessary for providers to recognize and manage cultural differences of patients and staff must be addressed. For example, communication barriers might occur when an Egyptian physician, a Russian nursing student, and a white American faculty member take care of a Mexican National patient receiving chemotherapy.

Accessibility to health care in the United States is linked to specific social strata. This challenges nurse leaders, managers, and followers who strive for worth, recognition, and individuality for patients and staff regardless of their ascribed economic and social standing. Beginning nurse leaders, managers, and followers may sense that the knowledge they bring to their job lacks "real-life" experiences that provide the springboard to address staff and patient needs. In reality, although lack of experience may be slightly hampering, it is by no means an obstacle to addressing individualized attention to staff and patients. The key is that if the nurse manager and staff respect people and their needs, economic and social standing becomes a moot point. Nurse managers must be cognizant of divergent views about health care as a right for all people rather than a privilege for a few.

Resources are a must for nurses to use to learn about working with culturally diverse staff and patients. D'Avanzo and Geissler (2003) wrote a fitting resource book about a variety of cultural groups, their differences in worldwide views and concepts of reality, and their variety of social, political, economic, religious values, and many concepts of health and illness. They noted that diversity exists both within and between groups, which may lead to intra-group and inter-group conflict. Lipson and Dibble (2005) indicated that culture is influenced by intersections of forces larger than the individual and by shared values of what constitutes ethical, professional practice. They provide an excellent set of general guidelines to alert nurses in the hospital or community settings to the similarities and differences within and among the cultural and ethnic groups. They have expanded the types of cultural and ethnic groups to include Roma (gypsies), former Yugoslavians, Russians, and other former Soviet Union people. All the cultural groups were selected based on their size according to the U.S. Census (each numbering at least 100,000) and/or on the lack of readily obtainable information elsewhere about a particular group. *Caring for women cross-culturally* (St. Hill, Lipson, & Meleis, 2003) is a rich, comprehensive resource of culturally relevant information about immigrant and minority women. Interspersed through each chapter are "notes to health providers." These notes purport to alert the provider to potential problems the nurse may encounter at certain developmental stages or when dealing with a particularly sensitive topic. The authors offer suggestions of helpful ways to approach these issues.

Meaning of Diversity in the Organization

The 2003 *Employment Status of the Civilian Population by Sex, Race and Ethnicity (No. 571)* provided important data for comparison (Table 8-1) of the civilian employment labor force (actual number and employment population ratio). There were 73,332,000 (56.1%) males; 64,404,000 (56.1%) females; 114,235,000 whites; 14,739,000 (83%) blacks; 5,756,000 (4%) Asians; and 17,372,000 (13%) Hispanics, including Mexicans, Puerto Ricans, and Cubans (U.S. Bureau of Labor Statistics, Bulletin 2307). By comparison, the registered nurse employment data (Table 8-2) reported a total employment of registered nurses as 2,449,000 of which approximately 93% were female, 7%

Table 8-1	CIVILIAN EMPLOYMENT [EMPLOYED] LABOR FORCE (WITH EMPLOYMENT POPULATION RATIO)—2003
Males	73,332,000 (69.1%)
Females	64,404,000 (56.1%)
Whites	114,235,000 (83%)
Blacks	14,739,000 (11%)
Asians	5,756,000 (4%)
Hispanics*	17,372,000 (13%)

*Includes Mexicans, Puerto Ricans, and Cubans.

Table 8-2	EMPLOYED CIVILIANS BY OCCUPATION, SEX, RACE, AND HISPANIC ORIGIN: REGISTERED NURSES, 2004
Total Employment—RNs 2,449,000	**Percentage of Total, %**
Females	93.0
Males	7.0
Blacks	10.0
Asian	7.0
Hispanic	3.9

were male; approximately 10% were black; 7% were Asian; and 4% were Hispanic in the *Employed Civilians By Occupation, Sex, Race, and Hispanic Origin. (No. 597)* (U.S. Census, 2004).

Health disparities between majority and racial ethnic minority populations are not new issues and continue to be problematic as they exist for multiple and complex reasons. Causes of disparities in health care include poor education, health behaviors of the minority group, inadequate financial resources, and environmental factors. Disparities in health care that relate to quality of care include provider/patient relationships, provider bias and discrimination, and patient variables of mistrust of the healthcare system and refusal of treatment (Baldwin, 2003). Health disparities in ethnic and racial groups are observed in cardiovascular disease, which is 40% higher in U.S. blacks than in U.S. whites; cancer with a death rate for all cancers is 30% higher in U.S. blacks than in U.S.

whites, and Hispanics with diabetes are twice as likely to die from this disease than non-Hispanic whites. In 2000, American Indians had a life expectancy that was 5 years less than the national average, whereas, Asian and Pacific Islanders were considered among the healthiest population groups. However, within the Asian Pacific Islanders, there was greater diversity within their population in regard to health outcomes. Solutions to health and healthcare disparities among ethnic and racial populations must be accomplished through research to improve care. Such research could include preventive services, health education and interventions, treatment services, and health outcomes (Baldwin, 2003). Consider how these disparities in disease and in healthcare services might impact the healthcare providers in the workplace in relationship to their ethnic or racial group. What should you know about the sick-leave policy based on acute or chronic disease/illness in your institution? Portillo (2003, p. 5) wrote that "our leadership efforts will have to move beyond the beginning to reduce health disparities. A better understanding of the strengths and limitations of the concepts of race and ethnicity is a priority of nursing." It is necessary to increase healthcare providers' knowledge so that they can more effectively manage and treat diseases related to ethnic and racial minorities, which might include themselves.

Leading and managing cultural diversity in an organization means managing personal thinking and helping others to think in new ways. Managing issues that involve culture—whether institutional, ethnic, gender, religious, or any other kind—requires patience, persistence, and much understanding. One way to promote this understanding is through shared stories that have symbolic power.

Exercise 8–1

Think of a recent event in your workplace, such as a project, task force, celebration, or something similar. What meaning did people give the event? Was it viewed as being a symbol of some quality of the workplace, such as its effectiveness, its values and beliefs, or its innovations?

Staff who know what is valuable to patients and to themselves can act accordingly and feel good about work. Having a clear mission, goals, rewards, and acknowledgment of efforts leads to a greater productivity and work effort from a culturally diverse staff that aspires to unity and uniqueness. When assessing staff diversity, the nurse leader or manager can ask these two questions:

- What is the cultural representation of the workforce?
- What kind of team-building activities are needed to create a cohesive workforce for effective healthcare delivery?

Box 8-1 lists some of the techniques that may be effective when managing a culturally diverse workforce.

CONCEPTS AND PRINCIPLES

What is *culture*? Does it exhibit certain characteristics? What is *cultural diversity,* and what do we think of when we refer to *cultural sensitivity*? Are *culture* and *ethnicity* the same? Various authors have different views. Spector (2000) specified that cultural background is a fundamental component of one's ethnic background. **Ethnicity** includes, but is not limited to, characteristics such as "migratory status, . . . race, . . . language and dialect, . . . an internal sense of distinctiveness, and . . . an external perception of distinctiveness" (p. 81).

Inherent characteristics of **culture** are often identified with the following four factors: (1) It develops over time and is responsive to its members and their familial and social environments, (2) its members learn it and share it, (3) it is essential for survival and acceptance, and (4) it changes with difficulty. For the nurse leader or manager, the characteristics of ethnicity and culture are important to keep in mind because the underlying thread in all of them is that staff's and patients' culture and ethnicity have been with them their entire lives. They view their cultural background as normal; the diversity challenge is for others to view it as normal also and to assimilate it into the existing workforce. **Cultural diversity** is the term currently used to describe a vast range of cultural differences among individuals or groups; whereas, **cultural sensitivity** describes the affective behaviors in individuals—the capacity to feel, convey, or react to ideas, habits, customs, or traditions unique to a group of people.

Based on the *Code of Ethics for Nurses* (ANA, 2001), nurses believe that they must care for all patients regardless of differences—whether it be cultural, economic status, or gender. Nursing a person or people from a culture other than one's own is a dynamic and complex experience. The experience according to Spence (2004) might

---

BOX 8-1

Techniques for Managing a Culturally Diverse Workforce

- Have patience. Treat all questions as equally important even though they may be common everyday knowledge to you.
- Be cognizant that foreign or minority staff may not consider themselves deprived or of lesser socioeconomic status than the majority.
- Do not treat gender bias or those with different lifestyles as needing intervening techniques to change behaviors. Assume they are happy with their choice.
- Do not assume emotional outbursts represent anger. This may be a natural communication style for different groups.
- Treat compliments from your staff with respect. Avoid feeling that they are trying to request a special favor from you. In some cultures, compliments are used quite often to demonstrate respect.

- Do not assume that physical features denote a specific race or ethnic identity. Some Hispanics demonstrate Asian features, whereas some Puerto Ricans or Jamaicans may be mistaken for African blacks.
- Take the time to know your colleagues. Make time for conversational chats that will facilitate learning about each other.
- Always remember that the less you know about your staff, the more difficult your job will be as an effective manager.
- Be aware that people in your workforce may at one time or another have actually felt a part of an oppressed group. Give them a feeling of value and dignity.

involve "prejudice, paradox and possibility." Using hermeneutic interpretation, her study consisted of accounts from 17 New Zealand nurses who delivered nursing care to patients in acute medical and surgical wards, public health centers, mental health settings and midwifery specialties. Spence used prejudice as conditions that enabled or constrained interpretation based on one's values, attitudes, and actions. By talking with people outside one's "circle of familiarity," one can enhance one's understanding of personally held prejudices.

Exercise 8-2

In a group, discuss the values and beliefs of justice and equality. As a nurse, you might have strong values and beliefs, but you may never have observed their application in health care. Consider language, skin color, dress, and gestures of patients and staff from other cultures. How will you learn and value what differences exist? Prejudices "enable us to make sense of the situations in which we find ourselves, yet they also constrain understanding and limit the capacity to come to new or different ways of understanding. It is this contradiction that makes prejudice paradoxical" (Spence, 2004, p. 163). Paradox, although it may seem incongruent with prejudice, describes the dynamic interplay of tensions between individuals or groups. It is our responsibility to acknowledge the "possibility of tension" as a potential for new and different understandings derived from our communication and interpretation. Possibility, therefore, presumes a condition for openness with a person from another culture (Spence, 2004).

The lack of mutual understanding between healthcare providers and immigrants, particularly children and adolescents, has been addressed by Choi (2001). She explored the concept of **cultural marginality,** which she defined as "situations and feelings of passive between-ness when people exist between two different cultures and do not yet perceive themselves as centrally belonging to either one" (p. 193). A model cultural marginality case of a 15-year-old high school student who moved to the United States from Korea when she was 14 years old is described by Choi.

Exercise 8-3

Reflect on your experiences with immigrant adolescents in which cultural marginality—the between-ness—was an existing challenge to them, as well as with their family members or peers. In what ways did values change as new generations of a culture group adopt the new country's views over time? Consider that first-generation groups very often have stronger ties to traditions and customs from their country of origin than second and third generations.

How do leaders, managers, or followers take all of the expanding information on the diversity of healthcare beliefs and practices and give it some organizing structure to provide culturally competent and culturally sensitive care to patients or clients? Purnell and Paulanka (2003), Campinha-Bacote (1999, 2002), Giger and Davidhizar (2002), and Leininger (2002a) provide an overview of each of their theoretical models to guide healthcare providers for delivering culturally competent and culturally sensitive care in the workplace.

Purnell and Paulanka's (2003) Model for Cultural Competence provides an organizing framework. The model uses a circle with the outer zone representing global society, the second zone representing community, the third zone representing family, and the inner zone representing the person. The interior of the circle is divided into 12 pie-shaped wedges delineating cultural domains and their concepts, for example, workplace issues, family roles and organization, spirituality, and healthcare practices. The innermost center circle is black, representing unknown phenomena. Cultural consciousness is expressed in behaviors from "unconsciously incompetent—consciously incompetent—consciously competent to unconsciously competent" (p. 10). The usefulness of this model is derived from its concise structure, applicability to any setting, and wide range of experiences that can foster inductive and deductive thinking when assessing cultural domains.

Campinha-Bacote's (1999, 2002) culturally competent model of care identifies five constructs: (1) awareness, (2) knowledge, (3) skill, (4) encounters, and (5) desire. She defined **cultural competence** as "the process in which the healthcare provider continuously strives to achieve the ability to effectively work within the cultural context of a client (individual, family, or community)" (1999, p. 203). Cultural awareness is the self examination and in-depth exploration of one's own cultural and professional background. It involves the recognition of one's bias, prejudices, and assumptions abut the individuals who are different (2002) "One's world view can be considered a paradigm or way of viewing the world and phenomena in it" (1999,

p. 204). Cultural knowledge is the process of seeking and obtaining a sound educational foundation about diverse cultural and ethnic groups. Obtaining cultural information about the patient's health-related beliefs and values will help to explain how he/she interprets his/her illness and how it guides his/her thinking, doing, and being (2002). The skill of conducting a cultural assessment is learned while assessing one's values, beliefs, and practices to provide culturally competent services. The process of cultural encounters encourages direct engagement in cross-cultural interactions with individuals from other cultures. This process allows the person to validate, negate, or modify his or her existing cultural knowledge. It provides culturally specific knowledge bases from which the individual can develop culturally relevant interventions. Cultural desire requires the intrinsic qualities of motivation and genuine caring of the healthcare provider to "want to" engage in becoming culturally competent (1999).

The Giger and Davidhizar Transcultural Assessment Model identifies phenomena in order to assess provision of care for patients who are of different cultures. Their model includes six cultural phenomena: communication, time, space, social organization, environmental control, and biological variations. Each one is described based on several premises, such as: culture is a patterned behavioral response that develops over time; is shaped by values, beliefs, norms, and practices; guides our thinking, doing and being; and implies a dynamic, everchanging, active or passive process.

Leininger's (2002a) central purpose in her theory of transcultural nursing care is "to discover and explain diverse and universal culturally based care factors influencing the health, well-being, illness, or death of individuals or groups" (p. 190). She uses her classic "Sunrise Model" to identify the mutlifaceted theory and provides five enablers beneficial to "teasing out vague ideas," two of which are The Observation, Participation, and Reflection Enabler and the Researcher's Domain of Inquiry. Nurses can use Leininger's model to provide culturally congruent, safe, and meaningful care to patients or clients of diverse or similar cultures.

Nurse leaders and managers who ascribe to a positive view of culture and its characteristics effectively acknowledge cultural diversity among patients and staff. This includes providing culturally sensitive care to patients while simultaneously balancing a culturally diverse staff. For example, cultural diversity might mean being sensitive to or being able to embrace the emotions of a large **multicultural** group comprising staff and patients. Unless we understand the differences, we cannot come together and make decisions that are in the best interest of the patient.

Transculturalism sometimes has been considered in a narrow sense as a comparison of health beliefs and practices of people from different countries or geographic regions. However, culture can be construed more broadly to include differences in health beliefs and practices by gender, race, ethnicity, economic status, sexual preference, age, and disability or physical challenge. Thus, when concepts of transcultural care are discussed, we should consider differences in health beliefs and practices not only between and among countries but also between genders and among, for example, races, ethnic groups, and different economic strata. This requires us to consider multiple factors about all individuals.

The range of attitudes toward culturally diverse groups can be viewed along a continuum of intensity (Lenburg et al., 1995, p. 4): hate → contempt → tolerance → respect → celebration/affirmation. Managers need to be aware of this continuum so that they are able to apply these strategies appropriately to the workforce—for example, contempt versus affirmation.

Two questions that are addressed by Lenburg and colleagues (1995) regarding becoming culturally competent should be considered by practicing nurses (p. 10):

1. What has more influence on health and illness behavior—a group's cultural characteristics or the political and economic context in which it exists?
2. Is it the cultural characteristics of patients that affect their behavior in the healthcare system or the knowledge and behavior of providers?

Variables that may influence the nurse's response may include how the illness is perceived by the culture and the cultural competency of the healthcare provider. Leininger (2002a) identified several major theoretical premises relating to transcultural nursing theory that nurse managers and staff can follow (see the Theory Box).

Theory Box

CULTURAL CARE THEORY

THEORY/CONTRIBUTOR	KEY IDEAS	APPLICATION TO PRACTICE
Leininger (2002a) is credited with developing and advancing a theory of transcultural nursing care since the mid-1950s.	The theory is explicitly focused on the close relationships of culture and care on well-being, health, illness, and death; it is holistic and multi-dimensional, generic (emic, folk) and professional (etic) care, and has a specifically designed research method (ethnonursing).	Care is the essence of nursing and culturally based care is essential for well-being, health, growth, survival, and in facing handicaps or death.

To understand, value, and use diversity, nurse managers need to approach every staff person as an individual. Although staff of different cultural groups may be diverse in appearance, values, beliefs, communication patterns, and mannerisms, they have many things in common. Staff members want to be accepted by others and to succeed in their jobs. With fairness and respect, nurse managers should openly support the competencies and contributions of staff members from all cultural groups with a goal of achieving quality patient care. Nurse managers hold the key to allowing the full potential of each person on the staff.

Sullivan and Decker (2001) described the importance of communication and how cultural attitudes, beliefs, and behavior affect communication. Body movements, gestures, verbal tone, and physical closeness when communicating are all part of a person's culture. For the nurse manager, understanding these cultural behaviors is imperative in accomplishing effective communication within the diverse workforce population. Tappen (2001) addressed differences across cultures that the nurse leader/manager needs to monitor. These differences include relationships to people in authority, spatial differences, eye contact, expressions of feelings, meaning of different language versions, thinking modes, evidence-based decision-making, and preferred leadership/management style. Nurses need to ensure that ineffective communication by staff with patients and others does not lead to misunderstandings and eventual alienation.

According to Parker and Nichols (2001), nurses who choose to work with the American Indian population must understand the complexities of tribal governance of American Indians and Alaska Natives in the United States to provide effective health care to their populations. *Trust, responsibility, tribal sovereignty, tribal politics,* and *self-governance* are commonly used terms in Indian communities, including in their healthcare programs; these concepts affect the nurses' roles when working in tribal settings. Cantone (2001) acknowledged that traditions vary from tribe to tribe and even among members of the same tribe who live in different regions. Basic American Indian beliefs about health that extend beyond tribal boundaries include the importance of prayer, the treatment received from the traditional medicine man or woman, and the reverence of elders for their life experiences and wisdom.

Exercise 8-4

Consider a culturally diverse patient who is admitted to the postpartum unit after delivery of her third baby. You see that the mother has no right forearm or hand due to surgical amputation. The patient is aware of your observation, and she comments, "We got our first daughter." What are your reactions to the mother's physical disability? What would you say in response to the patient's comment?

Failure to address cultural diversity leads to negative effects on performance and staff interactions. Nurse managers can find many ways to address this issue. For example, in relation to performance, a nurse manager can make sure messages about patient care are received. This might be accomplished by sitting down with the staff nurse and analyzing the situation to make sure that understanding has occurred. In addition, the nurse manager might use a communication notebook that allows the nurse to slowly "digest" information by writing down communication areas that may be unclear. For effective staff interaction, the nurse manager also can make a special effort to pair mentors and mentees who have different ethnic backgrounds. The use of a bilingual health professional interpreter can be an effective strategy when caring for non–English-speaking or limited English-speaking proficiency patients.

The current trend seems to be one of using interpreters rather than translators when speaking with non–English-speaking patients and clients. Why? Purnell and Paulanka (2003) advocate that trained healthcare providers as interpreters can decode words and provide the right meaning of the message. However, the authors also suggest being aware that interpreters might affect the reporting of symptoms, using their own ideas, or omitting information. It is important to allow time for translation and interpretation and to clarify information as needed. Purnell and Paulanka provided 21 guidelines for communicating with those who are non–English-speaking.

■ *Exercise 8–5*

During one of your group meetings, have everyone share one or two slang words that may have a different meaning for different groups of people. Following this meeting, have one in your group post a list of the words and meanings discussed in the meeting (similar to the list shown in Box 8-2). Allow everyone to continue to add slang words that patients or staff use that may create confusion or misunderstanding. Reviewing the list regularly allows staff to understand phrases and, in some instances, to gain a cultural perspective connected to the phrase.

INDIVIDUAL AND SOCIETAL FACTORS

Nurse managers must work with staff to foster respect of different lifestyles. To do this, nurse managers need to accept three key principles: **multiculturalism,** which refers to maintaining several different cultures; **cross-culturalism,** which

BOX 8-2

Slang Terms and Their Meanings

TERM	MEANING
"Circling the drain," Irish	Repeating behaviors with a downward outcome
"Pull up your socks," southern United States	Get on with it!
"Left to go up in the hollow", Appalachian	Death
"mija", Spanish	My daughter (from "mihija")
"I feel you," U.S. black	I sympathize with you
"Chill out; chillin," U.S. black	Relax; down time
"Running off," Appalachian	Diarrhea
"High blood," Appalachian	Hypertension
"Birds don't marry fishes," Japanese mother	Don't marry outside your race
"It's a disaster," various cultures	Chaos
"Fighting the fire within," white	Anger, hostility
"Lip lard," southern United States	Lipstick
"Lets leg it," England	Move on, walk faster
"Getting a husband is like catching a cold," common Ethiopian saying	Expected norm that every woman will get married at some point in her life
"Bakwas," India	Nonsense talk
"Vomiting the heart out and dripping the blood dry," Chinese	Making the ultimate sacrifice for a cause
"Puti," Philippines	White American
"Too little jam to spread over too much bread," United States	Not enough time, too many tasks
"Nip it in the bud", United States	Admonishment without embarrassment to keep information confidential
"On the down ramp of life," American	Aging and in decline

means mediating between/among cultures; and **transculturalism,** which denotes bridging significant differences in cultural practices.

Exercise 8-6

Consider doing a group exercise to enhance cultural sensitivity. Ask each group member to write down four to six cultural beliefs that he or she values. When everyone has finished writing, have the group members exchange their lists and discuss why these beliefs are valued. When everyone has had a chance to share lists, have a volunteer compile an all-encompassing list that reflects the values of your workforce. (The key to this exercise is that many of the values are similar or perhaps even identical.)

Cultural differences among groups should not be taken in the context that all members of a certain group or subgroup are indistinguishable. Tappen (2001) described this "indistinguishable" phenomenon and recommended that cultural differences be viewed as group tendencies. For example, in the area of gender differences, women are perceived to have a more participative management style; however, this does not mean that all male managers use an authoritative management model. Likewise, women managers may use multiple sources of information to make decisions, and this does not mean that all male managers make decisions on limited data. Thus, the norm for gender recognition should be that females and males be hired, promoted, rewarded, and respected for how successfully they do the job, not because of who they are, where they come from, or whom they know.

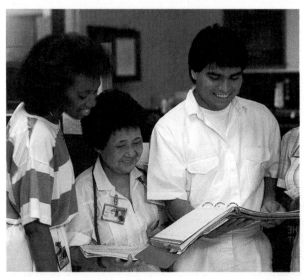

Respecting cultural diversity fosters cooperation and supports sound decision-making.

In today's workplace, female-male collaboration should provide efficacious models for the future. Gender does not determine response in any given situation. However, men reportedly seem to be better at deciphering what needs to be done, whereas women are best in collaborating and getting others to collaborate in accomplishing a task. Men tend to take neutral, logical, and objective stands on problems, whereas women become involved in how the problems affect people. It is important to recognize that women and men bring separate perspectives to resolving problems, which can help them function more effectively as a team on the nursing unit. Men and women must learn to work together and value the contributions of the other and the differences they bring to any situation.

Social capital is a relatively new concept that is described by Carlson and Chamberlain (2003). Their study was done to synthesize empirical findings using PubMed, CINAHL and applicable journals that link the concept of social capital to health outcomes and to identify implications for health disparities. The question that arises with this concept is: Is it an attribute of an individual, a social network, or a geographic space? People within geographic areas interact and develop social norms of behavior that can be transferred into the workplace by the healthcare providers. The rationale that social capital might be associated with racial and ethnic health disparities has remained relatively unexplored according to the authors.

Exercise 8-7

Read Carlson's and Chamberlain's article (2003) about social capital, which is defined as "the quality and quantity of the social relations embedded within community norms of interaction" (p. 325). Do a self analysis using the following questions, and decide whether you might have prejudices or biases toward people [staff, patients] of color or of your own ethnic or racial group. The attributes of social capital include trust and reciprocity. For trust, ask yourself: "Do you think most people [staff, patients] would try to take advantage of you if they got a chance, or would they try to be fair?" and "Generally speaking, would you say that most people [staff, patients] can be trusted or that you can't be too careful in dealing with people?" (p. 326). For reciprocity ask yourself, "Would you say that most of the time people [staff] try to be helpful, or are they mostly looking out for themselves?" (p. 326). Review the researchers' findings and conclusions. Consider their importance to your practice specialty.

Ethnocentrism "refers to the belief that one's own ways are the best, most superior, or preferred ways to act, believe, or behave" (Leininger, 2002b, p. 50), whereas, **cultural imposition** is defined as "the tendency of an individual or group to impose their values, beliefs, and practices on another culture for varied reasons" (p. 51). Such practices constitute a major concern in nursing and "a largely unrecognized problem as a result of cultural ignorance, blindness, ethnocentric tendencies, biases, racism or other factors" (p. 51).

Although the literature has addressed multicultural needs of patients, it is sparse in identifying effective methods for nurse managers to use when dealing with multicultural staff. Differences in education and culture can impede patient care, and uncomfortable situations may emerge from such differences. For example, staff members may be reluctant to admit language problems that hamper their written communication. They may also be reluctant to admit their lack of understanding when interpreting directions. Psychosocial skills may be problematic as well, because non-Westernized countries encourage emotional restraint. Staff may have difficulty addressing issues that relate to private family matters. Non-Asian nurses may have difficulty accepting the intensified family involvement of Asian cultures. The lack of assertiveness and the subservient physician-nurse relationships of some cultures are other issues that provide challenges for nurse managers. Unit-oriented workshops arranged by the nurse manager to address effective assertive techniques and family involvement as it relates to cultural differences are two ways of assisting staff with cultural work situations.

"Nurses migrating to Western nations, where nursing advocacy is a central tenet of practice and where malpractice actions are on the increase, may find themselves in a legal and cultural dilemma" (Priest, 2005, p. 20). The dominant culture in which the foreign-born nurse is trained is likely to impact the type of nursing care he/she provides to patients. Often, assertive advocacy and patients' rights are unfamiliar concepts to these nurses. They may perceive that their lack of assertiveness and advocacy skills could place them at "odds with their employing agency" (p. 22). Consider what might be influences or hindrances to cultural learning and the development of skills for foreign-born nurses to appropriately advocate on behalf of their patients.

Leininger (2002c) writes that "as the nurse discovers different transcultural ethical, moral, and legal care knowledge, several questions need to be considered, as examples: What specific ethical and moral values are universal or common among several cultures? Are there gender and class differences regarding who carries out ethical and moral duties or procedures?" (p. 273).

Providing quality of life and human care is difficult to accomplish if the nurse does not have knowledge of the recipient's culture as it relates to care. Leininger believes that "culture reflects shared values, beliefs, ideas, and meanings that are learned and that guide human thoughts, decisions, and actions. Cultures have *manifest* (readily recognized) and *implicit* (covert and ideal) rules of behavior and expectations. Human cultures have material items or symbols such as artifacts, objects, dress, and actions that have special meaning in a culture" (Leininger, 2002b, p. 48). Leininger states that her views of cultural care are, "a synthesized construct that is the foundational basis to understanding and helping people of different cultures in transcultural nursing practices" (Leininger, 2002b, p. 48). Accordingly, "quality of life" must be addressed from an emic (inside) cultural viewpoint and compared with an etic (outsider) professional's perspective. By comparing these two viewpoints, more meaningful nursing practice interventions will evolve. This comparative analysis will require nurses to include worldwide, global views in their cultural studies that take into account the social and environmental context of different cultures.

Exercise 8-8

As a small group activity, assess several clinical settings. Do these settings have programs related to cultural diversity? Why? What are the programs like? If there are no programs, why do you think they have not been implemented?

DEALING EFFECTIVELY WITH CULTURAL DIVERSITY

Wallace (2004) advocates doing an annual personal cultural audit. She wrote that honesty is essential when one does a personal audit, and it helps the person identify opportunities for developing skills that promote productivity and efficiency.

In developing intercultural relationships, she suggested that the person answer "yes" or "no" to several questions. Some of the questions were: "Are you able to tolerate and accept different views? Or do you tend to believe your view is right and others are simply misinformed? Did you place yourself in situations where you were in a minority by age, religion, ethnicity, or race? If so, did you gain from this experience? If you needed to hire an employee, would you select an applicant you feel is likely to agree with you or one likely to challenge you to grow?" (Section E, p. 2). If such a personal audit was done on an annual basis by the individual, the person could readily evaluate the amount of growth made over the year in managing cultural diverse relationships.

Jones, Cason, and Bond (2004) described cultural attitudes and skills in caring for patients from Hispanic and U.S. black backgrounds by healthcare providers who were white, Hispanic, U.S. blacks, or Asian-American. The study results suggested that the workers' knowledge of other cultures and how to care for them in culturally sensitive ways needed to be addressed more in depth.

The first individuals in the organizational structure who have to address cultural diversity are the leaders and managers. They have to give "unwavering" support to embracing diversity in the workplace rather than using a standard "cookie cutter" approach. Creating a culturally sensitive work environment involves a long-term vision, and financial and healthcare–provider commitment. Leaders and managers need to make the strategic decision to design services and programs especially to meet the needs of diverse cultural, ethnic, and racial differences of staff and patients. They need to focus first on building a knowledge base whereby employees are required to attend educational sessions to become familiar with cultural practices and to achieve a culture-friendly environment (Biggerstaff & Hamby, 2004).

Nurse managers hold the key to making the best use of cultural diversity. Managers have positions of power to begin programs that enrich the diversity among staff. For example, capitalizing on the knowledge that all staff bring to the patient is possible for better quality care outcomes. One method that can be used is to allow staff to verbalize their feelings about particular cultures in relationship to personal beliefs. Another is to have two or three staff members of different ethnic origins present a patient-care conference, giving their views on how they would care for a specific patient's needs based on their own ethnic values.

Establishing mentorship programs should be done so that all staff can expand their knowledge about cultural diversity. Mentors have specific relationships with their mentees. The more closely aligned a mentor is with the mentee (for example, same gender, age group, ethnicity, and primary language), the more effective the relationship. Programs that address the staff's cultural diversity should not try to make people of different cultures pattern their behavior after the prevailing culture. Nurse managers must carefully select those mentors who ascribe to transcultural, rather than ethnocentric, values and beliefs. A much richer staff exists when nurse managers build on the valuable culture of all staff and when diversity is rewarded. The pacesetter for the cultural norm of the unit is the nurse manager. For example, to demonstrate commitment to cultural diversity, a nurse manager might make a special effort to ensure that U.S. black, Asian-American, and Hispanic holidays or other cultural representations on the unit are recognized by the staff. Staff who are active participants in these programs can then be given positive reinforcement by the nurse manager. These activities promote a better understanding and appreciation of individuals' cultural heritage.

Nurse managers are aware of the increasing shortage of nurses, demanding work environment with its surrounding influences, and statistics indicating that almost 50% of all new nurses leave their first professional nursing position by the first year due to job dissatisfaction and level of stress. The Academy of Medical-Surgical Nurses (AMSN), as reported by Reeves (2004), developed a mentoring program for new graduates that is based on a foundation of "wisdom, caring, and confidence" and shared between new graduates and skilled, experienced nurses. The "N3" mentoring program provides supportive, encouraging relationships while guiding new nurses in their professional, personal, and interpersonal growth. It is a goal of this program to increase the retention of new nurses in the workplace.

Continuing-education programs should assist nurses in learning about the care of different ethnic groups. Meleis et al. (1995) identified 10 recommendations for enhancing the development of knowledge related to culturally competent care for diverse and marginalized populations (Box 8-3). For example, professional organizations related to cultural groups (Hispanic Nurses Association, Philippine Nurses Association, Black Nurses Association of America) and institutions might develop or sponsor a workshop or conference on cross-cultural nursing for nursing service staff and faculty in Schools of Nursing who have had limited preparation in the area of cultural care or cultural beliefs in healing.

Andrews, Burr, and Janetos (July 2004) identified selected examples of Internet sites that would enable nurses to quickly and effectively obtain information on a variety of topics related to transcultural nursing. When caring for culturally diverse patients, it becomes the nurse's responsibility to keep abreast of such information by using available computer-based tools as part of his/her "self-study" for continuing education. For example, Medline identifies topics through a formal system of medical subject headings, and it has two published indexes in print: *Index Medicus* and *International Nursing Index*. The *Cumulative Index to Nursing and Allied Health Literature* is another informative source for nurse managers and staff nurses to use when working with culturally diverse patients or other health care providers. Two common websites for retrieval of information include www.cinahl.com and the Educational Resources Information Center at www.eric.ed.gov.

Exercise 8–9

Identify a situation in which care to a culturally diverse patient had positive or negative outcomes of care. If a negative outcome resulted, what could you have done to make it a positive one?

Muslims are one of the fastest growing populations in the United States and worldwide. El Gindy (2004b) addressed the need for showing respect for accommodating Muslim nurses' dress requirements and understanding the role of Islam in their lives. For example, one Muslim nurse wore her hijab and became frustrated because the Infection Control staff consistently asked her to wear short sleeves or to roll up the sleeves. El Gindy stated the importance of the Islamic dress code as a way of life to obey Allah; therefore, it was mandatory. Healthcare providers should be made aware of this religious belief and respond to it in a positive way.

In another situation, El Gindy (2004a), using a question and answer format, wrote that at the

---

BOX 8-3

Recommendations for Action Related to Culturally Competent Care

1. Make a commitment to provide equitable, culturally competent care.
2. Sustain disciplinary culturally competent knowledge.
3. Identify mechanisms that allow integration of all existing knowledge pertaining to nursing care of different disadvantaged populations.
4. Develop a base of transdisciplinary knowledge that mirrors heterogeneous healthcare practices within cultural groups.
5. Develop knowledgeable health care for disadvantaged groups using appropriate theories and frameworks.
6. Explore organizational structures that create environments that foster cooperative working relationships and knowledge related to disadvantaged populations.
7. Use proven effective models when delivering care to disadvantaged populations.
8. Develop policies that support content addressing diversity in nursing curricula with the cooperation of curriculum committees and state regulatory bodies.
9. Develop methodologies to address adequate faculty and student preparation in culturally competent nursing practices on the local, regional, national, and international levels.
10. Work with ethnic minority nursing organizations to recruit and retain a diverse nurse population.

time of end-of-life care for patients and their families, diverse cultural needs become very significant. An intensive care unit nurse questioned the author concerning caring for a Hispanic/Latino patient who had to "face a crowd of family and friends all day," regardless of the visiting hours being posted in Spanish. Sometimes the families requested to place a special food next to the patient's bed. Like many institutions, our "inflexible unit policies" do not permit such policies. El Gindy's answer related the importance of having mutual communication to maintain a more positive environment for the patient and a better understanding of the unit policies by the family.

Sensitive or controversial issues are often addressed by behaviors that represent avoidance or coercion. The similarities or differences about the issue or person are not acknowledged, either subconsciously or consciously. Avoidance precludes any opportunities for open discussion and potential for change. Avoidance can be a powerful and controlling strategy, but situations do not vanish because they are avoided. Aspects of the situations may eventually resurface. If the situation becomes intolerable, frustration and anger most likely will occur. Various responses are possible, and insistence that the issue is no longer visible in the setting does not imply its resolution.

Coercion is acted out through the use of power or status to persuade people to act in specific ways. Although coercion is not a negative behavior, it can lead to negative consequences through the inequity of power. Coercive tactics limit choices and may result in powerlessness, although the importance of the outcome varies greatly. For example, the use of coercion in a situation may result in anger, which is a normal response to feelings of powerlessness that result from being or feeling controlled. Passivity and aggression often perpetuate the situation, and individuals may not recognize the effect of their actions.

Choices, decisions, and behaviors reflect learned beliefs, values, ideals, and preferences. The goal of communication is maintenance or restoration of personal integrity and recognition of worth and respect of individuals or groups.

The two scenarios described in Box 8-4 illustrate how problem-solving communication can promote mutual understanding and respect. The first scenario involves a compromise between staff members and a patient's family, and the second involves a nurse manager and a staff member from a different culture.

Exercise 8-10
Identify a situation involving a staff member in which a request for additional days leave was made that required a culturally sensitive decision. What religious or ethnic practices did you learn about in regard to this request and decision?

Passages of life that culminate in happy events also can challenge the nurse manager; for example, the quincineara observed by Hispanic families. This event is the celebration for 15-year-old girls to be introduced into society. The nurse whose daughter is celebrating this event must have time to make plans for this festive celebration. Because of the significance of the celebration and the pride that the parents take in their daughter, inviting "key" staff to the quincineara is common. Nurse managers who understand and value cultural rituals can help individuals meet their needs and help staff, in general, learn and accept various cultural practices and perspectives.

Exercise 8-11
Holiday celebrations have cultural significance. Select a specific holiday such as Chinese Lunar New Year (China and Chinatowns) or Araw Ng Mga Patay (Philippines) or Diwali (India). What is the cultural meaning of the specific holiday? How do staff of the respective culture celebrate the festive day? Does the nursing unit engage in recognition of special holidays? Table 8-3 provides examples of holiday celebrations.

Exercise 8-12
Form small groups representing various cultures to read, discuss, and share personal experiences as related to the excellent array of topics in Spector's (2000) book. Such topics of interest might include the magico-religious traditions used in healing; birth rights from a cross-cultural perspective; death, mourning, and after-death rituals; health traditions practices to ward off the "evil eye" (mal ojo); or objects and substances that protects one's health. Or such information could be reported by each group at a monthly unit in-service program that would benefit all staff or students in a clinical conference setting.

Implications in the Workplace
Considering culture from both the patient population and the nursing workforce perspective is a daunting task, one which can lead to a more solidly

BOX 8-4

Problem-Solving Communication: Honoring Cultural Attitudes Toward Death and Dying

Scenario 1: Staff and a Patient's Family

What nurses often call interference with the care of a patient commonly reflects family attitudes toward death and dying. Often, Hispanic families rush to the hospital as soon as they hear of a relative's illness. Because most Hispanics believe that death is the passing of an individual to a life that offers tranquility and everlasting happiness, being at the bedside offering prayers and encouragement is the norm rather than the unusual exception. The nurse manager in this situation, herself a non–American-educated nurse manager, had worked extensively at helping her staff to understand different cultures. A consensus compromise was worked out between the staff and one such Hispanic family. The family, consisting of three generations, was given the authority to decide what family members could stay at the loved one's side and for how long. By doing this, the family felt they had control of the environment and quickly developed a priority list of family members who could stay no more than 5 minutes at the patient's side. As the family member left the bedside, his or her task was to report the condition of the patient to other family members "camping" in the visitors' lounge. Although their loved one did not survive a massive intracranial hemorrhage, all of the family felt that they were a part of their loved one's "passage of life."

Scenario 2: A Nurse Manager and Another Staff Member

Eastern world cultures that profess Catholicism as their faith celebrate the death of a loved one 40 days after the death. The nurse manager needs to recognize that time off for the nurse involved in this celebration is imperative. Such an occurrence had to be addressed by a nurse manager of Asian descent. The nurse manager quickly realized that the nurse, whose mother died in India, did not ask for any time off to make the necessary burial arrangements, but rather waited 40 days to celebrate his mother's death. The celebration included formal invitations to a church service, as well as a dinner after the service. One day during early morning rounds, the nurse explained how death is celebrated by Eastern world Catholics. The Bible's description of the Ascension of the Lord into heaven 40 days after his death served as the conceptual framework for the loved one's death. The grieving family believed their loved one's spirit would stay on earth for 40 days. During these 40 days, the family held prayer sessions meant to assist the "spirit" to prepare for its ascension into heaven. When the 40 days have passed, the celebration previously described marks the ascension of the loved one's spirit into heaven.

Because this particular unit truly espoused a multicultural concept, the nurses had no difficulty in allowing the Indian nurse 2 weeks of unplanned vacation so that his mother's "passage of life" celebration could be accomplished in a respectful, dignified manner.

aligned service-community relationship. Even if the workforce is not as diverse as one might desire, learning about the cultures of the groups within the workforce is important. Making clear that diversity is valued, in fact celebrated, attracts others to engage in the complexity of care. One way is to make clear how patients are valued as people, not as representatives of some group. Showing respect to all patients irrespective of their cultural differences tells the staff that their differences also can be valued. The key is for managers and leaders to attend to the workforce issues with the same zest as they do the patient issues. Cultural differences enrich all of us when we make deliberate efforts to include them in our daily values.

Table 8-3 EXAMPLES OF HOLIDAY CELEBRATIONS OF CULTURAL SIGNIFICANCE

Term	Country	Date
Araw Ng Mga Patay	All Saints Day, Philippines	November 1
Chinese Lunar New Year	China, Chinatowns	January or February (varies with Chinese Calendar)
Cinco de Mayo	Independence Day, Mexico	May 5
Ramadan	Muslim/Islamic festival, India	Ninth month of Muslim year
Dipavali/Diwali	Hindu festival of lights, India	October–November
Hanukkah/Chanukah	Jewish festival of lights, U.S.	December
Christmas	Compare countries and dates	December 25 (United States)
Kwanzaa	U.S. Blacks	Between Christmas and New Year's Day, 7 days
Boxing Day	Worker's Recognition, Canada, Australia, Great Britain	December 26
Martin Luther King, Jr.	Civil rights, United States	January 20
Eid ul-Adha	Feast of Sacrifice, Muslim	January, 3-day feast
Day of Mourning for all manifestations of racism; ethnic discrimination (1969)	Various countries; holiday for Buddhists (Tibetan, Zen, Pure Land and Theravada)	January 4

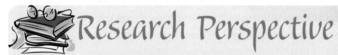

Research Perspective

DiCicco-Bloom, B. (2004, January) The racial and gendered experiences of immigrant nurses from Kerala, India. *Journal of Transcultural Nursing, 15*(1), 26-33.

This is a description of the experiences of a group of immigrant nurses who relate their life and work in a culture different from their own. Semi-structured, open-ended interviews were conducted in the homes at the requests of the 10 nurses. The nurses were born and educated in India and were actively employed as nurses in New Jersey and Pennsylvania. The researcher was conscious of her position as a middle-class white woman; however, for reasons of our "sameness" and "differences," they were eager to talk with me. These nurses told stories about (1) challenges of living between two cultures and countries, (2) racism they experienced, and (3) their marginalization as female nurses of color. The dominant themes that emerged from the content analysis were identified as (1) cultural displacement—a foot here (America), a foot there (India), a foot nowhere; (2) racial experiences/alienations in the work place and at home; and (3) intersections of categories—being a female nurse, an immigrant, and non-white. The researcher expressed her feelings that these women's stories about nursing incriminated the nursing profession and that their examples reflected the issues of racism in our larger society. Immigrant nurses are given responsibility without designated authority and salary differentiation. This study describes the experiences of a small group of immigrant women of color who are also nurses practicing in the United States. Thus, there are implications for nurses and nursing to address regarding cultural awareness and sensitivity in the work place.

IMPLICATIONS FOR PRACTICE
- Nurses need to be fully cognizant of how culture affects one's health and the delivery of health care.
- Nurses are at a vantage point to advocate for their immigrant colleagues in the work place and for those patients of another country and culture for whom they provide care.
- Nurses need to assess and use their capabilities to determine the challenges that immigrant women nurses face in functioning at their fullest potential in the work place.

The Solution

As nurse manager, I prefer to talk on a one-to-one basis. I had a meeting with the male staff member to learn from him, "what made you upset with the charge nurse when she made your assignment?" In our discussion, he told me "the charge nurse used words [slang] for which I did not know the meaning . . . I did not understand why she said it . . . she was trying to overpower me . . . I didn't like it . . . so I was defensive about it." We talked about being sensitive to cultural communication, the need to understand meanings of words and to ask for immediate clarification when such situations arise with members of two different cultures.

— Sally C. Fernandez

 Would this be a suitable approach for you? Why?

CHAPTER CHECKLIST

All potential or current nurse leaders or managers must acknowledge and address cultural diversity among staff and patients. Culture lives in each of us. It determines how we think, what we value, how we behave, and how we communicate with each other. In everyday work activities, the nurse manager must be able to do the following:

- Assess staff diversity and use techniques to manage a culturally diverse workforce.
- Lead staff with a clear understanding of principles that embrace culture, cultural diversity, and cultural sensitivity.
- Be able to communicate effectively with staff and patients from diverse cultural backgrounds:
  - Recognize slang terms that have different meanings in different cultures.
  - Understand that nonverbal behaviors also carry different connotations depending on one's culture.
- Select basic characteristics of any culture.
- Appraise factors, both individual and societal, inherent in cultural diversity:

- Three key principles relate to respect for different lifestyles:
  - Multiculturalism refers to maintaining several different cultures simultaneously.
  - Cross-culturalism refers to mediating between two cultures (one's own and another).
  - Transculturalism denotes bridging significant differences in cultural practices.

  Remember that sexual orientation and gender recognition are important factors to consider in dealing fairly with all patients and staff members.
- Use tools that clarify staff and patient cultural diversity effectively:
  - Mentoring programs can help staff expand their knowledge of cultural diversity.
  - Continuing education programs can help nurses learn about caring for different ethnic groups in ways that honor their beliefs.
  - Internet websites can assist nurses to quickly and effectively obtain information on cultural topics.
- Appreciate the cultural richness found among staff and patients.

TIPS FOR DEALING WITH CULTURAL DIVERSITY

Being a nurse manager in a country that views its strength in its population's cultural diversity requires special skills. The nurse manager needs to do the following:

- Ascribe to effective techniques for managing a culturally diverse workforce.
- Appreciate and encourage programs that address cultural diversity of staff.
- Assist staff in problem-solving special cultural needs of patients.
- Embrace three key principles relating to culture: multiculturalism, cross-culturalism, and transculturalism.

- Commit to lifelong learning about culture for self and staff.

TERMS TO KNOW

cross-culturalism
cultural competence
cultural diversity
cultural imposition
cultural marginality
cultural sensitivity
culture
ethnicity
ethnocentrism
multiculturalism
transculturalism

REFERENCES

American Nurses Association. (2001). *Code of ethics for nurses with interpretative statements*. Washington, DC: American Nurses Publishing.

ANA NursingWorld. (2005). Retrieved February 27, 2005 from www.nursingworld.org/readroom/position/ethics.

Andrews, M., Burr, J., & Janetos, D. H. (2004). Searching electronically for information on transcultural nursing and health subjects. *Journal of Transcultural Nursing, 15*(3), 242-247.

Baldwin, D. (2003). Disparities in health and health care: Focusing efforts to eliminate unequal burdens. *Online Journal of Issues in Nursing, 8*(1). Retrieved February 13, 2005 from http//nursingworld.org/ojin/topic20/tpc1.htm.

Biggerstaff, G., & Hamby, L. (2004, August). Diversity—An evolving leadership initiative. *Nurse Leader*. St. Louis: Elsevier.

Campinha-Bacote, J. (2002). The process of cultural competence in a delivery of healthcare services: A model of care. *Journal of Transcultural Nursing, 13*(3), 181-184.

Campinha-Bacote, J. (1999, May). A model and instrument for addressing cultural competence in health care. *Journal of Nursing Education, 38*(5), 203-207.

Cantone, J. A. (2001, Winter). Earth, wind, fire and water. *Minority Nurse*, 24-29.

Carlson, E. D., & Chamberlain, R. M. (2003). Social capital, health, and health disparities. *Journal of Nursing Scholarship, 35*(4), 325-331.

Castillo, H. M. (1996). Cultural diversity: Implications for nursing. In Torres, S. (Ed.) *Hispanic voices: Hispanic health educators speak out*. New York: NLN Press.

Choi, H. (2001). Cultural marginality: A concept analysis with implications for immigrant adolescents. *Issues in Comprehensive Pediatric Nursing, 24*, 193-206.

D'Avanzo, C. E., & Geissler, E. M. (2003). *Pocket guide to cultural health assessment* (3rd ed) St. Louis: Mosby.

DiCicco-Bloom, B. (2004, January). The racial and gendered experience of immigrant nurses from Kerata, India. *Journal of Transcultural Nursing, 15*(1), 26-33.

El Gindy, G. (2004a, Spring). Cultural competence: Death and dying. *Minority Nurse*, 54-56.

El Gindy, G. (2004b, Winter). Treating Muslims with cultural sensitivity in a post-9/11 world. *Minority Nurse*, 44-46.

Giger, J. N., & Davidhizar, R. (July 2002). The Giger and Davidhizar transcultural assessment model. *Journal of Transcultural Nursing, 13*(3), 185-188.

Hancock, C. (2004). Unity with diversity: ICN's framework of competencies. *Journal of Advanced Nursing, 47*(2), 119.

International Council of Nurses (2003). ICN framework of competence for the generalist nurse. ICN offers guidance on global nurse competencies. Retrieved March 25, 2005 from http://www.icn.ch/PR05_03.htm+competencies.

Jones, M. E., Cason, C., & Bond, M. L. (2004). Cultural attitudes, knowledge, and skills of a health workforce. *Journal of Transcultural Nursing, 15*(4), 283-290.

Leininger, M. (2002a). Cultural care theory: A major contribution to advance transcultural nursing knowledge and practice. *Journal of Transcultural Nursing, 13*(3), 189-192.

Leininger, M. (2002b). Essential transcultural nursing care concepts, principles, examples, and policy statements. Cited in Leininger, M. & McFarland, M. R. (2002). *Transcultural nursing: Concepts, theories, research & practice* (3rd ed) New York: McGraw-Hill Medical Publishing Division.

Leininger, M. (2002c). Ethical, moral, and legal aspects of trancscultural nursing. Cited in Leininger, M. &

McFarland, M. R. (2002). *Transcultural nursing: Concepts, theories, research & practice* (3rd ed). New York: McGraw-Hill Medical Publishing Division.

Lenburg, C. B., Lipson, J. G., Demi, A. S., Blaney, D. R., Stern, P. N., Schultz, P. R., & Gage, L. (1995). *Promoting cultural competence in and through nursing education: A critical review and comprehensive plan for action.* Washington, DC: American Academy of Nursing.

Lipson, J. G., & Dibble, S. L. (2005). *Culture & clinical care.* San Francisco, CA: UCSF Nursing Press.

Lowenstein, A. J., & Glanville, C. (1996). Cultural diversity and conflict in the health care workplace. *Nursing Economics, 13*(4), 203-209, 247.

Meleis, A. I., Isenberg, M., Koerner, J. E., Lacey, B., & Stern, P. (1995). *Diversity, marginalization, and culturally competent health care issues in knowledge development.* Washington, DC: American Academy of Nursing.

National Advisory Council on Nurse Education and Practice. (2000). *A national agenda for nursing workforce, racial/ethnic diversity.* Washington, DC: U.S. Department of Health and Human Services, Health Resources & Service Administration, Bureau of Health Professions.

Parker, J. G., & Nichols, L. A. (2001, Summer). Second opinion: Tribes know best. *Minority Nurse.* CASS Recruitment Media Publication.

Portillo, C. J. (January 2003). Health disparities and culture—Moving beyond the beginning. *Journal of Transcultural Nursing, 14*(1), 5.

Priest, C. (2005). Held liable. *Reflections in Nursing Leadership. 31*(1), 20-22, 36.

Purnell, L. D., & Paulanka, B. J. (2003). *Transcultural health care: A culturally competent approach* (2nd ed). Philadelphia: FA Davis.

Reeves, K. A. (December 2004). Nurses nurturing nurses: A mentoring program. *Nurse Leader, 2*(6), 47-49, 53.

Sayles-Cross, S. (1996). Aging, care giving effects and black family caregivers. In R. W. Johnson (Ed.), *African American voices: African American health educators speak out.* New York: NLN Press.

Spector, R. E. (2000). *Cultural diversity in health and illness* (5th ed). Upper Saddle River, NJ: Prentice Hall Health.

Spence, D. (2004). Prejudice, paradox and possibility: The experience of nursing people from cultures other than one's own. In Kavanaugh, K. H., & Knowlden, V. *Many voices: Toward caring culture in healthcare and healing.* Madison, WI: The University of Wisconsin Press.

Sullivan Commission. (2005). Retrieved on August 15, 2005 from http://admissions.duhs.duke.edu/sullivan-commission/index.cfm.

Sullivan, E. J., & Decker, P. J. (2001). *Effective leadership and management in nursing* (5th ed). Upper Saddle River, NJ: Prentice Hall.

Tappen, R. (2001). *Nursing leadership and management: Concepts and practice* (4th ed). Philadelphia: FA Davis.

U.S. Bureau of Labor Statistics, Bulletin 2307. Retrieved March 14, 2005 from www.bls.gov/cps/home.htm.

U.S. Census. (2004). Retrieved March 14, 2005 from www.census.gov/prod/2004pub/04statab/labor.pdf.

Wallace, L. S. (2004, December 12). The cultural coach: Honesty is essential in personal cultural audit. *Houston Chronicle*, E2.

SUGGESTED READINGS

Bonder, B., Martin, L., & Miracle, A. (2002). *Culture in clinical care.* Thorofare, NJ: Slack.

Corlese, I. B., Nicholas, P. K., & Nokes, K. M. (2001). Issues in cross-cultural quality-life research. *Journal of Nursing Scholarship, 33*(1), 15-20.

St. Hill, P., Lipson, J. G., & Meleis, A. I. (2003). *Caring for women cross-culturally.* Philadelphia: FA Davis.

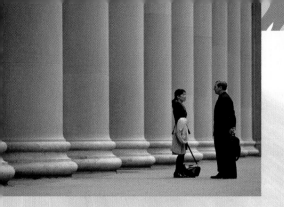

Chapter

9

Power, Politics, and Influence

Karen Kelly

*T*his chapter describes how power and politics influence the roles of leaders and managers. It focuses on contemporary concepts of power, empowerment, types of power exercised by nurses, key factors in developing a powerful image, personal and organizational strategies for exercising power, and the power of nurses to shape health policy and take action in the political arena of legislative politics. Having the opportunity to relate to politics in the workplace is critical for effective leadership and management.

Objectives

- Explore the concepts of professional and legislative politics related to nursing.
- Value the concept of power as it relates to leadership and management in nursing.
- Use different types of power in the exercise of nursing leadership.
- Develop a power image for effective nursing leadership.
- Choose appropriate strategies for exercising power to influence the politics of the work setting, professional organizations, legislators, and the development of health policy.

Questions to Consider

- What does the phrase "a powerful nurse" mean to you?
- How can you gain experience in the politics of nursing and in legislative politics?
- Do you ever think of yourself as a powerful nurse?
- What factors, persons, and events have influenced your development as a nurse?
- What kinds of behaviors do you observe in people that tell you whether they are powerful? Which are socially desirable? Which are undesirable? What are your behaviors?
- What behaviors or characteristics do you exhibit that tell people how powerful you are?
- What are your beliefs and values about power and politics in organizations?
- How can you shape health policy and legislative politics?

The Challenge

Gail Haller, MSN, RN
Former Chairperson, Illinois Nurses Association Political Action Committee, Illinois

As chairperson of the state nurses' association political action committee (PAC), I was involved in working with the state nurses association's (SNA) nurse-lobbyist on an amendment to the nurse practice act (NPA) to recognize certified registered nurse anesthetists (CRNAs) among advanced practice nurses. A hostile amendment to allow one anesthesia technician, with a bachelor's degree in anesthesia technology from a university in another state, was being offered by a legislator from the northern part of the state. The hostile amendment was a threat to the entire system of nursing licensure because it would legitimize the practice of a nonnurse as a CRNA.

The technician, on whose behalf the hostile amendment was offered, lived in the southern part of the state and was employed by an anesthesiology practice. The practice wanted her to work beyond the usual scope of practice of an anesthesia technician because of her previous work experience in another state where she was licensed and worked much like a CRNA. The hospital and anesthesia group had been unable to convince any local legislators in the area where she lived to sponsor this amendment; the legislators had a close working relationship with the district nurses' association and did not want to oppose their supporters' interests. The legislator from the northern part of the state was reported to have offered the amendment because of contacts with the family of the technician.

The key issue here focused on the hospital's willingness to credential this unlicensed individual. If the hospital's credentialing policy was allowed to override the state's licensure laws, the licensure system would be in chaos, and the door could be opened to institutional licensure. A hearing was scheduled before the Senate Licensed Activities Committee to determine support for the hostile amendment.

 What do you think you would do if you were this nurse?

INTRODUCTION

The profession of nursing developed in the United States at a time when women had limited legal rights (e.g., most were prohibited from voting, and many could not own property). Women were viewed as neither powerful nor political; in the late 19th century, feminine and powerful were practically contradictory terms. During the 20th century, as the status and role of women changed, so did the status and role of nurses. As the economic and social **power** of women evolved, so did the power of nurses. This is significant because nursing historically has been, and continues to be, a discipline comprised primarily of women.

As the healthcare environment continues to change in 21st century, the exercise of power by nurses is essential to a strong voice for nursing in shaping these changes. In an era of rapid and often unplanned change and of a growing nursing shortage like none before, nurses must exercise their power and flex their political muscles to create a preferred future for the healthcare system, healthcare consumers, and the profession of nursing.

HISTORY

The word "power" comes from the Latin word "potere," meaning "to be able." Simply defined, power is the ability to **influence** others in the effort to achieve goals. Power was once considered almost a taboo in nursing. In the profession's earliest years, the exercise of power was considered inappropriate, unladylike, and unprofessional. In nursing's earliest decades in America, many decisions about nursing education and practice were often made by persons outside of nursing (Ashley, 1976). Nurses began to exercise their collective power with the rise of early nursing leaders such as Lillian Wald, Isabel Stewart, Annie Goodrich, Lavinia Dock, M. Adelaide Nutting, Mary Eliza Mahoney, and Isabel

Hampton Robb and the development of organizations that evolved into the American Nurses Association (ANA) and the National League for Nursing (NLN).

Many social, technologic, scientific, and economic trends have shaped nursing and nurses and our ability to exercise power during the twentieth century. When the American Medical Association (AMA), in 1988, proposed a new category of healthcare worker (the Registered Care Technologist, or RCT) to replace nurses during a time of nursing shortage, nurses and nursing organizations responded powerfully. Leaders of nursing organizations came together in "summit meetings" to formulate powerful responses to the AMA and implemented a range of actions, including public education and the education of legislators. The new healthcare worker did not materialize from this proposal. Almost two decades later, nurses must be even more skilled and confident in exercising power to ensure the continuing development of the profession and that the voice of nurses will be heard in shaping the future of the healthcare system.

The media, politicians, organized medicine, some healthcare executives, and, sadly, some nurses have traditionally viewed nurses and nursing as powerless. That view began to change radically in the 1990s as nurses began to appear more often on local and national news and on talk shows as experts on health care, the changes occurring in the healthcare system, and the effect of these changes on the public. Nurses have become increasingly visible in political campaigns on the local, state, and national levels, both as candidates and as political influentials. In Missouri, for example, two nurses, one a Democrat, the other a Republican, ran in the primaries for two different Congressional seats in 2004 (Roberts, 2004). Lois Capps, RN, one of a handful of nurses in Congress, represents a California congressional district; she assumed the office held by her husband upon his death. A former school nurse, Congresswoman Capps has since been re-elected by her constituents to the House seat. Nurses and nursing have gained new respect in the political arena in recent years. Sheila Burke, RN, served as Chief of Staff for Senator Robert Dole while he was Senate Majority Leader in the United States Congress, making her one of the most powerful Congressional staff people in Washington. During the Clinton administration, nurse leaders

were prominent: two former ANA presidents, Virginia Trotter Betts and Beverly Malone served in roles that helped shaped health policy for the nation (Milstead, 2004).

Sadly, even today, as we enter a new and different era of nursing shortage, there are still a few nurses who see themselves as powerless and oppressed, demonstrating aspects of oppressed group behavior. Roberts (1983) addressed the historical evidence of oppressed group behavior among nurses, based on models developed from the study of politically and economically oppressed populations. Oppressed group behavior is apparent when a population is dominated by another group. This subordinate or oppressed group begins to take on the characteristics of the dominant group and reject the characteristics of their own group, although this behavior fails to create a balance of power with the dominant group (Roberts 1983, 2000). In later works, Roberts and her colleague (DeMarco & Roberts, 2003) noted that such behavior continues with harmful effects on nurses as individuals and on the profession as a whole. Among nurses, oppressed group behavior is manifested in low self-esteem ("I'm just a nurse"), passive aggressiveness, and distancing one's self from other nurses (e.g., the failure of nurses to join professional organizations), and engaging in intragroup conflicts (e.g., "infighting") (Roberts, 1983). Schools of nursing too often fail to socialize students to be activists. All nurses need to continue to expand their understanding of the concept of power and to develop their skills in exercising power. Avoiding involvement in the **politics** of nursing, in the workplace, in the profession at large, or in the area of public **policy** limits the power of the individual nurse and the profession as a collective whole.

Some nurses are still uncomfortable about politics and the use of power that politics demand. Some treat politics as if it were a dirty word. Historically, politics has been viewed with some disdain. Writer Robert Louis Stevenson noted, "Politics is perhaps the only profession for which no preparation is thought necessary." However, in view of contemporary nursing's need to thrive within a healthcare system, nursing education seems to be a most appropriate preparation for engaging in politics.

Politics can be defined in many ways. One simple definition of politics that this author uses, when teaching a course on health policy and politics in nursing, is "a process of human interaction within organizations." Politics permeates all organizations, including workplaces, legislatures, professions, and even families. Young children often learn that one parent is more likely than the other to give permission for special activities and more likely to buy toys and other desired items. They quickly learn to ask permission or ask for a desired item from that parent before asking the other. This is an unwritten political rule in many families. Political activism should be an unwritten rule in nursing.

The model of political activism, which is noted below, is based on merging elements of models of political activism offered by other authors (Kalisch & Kalisch, 1982; Leavitt, Chaffee, & Vance, 2002; Mason, Leavitt, & Chaffee, 2002). This model can be applied to the political development and activism of individual nurses related to both professional and legislative political arenas:

1. Apathy: no membership in professional organizations; little or no interest in legislative politics as they relate to nursing and health care
2. Buy-in: recognition of the importance of activism within professional organizations (without active participation) and legislative politics related to critical nursing issues
3. Self-interest: involvement in professional organizations to further one's own career; the development and use of political expertise to further the profession's self-interests
4. Political sophistication: high level of professional organization activism (e.g., holding office at the local and state level) moving beyond self-interests; recognition of the need for activism on behalf of the public
5. Leading the way: serving in elected or appointed positions in professional organizations at the state and national levels; providing true leadership on broad healthcare interests within legislative politics, including seeking appointment to policy-making bodies and election to political positions

FOCUS ON POWER

Nurses have sometimes viewed power as if it were something immoral, corrupting, and totally contradictory to the caring nature of nursing. However, the preceding definition (the ability to influence others in the effort to achieve goals) demonstrates the essential nature of power to nursing. Nurses regularly influence patients in an effort to improve their health status as an essential element of nursing practice. When nurses are providing health teaching to patients and their families, their goal is to provide needed information and to change behavior to promote optimal health. That is an exercise of power in nursing practice. Changing a colleague's behavior by instructing him or her about a new policy being implemented on the nursing unit is another example of how a nurse can exercise power. Coaching a nurse to improve his or her performance is an exercise of power. Serving as the chief nursing officer for a hospital, managing a multimillion dollar budget, demonstrates another exercise of power.

Exercise 9–1

Recall a recent opportunity when you had to observe the work of an expert nurse. Think about that nurse's interactions with patients, family members, nursing colleagues, and other professionals. What kinds of power did you observe this nurse using? What did the nurse do that told you: this is a powerful person?

Social scientists have studied the use and abuse of power in human organizations. They have analyzed and categorized the sources and applications of power in human experience. Hersey, Blanchard, and Natemeyer (1979) offer a classic formulation on the basis of social power. Sullivan (2004, p. 33) offers a revised view of types of power that readily apply to the efforts of nurses in the workplace, in professional organizations, and in politics (see the Theory Box). These types of power are not mutually exclusive. They are often used in concert to exert influence on individuals or groups.

Theory Box

TYPES OF POWER*

KEY CONTRIBUTORS	KEY IDEAS	APPLICATION TO PRACTICE
Types or bases of social power were formulated by Hersey, Blanchard, and Natemeyer (1979) to explain the personal use of power. Sullivan (2004) has reorganized these types, eliminating much of the overlap in the original categories.	**Personal power:** Based on one's reputation and credibility.	The leader of a state nurses association (SNA) may have access to the leaders of the state legislature based on the leader's personal power that is based on years of work with members of the legislature. The SNA president has always delivered on promises of support and provided useful information to legislators on matters of health policy.
	Expert power: Results from the knowledge and skills one possesses that are needed by others.	An advanced practice nurse is viewed as the clinical expert on a nursing unit and as a powerful person.
	Position power: Possessed by virtue of one's position within an organization or status within a group.	The Dean of a College of Nursing is viewed on campus as powerful, because this Dean leads the fastest growing academic unit on campus.
	Perceived power: Results from one's reputation as a powerful person.	A nursing student seeks a certain nurse manager as a preceptor during a senior clinical practicum because of the manager's reputation as an effective manager within the organization.
	Information power: Stems from one's possession of selected information that is needed by others.	A staff nurse demonstrates great skill in teaching patients difficult self-care activities and is sought out by colleagues to help them teach their patients.
	Connection power: Gained by association with people who have links to powerful people.	At a Nurses' Week celebration, nurses take advantage of the opportunity to have extended, informal conversations with those who report to the chief nursing officer.

*These categories help explain how we use power to influence others. The categories are not mutually exclusive and usually are used in concert with one another.

Nurses commonly use all of these types of power while implementing a wide range of nursing activities. Nurses who teach parents about the care of their newborn use expert and information power by virtue of the information they share with parents; they also exercise position power because they are registered nurses and therefore are accorded a certain status by society. Members of a state nurses' association who lobby their members of the state legislature use expert and position power when trying to gain legislators' support for a piece of healthcare legislation. New graduates, who are employed on probationary status until they successfully meet and demonstrate the initial clinical competencies of a position, may view the nurse manager as exercising both position and expert power related to their evaluation for continued employment. Nursing faculty and skilled clinicians often serve as role models to nursing students. The faculty and clinicians exercise expert and perceived power as students emulate their behavior. Examples of connection power are evident at any kind of social gathering in the workplace. People of high status (e.g., vice presidents, directors, deans) within an organization may be sought out for conversation by those who want to move up the organizational hierarchy. Nurses elected to state or federal legislatures may use informational, expert, perceived, and personal power as they work to gain passage of healthcare legislation.

Having a high-status position in an organization immediately provides stature, but power depends on the ability to accomplish goals from that position. Although some may think that "knowledge is power," acting on that knowledge is where the real power lies. Sharing knowledge expands one's power and, in turn, empowers colleagues by giving them information or skills that they need to take action in a situation.

Nursing's early history in the United States was marked by powerlessness (Sullivan, 2004). Nurses were absent from the decision-making processes about their education, practice, and employment. As the social, political, and economic status of women and nurses changed, so did the exercise of power by nursing as a profession and nurses as individuals. Powerlessness, a behavior still exhibited by some nurses, results in negative emotions such as apathy and anger. This can result in a workplace culture that is marked by conflict, anger, and other dysfunctional behaviors. Sharing power and facilitating the **empowerment** of colleagues so that they exercise their power are strong forces in creating revitalized workplace cultures.

Influence is the process of using power. Influence can range from the punitive power of coercion to the interactive power of collaboration. Coaching a new graduate nurse in orientation to complete a complicated nursing procedure successfully vividly demonstrates the ability of the experienced nurse to influence that orientee. The coach uses expert, position, perceived, and information power to influence the orientee not only at that moment but also perhaps over the span of a career. A nurse who testifies before a legislative committee uses expertise, information, and perceived power to encourage support for a bill to expand health-

care services to the children of the working poor. Nurses can use personal, expert, and perceived power while working on the campaigns of legislators who support nursing and healthcare issues; they also use perceived, expert, and connection power by avoiding the campaigns of those legislators who are not supportive of such issues.

EMPOWERMENT

Empowerment is a term that has come into common usage in nursing in recent years. It has been used extensively in the nursing literature related to administration and management; it is also highly relevant to the domain of clinical practice. Empowerment is a process of gaining control to exercise one's power (Tomey, 2004). Empowerment is also the process by which we facilitate the participation of others in decision-making and taking action within an environment where they are free to exercise power (Tomey, 2004; Mason, Leavitt, & Chaffee, 2002). Empowerment is consistent with the contemporary view of leadership, a paradigm that is exemplified by behaviors characteristic of nurses: facilitator, coach, teacher, and collaborator. These leadership skills are an essential component of professional nursing practice, whether a nurse is a clinician, an educator, a researcher, or an administrator/manager (Porter-O'Grady & Malloch, 2003). Nursing leaders, whether in the employment setting or in professional organizations, exercise power in making professional judgments as they do their daily work.

These leadership skills are essential to effective followers, too. Powerful nurse managers enable their staffs to exercise power, influencing them to grow professionally. Powerful nurses support their patients and families so they can participate actively in their care. Hence, these leadership skills can be viewed as an essential component of professional nursing practice whether one is a clinician, an educator, a researcher, or an executive/manager.

Empowerment is the process by which power is shared with colleagues and patients as part of the nurse's exercise of power. This is in sharp contrast to traditional conceptualizations of power, a patriarchal model of power, which relies on coercion, hierarchy, authority, control, and force. Viewed with a feminist perspective, empowerment is supported through collaboration, not competition and power plays (Sullivan, 2004).

Nurses have too often viewed power as a finite quantity: "If I give you some of my power, I will have less." Empowerment emphasizes the notion that power grows when shared. If one can conceptualize the exercise of shared power along a spectrum from low to high levels of sharing, the ends of the spectrum can be characterized by two very different groups of nurses:

- Nurses who view power as finite will avoid cooperation with their colleagues and refuse to share their expertise; and
- Nurses who conceptualize power as infinite are strong collaborators who gain satisfaction by helping their colleagues expand their expertise and their power base.

Empowered nurses make truly professional practice possible, the kind of professional practice that is satisfying to all nurses. Empowered clinicians are essential for effective nursing management, just as empowered managers set the stage for excellence in clinical practice. Encouraging a reticent colleague to be an active participant in committee meetings serves to empower that nurse and to shape practice policy with the institution. Guiding a novice nurse in exercising professional judgment empowers both the senior nurse and the novice clinician. Coaching a patient on how to be more assertive with a physician who is reluctant to answer the patient's questions is another form of empowerment.

Exercise 9–2

Think about a recent clinical experience when you empowered a patient. What did you do for and/or with the patient (and family) that was empowering? How did you feel about your own actions in this situation? How did the patient (or family) respond to your efforts?

Strategies for Developing a Powerful Image

As Margaret Thatcher, former prime minister of Great Britain, said, "Being powerful is like being a lady. If you have to tell people you are, you aren't."

The most basic power strategy is the development of a powerful image. Lady Thatcher's statement emphasizes the importance of this powerful image. If nurses think they are powerful, others

will view them as powerful (perceived power); if they view themselves as powerless, so will others. A sense of self-confidence is a strong foundation in developing one's "power image," and it is essential for successful political efforts in the workplace, within the profession, and within the public policy arena. Several key factors contribute to one's power image:

- Self-image: thinking of oneself as powerful and effective
- Grooming and dress: ensuring that clothing, hair, and general appearance are neat, clean, and appropriate to the situation
- Good manners: treating people with courtesy and respect
- Body language: maintaining good posture, using gestures that avoid too much drama, maintaining good eye contact, and being confident in your movement
- Speech: using a firm, confident voice; good grammar and diction; an appropriate vocabulary; and strong communication skills

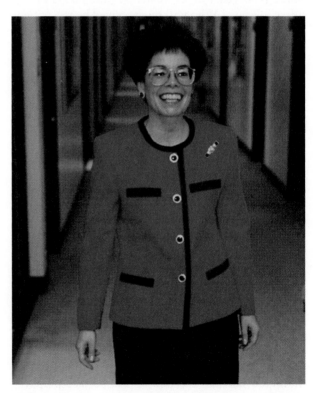

A powerful image is needed when representing the profession of nursing.

■ *Exercise 9-3*

Think about a powerful public figure whom you admire. What key factors contribute to this person's powerful image? Think about a powerful nurse you have met. Identify this person's key image factors. Think about nurses who work in wrinkled scrubs, hair pulled back haphazardly into ponytails, who fail to make eye contact with patients or their family members. What kind of powerful image message does she/he send?

Concern about a powerful image may seem superficial. However, the impressions we make on people influence the way they view us now and in the future and how they value what we do and say. First impressions are important; we do not get a second chance to make a first impression. Given similar educational and experiential backgrounds, who is more likely to be hired for a nursing position: the candidate who comes dressed in a suit or the candidate who arrives in jeans and sandals? Who will be seen as the more competent professional by a patient: the nurse in wrinkled scrubs or the nurse in neat street clothes and a freshly laundered lab coat? Who will have a greater positive impact on a member of the state legislature: the nurse who visits in a sweatshirt and shorts or the nurse in a suit? Who will be perceived by the patient as the more competent caregiver: a nurse with multiple body piercings and 4-inch acrylic nails or the neatly groomed nurse? A powerful image signals to others that one is professionally competent, influential, powerful, and capable of exercising appropriate judgments.

Attitudes and beliefs are other important aspects of a powerful image; they reflect one's values. Believing that power is a positive force in nursing is essential to one's powerful image. A firm belief in nursing's value to society and the centrality of nursing's contribution to the healthcare delivery system is also important. Powerful nurses do not allow the phrase "I'm just a nurse" in their vocabulary. Behavior reflects one's pride in the profession of nursing. This not only increases a nurse's own power but also helps empower nursing colleagues.

Make a Commitment to Nursing as a Career
Nursing is a profession; professions offer careers, not just a series of jobs. For a long time, nursing marketed itself to recruits as the perfect preparation for marriage and family. Even some contemporary job advertisements hint at romance as an outcome of employment at the agency featured. Some people still view nurses only as members of an occupation who drop in and out of employment, not as members of a profession with a long-term career commitment. Having a career commitment does not preclude leaving employment temporarily for family, education, or other demands. Having a career commitment implies that nurses view themselves first and foremost as members of the discipline of nursing with an obligation to make a contribution to the profession. Status as an employee of a particular hospital, home health agency, long-term-care facility, or other venue is secondary to one's status as a member of the profession of nursing.

Value Continuing Nursing Education Valuing education is one of the hallmarks of a profession. The continuing development of one's professional skills and knowledge is an empowering experience, preparing the nurse to make decisions with the support of an expanding body of knowledge. Seminars, workshops, and conferences offer opportunities for continued professional growth and empowerment. Returning to school for advanced degrees or post-baccalaureate or post-graduate certificates is also a powerful growth experience and reflects commitment to the profession of nursing. For several decades, some nurses thought the best way to get ahead in nursing was to seek education outside of nursing at the baccalaureate and graduate level. To develop expertise in the science and art of nursing, one needs to be educated in the discipline of nursing.

Change will continue in the healthcare system, necessitating continuing education to empower nurses to be proactive, not just reactive. A well-educated nursing workforce is essential if nursing is to have a strong voice in shaping the changes in health care. An additional advantage of participating in educational experiences is that it creates opportunities for networking, a strategy that is discussed later in this chapter.

PERSONAL POWER STRATEGIES

Developing a collection of power strategies, or power tools, is an important aspect of personal empowerment. These strategies should be used in situations that demand the exercise of leadership.

Such strategies are techniques for building a professional power base and for developing political skills within an organization (Boxes 9-1 and 9-2). They also indicate to others that one is a powerful nurse and a leader. These boxes identify personal power strategies beyond those discussed in this section. These "power tools" have been developed and collected by this author during nearly 30 years of nursing experience and observation of successful, effective, powerful nurses.

Communication Skills

The most basic tool is effective verbal communication skills, which help define a power image. These are the same communication skills nurses learn to ensure effective interaction with patients and families. Listening skills are essential leadership skills. Just as the clinician listens to the patient to collect assessment data, the manager uses listening skills to assess and evaluate. Managers who are good listeners develop reputations for being fair and consistent. Listening to recurring themes related to minor issues of staff dissatisfaction in informal conversations can enable the manager to take action before a staff crisis occurs.

Verbal and nonverbal skills are important personal power strategies; the ability to assess these messages is a critical power strategy. Experts in communication estimate that 90% of the messages we communicate to others are nonverbal. When nonverbal and verbal messages are in conflict, the nonverbal message is always more powerful. The basic lessons on the power of nonverbal communication that most nurses learn in an introductory psychiatric course are relevant in all areas of nursing!

BOX 9-1

Strategies for Developing a Powerful Image

- Self-image
- Grooming and dress
- Speech
- Body language
- Belief in power as a positive force
- Belief in the value of nursing to society
- Career commitment
- Continuing professional education

Exercise 9-4

You encounter an old friend at a nursing conference. You greet one another warmly, each stating how good it is to see the other. Yet your friend visibly backs away when you extend your arms to embrace. What is your immediate reaction? Despite the warm words of greeting, do you question your old friend's sincerity because of the strong nonverbal message regarding physical contact? Consider other situations you have experienced recently when words and actions contradict one another. Which message, the verbal or the nonverbal, did you accept as the person's "real" communication to you? Practice with a friend: Pretend you are greeting a visitor to your home, a colleague, or a patient. In the first trial, state your greeting warmly, extend your hand to shake the other person's hand, smile, and make eye contact. In the second trial, use the same words of greeting, but use an angry tone of voice, avoid eye contact, and fold your arms across your chest while moving one step back from the other person. Observe the physical actions and listen carefully, especially to the tone of voice. Repeat the exercise, switching roles. Discuss your response to these interactions.

Networking

Networking is an important power strategy and political skill. A **network** is a deliberate outcome of identifying, valuing, and maintaining relationships with a system of individuals who are sources of information, advice, and support. Networking

BOX 9-2

Additional Personal Power Strategies

- Be honest.
- Be courteous; it makes other people feel good!
- Smile when appropriate; it puts people at ease.
- Accept responsibility for your own mistakes, and learn from them.
- Be a risk taker.
- Win and lose gracefully.
- Learn to be comfortable with conflict and ambiguity; they are both normal states of the human condition.
- Give credit to others where credit is due.
- Develop the ability to take constructive criticism gracefully; learn to let destructive criticism "roll off your back."
- Use business cards when introducing yourself to new contacts and collect the business cards of those you meet when networking.
- Follow through on promises.

supports the empowerment of participants through interaction and the refinement of their interpersonal skills. Most nurses have relatively limited networks within the organizations where they are employed. They tend to have lunch or coffee with those people with whom they work most closely. One strategy to expand a workplace network is to have lunch or coffee with someone from another department, including managers from nonnursing departments, at least two or three times a month.

Active participation in nursing organizations is the most effective method of establishing a professional network outside one's place of employment. Although only a minority of nurses actively participate in professional organizations, such participation can propel a nurse into the politics of nursing, including involvement in shaping health policy. State and district nurses' associations offer excellent opportunities to develop a network that includes nurses from various clinical and functional areas. Membership in specialty organizations, especially organizations for nurse managers and executives, provides the opportunity to network with nurses with similar expertise and interests. In addition, membership in civic, volunteer, and special interest groups and participation in educational programs (e.g., formal academic programs and conferences) also provide networking opportunities.

The successful networker identifies a core of networking partners who are particularly skilled, insightful, and eager to support the development of colleagues. These partners need to be nurtured through such strategies as sharing information with them that relates to their interests, introducing them to persons who have comparable interests or who are connected with others of influence, staying connected through notes, e-mail, calls, or instant messages, and planning to meet at important events. Successful networkers are not a burden to others in making requests for support and they do not refute support that is provided.

Mentoring

In recent years, mentoring has become a driving force in nursing. Mentors are competent, experienced professionals who develop a relationship with a novice for the purpose of providing advice, support, information, and feedback to encourage the development of another individual. Mentoring has been an important element in the career devel-

opment of men in business, academia, and selected professions. Mentoring has become a significant power strategy for women in general and for nurses in particular during the past 30 years. Mentoring provides novices with expanded access to information, power, and career opportunities. Mentors have historically been a critical asset to novices trying to negotiate workplace and professional politics. Effective mentoring in nursing benefits both the mentor and the mentee by helping each to develop professionally (McKinley, 2004; Reeves, 2004).

The mentors benefit by supporting their own professional development and that of their colleagues, improving their own self-awareness, experiencing the intrinsic benefits of teaching another, nurturing their own interpersonal skills, and expanding their political savvy. Mentees receive one-on-one nurturing from the mentor; gain insight about the political rules of the organization and learn about organizational culture from an insider; can expand their self-confidence in a supportive relationship; receive career development advice; profit from the mentor's professional network; and have a unique opportunity for individualized professional development (Reeves, 2004, p. 49).

Mentoring is an empowering experience for both mentors and novices. The process of seeking out mentors is an exercise in growth for novices or protégés. Mentors often come from one's professional networks. Some mentors select their protégés; other times the reverse is true.

Novices learn new skills from influential mentors and gain self-confidence. Mentors share their influence through the influence of the novices they mentor and gain satisfaction by experiencing the evolution of a novice into an experienced nurse.

Goal-Setting

Goal-setting is another power strategy. Every nurse knows about setting goals. Students learn to devise patient care goals or patient outcomes as part of the care-planning process. Nurses may be expected to write annual goals for performance reviews at work. Even a project at home (e.g., painting rooms) may necessitate setting goals (e.g., painting a room each day of one's vacation). Goals help one to know if what was planned was actually accomplished. Likewise, a successful nursing career needs goals to define what one wants to achieve as a nurse.

Without such goals, one can wander endlessly through a series of jobs without a real sense of satisfaction. To paraphrase what the Cheshire Cat told Alice during her trip through Wonderland: Any road will take you there if you don't know where you are going.

Well-defined, long-term goals may be hard to formulate early in a career. For example, few new graduates know specifically that they want to be chief nurse executives, deans, managers, or researchers, yet, eventually, some will choose those career paths. However, developing such a vision early in a career is an important personal power strategy. Once this career vision is developed, one must create opportunities to move toward that vision. Such planning is empowering; it puts the nurse in charge, rather than letting a career unfold by chance. Having this sense of vision is consistent with the commitment to a career in nursing that is part of developing a power image. This vision is always subject to change as new opportunities are experienced, and new interests, knowledge, and skills are gained. Education and work experiences are tools for achieving the vision of one's career.

Developing Expertise

As noted earlier in this chapter, expertise is one of the bases of power. Developing expertise in nursing is an important power strategy. Expertise must not be limited to clinical knowledge. Leadership and communication skills, for example, are essential to the effective exercise of power in a range of nursing roles. Education and practice provide the means for developing such expertise in any of the domains of nursing: clinical practice, education, research, and management. Developing expertise expands one's power among nursing colleagues, other professional colleagues, and patients. A high level of expertise can make one nearly indispensable within an organization. This is a powerful position to have within any organization, whether it is the workplace or a professional association. A high level of expertise can also lead to a high level of visibility within an organization.

High Visibility

The strategy of high visibility within an organization also requires volunteering to serve as a member or the chairperson of committees and task forces. High visibility can be nurtured by attending the open meetings of committees and other groups, including those for which you are not a member, in the workplace, professional associations, or the community. This is especially true of meetings that deal with local health issues. Review the agendas of these meetings if agendas are circulated ahead of the meeting. Use opportunities both before and after meetings to share your expertise, providing valuable information and ideas to members and leaders of such groups. Share this expertise at open meetings when appropriate. Speak up confidently, but have something relevant to say. Be concise and precise; members of the committee will ask for more information if they need it. Create your own business cards using a computer and sheets of business card stock (purchased at any office supply store). Give members of these committees your personal card so that they can contact you later for information.

EXERCISING POWER AND INFLUENCE IN THE WORKPLACE AND OTHER ORGANIZATIONS: SHAPING POLICY

To use influence effectively in any organization, one must understand how the system works and develop organizational strategies. Developing organizational savvy includes identifying the real decision-makers and those persons who have a high level of influence with the decision-makers. Recognize the informal leaders within any organization. In the workplace an influential senior staff nurse may have more decision-making power than the nurse manager on significant aspects of the nursing unit's operations. The senior staff nurse may have more clinical expertise and a greater wealth of knowledge about the history of the unit and its personnel than a nurse manager with excellent management and leadership skills who is new to the unit.

Office staff of chief nursing officers (CNOs), for example, are usually very powerful people, although they are not always recognized as such. The CNO's assistant has a great deal of control over information, making decisions about who gets to meet with the nurse executive and when, screening incoming and outgoing mail, letting the CNO know when a letter or memo needs immediate attention, or placing a memo on the bottom of the stack of mail for review at a later time.

Collegiality and Collaboration

Nursing does not exist in a vacuum, nor do nurses work in isolation from one another, other professionals, or support personnel. Nurses function within a wide range of organizations, such as schools, hospitals, community health organizations, government agencies, professional associations, and universities. Nurses have been characterized for too long as divided over educational level for entry into practice and for their failure to join nursing organizations. Developing a sense of unity requires each nurse to act collaboratively and collegially in the workplace and in other organizations (e.g., professional associations). Collegiality demands that nurses value the accomplishments of nursing colleagues and express a sincere interest in their efforts. Turning to nursing colleagues for advice and support empowers them and expands one's own power base at the same time. Unity of purpose does not contradict diversity of thought. One does not have to be a friend to everyone who is a colleague. Collegiality demands mutual respect, not friendship.

Collaboration and collegiality require that nurses work collectively to ensure that the voice of nursing is heard in the workplace and the legislature. Volunteer to serve on committees and task forces in the workplace, not only within the nursing department but also on organization-wide committees. Become an active member of nursing organizations, especially one's state nursing organization (affiliates of the ANA) and a specialty organization consistent with one's clinical specialty (e.g., American Association of Critical Care Nurses [AACN]) or functional role (e.g., American Organization of Nurse Executives [AONE]). If eligible, become a member of a chapter of Sigma Theta Tau International Nursing Honor Society. Get involved in the politics of the organization, whether in the workplace or through a professional association. If a workplace organization uses shared governance or continuous quality improvement models, get involved in these councils, committees, task forces, and work groups to share your energy, ideas, and expertise. Many organizations have instituted joint practice committees that bring together nurses and physicians to improve the quality of interdisciplinary collaboration and, in turn, the quality of patient care. Become an active, productive member of such groups within the workplace and in the professional associations and community groups dealing with healthcare issues and problems.

An Empowering Attitude

Demonstrate a positive and professional attitude about being a nurse to nursing colleagues, patients and their families, other colleagues in the workplace, and the public, including legislators. This attitude is very contagious and can facilitate the exercise of power among colleagues while educating others about nurses and nursing. A powerful image is an important aspect of demonstrating this positive professional attitude. The current practice of nurses to identify themselves by first name only may decrease their power image in the eyes of physicians, patients, and others. Physicians are always addressed as "Doctor"; when they address others by their first names, inequality of power and status is evident. The use of first names among colleagues is not inappropriate so long as everyone is playing by the same rules. Managers may want to enhance the empowerment of their staffs by encouraging them to introduce themselves as "Dr.," "Ms.," or "Mr." Arriving at work, appointments, or meetings on time; looking neat and appropriately attired for the work setting or other professional situation; and speaking positively about one's work are examples of how easy it is to demonstrate a positive, powerful, and professional attitude.

Kovach and Morgan (2003) question the use of the phrase "doctor's orders" as it relates to a section of the patient's healthcare record. They view this phrase as disempowering to nurses and other healthcare professionals with the implied assumption that physicians must give "orders" to nurses for nurses to exercise power to carry out patient care. The phrase also negates the reality that disciplines, other than medicine, write "orders" and observations on those same pages, whether in an electronic or paper format.

Magnet™ institutions, as recognized by the American Nurses Credentialing Center, are characterized by work environments that empower nurses (Kramer & Schmalenberg, 2004). Leadership activities have been identified by staff nurses in Magnet hospitals as a critical element of the work culture. Kramer and Schmalenberg identify leadership activity as one of the "essentials of magnetism" (see the Research Perspective.).

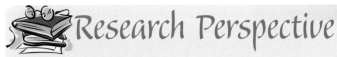

Research Perspective

Kramer, M., & Schmalenberg, C. (2004). Development and evaluation of essentials of magnetism tool. *Journal of Nursing Administration, 34*, 365-378.

Magnet facilities have become the gold standard for professional nursing practice environments. Magnet facilities attract and retain nurses and support nurses efforts to give quality care. Nurses in Magnet facilities work in empowering environments.

This study sought to identify key elements of the magnetic work environment to create a diagnostic tool to use in identifying what is needed in a workplace environment to produce quality patient care. An earlier tool developed some 20 years ago by the same authors in the earliest study of Magnet hospitals was considered outdated. To develop the Essentials of Magnetism Tool, the authors identified the essential elements of magnetism through participant observations and interviews. In this qualitative study, the authors visited 14 Magnet hospitals and conducted individual interviews with staff nurses, directors of education, and chief nursing officers, as well as group interviews of nurse managers and clinical directors, for a total of 289 participants (p. 366). Using a grounded theory approach, the authors sought definitions, dimensions, and examples of the eight essentials of magnetism.

The Essentials of Magnetism Tool (EOM) was then administered to 3602 staff nurses in 26 hospitals (16 Magnet, 10 nonmagnet hospitals) to establish the psychometric properties of the tool. Using factor analysis, factors identified in the interviews were clustered around the eight essential elements of magnetism, and content validity was established. The tool included 54 items, with 3 to 11 items included under each EOM factor.

ESSENTIALS OF MAGNETISM
- Adequacy of staffing
- Support for education
- RN-MD relationships
- Working with clinically competent nurses
- Autonomy
- Control over nursing practice
- Values
- Nurse manager support

SIGNIFICANT DIFFERENCES IN MAGNET AND NONMAGNET HOSPITALS
Nurses from Magnet hospitals ($n = 2355$) reported that their work environments were characterized by the EOM characteristics at higher levels than the nurses from nonmagnet hospitals ($n = 1247$) along all elements except nurse manager support ($P \leqq 0.05$).

IMPLICATIONS FOR PRACTICE
Magnet hospitals provide an environment that empowers nurses to provide high-quality care. The Magnet environment also supports the professional development and empowerment of nurses through support of education and nurse manager support. Magnet facilities offer nurses the opportunity to exercise their power in the pursuit of high-quality nursing care. The EOM Tool identified workplace characteristics that reflect the exercise of power by staff nurses, nurse managers, and nurse administrators.

Exercise 9–5
How do you routinely introduce yourself to patients, families, physicians, and other colleagues? A powerful and positive approach involves making eye contact with each individual, shaking hands, and introducing yourself by saying, "I'm Terry Jones, a registered nurse [or nursing student]." If you do not currently use this technique, try it out. Note any difference in the responses of people whom you meet using this technique in comparison with a less formal approach.

Developing Coalitions

The exercise of power is often directed at creating change. Although an individual can often be effective at exercising power and creating change, creating certain changes within most organizations requires collective action. Coalition building is an effective political strategy for collective action. **Coalitions** are groups of individuals or organizations that join together temporarily around a common goal. This goal often focuses on an effort to effect change. The networking between organizations that results in coalition-building requires members of one group to reach out to members of other groups. This often occurs at the leadership level and may come through formal mechanisms, such as letters that identify an issue or problem—a shared interest—around which a coalition could be built. For example, a state nurses' association may invite the leaders of organizations interested in child health (e.g., organizations of pediatric nurses, public health nurses and physicians, elementary school teachers, day-care providers) and consumers (e.g., parents) to discuss collaborative support for a legislative initiative to improve access to immunization programs in urban and rural areas. Such coalitions of professionals and consumers are powerful in influencing public policy related to health care.

Collaboration among groups and individuals with common interests and goals often results in greater success in effecting change and exercising power in the workplace and within other organizations, including legislative bodies. For example, in Illinois, a coalition of nursing organizations and individuals concerned about the nursing shortage was founded. The Illinois Coalition for Nursing Resources (n.d.) brings together a diverse group of nursing and healthcare organizations and individuals to prevent a nursing shortage crisis and to maximize nursing resources in the state. Expanding networks in the workplace, as suggested earlier in this chapter, facilitates creating a coalition by developing a pool of candidates for coalition building before they are needed. Invite people with common goals to lunch or coffee to begin building a coalition around an issue. Discuss this shared interest and gain the commitment of the individuals. Meet over lunch or coffee with members of the committee or task force that is working on this issue. Attend the open meetings of professional groups that share the same interests as the organization to which you belong. Share ideas on how to create the desired change most effectively as one builds coalitions.

Coalition building is an important skill for involvement in legislative politics. Nursing organizations often use coalition building, such as the development of Illinois Coalition for Nursing Resources, when dealing with state legislatures and Congress. Changes in nurse practice acts to expand

opportunities for advanced nursing practice have been accomplished in many states through coalition building. State medical societies or the state agencies that license physicians often oppose such changes. Efforts by a single nursing organization (e.g., a state nurses' association or a nurse practitioners' organization), representing a limited nursing constituency, often lack the clout to overcome opposition by the unified voice of the state's physicians. However, the unified effort of a coalition of nursing organizations, other healthcare organizations, and consumer groups can be powerful in effecting change through legislation.

Negotiating

Kritek (2002) points out nursing's vulnerability in the title of her book Negotiating at an Uneven Table. **Negotiating,** or bargaining, is a critically important skill for organizational and political power. It is a process of making trade-offs. Children are natural negotiators. Often, they will initially ask their parents for more than what they are willing to accept in the way of privileges, toys, or activities. The logic is simple to children: Ask for more than is reasonable and negotiate down to what you really want!

Negotiating often works the same way within organizations. People will sometimes ask for more than what they want and be willing to accept less. In other situations, both sides will enter a negotiation asking for radically different things, but each may be willing to settle for a position that differs significantly from their original positions. In the simplest forms of bargaining, each participant has something that the other party values: goods, services, or information. At the "bargaining table" each party presents an opening position, and the process moves on until they reach a mutually agreeable result or until one or both parties walk away from the unsuccessful process.

Bargaining may take many forms. Individuals may negotiate with a supervisor for a more desirable work schedule or with a peer to effect a schedule change so that the nurse can attend an out-of-town conference. A nurse manager may sit at the bargaining table with the department director during budget planning to expand training hours for the nursing unit in the next year's budget. Representatives of a coalition of nursing organizations meeting with a legislator may negotiate with the legislator over sections of a proposed healthcare–related bill in an effort to eliminate or modify those sections not viewed by the nursing coalition as in the best interests of nurses, patients, or the healthcare system. Or a group of nurses may bargain with nursing and hospital administration over wages, staffing levels, other working conditions, and the conditions and policies that govern clinical practice. This is called collective bargaining, a specific type of negotiating that is regulated by both state and federal labor laws and that usually involves representation by a state nurses' association or a nursing or nonnursing labor union (see Chapter 18).

Successful negotiators are well informed about not only their own positions but also those of the opposing side. Successful negotiators must be able to discuss the pros and cons of both positions. They are able to assist the other party in recognizing the costs versus the benefits of each position. These skills are also essential to exercising power effectively with the arenas of professional and legislative politics. When lobbying a member of the legislature to support a bill that is desired by nurses, one must understand the position of those opposed to the bill to respond effectively to questions that the legislator may ask.

Exercise 9–6

Consider a situation in which you engaged in bargaining or negotiating. Have you ever bought a car? Negotiating the price of the car is a great American tradition. Few people enter into the purchase of a car intending to pay the sticker price. The manufacturer sets most sticker prices at a level that gives the dealer room to negotiate the price down; a few makes of automobiles have firm sticker prices with no room for negotiation. Have you ever negotiated a schedule change at work or school? Have you ever negotiated a raise in your salary? What was the trade-off you made in the process? How far did the other person move from his or her original position? What factors led to your success or failure in this negotiation?

Taking Political Action to Influence Policy

In the 1990s, Carolyn McCarthy was a licensed practical nurse (LPN) from New York when a tragedy turned her life around. Her husband was killed and her son injured by a gunman on the Long Island Railroad. She sought the support of her congressman on gun control legislation as a result of her personal tragedy. He refused to support such

legislation. She took extraordinary action, changing her party affiliation from Republican to Democrat and then running against the incumbent for his seat in Congress. Today she is still an LPN, but she is also Congresswoman Carolyn McCarthy (D-NY). Taking action may include such simple acts as working in a legislative campaign or volunteering to work on a church committee to establish a parish health ministry. Extraordinary actions like those taken by Carolyn McCarthy are also essential for nursing's voice to be heard loudly and clearly in the uncertain future.

Developing political skills, like any other skill set, is a developmental process. Some suggested strategies for developing political skills include:

- Build a working relationship with a legislator, such as one's state senator or representative or member of the U.S. Congress and the legislative staff members.
- Join and be an active member of your state nurses association affiliate of the ANA.
- Invite a legislator to a professional organization meeting.
- Invite a legislator or staff person from the legislator's office to spend a day with you at work.
- Register to vote and vote in every election.
- Join your state nurses association's government relations or legislative committee and political action committee (PAC); join ANA's political action committee.
- Be in touch with your federal and state legislators on nursing and healthcare issues, especially related to specific bills, by letter writing, telephone calls, or e-mails.
- Participate in nurse lobby day and meet with your state legislators.
- Work on a federal or state legislative campaign.
- Visit your U.S. senators and member of Congress if visiting in the Washington, DC, area to discuss federal legislation related to nursing and health care.
- Get involved in the local group of your political party.
- Run for office at the local, county, state, or congressional level.
- Enhance the image of nursing in all your policy efforts.
- Communicate your message effectively and clearly.
- Develop your expertise in shaping policy.

BOX 9-3

Political Astuteness Inventory

Place a check mark (√) next to those items for which your answer is yes. Then give yourself one point for each yes. After completing the inventory, compare your total score with the scoring criteria at the end of the inventory.

1. I am registered to vote.
2. I know where my voting precinct is located.
3. I voted in the last general election.
4. I voted in the last two elections.
5. I recognized the names of the majority of the candidates on the ballot and was acquainted with the majority of issues in the last election.
6. I stay abreast of current health issues.
7. I belong to the state professional or student nurse organization.
8. I participate (e.g., as a committee member, officer) in this organization.
9. I attended the most recent meeting of my district nurses' association.
10. I attended the last state or national convention held by my organization.
11. I am aware of at least two issues discussed and the stands taken at this convention.
12. I read literature published by my state nurses' association, a professional journal/magazine/newsletter, or other literature on a regular basis to stay abreast of current health issues.
13. I know the names of my senators in Washington.
14. I know the name of my representative in Washington.
15. I know the name of the state senator from my district.
16. I know the name of the state representative from my district.
17. I am acquainted with the voting record of at least one of the above in relation to a specific health issue.
18. I am aware of the stand taken by at least one of the above in relation to a specific health issue.
19. I know whom to contact for information about health-related issues at the state or federal level.
20. I know whether my professional organization employs lobbyists at the state or federal level.
21. I know how to contact these lobbyists.
22. I contribute financially to my state and national professional organization's political action committee (PAC).
23. I give information about effectiveness of elected officials to assist the PAC's endorsement process.
24. I actively supported a senator or representative during the last election.
25. I have written to one of my state or national representatives in the last year regarding a health issue.
26. I am personally acquainted with a senator or representative or member of his or her staff.
27. I serve as a resource person for one of my representatives or his or her staff.
28. I know the process by which a bill is introduced in my state legislature.
29. I know which senators or representatives are supportive of nursing.
30. I know which House and Senate committees usually deal with health-related issues.
31. I know the committees of which my representatives are members.
32. I know of at least two health issues related to my profession that are currently under discussion.
33. I know of at least two health-related issues that are currently under discussion at the state or national level.
34. I am aware of the composition of the state board that regulates my profession.
35. I know the process whereby one becomes a member of the state board that regulates my profession.
36. I know what DHHS stands for.
37. I have at least a vague notion of the purpose of the DHHS.
38. I am a member of a health board or advisory group to a health organization or agency.
39. I attend public hearings related to health issues.
40. I find myself more interested in political issues now than in the past.

Scoring:

 0-9   Totally unaware politically/apathetic
10-19   Slightly more aware of the implications of the politics of nursing/buy-in
20-29   Beginning political astuteness/self-interest to political sophistication
30-40   Politically astute, an asset to nursing/leading the way

From Goldwater, M., & Zusy, M. J. L. (1990). *Prescription for nurses: Effective political action.* St. Louis: Mosby; with permission.

- Seek appointive positions or elective office to shape policy more effectively.

The personal power strategies mentioned earlier in this chapter are also important for building one's political power. Nurses can no longer be passive observers of the political world; political involvement is a professional responsibility, not just a privilege (Boswell, Cannon, & Miller, 2005).

The Political Astuteness Inventory (Goldwater & Zusy, 1990) is a helpful tool in determining how well-prepared you are to influence legislative politics and public policy, especially public policy related to health care (Box 9-3).

The Solution

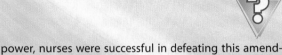

The SNA lobbyist and I put out an action alert by mail, e-mail, and telephone to alert members to this situation. This alert resulted in hundreds of calls to members of the senate committee from SNA members, other registered nurses, and student nurses. The members of the committee were overwhelmed with calls in opposition to the hostile amendment. In addition, the executive director of the SNA testified at the hearing about the disastrous results that this hostile amendment would hold for quality health care in the state. By using their collective power, nurses were successful in defeating this amendment, thus shaping public policy related to the integrity of the state's nursing practice act and other licensing laws. This issue has re-appeared in the legislature in a later session and was again defeated because of the visibility of the state nurses association.

— Gail Haller

 Would this be a suitable approach for you? Why?

CHAPTER CHECKLIST

Power was once a taboo issue in nursing. The exercise of power in nursing conflicted sharply with the historic feminine stereotypes that surrounded nursing. The evolving social and political status of women has also opened nursing to the exercise of power. Power is essential to the effective implementation of both the clinical and the managerial roles of nurses.

- Contemporary concepts of power focus on power as influence and a force for collaboration rather than coercion, an infinite quality rather than a finite quantity.
- Empowerment is a feminine-feminist process of power-sharing and leadership.
- Contemporary views of leadership in social systems are consistent with the concept of empowerment.
- Six types of power exercised by nurses include:
  - Position
  - Perceived
  - Expert
  - Personal
  - Information
  - Connection

- Key factors in developing a powerful image include:
  - Self-confidence
  - Body language
  - Self-image
  - Career commitment
  - Grooming and dress
  - Speech
  - Attitudes, beliefs, and values
  - Continuing professional education
- Key personal and organizational strategies for exercising power include:
  - Communication skills
  - Career goal-setting
  - High visibility
  - A sense of unity
  - Coalition-building
  - Networking
  - Expertise
  - Organizational savvy
  - Collaboration and collegiality
  - Negotiation skills
  - Mentoring
  - An empowering attitude

TIPS ON POWER AND POLITICS

- Remember that power is not a "dirty word," nor is it an undesirable professional characteristic for nurses; it is the ability to influence others effectively.
- By exercising power in the workplace and other professional activities, you empower patients, families, and colleagues to accomplish their goals.
- Believing in your own ability to create change (i.e., exercise power), valuing the exercise of power, and projecting a powerful image (e.g., grooming, manners, body language, verbal communication skills) are essential to functioning as an influential professional nurse.
- Participating in networking and mentoring, setting clear career goals, and developing your expertise are key power strategies.
- Shaping policy is an extension of nursing practice, part of the nurse's advocacy role.

TERMS TO KNOW

coalitions	policy
empowerment	politics
influence	power
negotiating	

REFERENCES

Boswell, C., Cannon, S., & Miller, J. (2005). Nurses' political involvement: Responsibility vs. privilege. *Journal of Professional Nursing 21*, 5-8.

DeMarco, R. F., & Roberts, S. J. (2003). Negative behaviors in nursing: Looking in the mirror and beyond. *American Journal of Nursing, 103*(3), 113, 115-116.

Goldwater, M., & Zusy, M. J. L. (1990). *Prescription for nurses: Effective political action.* St. Louis: Mosby.

Hersey, P., Blanchard, K., & Natemeyer, W. (1979). Situational leadership, perception and impact of power. *Group and Organizational Studies, 4*, 418-428.

Illinois Coalition for Nursing Resources. (n.d.). *About us.* Retrieved February 24, 2004, from www.ic4nr.org.

Kalisch, B. J., & Kalisch, P. A. (1982). *Politics of nursing.* Philadelphia: JB Lippincott.

Kovach, C. R., & Morgan, S. W. (2003). Doctor's orders: Rethinking language and intent. *Journal of Nursing Administration, 33*, 563-564.

Kramer, M., & Schmalenberg, C. (2004). Development and evaluation of an essentials of magnetism tool. *Journal of Nursing Administration, 34*, 365-378.

Kritek, P. B. (2002). *Negotiating at an uneven table: A practical approach to working with differences and diversity* (2nd ed.). San Francisco: Jossey-Bass.

Leavitt, J. K., Chaffee, M. W., & Vance, C. (2002). Learning the ropes of policy and politics. In D. J. Mason, J. K. Leavitt, & M. W. Chaffee (Eds.). *Policy & politics in nursing and health care* (4th ed., pp. 31-43). St. Louis: Saunders.

Mason, D. J., Leavitt, J. K., & Chaffee, M. W. (2002). *Policy & politics in nursing and health care* (4th ed.). St. Louis: Saunders.

McKinley, M. G. (2004). Mentoring matters: Creating, connecting, empowering. *AACN, 15*, 205-214.

Milstead, J. A. (2004). Advanced practice nurses and public policy, naturally. In J. A. Milstead (Ed.), *Health policy and politics: A nurse's guide* (2nd ed., pp. 1-36). Sudbury, MA: Jones and Bartlett.

Porter-O'Grady, T., & Malloch, K. (2003). *Quantum leadership: A textbook of new leadership.* Sudbury, MA: Jones and Bartlett.

Reeves, K. A. (2004). Nurses nurturing nurses: A mentoring program. *Nurse Leader, 2*(6), 47-49, 53.

Roberts, K. (2004). Profiles: On the campaign trail. *American Journal of Nursing, 104*(2), 102-103.

Roberts, S. J. (1983). Oppressed group behavior: Implications for nursing. *Advances in Nursing Sciences, 5*, 21-30.

Roberts, S. J. (2000). Development of a positive professional identity: Liberating oneself from the oppressor within. *Advances in Nursing Science, 22*(4), 71-82.

Sullivan, E. J. (2004). *Becoming influential: A guide for nurses.* Upper Saddle River, NJ: Pearson Education.

Tomey, A. M. (2004). *Guide to nursing management and leadership* (7th ed.). St. Louis: Mosby.

SUGGESTED READINGS

Ashley, J. A. (1976). *Hospitals, paternalism, and the role of the nurse.* New York: Teachers College Press.

Ashley, J. A. (1980). Power in structured misogyny: Implications for the politics of care. *Advances in Nursing Science, 2*, 3-22.

Borman, J., & Biordi, D. (1992). Female nurse executive: Finally, at an advantage? *Journal of Nursing Administration, 22*(9), 37-41.

Campbell-Heider, N., & Hart, C. A. (1993). Updating the nurse's bedside manner. *Image: Journal of Nursing Scholarship, 25*, 133-139.

Chinn, P. L. (2001). *Peace and power: Building communities for the future* (5th ed.). Sudbury, MA: Jones and Bartlett.

Cohen, S. S., Mason, D. J., Kovner, C., Leavitt, J. K., Pulcini, J., & Sochalski, J. (1996). Stages of nursing political development: Where we've been and where we ought to go. *Nursing Outlook, 44,* 259-266.

Cunningham, M. P. (2000). Breaking the mold: The many legacies of nurses in progressive movements. *American Journal of Nursing, 100*(10), 121, 123-124, 126, 129, 131, 133, 135-136.

del Bueno, D. (1986). Power and policy in organizations. *Nursing Outlook, 34,* 124-128.

Dobos, C. (1997). Understanding personal risk taking among staff nurses: Critical information for nurse administrators. *Journal of Nursing Administration, 27*(1), 12-13.

Fisher, R., Ury, W., & Patton, B. (1991). *Getting to yes: Negotiating agreement without giving in* (2nd ed.). New York: Penguin.

Gebbie, K. M., Wakefield, M., & Kerfoot, K. (2000). Nursing and health policy. *Journal of Nursing Scholarship, 32,* 307-315.

Greene, R. (2000). *The 48 Laws of Power.* New York: Penguin Books.

Heim, P., & Goliant, S. K. (1993). *Hardball for women: Winning at the game of business.* Los Angeles: Plume Books.

Holloran, S. D. (1993). Mentoring: The experience of nursing service executives. *Journal of Nursing Administration, 23*(2), 49-54.

Kippenbrock, T. A. (1992). Power at meetings: Strategies to move people. *Nursing Economics, 10,* 282-286.

Laschinger, H. K. S., & Havens, D. S. (1996). Staff nurse work empowerment and perceived control over nursing practice: Conditions for work effectiveness. *Journal of Nursing Administration, 26*(9), 27-35.

Schutzenhofer, K. K. (1992). Essential for the year 2000. *Nursing Connections, 5*(1), 15-26.

Schutzenhofer, K. K. (1995). Networking and professionalism. In M. Strader & P. J. Decker (Eds.), *Role transition to patient care management.* Norwalk, CT: Appleton & Lange.

Schutzenhofer, K. K., Shelley, S. R., & Pontious, S. L. (1992). Communication systems. In P. J. Decker & E. J. Sullivan (Eds.), *Nursing administration: A micro/macro approach for effective nurse executives.* Norwalk, CT: Appleton & Lange.

Stanhope, M. (1999). Health policy: Strategies for analysis and influence. In J. Lancaster (Ed.), *Nursing issues in leading and managing change.* St. Louis: Mosby.

Stewart, B. M., & Kruger, L. E. (1996). An evolutionary concept of mentoring in nursing. *Journal of Professional Nursing, 12,* 311-321.

Vance, C. N. (1985). Political influence: Building effective interpersonal skills. In D. J. Mason & S. W. Talbott (Eds.), *Political action handbook for nurses: Changing the workplace, government, and organizations, and community.* Menlo Park, CA: Addison-Wesley.

Wakefield, M. (1999). Nursing future in health care policy. In E. J. Sullivan (Ed.), *Creating nursing's future: Issues, opportunities, and challenges.* St. Louis: Mosby.

Wolf, G. A. (1989). The effective use of influence. *Journal of Nursing Administration, 19*(11), 8-9.

Part 2

Managing Resources

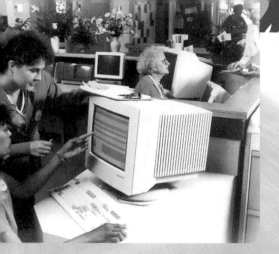

Chapter 10

Managing Information and Technology: Caring and Communicating with Computers

Karen S. Cox
Cheri Hunt

This chapter describes current applications of information and information technology that allow nurses to use the data gathered at the point of care most effectively and efficiently. It discusses nurses as knowledge workers, the science of informatics, evidence-based practice, informatics competencies, various types of information technologies, standardized nursing terminologies, and future trends. Nurses need to build knowledge from practice by comparing and contrasting not only current patient data with previous data for the same patient but also data across patients with the same diagnosis. Information tools and skills are essential for these decision-making processes now and in the future.

Objectives

- Analyze the core components of informatics: data, information, and knowledge.
- Evaluate a model to change accepted practice into evidence-based practice.
- Describe three types of healthcare information technology trends.
- Apply one structured nursing language to a nursing scenario.
- Analyze three types of technology for capturing data at the point of care.
- Discuss decision support systems and their impact on patient care.

- Explore the issues of nurse ethics and patient privacy and security in information technology.

- Value the use of the Internet for healthcare information.

Questions to Consider

- What types of technology promote safe and effective patient care?
- How do you transform patient data into information and then knowledge for knowledge-based decisions?
- How can technology enhance efficiency, effectiveness, and timeliness?
- What competencies are needed to process information effectively and utilize new information technology?
- How can you facilitate the use of informatics and technology in patient-care delivery?

The Challenge

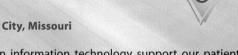

Cheri Hunt, RN, MHA
Chief Nursing Officer, Children's Mercy Hospitals and Clinics, Kansas City, Missouri

The nursing leadership team in my specialty hospital is collaborating with the hospital's medical staff, information system, and allied health managers to select a clinical information system and to evaluate information technology solutions that support clinical decision-making, communication, outcomes, and financial and administrative processes. I have several questions to consider:

1. How can clinicians be actively involved in the selection phase of the project?
2. Is one type of device strategy appropriate for all care settings?

3. Can information technology support our patient safety initiatives?
4. Do we automate our paper forms and simply replicate our current computer screens/functions or do we take this opportunity to transform work processes?

 What do you think you would do if you were this nurse?

INTRODUCTION

Technology surrounds us! Computers are being used at the bank, at the grocery checkout, in our cars, and in almost every other aspect of daily living, including the provision of health care. Health care is an information-intensive business; therefore, how the nurse gathers, manages, and uses information and the supporting information technologies will determine his or her success.

In the hospital of the future, technology will likely be the foundation for how care is planned, organized, and delivered (Parker, 2005). Underuse, overuse, and misuse of resources are cited by the Institute of Medicine in the report, "Crossing the Quality Chasm" as widespread in the U.S. health system. Many leaders in health care also see technology as a means to improve efficiency and thereby decrease costs (IOM, 2001). If appropriately deployed and fully integrated, technology has the potential to improve the practice environment for nurses and safety for patients.

Nurses are **knowledge workers.** Knowledge workers need **data** and **information** to do their jobs effectively. Knowledge work is nonrepetitive, nonroutine work that requires considerable levels of cognitive activity (Drucker, 1993). The core activity of knowledge work is critical thinking, and the outcome is shared expertise.

Nurse knowledge workers need support from information technologies. Data and information must be accurate, reliable, and presented in an actionable form. Information technologies should facilitate and extend the nurses' decision-making abilities. They should support nurses in the following areas: (1) storing clinical data, (2) translating clinical data into information, (3) linking clinical data and domain knowledge, and (4) aggregating clinical data (Snyder-Halpern, Corcoran-Perry, & Narayan, 2001).

INFORMATICS

Informatics is "a science that combines a domain science, computer science, information science, and cognitive science" (Hunter, 2001, p. 180). In this case, the domain science is nursing. In 1989, Graves and Corcoran published a classic work that describes the study of nursing informatics. Their initial model has subsequently been expanded and is depicted in Figure 10-1 (Graves, Amos, Huether, Lange, & Thompson, 1995).

The core of this model is the transformation of data into information and then into **knowledge.** This transformation occurs to facilitate decision-making, new discoveries, and the creation of designs. Information and computer literacy, as well

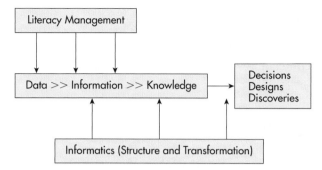

Figure 10-1 Nursing informatics conceptual model. (From Graves, J. R., Amos, L. K., Huether, S., Lange, L. L., & Thompson, C. B. [1995]. Description of a graduate program in clinical nursing informatics. *Computers in Nursing, 13* [2], 60-70.)

as the informatics infrastructure, influence this transformation of data into knowledge.

Data are discrete entities that describe or measure something without interpreting it. Numbers are data; for example, the number 30, without interpretation, means nothing. Information consists of interpreted, organized, or structured data. The number 30 interpreted as milliliters or as a length of time in minutes or hours has meaning. Knowledge refers to information that is combined or synthesized so that interrelationships are identified. For example, the number 30, when included in the statement "all patients who had indwelling catheters for longer than 30 days developed infections" becomes knowledge, something that is known.

The progression from data to information to knowledge can occur quickly in practice as data are interpreted and compared with previous information about the patient to provide knowledge. Much of the value is lost, however, if these data are not stored where others might retrieve and use them in a timely manner to synthesize new knowledge. Box 10-1 provides an example that illustrates combining and interpreting data to provide information, which, when synthesized, provides new knowledge. Because of informatics, nurses are now better able to practice from an evidence-based perspective.

So much work now is focused on evidence. Without it, we are doing our best; but the evidence either reassures us that our thoughts are correct, or the evidence redirects our thinking. Technology has changed the way we approach using evidence because it is now readily available.

BOX 10-1

Using the Information Triad

Several patients in the coronary care unit had fallen at night in the previous 3 weeks. This was very unusual because patients with heart conditions do not usually become disoriented at night. The newly assigned charge nurse became concerned about this and began to look for commonalities among the patients who had fallen. She found that they were all taking the same sleeping medication. She mentioned this at a meeting and found that several other nurses had noticed the same situation. Together, they contacted the pharmacist, who contacted the pharmaceutical representative. He found that the medication dosage had been tested on college students and that the dose was too high for older, less healthy patients. This is an example of combining data to provide information that, when aggregated and processed, becomes new knowledge.

EVIDENCE-BASED PRACTICE

Evidence-based practice (EBP) originated from evidence-based medicine (EBM) in the late 1990s (Schlosser, 2004). EBP is an integration of current evidence, clinical expertise, and patient values to optimize the patients' outcomes as well as their quality of life (Sackett, Straus, Richardson, Rosenberg, & Haynes, 2000). With the rapid research advancements, the traditional nursing strategies are inadequate in keeping pace. Practitioners may lack the skills to access and appraise the available scientific knowledge. This creates a barrier in translating research into clinical practice. Realizing this need, nursing has started to incorporate EBP principles into its curricula as well as its practices (Melnyk, Fineout-Overholt, Feinstein, Small, Wilcox, et al. 2004). In doing this, nurses will be trained to practice EBP, and this knowledge will empower them to create practices based in evidence. There are several EBP models, all of which are based on five key elements in EBP:

1. Ask a clinical question
2. Acquire the evidence
3. Appraise the evidence

4. Apply the evidence and
5. Assess the outcomes (Moyer, Elliott, 2004).

Informatics plays an important role in three of these five elements.

Ask a Clinical Question

To change the nursing paradigm, nurses must first realize they have an information need. Once the information need is established, nurses need to develop a four-part clinical question using the PICO (population, intervention, comparison, outcome) acronym. The PICO acronym is used to assist nurses in identifying what type of question is being asked (diagnosis, prognosis, etiology/harm, or therapy), which will assist them in identifying key search components and what type of research methodology (e.g., case control, cross-sectional survey, cohort study, or randomized control trials) would be appropriate to answer this question (Richardson, Wilson, Nishikawa, & Hayward, 1995).

P	Population
I	Intervention
C	Comparison
O	Outcome

Acquire the Evidence

The evidence must be available for nurses via technology. When clinicians identify a need for information, they must be able to search current literature. Haynes & Wilczynski (2004, pp 1162-1163) identified that as of May 1, 2004, Medline had "over 11 million articles from over 4500 journals." Doing a search in a non-electronic format would be impossible!

Clinicians should have versions of electronic summaries, such as Clinical Evidence (http://www.clinicalevidence.com/) and BestBETs (http://www.bestbets.org/). These summary sites review the literature and identify for the clinician a "clinical bottom line." The Cochrane Collection reviews current literature and offers an academic interpretation of the literature. And finally, if there are no summaries, clinicians should be able to access relevant electronic databases, such as CINAHL, EMBASE, MedLine, OVID, and PsycLIT, to retrieve individual studies to assist them in answering their question (Moyer & Elliott, 2004).

Appraise the Evidence

For any type of evidence found, the Oxford Centre for Evidence-Based Medicine recommends that the clinician reviews the evidence and answers three questions:

1. Is it valid?
2. Is it important?
3. Is it important to the patient (www.cebm.net/critical_appraisal.asp)?

Because there are different kinds of research, there are different assessment tools to review methodologic validity. These tools can be accessed and downloaded from the Centre's website (www.cebm.net/critical_appraisal.asp). Initially, these assessments seem very complex and time consuming; however, with practice, the literature search and assessment should take no longer than 10 minutes. This step is important for the process of building of the evidence basis for the practice of nursing continues. Knowing what others have done to date is key so that valuable time and resources are not used redoing work previously completed. However, careful review must still be done to ensure validity of past work.

Apply the Evidence

If clinicians have identified either a summary or individual studies that answer their question, they must address a practice change with the appropriate governing body (e.g., nurse practice council). This governing body would then evaluate the information and incorporate appropriate changes into the appropriate policies, procedures, and standards of care. Additionally, communication would occur with all nurses, and quality measurements would be identified.

Assess the Outcomes

Outcome measurement is a key step in this entire process. Informatics plays a key role in this validation process. Informatics provides "a mechanism by which nurses can view the effectiveness of application of evidence in practice over time" (Bakken & McArthur, 2001; pp. 289-290).

Measuring daily practice against evidence-based protocols/standards is not a one-time activity. It must be hard-wired into a system, whether it is a small primary care office or large hospital.

Using technology, real time reports can generate the variance from standards by service, department, or individual practitioner. A regular review must take place to evaluate the findings of these reports. This review will reveal whether there were important reasons to vary, barriers to practice the accepted standard, or new evidence supporting a review of the practice (DePalma, 2002).

Exercise 10-1

Think about the data that you gather every day: vital signs, intake and output, and the symptoms that you communicate during shift report. What data did you automatically combine or reorganize to help you make a decision regarding patient care? How did you use this information to improve your patient's outcome? How did technology combine or organize data?

For example, you are charting vital signs and notice that a patient's blood pressure is lower than it was the day before. He is also complaining of nausea and light-headedness. You check his medications and see that he is receiving hydralazine (Apresoline). Based on your processing of the data that you have collected, you make a note to check his blood pressure and other symptoms again and notify the physician if the situation has not changed.

TYPES OF TECHNOLOGIES

As nurses, we commonly use and manage three types of technologies: biomedical technology, information technology, and knowledge technology. **Biomedical technology** involves the use of equipment in the clinical setting for diagnosis, physiologic monitoring, testing, or administering therapies to patients. **Information technology** entails recording, processing, and using data and information, in this case, for the purpose of delivering patient care. **Knowledge technology** is the use of expert and decision-support systems to assist nurses in making decisions about patient care. These systems are designed to mimic the reasoning of nurse experts in making such decisions.

Biomedical Technology

Biomedical technology is used for (1) physiologic monitoring, (2) diagnostic testing, (3) drug admin-

istration, and (4) therapeutic treatments. Physiologic monitoring systems measure heart rate, blood pressure, and other vital signs. They also monitor arrhythmias, record pressures such as central venous pressure or pulmonary wedge pressure, and analyze oxygen and carbon dioxide levels in the blood. Continuous arrhythmia monitors and electrocardiograms (ECGs) are used to provide visual representation of electrical activity in the heart. Two types of arrhythmia systems are detection surveillance and diagnostic, or interpretive, systems. In the detection system, the criteria for a normal cardiac rhythm are programmed into the computer, which then continuously surveys the patient's cardiac rhythm for normal and abnormal waveforms. The detection systems also monitor rhythm, rate, and pacemaker artifacts. The computer can audibly and visually alert the nurse when a preset number of abnormal waveforms is reached or when deviations from any other preset limit occurs. These data are stored so that the patient's history can be retrieved.

These systems can also be diagnostic. The computer, after processing the ECG, generates an analysis report. The ECG tracings may be transmitted over telephone lines from remote sites, such as the patient's home, to the physician's office or clinic. Patients with implantable pacemakers can have their cardiac activity monitored without leaving home.

Many hospitals are using oximetry to monitor arterial oxygenation continuously. This is a simple, noninvasive procedure that can detect any trend in the patient's oxygenation status within seconds. The oximeter can measure oxygenation through ear, pulse, or nasal septal oximetry. Ear oximetry measures the arterial oxygen saturation by monitoring the transmission of light waves through the vascular bed of the earlobe. If low cardiac output causes insufficient arterial perfusion in the earlobe, a pulse oximeter may be used to measure the wavelengths of light transmitted through a pulsating vascular bed, such as a fingertip. As the pulsating bed expands and relaxes, the light path length changes, producing a waveform. Because the waveform is produced from arterial blood, the pulse oximeter calculates the arterial oxygen saturation for every heartbeat without interference from surrounding tissues. If the patient has reduced peripheral vascular pulsations or is taking vasoactive drugs, a nasal probe may be used. This device fits around the septal anterior ethmoidal artery to detect vascular pulsations.

Systems for diagnostic testing include blood gas analyzers, pulmonary function systems, and intracranial pressure monitors. Blood gas analyzers use arterial blood to sense and calculate arterial blood gases, saturation curves, and buffer curves from normal data. These analyzers measure the partial pressures of oxygen and carbon dioxide and the pH of the arterial blood used in the test, enter primary results as soon as they are available, communicate the results quickly, and generate trend analysis for patients throughout their hospitalization.

Pulmonary function systems automate and simplify routine lung mechanics, lung volume, and diffusion capacity measurements. They can store data, calculate results, generate a numeric report, and display volumes graphically.

Intracranial pressure (ICP) monitoring systems monitor the cranial pressure in patients with closed head injuries or postoperative craniotomy patients. The ICP, along with the mean arterial blood pressure, can be used to calculate perfusion pressure. This allows assessment and early therapy as changes occur. When the ICP exceeds a set pressure, some systems allow ventricular drainage. These systems supplement rather than replace nursing observations of the patient.

Drug administration systems are often used with implantable infusion pumps that administer medications. This equipment can be programmed to deliver medication at a predetermined rate for a defined period. These pumps are commonly used for hormone regulation; treatment of hypertension, chronic intractable pain, diabetes, and thrombosis; and cancer chemotherapy.

Therapeutic treatment systems may be used to regulate intake and output, regulate breathing, and assist with the care of the newborn. Intake and output systems are linked to infusion pumps that control arterial pressure, drug therapy, fluid resuscitation, and serum glucose levels. These systems calculate and regulate the intravenous drip rate.

Ventilators are used to deliver a prescribed percentage of oxygen and volume of air to the patient's lungs and to provide a set flow rate, inspiratory-to-expiratory time ratio, and various other complex functions. Ventilators also provide sophisticated, sensitive alarm systems for patient safety. Some computer-assisted ventilators are electromechanically controlled by a closed-loop feedback system to analyze and control lung volumes and alveolar gases by a preset inspiratory pressure.

In the newborn nursery, computers monitor the heart and respiratory rates of the babies. In addition, these newborn nursery systems can regulate the temperature of the isolette by sensing the infant's temperature and the air of the isolette. Alarms can be set to notify the nurse when preset physiologic parameters are exceeded. Newer systems are used to monitor fetal activity before delivery; these systems monitor the ECGs of the mother and baby and the pulse oximetry, blood pressure, and respirations of the mother.

Developments in biomedical technology include the use of implantable devices, such as automated defibrillators, artificial organ transplants, gene therapy, and the use of robot servants for people who are disabled. Biomedical technology affects nursing care because nurses assume responsibility for monitoring the data generated by these devices and assessing their effectiveness.

Nurse leaders must be aware of how these technologies fit into the delivery of patient care and the strategic plan of the organization they work in. They must have a vision for the future and be ready to suggest solutions that will assist nurses across specialties and settings.

Exercise 10–2

List the types of biomedical technology available for patient care in your organization. List ways that you currently use the information gathered by these systems. How does this information help you care for patients? Can you think of other ways to use the technology? Can you think of other ways to use the information? For example, patients with respiratory problems often have frequent arterial blood gases drawn to assess the effectiveness of treatment. Are there instances when the noninvasive pulse oximetry might be used? Nurses spend many hours learning to use the devices and to interpret the information gained from them. Have we come to rely on technology rather than on our own judgment?

Nurse managers must be aware of the latest technologies for monitoring patients' physiologic status, diagnostic testing, drug administration, and therapeutic treatments. It is important to identify the data to be collected, the information that might be gained, and the many ways that these data might be used to provide new knowledge. More importantly, nurses must remember that these systems are tools for our use and do not replace our responsibility for assessing and monitoring the patient. Box 10-2 describes the development of informatics skills from novice to expert.

Information Technology

Computers offer the advantage of storing, organizing, retrieving, and communicating digital data with accuracy and speed. Patient care data can be entered once, stored in a database called a central data repository, and then quickly and accurately retrieved many times and in many combinations by healthcare providers and others. A **database** is a collection of data elements organized and stored together. Data processing is the structuring, organizing, and presenting of data for interpretation as information. For example, vital signs for one patient can be entered into the computer and communicated on a graph; the vital signs of several patients can be compared with the number of doses of antiarrhythmic medication. Vital signs for male patients between the ages of 40 and 50 years can be correlated and used to show a relationship between blood pressures and use of hypertensive medications.

Nurses process data continuously, but in an analog form. Computers process data in a digital form, process data faster and more accurately than humans, and provide a method of storage so that the data can be retrieved as needed. The Theory Box provides key ideas about information processing.

BOX 10-2

Development of Informatics Skills From Novice to Expert Practice

Novice nurses focus on learning what data to collect, the process of collecting and documenting the data, and how to use this information. They learn what clinical applications are available for use and how to use them. Computer and informatics skills focus on applying concrete concepts.

As nurses grow in expertise, they look for patterns in the data and information. They aggregate data across patient populations to look for similarities and differences in response to interventions. Expert nurses integrate theoretical knowledge with practical knowledge gained from experience.

Expert nurses know the value of reflection on knowledge gained and synthesis and evaluation of information for discovery and decision-making.

Theory Box

INFORMATION THEORY

KEY CONTRIBUTORS	KEY IDEAS	APPLICATION TO PRACTICE
Tan (1995) describes the elements of information theory as source, transmitter, channel, receiver, and destination.	The information source selects the message or information to be transmitted. An underlying code or set of characters represents the message to be processed by the computer. The transmitter has an encoding function that converts the message to be sent. The communication channel (cable, air waves) provides the medium necessary for the information to be transmitted over distance. The receiver converts the information from its transmitted form, and the destination is the final stage of reception, in which the message is decoded to be understandable.	The physician enters an order for laboratory tests (source, message). The computer program converts the message (transmitter). The converted order is sent over the computer network (communication channel) to the laboratory (receiver), where it is converted and read by the computer system in the laboratory (destination).

Structured Nursing Terminologies The **nursing minimum data set (NMDS)** was defined to establish uniform standards for the collection of comparable essential patient data. Collecting a set of basic data from every healthcare encounter makes sense because comparisons can be made among many patients, institutions, or countries, almost in any combination imaginable, as well as across time. The NMDS is based on the concept of the uniform minimum health data set (UMHDS), a minimum set of items of information with uniform definitions and categories that meets the needs of multiple data users. UMHDSs have been developed for long-term care, hospital discharge, and ambulatory care.

In their classic work, Werley and Lang (1988) developed the NMDS, which represents nursing's first attempt to standardize the collection of nursing data. It follows UMHDS criteria in that (1) data items included in the set must be useful to healthcare professionals and administrators and to local, state, and federal planning, regulatory, and legislative bodies; (2) data items must be collected readily and with reasonable accuracy; (3) data items should not duplicate data available from other sources; and (4) confidentiality must be protected.

The purposes of the NMDS are to (1) establish the comparability of patient care data across clinical populations, settings, geographic areas, and time; (2) describe the care of patients and families in various settings; (3) provide a means to mark the trends in the care provided and the allocation of nursing resources based on health problems or nursing diagnosis; (4) stimulate nursing research through links to existing data; and (5) provide data about nursing care to influence and facilitate healthcare policy decision-making. Box 10-3 lists the elements of the nursing minimum data set.

Some NMDS elements (e.g., interventions and outcomes) are not collected as easily as the demographic and service elements, many of which are captured at patient registration or discharge, because of the lack of a uniform or unified **structured nursing language.** Significant efforts have been made to bridge this gap. Thirteen classification systems have been recognized by the American Nurses Association (ANA) (Elfrink, Bakken, Coenen, McNeil, & Bickford, 2001) based on the following criteria (Bakken et al., 2001):

- Support for nursing practice by providing clinically useful terminology (e.g., nursing diagnoses,

---

BOX 10-3

Elements of the NMDS

Nursing Care Elements
1. Nursing diagnosis
2. Nursing intervention
3. Nursing outcome
4. Intensity of nursing care
5. Patient demographic elements

Personal identification*
6. Date of birth*
7. Sex*
8. Race and ethnicity*
9. Residency*

Service Elements
10. Unique facility or service agency number*
11. Unique health record number of the patient
12. Unique number of the principal registered nurse provider
13. Episode, admission, or encounter date*
14. Discharge or termination date*
15. Disposition of patient or client*
16. Expected payer for most of the bill

From Werley, H. H., & Lang, N. M. (1988). The consensually derived nursing minimum data set: Elements and definitions. In H. H. Werley & N. M. Lang (Eds.), Identification of the nursing minimum data set (pp. 402-411). New York: Springer.
*Elements comparable to those in the UMHDS.

---

nursing interventions) and rationale for development
- A level of development beyond an application, adaptation, or synthesis of currently recognized ANA vocabulary/classification schemes or presentation of an explicit rationale for seeking recognition for synthesis, application, or adaptation of existing schemes
- Clear and unambiguous terms
- Documented testing of reliability, validity, and utility in practice
- A systematic method of development
- A named entity responsible for a formal process of documenting evolving development and maintenance, including tracking of deleted terms and version control

- A coding scheme that provides a unique identifier for each term
- Identification of pertinent data elements as the variables of interest to whom and within what context
- Definition of the set of possible values for each variable
- A clear description of a defined structure or architecture with explicit principles of division
- Terms that can be combined to represent more complex concepts
- A classification structure that supports multiple parents and multiple children as relevant
- Preestablished rules for combining the terms

These recognized classification systems differ in specialty focus and included components. Some contain vocabularies for diagnosis, interventions, and outcomes, whereas others focus only on one or two of these groups. Some terminologies are specialty specific, such as the perioperative nursing data set. Table 10-1 lists the recognized standardized languages, with included components and a reference for each. An example of outcomes research being conducted using the NMDS and a structured nursing terminology can be found in the Research Perspective box.

Table 10-1 ANA-RECOGNIZED TERMINOLOGY THAT SUPPORTS NURSING PRACTICE

Terminology and Website or E-mail Contact	Type of Terminology	Recognition Date
NANDA International www.nanda.org	Interface	1992
Nursing Interventions Classification (NIC) www.nursing.uiowa.edu/centers/cncce	Interface	1992
Home Health Care Classification (HHCC) www.sabacare.com	Interface	1992
Omaha System www.omahasystem.org	Interface	1992
Nursing Outcomes Classification (NOC) www.nursing.uiowa.edu/centers/cncce	Interface	1997
Nursing Management Minimum Data Set (NMMDS) e-mail: connie-delaney@uiowa.edu	Data set framework	1998
Patient Care Data Set (PCDS) e-mail: judy.ozbolt@vanderbilt.edu	Interface	1998
PeriOperative Nursing Data Set (PNDS) www.aorn.org/research/pnds.htm	Interface	1999
SNOMED CT® www.snomed.org/clinical/nursing.html	Reference and interface	1999
Nursing Minimum Data Set (NMDS) www.nursing.uiowa.edu/NI/collabs_files/collaborations.asp#nmds	Data set framework	1999
International Classification of Nursing Practice (ICNP®) www.icn.ch/icnp.htm	Interface	2000
ABC Codes www.alternativelink.com/ali/abc_codes/	Interface	2000
Logical Observation Identifiers names and Codes (LOINC®) www.loinc.org	Reference and interface	2002

From Lunney M., Delaney C., Duffy M., Moorhead S., & Welton J. (2005). Advocating for standarized nursing languages in electronic health records. *Journal of Nursing Administration, 35*(1), 1-3.

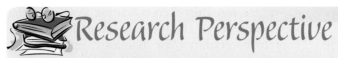
Research Perspective

Miller K., Ward-Smith P., Cox K., Jones E., & Portnoy, J. (2003, November). Development of an Asthma Disease Management Program in a Children's Hospital". *Current Allergy Asthma Report, 3*(6), 491-500.

A multidisciplinary team caring for children with asthma initiated a Quality Improvement project. Using data collected through the electronic medical record, they found that a small number of children were high users of emergency department care and had limited encounters with primary providers. Subsequently, they developed a disease-management model focusing on intense case management and education. This approach resulted in a decrease in emergency department visits and hospital admissions as well as improved caregiver quality of life.

IMPLICATIONS FOR PRACTICE
This study shows the importance of organized and systematic data collection in evaluating the care delivery process. The clinical team was able to assess current outcomes and design a new process objectively. Using information technology in this manner will allow ongoing quality improvement.

Nurse managers must advocate for use of structured nursing terminologies so that data can be collected and aggregated within and across patient populations to build evidence from practice and to use evidence in practice. These data are also needed to quantify and describe nursing practice and its effect on patient outcomes and the quality of care delivered.

Nurses must be able to quantify their contributions to patient care. Clark & Lang (1992, p. 109) found that "If we cannot name it (nursing), we cannot control it, practice it, research it, teach it, finance it or put it into public policy."

Exercise 10–3

Examine the elements of the NMDS. Which of them would be collected by patient registration? What information do you as a nurse need to collect? For example, in an acute-care setting, you have given pain medication several times today. The nursing diagnosis was alteration in comfort due to pain. You charted the medication given and the patient's quantitative rating of pain 30 minutes after medicating him. You have documented an intervention and an outcome, two nursing care elements of the NMDS. Can you locate the service elements in the patient record?

Information Systems   An information system may be manual or automated. Automated systems are needed to manage large volumes of data. They use computer hardware and software to process data into information needed to examine patterns and trends, solve problems, and answer questions. Data should be gathered at the point of care, and information should be made available to healthcare providers when and where it is needed. This is accomplished by networking computers both within and between organizations to form larger systems. These networked systems might encompass several hospitals, clinics, hospice centers, home health agencies, and/or physician practices. Data from all patient encounters with the healthcare system are stored in a central data repository, where they are accessible to authorized users located anywhere in the world. These have the potential to become the automated patient records, which contain health data from birth to death.

Nursing leaders must influence and make choices that will benefit the staff and patients. Box 10-4 lists elements of the ideal hospital information system for consideration in choosing a system for an institution. These systems must make sense to the people who use them and not increase the workload. Nurse leaders and staff should be members of the selection team so that the systems chosen reflect the work being done. Remember: All nurses as knowledge workers need information to deliver effective patient care.

BOX 10-4

Elements of the Ideal Hospital Information System

- Data are standardized and support a common lexicon/nomenclature.
- The system is reliable—minimal scheduled or unscheduled downtime.
- Applications are integrated across the system.
- Data are collected at the point of care.
- The database is complete, accurate, and easy to query.
- The infrastructure is interconnected and supports accessibility.
- Data are gathered by instrumentation whenever possible so that only minimal data entry is necessary.
- The system has a rapid response time.
- The system is intuitive and reflective of patient care delivery models.
- The location facilitates functionality, security, and support.
- Screen displays can be configured by user preference.
- The system supports outcomes and an evidence-based approach to care delivery.

Exercise 10-4

Select a hospital with which you are familiar. What information systems are used? Make a list of the names of these systems and the information that they provide. How do they help you in caring for patients or in making management decisions? Think about the communication of data and information between departments. Do the systems communicate with each other? If you do not have computerized systems, think about how data and information are communicated. How might a computer system help you be more efficient?

As an example, assume that a barium enema has been ordered. Handwritten requisitions are sent to nutrition services, the pharmacy, and the radiology department. With a computerized system, the barium enema is ordered, and the requests for dietary changes, bowel preparation medications, and the barium enema itself are automatically sent to the appropriate departments. Radiology will compare its schedule openings with the patient's schedule and automatically place the date and time

for the barium enema on the patient's automated plan of care.

Selection of a software partner may be one of the most important legacies of a chief nursing officer and his/her leadership team (Simpson, 2003). Box 10-5 identifies key considerations necessary for selecting software. It is imperative that site visits are made to organizations that already have the software in use. Nurses at all levels should actively participate and have a voice in the decision-making. Discussions should include not just utility of the software but also customer service and responsiveness.

Nurse leaders have a responsibility to ensure that cost-effective, quality patient care is being delivered by the nursing staff under their supervision. Nursing databases that support decision-making for this purpose are needed. Both clinical data and management data are required. Administrative databases assist in the development of the organization's information infrastructure, which ultimately allows for links between management and clinical outcomes. Table 10-2 lists the essential components of a nursing administration information system.

Once these data are available on the computer, nurse leaders can use this information to monitor staff performance, patient safety, unit error rates (e.g., from incident reports), patient acuity levels, and staffing and scheduling patterns in relation to budget and census. Computerized personnel files could be used to generate reminders for license renewal and track position changes to produce reports for budgeting and forecasting purposes. Staffing levels and skill mix could be correlated with patient outcome data.

Quality management and the measurement of efficiency, effectiveness, and patient care outcomes have become necessary for the accreditation and licensing of healthcare organizations. This can be accomplished through documentation of the patient care processes and outcomes. The computerized plan of care outlines what patient care needs to occur, orders are executed to make the prescribed care happen, nursing documentation confirms that it was done, and then the computer can be used to aggregate the data and evaluate patient outcomes.

Beginning with the 1994 Accreditation Manual, the Joint Commission on Accreditation of Healthcare Organizations (JCAHO) has provided a separate chapter that addresses management of

BOX 10-5

Vendor Selection Checklist

Management Considerations

- What is the ability of the vendor to meet its schedule and budget commitments? What is its track record in meeting commitments?
- What are the satisfaction levels of the vendor's current customers, including long-term customers? Does the vendor have any long-term customers?
- What are the vendor's project management capabilities? Does it have expertise in all aspects of software project management including size estimation, cost estimation, project planning, project tracking, and project control?
- Can you trust the confidentiality of the vendor? Does the vendor also serve your competitors?
- Who will provide product support, you or the vendor? Do you want the vendor to provide support to your customers?
- Is any litigation pending against the vendor?

Technical Considerations

- What is the vendor's ability to rise to the technical challenges of the project?

- Has the vendor's software development capability been evaluated by your technical staff or a third party? Were both technical work products and development processes included in the evaluation?
- What is the level of the vendor's expertise in the application area?
- What is the level of the vendor's expertise in the implementation environment?
- Is the quality of the vendor's other software acceptable? Does the vendor have quantitative data to support its quality of claims?
- Is the quality of the vendor's work sufficient to support future enhancements?

General Considerations

- Is the vendor financially stable? What would happen to your project if the vendor encountered a severe financial downturn?
- Has the vendor developed software in an outsourcing capacity before? Is building outsourced software its primary business? What is the level of the vendor's commitment to outsourcing?

information. Within these standards, the goals of information management are to obtain, manage, and use information to improve patient outcomes and individual and organizational performance in patient care, as well as to improve performance in other organizational processes. The standards address the identification, design, capture, analysis, communication, integration, and use of information. Four areas of management of information are reviewed: (1) patient-specific data and information, (2) aggregate data and information, (3) expert knowledge–based information, and (4) comparative performance data and information (JCAHO, 2005).

In 1997, JCAHO introduced the ORYX initiative, which integrated outcome and performance measurement data into the accreditation review process. Organization-specific performance data are used to guide the accreditation survey process and to monitor performance between surveys when indicated. In addition, core performance measures, categorized by type of institution, have been selected to begin a process of comparing performance across organizations (JCAHO, 2001).

Communication networks are used to transmit information that is entered at one computer and received by another. These networks are usually part of the integrated system and reduce the clerical functions of nursing. They can provide patient census and locations, results from tests, and lists of medications. Nursing policies and procedures may be entered onto a communication network to be accessible to authorized personnel.

Discussion has focused on information systems for acute care institutions, but many patients are cared for in outpatient or community settings. Nursing focus in these settings involves health promotion, maintenance, and education, as well as coordinated continuity of care and monitoring chronic conditions. Information systems also support nursing functions in these settings. They are used for financial management and billing,

Table 10-2 ESSENTIAL COMPONENTS OF A NURSING ADMINISTRATION INFORMATION SYSTEM

Level	Administrative Data	Clinical Data
Interinstitution	Nursing management minimum data set (NMMDS)	Nursing minimum data set (NMDS)
Organization	Organizational productivity measures Referral patterns Cost per drug or procedure; profit calculations Case mix analysis Achievement of accrediting body standards Strategic planning data (e.g., forecasting market share, patient distribution by county of residence)	Site of care (e.g., inpatient, outpatient, skilled-care facility, home care, community-based site) Outcomes research findings Number of caregivers per patient Aggregate patient profile (e.g., volume, type, diagnosis by service, outcomes, utilization rates)
Department or discipline	Staffing profile (skill mix, educational mix, experience mix) Employee satisfaction Chief nurse executive profile Salary—total and distribution	Research studies with findings Clinical knowledge Number of caregivers per patient Standards of care Average patient intensity Patient satisfaction
Division or product line	Type of division/product line Staffing profile (skill mix, educational mix, experience mix) Salary—total and distribution Units of service (patient days, procedures, visits) Size of division (number of beds available, operational, and occupied) Budget Nursing resources (FTEs—total and by skill level) Activity levels (admission, discharge, and transfer) Costs—direct and indirect expenses Resources (equipment, supplies) Nursing turnover Employee satisfaction Profile of the director	Average intensity (e.g., HPPD, HPWI) Patient satisfaction Division profile (e.g., volume, type, diagnosis by service, outcomes, utilization rates) Standards of care
Unit or patient population/ service	Type of unit Care delivery system (e.g., primary, team, functional, care partners) Nurse manager profile Staff mix Units of service (patient days, procedures, visits) Size of unit (number of beds available, operational, and occupied) Budget Nursing resources (FTEs—total and by skill level) Activity levels (admission, discharge, and transfer) Costs—direct and indirect expenses Resources (equipment, supplies) Administrative standards Nursing turnover	Standards of care Patient educational information Aggregate patient profile (histories, diagnoses, interventions, outcomes, volume, patterns of care/day, educational needs, LOS, discharge disposition and summary) Modeling of preferred care Average intensity (e.g., HPPD or HPWI)

Continued

Level	Administrative Data	Clinical Data
	Nonfunctional positions by pay period (vacancy rate by job category, orientation time, unfilled positions because of LOAs or employees offered positions but not here yet)	
Individual	Salary (base, differentials, and bonuses) and salary plan (e.g., regular, Baylor, per diem)	Individual patient intensity score
	Skill level	Individual nurse assignment
	Credentials (license type, number, and expiration date; educational preparation; experience; work history—FT and PT; certification types, numbers, and expiration dates)	Each patient medical record (patient history, diagnosis, plan of care, interventions, outcomes, primary nurse, demographic data, LOS, discharge disposition, and summary)
	Current work history (hire date, change in positions and salary, termination date)	Patient satisfaction
	Clinical ladder appointment(s)	Incident reports by patient and by nurse
	Clinical privileges	Uniform billing information (cost per patient)
	Performance evaluation	
	Demographic data (SSN, name, position, number, gender, date of birth, address, race, phone number)	
	Continuing education programs and hours	
	Cost center	
	Position title	
	Appointment fraction	
	Schedule (include shift length)	
	Nonproductive time (e.g., LOAs, sick, vacation)	
	Employee satisfaction	
	Audits of practice by nurse	

Table 10-2 ESSENTIAL COMPONENTS OF A NURSING ADMINISTRATION INFORMATION SYSTEM—cont'd

From Curran, C. R. (1995). Data requirements of the nurse executive. Unpublished paper.
DRG, Diagnosis-related group; *FT,* full-time; *FTE,* full-time equivalent; *HPPD,* hours per patient day; *HPWI,* hours per workload index; *LOA,* leave of absence; *LOS,* length of stay; *PT,* part time.

statistical reporting, and patient care information systems. These systems can be used within the agency or at the point of care to connect the nurse to an enterprise-integrated data network that allows access to the computerized patient record.

Links can be provided between the patient's home, hospital, and/or physician office with patient-side computers, handheld technologies, voice-activated systems, or laptop computers. Day-to-day events can be recorded on these devices and downloaded into the patient record remotely or back at the office at the end of the day.

Nurses caring for patients in the home health-care industry have many government and insur-ance requirements for documentation completion. Computers offer a means of reducing this paperwork burden by allowing direct entry of data in the required format. Portable and wireless computers have made recordings of patient care information more efficient and have improved personnel productivity.

These portable computers are used to download files of the patients to be seen during the day from the main database. During each visit, the computer prompts the nurse for vital signs, assessments, diagnosis, interventions, long- and short-term goals, and medications based on previous entries in the medical record. The nurses then enter any new data, modifications, or nursing information directly into the portable computer. Entries related to patient care can be transmitted by telephone line to the main computer at the office or downloaded from the device at the end of the day. This action automatically updates the patient record and any verbal order entry records, home visit reports, federally mandated treatment plans, productivity and quality improvement reports, and other documents for review and signature.

The elimination of the paper trail has been partially accomplished by the placement of computers at the patients' sides or through the use of handheld devices. In this way, information can be entered once at the point of care and accessed over and over again. Documentation of the patient assessment at the patient-side saves time, gives others access to more timely access to the data, and decreases the likelihood of forgetting to document vital information. Point-of-care systems that adapt to the nurse's workflow, personalize patient assessments, and simplify care planning are available. Patient care areas with point-of-care computers have improved the quality of patient care by decreasing errors of omission, providing greater accuracy and completeness of documentation, reducing medication errors, providing more timely responses to patient needs, and improving discharge planning and teaching. These systems shorten or eliminate shift-to-shift communication and eliminate redundant charting of data.

Wireless (WL) messaging has changed the way we work. WL communication is an extension of an existing wired network environment and uses radio-based systems to transmit data signals through the air without any physical connections. Nurses can communicate with offices/departments, other healthcare team members, and patients through the use of pagers, cellular phones, or **personal digital assistants (PDAs)**. These devices can send and receive alphanumeric data. Nurses can send and receive **e-mails,** clinical data, and other textual messages. They can also access the **Internet** on these devices.

WL systems are being used by emergency medical personnel to request authorization for the treatments or drugs needed in emergency situations. Laboratories use WL technology to transmit laboratory results to physicians; patients awaiting organ transplants are being provided with WL pagers so that they can be notified if a donor is found; and parents of critically ill children carry them when they are away from a phone. Visiting nurses using a home monitoring system employ WL technology to enter vital signs and other patient-related information. Inpatient nurses can send messages to the admissions department when a patient is being transferred to another unit without having to wait for someone to answer the telephone.

Voice technology will also enhance the use of computer systems when this technology is further developed. Voice technology is the ability to control a computer system through voice input by the user. The machine gathers, processes, interprets, and executes audible signals by comparing the spoken words with a template already resident in the system. If the patterns match, recognition occurs, and a previously stored command is executed by the computer. This allows untrained personnel or those whose hands are busy to work in computer-based environments without touching the computer. Voice technology will also allow quadriplegic and other physically challenged individuals to function more efficiently when using the computer.

These systems recognize a large number of words but are still immature. The speaker must use staccato-like speech, pausing about one tenth of a second between each clearly spoken word, and these systems must be programmed for each user so that the system recognizes the user's voice patterns.

Technology has both advantages and disadvantages. The use of handheld devices is less expensive because each caregiver on a shift can be equipped with a device rather than placing a stationary computer in each patient room. They allow access to information at the point of care, both for retrieval of information and entry of patient data. Disadvantages of handheld technology stem from their size and portability; they can be put down and forgotten, or dropped and broken, and are a target for theft. There must also be a convenient and adequate place to store them when they are not in use and to charge their batteries if needed. These computers have a small display screen, which limits the amount of data available on the screen and the size of the text.

Patient-side computers must be suited to patient rooms. They must be lighted to be viewed in the dark and must be either mounted on the wall or placed on portable stands. In addition, automating the healthcare delivery process is not an easy task.

Processes are not standardized across settings, and most vendors cannot customize applications for each organization. Some current versions of the electronic patient record have merely automated the existing schema of the chart rather than considering how computers could permit data to be viewed or used differently from the previous manual method.

Management of these technologies is important. Nurse leader and managers must make knowledgeable decisions about the type of technology to use, the education needed, and the proper care and maintenance of the equipment. Important questions to ask include the following: What data and information do we need to gather? When and where should it be gathered? How difficult is the equipment to use? Has the technology been tested sufficiently to ensure purchase of a dependable product?

Exercise 10-5

Think about the data you gather as you go through the day. How do you communicate the information and knowledge gleaned about your patient to others? Does the information system support the way you need this information organized, stored, retrieved, and presented to other healthcare providers? For example, if a patient's pain medication order is about to expire and you want to assess the patient's use and response to the pain medication during the past 24 hours, can the information system generate a graph for this patient comparing the time, dose, and pain score for this period? If your assessment is that the medication needs to be renewed, can you leave an electronic message for the physician to renew this medication—is there an "electronic sticky note" function?

Knowledge Technology

Knowledge technology consists of systems that generate or process knowledge and provide clinical decision support. Knowledge technology involves decision support systems. A **decision support system** is a computer program that mimics the inductive or deductive reasoning of a human expert. These programs process knowledge to produce decisions by means of a knowledge base and a software application that controls the use of the knowledge (an inference engine). To automate this process, the necessary data elements must be identified and rules for combining the data established. The same data elements are always required, and the same formula or rule is applied in the same way to the same data. The knowledge base contains the knowl-

edge (rules, heuristics) that an expert nurse would apply to the data and information to solve a problem. The inference engine controls the use of the knowledge by providing the logic for its use. Box 10-6 illustrates the use of an expert system for giving a maximum dose of pain medication. The knowledge base contains eight items that are to be considered when giving the maximum dose. The inference engine controls the use of the knowledge base by applying logic that an expert nurse would use in making the decision to give the maximum dose.

This decision frame states that if pain is severe (A) or a painful procedure is planned (B), and there is an order for pain medication (C) and the time since surgery is less than 48 hours (H) and the time since the last dose is greater than 3 hours (G), and there are no contraindications to the medication (D) or history of allergy (E) or contraindication to the maximum dose (F), then the "decision" would be to give the dose of pain medication. The rule, or heuristics, appearing in this logic are those that expert nurses would apply in making the decision to give pain medication. The inference engine controls the "if" logic or knowledge.

BOX 10-6

Expert Decision Frame for "Give Maximum Dose of Pain Medication"

The Knowledge Base
A. Pain score
B. Invasive procedure scheduled
C. Opiate analgesia ordered
D. Contraindications to the medication
E. History of allergic reaction to opiate analgesics
F. Contraindication to maximum dose of opiate analgesic
G. Time since last dose of opiate analgesia administered
H. Time since surgical procedure

The Inference Engine
Give the maximum dose of pain medication if (A or B) and (C and H < 48 hours and G > 3 hours) and not (D or E or F)

    or:

(C and H < 48 hours and G > 4 hours) and not (D or E or F)

One of the benefits of decision support systems is that they outperform nonexpert human clinicians by assisting with the decision-making for novices and nurses working outside their areas of expertise and help orientees with validation of decisions by expert nurses with heavy caseloads. Because the systems obtain their information directly from patient care documentation, the computer never forgets when a patient needs pain medication or the effectiveness of the last treatment. If the expert decision support system is used in conjunction with an information system, the documentation of observations, care, and patient outcomes can be expected to increase significantly and improve the quality of care (Simpson, 2005).

A critical use of information has been in the area of the medication management process. Medications are a high risk and high volume activity (Malashock, Smith-Schull, & Gould, 2004). New applications provide support for all aspects of the process, thereby improving safety and efficiency (Box 10-7).

Nurse managers must be aware of the usefulness of decision support systems for nursing. By helping to develop the logic used in the knowledge base through the use of critical-thinking skills, changes in current practice can be made for the improvement of patient care.

> ### Exercise 10-6
> Mr. Jones's heart rate is 58 beats per minute. Tony is about to give Mr. Jones his atenolol (Tenormin). When Tony enters Mr. Jones's identification number and the medication name, the computer warns him that atenolol should not be given for a heart rate less than 60 beats per minute. What should Tony do?

PROFESSIONAL ISSUES AND FUTURE TRENDS

Because of escalating healthcare costs, insurance companies (third-party payers) and the federal government are supporting new technologies to reduce costs. Longitudinal computerized patient records, telecommunications, and WL devices that store health history data are technologies that will grow in the future. Use of the Internet and **World Wide Web (WWW)** will also provide new exciting options for health care. Use of robotics will be common-

place. Miniaturization of devices will continue, and wearable computers are in development.

Electronic Medical (Patient) Records

Managed care is an effort by the insurance companies, the payers for health care, to manage healthcare costs by limiting the care provided for each diagnosis. In the hospital, this means that the number of days a patient is permitted to stay is limited, depending on the diagnosis. If the patient remains longer than the permitted days, the health insurer will not reimburse the costs of the care for the unapproved days. The concept of managed care has resulted in the redesign of patient care plans to clinical pathways that detail the interventions needed day by day to achieve the outcome of discharge by the final approved day. Data from the clinical pathway form the basis of the episode of care in the endorsed widespread adoption of the **electronic medical record (EMR)**. The federal government has endorsed widespread adoption of the EMR.

Credit card–like devices called **smart cards** store a limited number of pages of data on a computer chip. The implementation of computer-based health information systems will lead to computer networks that will store health records across local, state, national, and international boundaries. The smart card serves as a bridge between the clinician terminal and the central repository, making patient information available to the caregiver quickly and cheaply at the point of service because the patients bring it with them. This will help coordinate care; improve quality-of-care decisions; and reduce risk, waste, and duplication of effort. Patients are mobile and consult many practitioners, thereby causing their records to be fragmented. With the electronic smart card, patients, providers, and notes can be brought together in any combination at any place. Box 10-8 provides examples of the kinds of data that are recorded on smart cards.

Telecommunications

Telecommunications and systems technology facilitate clinical oversight of health care via telephone or cable lines, remote monitoring, information links, and the Internet. **Telehealth** is the use of modern telecommunications and information technologies for the provision of health care to individuals at a distance and the transmission of information to provide that care. This is

BOX 10-7

Information Technology: Trends in the Medication Management Process

Various IT devices and software applications are designed to support the medication management process. Each has unique functionality and targets a specific phase of the medication process.

Computerized Prescriber Order Entry (CPOE)

- Decision support and clinical warnings (alerts the provider of allergies, pertinent laboratory data, drug-drug and drug-food interactions, etc.)
- Automatic dose calculation
- Link to up-to-date drug reference material
- Automatic order notification
- Standardized formulary compliant order sets
- Legible, accurate, and complete medication orders
- Decreased variations in practice
- Less time clarifying orders
- Fewer verbal orders
- No manual transcription errors

Electronic Medication Administration Record (e-MAR)

- Integration with clinical documentation (in the electronic record)
- Link to up-to-date drug reference material
- Automatic reminders and alarms for approaching or missed medication administration times
- Prompts for associated tasks or additional documentation requirements
- Alert when cumulative dosing exceeds maximum
- Legible record
- Accessible to multiple users
- Improved accuracy of pharmacokinetic monitoring (administration times are reliable)
- Record matches the pharmacy profile
- Generated reports to track medication errors + provides visibility to near misses
- Perpetual interface with pharmacy inventory system
- Increased the accuracy of charge capture (at the time of administration versus when drug is dispensed)

Bar Coding and RFID Scanning

- Medication documentation captured electronically at the time of administration (populates the e-MAR)
- Five rights verified
- Positive patient identification

- Clinician alerted to discrepancies (wrong drug, wrong dose, wrong time, wrong patient, expired drug, etc.).
- Automatic tracking of medication errors + provides visibility to near misses

"Smart" Infusion Pumps (Medication Infusion Delivery System)

- Reduced the need for manual dose/rate calculation
- Institution defined standardized drug library (drugs, concentrations, dosing parameters)
- Software filter prevention of programming errors/ programming is within pre-established minimum and maximum limits before the infusion can begin
- Device infusion parameter limits based on patient type or care area
- Interface with the patient's pharmacy profile with capabilities to program the pump electronically
- User alerted to pump setting errors, wrong channel selection, and mechanical failures
- Electronic notification to pharmacy when fluids/medications need to be dispensed
- Interface with the patient's e-MAR (accurate documentation of administration times and volumes infused)
- User alerted to pump setting errors, wrong channel selection, and mechanical failures
- Memory functions for settings and alarms with a retrievable log
- Electronic recording of reprogramming and limit override activity

Automated Dispensing Unit/Cabinets

- Secure drug storage
- Controlled user access—biometric identification
- Interface with the pharmacy profile—access restricted until order reviewed
- Quick access once medication order reviewed by pharmacist
- Ability to monitor controlled substance waste and utilization patterns
- Perpetual interface with pharmacy inventory

Pharmacy Automation and Robotics

- Increased accuracy and speed of dispensing

From Schlosser, R. W. (2004, June 22). Evidence-based practice in AAC: 10 points to consider. Retrieved August 5, 2005, from www.asha.org/about/publications/leader-online/archives/2004/040622/f040622b.htm; Bell, M.J., (2005, February). Nursing Information of Tomorrow. *Healthcare Informatics, 22*(2), 74-78; and Larrabee, S., & Brown, M. M. (2003, July). Recognizing the Institutional Benefits of Bar-Code Point-of-Care Technology. *Joint Commission Journal on Quality and Safety, 29*(7), 345-353.

BOX 10-8

Smart Cards

1. Patient demographics/photo identification
2. ICE—In Case of Emergency—contact and other key information
3. Patient medical history: allergies, medications, immunizations, laboratory results, etc.
4. Past care encounter summaries, including surgical procedures
5. Patient record locations and electronic address information
6. Ability to upload or download patient information

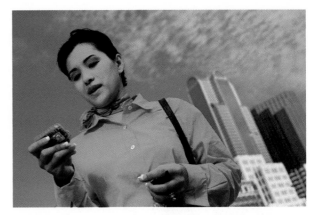

Nurses working in the community often use cellular phones and other technologies (e.g., personal digital assistants) to communicate and remain connected with their offices.

accomplished through the use of two-way interactive video-conferencing and high-speed telephone lines, fiberoptic cable, and satellite transmissions. Patients sitting in front of the teleconferencing camera can be diagnosed, treated, monitored, and educated by nurses and physicians. ECGs and radiographs can be viewed and transmitted. Sophisticated electronic stethoscopes and dermascopes allow nurses and physicians to hear heart, lung, and bowel sounds and to look closely at wounds, eyes, ears, and skin. Ready access to expert advice and patient information is available no matter where the patient or information is located. Patients in rural areas and prisons especially benefit from this technology.

Internet

Another vehicle for health information is the Internet. The Internet, which can provide health education and other health information, is a worldwide network of computers that fosters communication, collaboration, resource sharing, and information access. It is a multicultural library that is open all day, every day to ordinary computer users.

The main uses of the Internet are sending and receiving electronic mail (e-mail) and browsing the WWW. Mail may be sent to individuals in any part of the world through e-mail if they have an e-mail address, or e-mail of particular interest may be obtained by subscribing to a listserv. A listserv is a group of people who have similar interests. Subscribers to a listserv become part of the "conversation." All messages sent to the listserv are forwarded to all subscribers, who can then read and respond to them.

E-mail is rapidly becoming a preferred communication method between healthcare providers and patients. This asynchronous mode of communication allows timely responses to nonemergent healthcare issues at the convenience of both the patient and provider. It prevents "telephone tag" and avoids the interruptions often encountered when paging healthcare providers. However, reimbursement for these "virtual office visits" is rarely supported. Third-party payers need to support this method of care delivery financially to improve access and decrease cost.

E-mail can be a very effective means of delivering health services to people. It provides documentation of the patient-provider communication and gives patient instructions in writing. E-mails can have embedded links to information on the WWW. Box 10-9 presents guidelines for the use of e-mail between patients and providers.

The WWW is a network of information in the form of text, pictures, video, and sound. Web pages contain text and "links" to other documents filled with information. Links are highlighted or underlined words that are clicked on with the mouse to activate another linked document. Web servers are located all over the world, and information can be retrieved from linked web pages without knowledge of whether the server is located in Australia, Europe, or California. A software program called a browser is needed to view web pages. Box 10-10 lists websites of interest to nurses.

BOX 10-9

Patient-Provider E-mail Communication Guidelines

Patient Responsibilities and Expectations

- Include patient's name in the body of the e-mail
- Include the category or type of message in the subject line
- Review the e-mail to make sure it is clear and that all relevant information is provided before sending to provider
- Follow-up with the provider as needed to determine whether the intended recipient received the e-mail and when the recipient will respond
- Take precautions to preserve the confidentiality of the e-mail
- Inform the provider of e-mail address changes
- Inform the provider of the types of information the patient does not want to be sent by e-mail

Provider Responsibilities and Expectations

- Use an encrypted security system
- Obtain informed consent from the patient before using e-mail communication
- Establish acceptable types of e-mail messages and provide clear guidelines regarding emergency subject matter
- Develop a system for integrating e-mail contact into the patient's record
- Establish an expected response time for messages

Web users need to evaluate the quality of healthcare information found on the WWW. Websites can be created but may not be updated. Links are often "broken" when websites relocate to another address. How does one evaluate the credentials of the author of the information or site? Several texts and articles suggest criteria for the evaluation of websites related to health (Goldsborough, 1999; Hollaway, Kripps, Koepke, & Skiba, 2000; Nicoll, 2001). Box 10-11 lists criteria for evaluation of these sites.

Search engines are often used to look up information on the WWW. Even the best search engines are currently not very effective; a recent study found that only about one third of all available information on a topic was typically retrieved (Lawrence & Giles, 1998). Thus, the data retrieved should be considered a starting point and not an end point of possible information on the subject.

Data Privacy and Security

Patients' rights to privacy of their data must be maintained whether in a manual or automated system. Converting the patient record to a computer-generated document increases the likelihood that a breach in confidentiality will have broader implications. With manually generated documents, there is only one copy of the data, and caregivers access the chart individually and in a geographically limited place. With computerized data, any person with the proper permission may access the information anywhere in the world, and multiple people can do so simultaneously. Data can also be inadvertently sent to the wrong individual or site.

System users must never share the passwords that allow them access to information in the computerized database. Each password uniquely identifies a user to the system by name and title, gives approval to carry out certain functions, and provides access to data appropriate to the user. When a nurse signs on to a computer, all data and information that are entered or reviewed can be traced to that password. Therefore, you are accountable for all actions taken using your password.

A firewall protects the information in the central data repository from access by unauthorized users. It is a network security measure that keeps electronic intruders from accessing an organization's data on its private network while allowing members of the organization to reach the Internet. Organizational policies on the use, security, and accuracy of data must be developed and monitored for compliance.

Ethics

Ethics is a form of thinking about morality, moral problems, and moral judgments. Principles are general action guides for judgment; an ethical principle might be to prevent harm and promote the highest level of health possible. Despite security measures available in computerized systems, the integrity and ethical principles of the users of these systems provide the only safeguard of patients' welfare, privacy, and confidentiality of data.

Because of the increasing ability to preserve and maintain human life via technologic interventions, questions become complex: both conceptually and ethically. Conceptually, it becomes more

BOX 10-10

Health-Related Website Uniform Resource Locators (URLs)

DESCRIPTION	URL
Agency for Health Care Research and Quality (AHRQ)	www.ahrq.gov
American Heart Association	www.americanheart.org
American Hospital Association (AHA)	www.aha.org
American Nurses Association (ANA)	www.nursingworld.org
American Nurses Credentialing Center (ANCC)	www.nursecredentialing.org
American Organization of Nurse Executives (ANOE)	www.aone.org
Centers for Disease Control and Prevention	www.cdc.gov
Guide to Evidence Based Practice	www.cebm.utoronto.ca/
Health on the Net	www.hon.ch/
Healthfinder—Department of Health/Human Services	www.healthfinder.gov
Institute of Health Care Improvement (IHI)	www.ihi.org
Joint Commission on Accreditation of Health Care Organizations (JCAHO)	www.jcaho.org
Nursing and healthcare resources	http://nmap.ac.uk/
Resources for nurses and families	http://pegasus.cc.ucf.edu/%7Ewink
World Health Organization	www.who.int/

BOX 10-11

Ten C's for Evaluating Internet Sources

1. Content	What is the intent of the content?
	Are the title and author identified?
	Is the content "juried"?
	Is the content "popular" or "scholarly," satiric or serious?
	What is the date of the document or article?
	Is the "edition" current?
	Do you have the latest version?
2. Credibility	Is the author identifiable and reliable?
	Is the content credible? Authoritative? Should it be?
	What is the purpose of the information (i.e., is it serious, satiric, or humorous)?
	Is the URL extension .edu, .com, .gov, .org, .net, or .info?
	What does this information tell you about the "publisher"?
3. Critical Thinking	How can you apply critical thinking skills, including previous knowledge and experience, to evaluate Internet resources?
	Can you identify the author, publisher, edition, etc. as you would with a "traditionally" published resource?
	What criteria do you use to evaluate Internet resources?
4. Copyright	Even if the copyright notice does not appear prominently, someone wrote, or is responsible for, the creation of a document, graphic, sound or image, and the material falls under copyright conventions. "Fair use" applies to short, cited excerpts, usually as an example for commentary or research.
	Materials are in the "public domain" if this is explicitly stated. Internet users, as users of print media, must respect copyright.

Continued

BOX 10-11

Ten C's for Evaluating Internet Sources—cont'd

5. Citation	Internet resources should be cited to identify sources used, both to give credit to the author and to provide the reader with avenues for further research. Standard style manuals (print and online) provide some examples of how to cite Internet documents, although these standards are not uniform.
6. Continuity	Will the Internet site be maintained and updated? Is it now and will it continue to be free? Can you rely on this source over time to provide up-to-date information? Some good .edu sites have moved to .com, with possible cost implications. Other sites offer partial use for free, and charge fees for continued or in-depth use.
7. Censorship	Is your discussion list "moderated"? What does this mean? Does your search engine or index look for all words or are some words excluded? Is this censorship? Does your institution, based on its mission, parent organization or space limitations, apply some restrictions to Internet use? Consider censorship and privacy issues when using the Internet.
8. Connectivity	If more than one user will need to access a site, consider each user's access and "functionality." How do users connect to the Internet and what kind of connection does the assigned resource require? Does access to the resource require a graphical user interface? If it is a popular (busy) resource, will it be accessible in the time frame needed? Is it accessible by more than one Internet tool? Do users have access to the same Internet tools and applications? Are users familiar with the tools and applications? Is the site "viewable" by all Web browsers?
9. Comparability	Does the Internet resource have an identified comparable print or CD ROM data set or source? Does the Internet site contain comparable and complete information? Do you need to compare data or statistics over time? Can you identify sources for comparable earlier or later data? Comparability of data may or may not be important, depending on your project.
10. Context	What is the context of your research? Can you find "anything" on your topic, that is, commentary, opinion, narrative, statistics and your quest will be satisfied? Are you looking for current or historical information? Definitions? Research studies or articles? How does the Internet information fit in the overall information context of your subject? Before you start searching, define the research context and research needs and decide what sources might be best to use to successfully fill information needs without data overload.

The Ten C's were developed 1991-1996 by the University of Wisconsin—Eau Claire; a revision was made June 19, 2003.

difficult to define extraordinary treatment and human life because technology has changed our concepts of living and dying. The ethics problem becomes one of precedence, such as the dilemma of how to relieve pain without hastening death.

A frequent source of ethical dilemmas is the use of invasive technological treatment to prolong life for patients with limited or no decision-making capabilities. Healthcare institutions that use technology strive for efficiency and cost-effectiveness with an ethical mandate of the greatest good for the greatest number. The nursing profession holds a holistic orientation and is concerned with individual patient welfare and effect of technological intervention as it affects the immediate and long-term quality of the patients and their families. Patient advocacy remains an important function of the professional nurse.

Nurse leaders must promote the existence and use of an ethics committee in their institutions and assign knowledgeable nurses to serve on these committees. Nurse managers must ensure that policies and procedures for collecting and entering data and the use of security measures (e.g., passwords) are established to maintain confidentiality of patient data and information. Nurse managers must also be knowledgeable patient advocates in the use of technology for patient care by referring ethical questions to the organization's ethics committee. Staff nurses must be aware of their responsibilities for the confidentiality and security of the data they gather and for the security of their passwords.

Exercise 10-7

Think about the use of the WWW in health care. How do you use it to look up healthcare information? How would you advise a patient to select appropriate sites? (Hint: See Box 10-10.)

SUMMARY

We have discussed the advances of technology that link wellness, health promotion, and illness management, as well as linking local and global communities. Care in this new era will focus on empowering patients and their families through information and education. Health care in the future will emanate from wherever the client is located. Technology has become the bond that links people and information together in a rapidly changing world of health care, and with technology comes the need for a new set of competencies. We need to ensure nursing's participation in designing this exciting future.

The Solution

I knew successful implementation of an integrated clinical information system requires active participation of the clinical staff during all phases of the project, including the selection, design, build, and training phases. I made sure each care setting was represented by all types and levels of care providers. Installing a new clinical information system provides an opportunity to transform processes so that the provision of care is more efficient and effective. We used this approach even though it extended the project's completion timeline. The solution was progressive and enthusiastically embraced by users.

One device solution does not meet the needs of a diverse user group working with different software applications. So, we provided a variety of device options at the point of care. Because this approach is more expensive at the initial outlay, we were somewhat reluctant to fund it. However, our project leaders demonstrated how the efficiencies gained in the clinician's daily work flow quickly offset the extra expense.

Information technology is an essential component of a patient safety program. The positive impact of technology is clearly illustrated when applied to the complex medication process. The software enhancements we made provided decision support, patient identification verification, device programming safeguards, accurate automated drug dispensing, alerts and integrated monitoring systems.

Cheri Hunt, RN, MHA

 Would this be a suitable approach for you? Why?

CHAPTER CHECKLIST

Nurses are the key personnel in the healthcare system to mediate the interaction among science, technology, and the patient because of our unique holistic viewpoint and "24 by 7" role of vigilant healthcare providers who preserve the patients' humanity, optimal functioning, and promotion of health. The challenge for the profession is to continue to provide patient-centered care in a technological society that strives for efficiency and cost-effectiveness. Nurse administrators, managers, and staff must provide leadership in managing information and technology to meet the challenge.

- Nurses are knowledge workers.
- Informatics is the transformation of data into knowledge. It consists of three core components:
  - Data
  - Information
  - Knowledge
- Evidence-based practice involves both the application of evidence to practice and the building of evidence from practice.
  - Ask a clinical question
  - Acquire the evidence
  - Appraise the evidence
  - Apply the evidence
  - Assess the outcomes
- Nurses commonly manage three types of information technology:
  - Biomedical
  - Information
  - Knowledge
- Biomedical technology includes the use for the following:
  - Physiological monitoring
  - Diagnostic testing
  - Medication administration
  - Therapeutic interventions
- Information technology refers to computers and programs that are used to process data and information.
- Using a central data repository, the data can be entered, stored, organized, retrieved and communicated with accuracy and speed
- Use of nursing minimum data sets was established to standardize the collection of essential patient data

- Use of structured nursing languages provides standards for gathering data so that they can be retrieved and compared across time and place.
- Goals of information management
  - Obtain, manage, and use information to improve patient outcomes
  - Improve individual and organizational performance in patient care
  - Improve performance in other organizational processes
- Areas of management of information
  - Patient-specific data and information
  - Aggregate data and information
  - Expert knowledge-based information
  - Comparative performance data and information
- Transmission of information communication networks are used
- Information systems can be used for:
  - Reduction of clerical nursing
  - Providing patient census and location
  - Obtaining results from tests and list of medications
  - Accessing nursing policies and procedures
  - Coordinating patient care
  - Monitoring chronic conditions
  - Managing financial billing and statistical reporting
- Placement of computers at the patient's side or using hand-held devices has many advantages
  - Saves time
  - Improves communication by providing more timely access by others
  - Decreases likelihood of documentation omission
  - Adapts to nurse's workflow
  - Personalizes patient assessment
  - Simplifies care planning
- Knowledge technology involves decision support systems that are used to mimic the informational processing of an expert nurse
- Privacy and security issues have become important with increased access to, and, therefore, potential broad misuse of, patient care data.
- Ethical decision in health care becomes more complex with the increasing medical technology
- The electronic health record contains healthcare information for an individual from birth to death, allowing immediate access to comprehensive health information

- Smart cards are credit card–like devices that store a limited amount of data. These cards and the demographic, medical and emergency contact information they provide help coordinate care across local, state, national, and international boundaries—wherever patients may need access to health care.
- Telehealth is the process of using modern telecommunication and information technologies to provide health care to patients in remote locations.
- The Internet is a worldwide network of compu-ters that fosters communication, collaboration, resource sharing, and information access. It is a multicultural library that is open all day, every day to ordinary computer users. The main uses of the Internet are sending and receiving electronic mail (e-mail) and browsing the WWW.

TIPS FOR MANAGING INFORMATION AND TECHNOLOGY

- Create a vision for the future.
- Match your vision to the institution's mission and strategic plan.
- Learn what you need to know to fulfill the vision.
- Join initiatives that are moving in the direction of your vision.
- Be prepared to initiate, implement, and support new technology.
- Use automated dispensing system.
- Use biometric technology.
- Use bar coding systems/bar code technology
- Never stop learning, or you will always be behind.

TERMS TO KNOW

bar coding systems/bar code technology
biomedical technology
computerized prescriber order entry (CPOE)
data
database
decision support systems
disease management
e-learning
e-mail
electronic medical record (EMR)
electronic medication administration record (e-MAR)
evidence-based practice
expert system
Health Insurance Portability and Accountability Act (HIPAA)
informatics
informatics competencies
information
information technology
Internet
knowledge
knowledge technology
knowledge worker
nursing minimum data set (NMDS)
personal digital assistant (PDA)
radio frequency identification (RFID)
smart card
structured nursing language
telehealth
voice technology
wireless (WL) messaging
World Wide Web (WWW)

REFERENCES

Anderson, M. A., & Wilson, J. (2004, October). Casting Electronic Safety Nets Across Care Continuums. *IT Solutions*, 35(supplement 5), 4-7.

Ash, J. S., Gorman, P. N., Seshadri, V., & Hersh, W. R. (2004). Computerized physician order entry in U.S. hospitals: Result of a 2002 survey. *Journal of the American Medical Informatics Association, Mar-Apr*(2), 121-124.

Bakken, S., Button, P., Konicek, D., Matney, S., McCormick, K., Ozbolt, J. G., Saba, V. K., Warren, J. J., & Westra, B. (2001). Standardized terminologies for nursing concepts: Collaborative activities in the United States. In *NI 2000 Postconference Proceedings*. Rotorua, New Zealand: Premier Press.

Bakken, S., & McArthur, J. (2001). Evidence-based nursing practice: A call to action for nursing informatics. *Journal of the American Medical Informatics Association, 8*(3), 289-290. Retrieved August 7, 2005, from PubMed database.

Bell, M. J., (2005, February). Nursing information of tomorrow. *Healthcare Informatics, 22*(2), 74-78.

Clark, J. & Lang, N. (1992). Nursing's next advance: An International Classification for Nursing Practice. *International Nursing Review, 39*(4), 109-112.

Contrux Software Builders (n.d.) Vendor Selection. Retrieved October 20, 2005 from www.construx.com/survivalguide/doc/chk27.htm.

Critical appraisal. (n.d.) In Centre for evidence based medicine. Retrieved August 05, 2005 from http://www.cebm.net/critical_appraisal.asp.

Curran, C. R. (1995). Data requirements of the nurse executive. Unpublished paper.

DePalma, J. (2002). Proposing an evidence-based policy process. *Nursing Administration Quarterly, 26*(4), 55-61.

Drucker, P. (1993). Post capitalist society. New York: Harper Business Publishers.

Elfrink, V., Bakken, S., Coenen, A., McNeil, B., & Bickford, C. (2001). Standardized nursing vocabularies: A foundation for quality care. *Seminars in Oncology Nursing, 17*(1), 18-23.

Goldsborough, R. (1999). Information on the net often needs checking. *RN, 62*(5), 22, 24.

Graves, J. R., Amos, L. K., Huether, S., Lange, L. L., & Thompson, C. B. (1995). Description of a graduate program in clinical nursing informatics. *Computers in Nursing, 13*(2), 60-70.

Graves, J. R., & Corcoran, S. (1989). The study of nursing informatics. *Image: Journal of Nursing Scholarship, 21*(4), 227-231.

Haynes, R. B., & Wilczynski, N. L. (2004). Optimal search strategies for retrieving scientifically strong studies of diagnosis from Medline: Analytical survey. *British Medical Journal, 328*(7447), 1162-1163. Retrieved on April 30, 2004 from the bmj.com database.

Hollaway, N., Kripps, B., Koepke, K., & Skiba, D. J. (2000). Evaluating health care information on the Internet. In J. Fitzpatrick & K. S. Montogomery (Eds.), *Internet resources for nurses*. New York: Springer.

Hunter, K. M. (2001). Nursing informatics theory. In V. K. Saba & K. A. McCormick (Eds.), *Essentials of computers for nurses: Informatics for the new millennium* (pp. 179-190). New York: McGraw-Hill.

Institute of Medicine. (2001, July). Crossing the quality chasm. A new health system for the 21st century/ Committee on Quality Health Care in America. Washington, DC: National Academy Press.

Joint Commission on Accreditation of Healthcare Organizations. (1994). *JCAHO accreditation manual.* Chicago: Author.

Joint Commission on Accreditation of Healthcare Organizations. (2001). *JCAHO accreditation manual.* Chicago: Author.

Joint Commission on Accreditation of Healthcare Organizations. (2005). *JCAHO accreditation manual.* Chicago: Author.

Larrabee, S., & Brown, M. M. (2003, July). Recognizing the institutional benefits of bar-code point-of-care technology. *Joint Commission Journal on Quality and Safety, 29*(7), 345-353.

Lawrence, S., & Giles, C. L. (1998). Searching the World Wide Web. *Science, 280*, 98-100.

Lunney, M., Delaney, C., Duffy, M., Moorhead, S., & Welton J. (2005). Advocating for standarized nursing languages in electronic health records. *Journal of Nursing Administration, 35*(1), 1-3.

Malashock, C., Smith-Shull, S., & Gould, D. A. (2004, May). Effect of smart infusion pumps on medication errors related to infusion device programming. *Hospital Pharmacy, 39*(5), 460-469.

Melnyk, B. M., Fineout-Overholt, E., Feinstein, N. F., Li, H., Small, L., Wilcox, L., et al. (2004). Nurses' perceived knowledge, beliefs, skills, and needs regarding evidence-based practice: Implications for accelerating the paradigm shift. Worldviews on evidence-based nursing (3rd quarter), 185-192.

Miller, K., Ward-Smith, P., Cox K., Jones, E, & Portnoy, J. (November 2003). Development of an asthma disease management program in a children's hospital. *Current Allergy and Asthma Reports, 3*(6), 484-490.

Moyer, V. A. & Elliott, E. J. (Eds.). (2004). *Evidence-based pediatrics and child health* (2nd ed.). London: BMJ Publishing Group.

Nicoll, L. H. (2001). *Nurses' guide to the Internet* (3rd ed.). Philadelphia: Lippincott.

Parker, P. J. (2005). One nurse informatics specialist views the future technology in the crystal ball. *Nursing Administration Quarterly, 29*(2), 123-124.

Richardson, W. S., Wilson, M. C., Nishikawa, J., & Hayward, R. S. (1995). The well-built question: A key to evidence-based decisions. *ACP Journal Club, 123,* A-12.

Sackett, D. L., Straus, S. E., Richardson, W. S., Rosenberg, W., & Haynes, R. B. (2000). *Evidence based medicine: How to practice and teach EBM* (2nd ed.). New York: Churchill Livingstone.

Schlosser, R. W. (2004, June 22). *Evidence-based practice in AAC: 10 points to consider.* Retrieved August 5, 2005, from www.asha.org/about/publications/leader-online/archives/2004/040622/f040622b.htm

Simpson, R. (2003, July-August). Everything a CNO needs to know about managing information technology. *Nurse Leader 1*(4), 43-45.

Simpson: HR.L. (2005, January-March). Patient and nurse safety: How information technology makes a difference. *Nursing Administration Quarterly*, 27(4), 97-101.

Snyder-Halpern, R., Corcoran-Perry, S., & Narayan, S. (2001). Developing clinical practice environments supporting the knowledge work of nurses. *Computers in Nursing*, 19(1), 17-23.

Tan, J. (1995). *Health management information systems: Theories, methods, applications*. Gaithersburg, MD: Aspen.

University of Wisconsin—Eau Claire. (2003). The ten C's for evaluating Internet resources. Retrieved October 10, 2005 from http://www.uwec.edu/Library/guides/tencs, html

Werley, H. H., & Lang, N. M. (Eds.). (1988). *Identification of the nursing minimum data set*. New York: Springer.

SUGGESTED READINGS

American Nurses Association. (1999). *Core principles on telehealth*. Washington, DC: Author.

Ash, J. S., Gorman, P. L., Seshadri, V., & Hersh, W. R. (2004, March-April). Computerized Physician Order Entry in U.S. hospitals: Results of a 2002 survey. *Journal of the American Medical Informatics Association*, 11(2), 95-99.

Averill, C. B., Marek, K. D., Zielstorff, R., Kneedler, J., Delaney, C., & Milholland, D. K. (1998). ANA standards for nursing data sets in information systems. *Computers in Nursing*, 16(3), 157-161.

Douglas, J., & Larrabee, S. (2003, May). Implement information technology to track and reduce medication errors. *Nursing Management*, 37-40.

Dochterman, J. M., & Bulecheck, G. M. (2004). *Nursing Interventions Classification* (NIC) (4th ed.). Philadelphia: Elsevier's Health Sciences, 506-507.

Person, S. D., Allison, J. J., Kiefe, C. I., Weaver, M. T., Williams, O. D., Centor, R. M., & Weissman, N. W. (2004). Nurse staffing and mortality for medicare patients with acute myocardial infarction. *Med Care*, 42, 4-12.

Rosow, E., Grimes, S. L., (2003, October-December). Technology's implications for health care quality: A clinical perspective. *Nursing Administration Quarterly*, 27(4), 307-317.

Saba, V. K., & McCormick, K. A. (2001). *Essentials of computers for nurses: Informatics for the new millennium* (3rd ed.). New York: McGraw-Hill.

Scalise, D. (2005, August). Where the patient and technology meet. *Hospitals and Health Network*, 79(8), 34-42.

Sensmeier, J. (2004, December). Medication safety—Transform workflow through selective implementation. *2005 Guide to Technology*, 35(12), 46-51.

Smith, C. (2004, April-June). New technology continues to invade health care. What are the strategic implications/outcomes? *Nursing Administration Quarterly*, 8(2), 92-98.

Staggers, N., Thompson, C. B., & Synder-Halpern, R. (2001). History and trends in clinical information systems in the United States. *Journal of Nursing Scholarship*, 33(1), 75-81.

Sullivan, M., & Wilson, K., (2004, January 15). Preventing medication errors with smart infusion technology. *American Journal of Health System Pharmacy*, 61(2).

Vahey, D. C., Corser, W. D., & Brennan, P. F. (2001). Publicly available health care databases for administrative strategic planning. *Journal of Nursing Administration*, 31(1), 9-15.

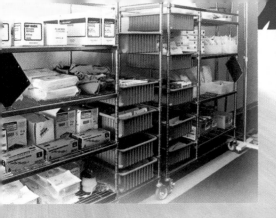

Chapter

11

Managing Costs and Budgets

Trudi Stafford

T his chapter focuses on methods of financing health care and specific strategies for managing costs and budgets in patient-care settings. Factors that escalate healthcare costs, sources of healthcare financing, reimbursement methods, cost-containment and healthcare reform strategies, and implications for nursing practice are discussed. Various budgets and the budgeting process are explained. In addition to clinical competency and caring practices, understanding the cost issues in healthcare delivery and the ethical implications of financial decisions are essential for nurses to contribute fully to the health and healing of patients and populations.

Objectives

- Explain several major factors that are escalating the costs of health care.
- Evaluate different reimbursement methods and their incentives to control costs.
- Differentiate costs, charges, and revenue in relation to a specified unit of service, such as a visit, hospital stay, or procedure.
- Value why all healthcare organizations must make a profit.
- Give examples of cost considerations for nurses working in managed care environments.

- Discuss the purpose of and relationships among the operating, cash, and capital budgets.

- Explain the budgeting process.
- Identify variances on monthly expense reports.

Questions to Consider

- *How can you stay abreast of changes in the healthcare system and what they mean for the practice of nursing?*
- *What are the typical nursing care activities and supplies charges?*
- *Who are the major payers to your organizations? What is their method of payment or reimbursement?*
- *Does the organization recoup all of the charges? If not, what portion of the charges do they get for various patient groups?*
- *How is nursing reimbursed in your organization?*
- *How can you increase your cost-effectiveness as a nurse?*
- *Do the nursing practices in your organization add value for patients?*

The Challenge

Robin Stoupa, RN, MSN
Director of Ambulatory Services, University of Nebraska Medical Center, Omaha, Nebraska

The Internal Medicine Clinic (IMC) consists of one primary care section and eight specialty sections. The IMC is one of many clinics owned and managed by a physician group. Professional fees are the sole source of revenue for the IMC and are pooled into one fund. Professional fees are received for physician services provided in the hospital, in special procedure laboratories, and in the ambulatory clinic.

For the past 3 years, the IMC has experienced a 15% to 18% increase in ambulatory visit volume. At the same time, IMC revenues have declined. However, administrators want to stay budget neutral. As payers decrease payment in all areas, it is easy for administrators to assume that the areas of greatest activity are the areas

losing money. The next logical step is to require that variable expenses in that area be reduced. Because nursing personnel are the greatest variable expense in the clinic, such thinking often leads to demands to reduce nursing staff or to substitute lower-paid personnel. As the nurse manager of the IMC, my goal is to maintain a high-quality, high-performance work team that adds value for patients. In this situation, what steps can be taken before reducing staff in the IMC ambulatory clinic? How can I justify that the amount spent currently for staff keeps the clinic functioning in the black?

What do you think you would do if you were this nurse?

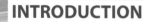

INTRODUCTION

Healthcare costs in the United States continue to rise at a rate greater than general inflation. In 1999, for example, Americans spent $1.2 trillion for health care, approximately 13% of the gross domestic product (GDP). This equals $4368 per person and surpasses the per capita expenditures of other Western nations by almost 50%. The health share of the GDP is projected to increase to 18% in 2013 (Heffler, Smith, Keehan, Clemens, Zezza, & Truffer, 2004). Yet millions of uninsured and underinsured Americans do not have access to basic healthcare services. With the exception of South Africa, the United States is the only industrialized nation where health care is a privilege rather than a right.

Despite our huge expenditures, major indicators reveal significant health problems in the United States, as well as large disparities in health status related to gender, race, and socioeconomic status *(Healthy People 2010)*. Our infant mortality rate is among the highest of all industrialized nations, and black infants die at more than twice the rate of white infants. Average life expectancy is lower than that in most developed countries,

and men have a life expectancy that is 6 years less than that of women. One in eight women will develop breast cancer during their lifetime, with black and American Indian women experiencing a much higher death rate than white women. Violence-related injuries are on the rise, and unintentional injuries, such as motor vehicle accidents, are a leading cause of death. Clearly, we are not receiving a high value return for our healthcare dollar.

The large portion of the GDP that is spent on health care poses problems to the economy in other ways, too. Funds are diverted from needed social programs such as childcare, housing, education, transportation, and the environment. The **price** of goods and services is increased, and, therefore, the country's ability to compete in the international marketplace is compromised. One illustration is that up to 10% of the cost of a new American car is allocated to pay for the healthcare costs of automobile workers. As the amount of the GDP devoted to healthcare expenses rises, the more vulnerable the healthcare industry is to external influences. This creates a major concern for an industry that already expresses concerns about being over-regulated.

WHAT ESCALATES HEALTHCARE COSTS?

Total healthcare **costs** are a function of the prices and the **utilization** rates of healthcare services (Costs = Price × Utilization) (Table 11-1). *Price* is the rate that healthcare **providers** set for the services they deliver, such as the hospital rate or physician fee. *Utilization* refers to the quantity or volume of services provided, such as diagnostic tests provided or number of patient visits.

Price inflation and administrative inefficiency are leading contributors to increasing prices for health services. In recent decades, rises in healthcare prices have dramatically outpaced general inflation. Examples of factors that stimulate price inflation are physician incomes that rise faster than average worker earnings and the high prices of prescription drugs, which are often 50% higher than prices in other nations (Bodenheimer & Grumbach, 2005). Administrative inefficiency or waste is primarily a result of the large numbers of clerical personnel whom organizations use to process reimbursement forms from multiple **payers.** U.S. hospitals spend an average of 20% of their **budgets** on billing administration alone! This single fact indicates why some hospital administrators advocate for the elimination of multiple payers.

Several interrelated factors contribute to increased utilization of medical services. These include unnecessary care, consumer attitudes, healthcare financing, pharmaceutical usage, and changing population demographics and disease patterns. There are substantial amounts of unnecessary care that do not add health benefits for patients. Inappropriate or ineffective medical procedures are also prevalent and have led to national initiatives to demonstrate efficacy of interventions and to decrease variations in physician practice.

Our attitudes and behaviors as consumers of health care also contribute to rising costs. In general, we prefer to "be fixed" when something goes wrong rather than to practice prevention. When we need "fixing," expensive high-tech services typically are perceived as the best care. Many of us still believe that the physician knows best, so we do not seek much information related to costs and effectiveness of different healthcare options. When we do seek information, it is not readily available or understandable. Also, we are not accustomed to using other, less costly, healthcare providers, such as nurse practitioners.

The way health care is financed contributes to rising costs. When health care is reimbursed by third-party payers, consumers are somewhat insulated from personally experiencing the direct effects of high healthcare costs. For example, the huge rise in consumer demand for prescription drugs since 1995 was fueled by low copayments for drugs required by most insurance companies (Heffler et al., 2004). As consumer out-of-pocket expenses for drugs increase, consumer demand should decrease. In most instances, however, consumers do not have many incentives to consider costs when choosing among providers or using services. In addition, the various methods of reimbursement have implications for how providers price and use services.

Evidence of pharmaceutical usage can be seen in advertisements in magazines and on television. No longer do pharmaceutical companies attempt to influence the prescribers only. They go directly to the consumer, who then goes to the prescriber. Because of some typical drug benefit programs, the consumer often is unaware of the total cost of a

Table 11-1 RELATIONSHIP OF PRICE AND UTILIZATION RATES TO TOTAL HEALTHCARE COSTS				
Price	× Utilization Rate	=	Total Cost	% Change
$1.00	100		$100.00	0
$1.08*	100		$108.00	+8.0%
$1.08	105†		$113.40	+13.4%
$1.08	110‡		$118.80	+18.8%

*8% increase for inflation.
†5% more procedures done.
‡10% more procedures done.

medication, which may be a "quick fix" (described previously) or a lifestyle enhancement, such as sexual enhancers or skin conditioning.

Changing population demographics also are increasing the volume of health services needed. For example, chronic health problems increase with age, and the number of elderly Americans is rising. The fastest growing population is the group aged 85 or older, and Baby Boomers are beginning to move into their senior years. Infectious diseases such as AIDS and tuberculosis, as well as the growing societal problems of homelessness, drug addiction, and violence, increase demands for health services.

HOW IS HEALTH CARE FINANCED?

Health care is paid for by four sources: government (36%), private insurance companies (41%), individuals (19%), and other, primarily philanthropy (4%) (Figure 11-1). Three fourths of the government funding is at the federal level. Federal programs include Medicare and health services for members of the military, veterans, American Indians, and federal prisoners. Medicare, the largest federal program, was established in 1965 and pays for care provided to people 65 years and older and some disabled individuals. Medicare Part A is an insurance plan for hospital, hospice, home health, and skilled nursing care that is paid for through

Social Security taxes. Nursing home care that is mainly custodial is not covered. Medicare Part B is an optional insurance that covers physician services, medical equipment, and diagnostic tests. Part B is funded through federal taxes and monthly premiums paid by the recipients. Medicare does not cover outpatient medications, eye or hearing examinations, or dental services. The drug benefit plan, effective in 2006, has been viewed as beneficial and very difficult to understand.

Medicaid, a state-level program financed by federal and state funds, pays for services provided to persons who are medically indigent, blind, or disabled and to children with disabilities. The federal government pays between 50% and 83% of total Medicaid costs based on the per capita income of the state. Services funded by Medicaid vary from state to state but must include services provided by hospitals, physicians, laboratories, radiology departments; prenatal and preventive care; and nursing home and home healthcare services.

Private insurance is the second major source of financing for the healthcare system. Most Americans have private health insurance, which usually is provided by employers through group policies. Individuals can purchase health insurance, but typically the rates are very high and provide minimal coverage. Health insurance that is so intertwined with employment is problematic and contributes to the number of uninsured and underinsured Americans. Many of the uninsured workers are employed in small businesses that cannot afford to provide group insurance, or they have part-time, seasonal, or service positions.

Individuals also pay directly for health services when they do not have health insurance or when insurance does not cover the service. Costs paid by individuals are called out-of-pocket expenses and include deductibles, copays, and coinsurance. Health insurance benefits often do not cover preventive care or things such as eyeglasses, non-prescription medications, cosmetic surgeries, or alternative healthcare therapies.

REIMBURSEMENT METHODS

Four major payment methods are used for reimbursing healthcare providers: charges, **cost-based reimbursement**, flat-rate reimbursement, and capi-

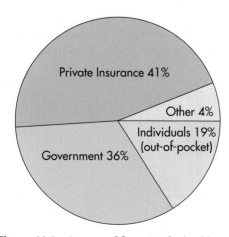

Figure 11-1   Sources of financing for health care.

BOX 11-1

Major Reimbursement Methods

- Charges
- Cost-based (retrospective)
- Flat rate (prospective)
- Capitated

Exercise 11–1

What is the contractual allowance when a hospital charges $800 per day to care for a ventilator-dependent patient and an insurance company reimburses the hospital $685 per day? What is the impact on hospital income (**revenue**) if this is the reimbursement for 2500 patient days?

tated payments (Zelman, McCue, Millikan, & Glick, 2003). These methods are summarized in Box 11-1. Health-service researchers do not agree on the exact effects of these reimbursement methods on cost and quality. However, considering these effects is important because changes in payment systems have implications for how care is provided in healthcare organizations.

Charges consist of the cost of providing a service plus a markup for **profit.** Third-party payers often put limitations on what they will pay by establishing usual and customary charges by surveying all providers in a certain area. Usual and customary charges rise over time as providers continually increase their prices. In cost-based reimbursement, all allowable costs are calculated and used as the basis for payment. Each payer (government or insurance company) determines what the allowable costs are for each procedure, visit, or service. Charges and cost-based reimbursement are retrospective payment methods because the amount of payment is determined after services are delivered. When the reimbursed costs are less than the full charge for the service, a **contractual allowance** or discount exists. Charges and cost-based reimbursement were the predominant payment method in the 1960s and 1970s but have been largely supplanted by payer fee schedules determined before service delivery.

Flat-rate reimbursement is a method in which the third-party payer decides in advance what will be paid for a service or episode of care. This is a **prospective reimbursement** method. If the costs of care are greater than the payment, the provider absorbs the loss. If the costs are less than the payment, the provider makes a profit. In 1983, Medicare implemented a prospective payment system (PPS) for hospital care that uses diagnosis-related groups (DRGs) as the basis for payment.

DRGs, a classification system that groups patients into categories based on the average number of days of hospitalization for specific medical diagnoses, considers factors such as the patient's age, complications, and other illnesses. Payment includes the expected costs for diagnostic tests, various therapies, surgery, and length of stay (LOS). The cost of nursing services is not explicitly calculated. With a few exceptions, DRGs do not adequately reflect the variability of patient intensity or acuity within the DRG. This is problematic for nursing because the amount of resources (nurses and supplies) used to care for patients is directly related to the patient acuity. Therefore, many nurses believe that DRGs are not good predictors of nursing care requirements. Recently, Medicare also began reimbursing home health agencies, nursing homes, and ambulatory care providers through a PPS.

In addition to Medicare, some state Medicaid programs and private insurance companies use a DRG payment system. Although DRGs are not currently used for specialty hospitals (pediatric, psychiatric, and oncology), they are a dominant force in hospital payment. Implementation of a PPS with DRGs resulted in increased patient acuity and decreased LOS in hospitals, along with a greater demand for home care. The need for hospital and community-based nurses also increased.

The resource-based relative value scale (RBRVS) is a flat-rate reimbursement method the federal government uses to pay physicians. Fees in this system are set by estimating the time, cognitive and technical skills, and physical effort required to provide the specific service. Another common flat-rate method is the discounted payments payers negotiate with providers in preferred provider organizations (PPOs).

Capitated payments are based on the provision of specified services to an individual over a set period such as 1 year. Providers are paid a per-person-per-year (or per-month) fee. If the services cost more than the payment, the provider absorbs the loss. Likewise, if the services cost less than the payment, the provider makes a profit. **Capitation** is the mode of payment characteristic of health maintenance organizations (HMOs) and other **managed care** systems.

Exercise 11-2

Medicare reimburses a hospice $70 for home visits. For one particular group of patients, it costs the hospice an average of $98 per day to provide care. What are the implications for the hospice? What options should the hospice nurse manager and nurses consider?

THE CHANGING HEALTHCARE ECONOMIC ENVIRONMENT

Health care is a major public concern, and rapid changes are occurring in an attempt to reduce costs and improve the health and wellness of the nation. As shown in Box 11-2, strategies shaping the evolving healthcare delivery system include managed care; **organized delivery systems (ODSs)**; and competition based on price, patient outcomes, and service quality. These strategies affect both the pricing and use of health services.

Exercise 11-3

For each reimbursement method, think about the incentives for healthcare providers (individuals and organizations) regarding their practice patterns. Are there incentives to change the quantity of services used per patient or the number or types of patients served? Are there incentives to be efficient? List the incentives. How might each method affect overall healthcare costs? (Think in terms of effect on utilization and price.) What do you think the effect on quality of care might be with each payment method?

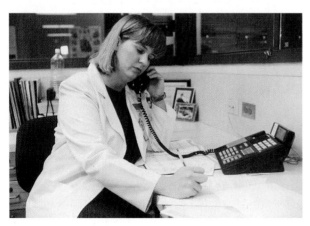

Nurses in ambulatory care settings often work directly with insurance companies to plan patient care.

BOX 11-2

Healthcare Delivery Reform Strategies

- Managed care
- Organized delivery systems
- Competition based on price, patient outcomes, and service quality

Managed care is a health plan that brings together the delivery and financing function into one entity, in contrast with a traditional fee-for-service plan, in which insurers pay providers based on costs (Finkler, 2001). A major goal of managed care is to decrease unnecessary services, thereby decreasing costs. Managed care also works to ensure timely and appropriate care. HMOs are a type of managed care system in which the primary physician serves as a gatekeeper who determines what services the patient uses. Because HMOs are paid on a capitated basis, it is to their advantage to practice prevention and use ambulatory care rather than more expensive hospital care. In other forms of managed care, a nonphysician case manager arranges and authorizes the services provided. Many insurance companies have used case managers for years. Nurses who work in home health and ambulatory settings often communicate with insurance company case managers to plan the care for specific patients. PPOs and point-of-service (POS) plans are other types of managed care plans that give the patient more options than traditional HMOs for selecting providers and services.

ODSs comprise networks of healthcare organizations, providers, and payers. Typically, this means hospitals, physicians, and insurance companies. The aim of such joint ventures is to develop and market collectively a comprehensive package of healthcare services that will meet most needs of large numbers of consumers. Hospitals, physicians, and payers will share the financial risks of the enterprise. Although hospitals share some risk now with prospective payment, physicians have not generally shared the risk. This risk-sharing is expected to provide incentives to eliminate unnecessary services, use resources more effectively, and improve quality of services.

Competition among healthcare providers increasingly is based on cost and quality outcomes.

Decision-making regarding price and utilization of services is shifting from physicians and hospitals to payers, who are demanding significant discounts or lower prices. Scientific data that demonstrate positive health outcomes and high-quality services are required. Providers who are unable to compete on the basis of price, patient outcomes, and service quality will find it difficult to survive as the system evolves.

WHAT DOES THIS MEAN FOR NURSING PRACTICE?

What does the healthcare economic environment mean for the practicing professional nurse? We must value ourselves as providers and think of our practice within a context of organizational viability and quality of care. To do this, we must add "financial thinking" to our repertoire of nursing skills, and we must determine whether the services we provide add value for patients. Services that add value are of high quality, affect health outcomes positively, and minimize costs. The following sections help develop financial thinking skills and ways to consider how nursing practice adds value for patients by minimizing costs.

WHY IS PROFIT NECESSARY?

Private, nongovernmental healthcare organizations may be either for-profit (FP) or not-for-profit (NFP). This designation refers to the tax status of the organization and specifies how the profit can be used. Profit is the excess income left after all expenses have been paid (Revenues – Expenses = Profit). FP organizations pay taxes, and their profits can be distributed to investors and managers. NFP organizations, on the other hand, do not pay taxes and must reinvest all profits in the organization to better serve the public.

All private healthcare organizations must make a profit to survive. If expenses are greater than revenues, the organization experiences a loss. If revenues equal expenses, the organization breaks even. In both cases, nothing is left over to replace facilities and equipment, expand services, or pay for inflation costs. Some healthcare organizations are able to survive in the short run without making a profit because they use interest from investments to supplement revenues. The long-term viability of any private healthcare organization, however, is dependent on consistently making a profit. Box 11-3 presents a simplified example of an income statement from a neighborhood nursing center.

BOX 11-3

Income Statement of Revenues and Expenses from a Neighborhood Nursing Center: FYE December 31, 2005

Revenues		
Patient revenues	$115,700	
Grant income	60,000	
Other operating revenues	5,300	
TOTAL	$181,000	$181,000
Expenses		
Salary costs	$130,500	
Supplies	14,400	
Other operating expenses (rent, utilities, administrative services, etc.)	29,900	
TOTAL	$174,800	174,800
Excess of revenues over expenses [profit]*		$6,200

FYE, Fiscal year ending.
*Loss would be shown in parentheses ( ) or brackets.

Nurses and nurse managers directly affect an organization's ability to make a profit. Profits can be achieved or improved by decreasing costs or increasing revenues. In tight economic times, many managers think only in terms of cutting costs. Although cost-cutting measures are important, especially to keep prices down so that the organization will be competitive, ways to increase revenues also need to be explored.

Exercise 11-4

Obtain a copy of an itemized patient bill from a healthcare organization, and review the charges. What was the source and method of payment? How much of these charges was reimbursed? How much was charged for items you regularly use in clinical care?

COST-CONSCIOUS NURSING PRACTICES

Understanding What Is Required to Remain Financially Sound

Understanding what is required for a department or agency to remain financially sound requires that nurses move beyond thinking about costs for individual patients to thinking about income and expenses and numbers of patients needed to make a profit. In a fee-for-service environment, revenue is earned for every service provided. Therefore, increasing the volume of services, such as diagnostic tests and patient visits, increases revenues. In a capitated environment where one fee is paid for all services provided, increasing the overall number of patients served and decreasing the volume of services used is desirable. With capitation, nurses must strive to accomplish more with each visit to decrease return visits and complications. Many healthcare organizations function in a dual-reimbursement environment, part capitated and part fee-for-service. Nurses need to understand their organization's reimbursement environment and strategy for realizing a profit in its specific circumstances.

Knowing Costs and Reimbursement Practices

As direct caregivers and case managers, nurses are constantly involved in determining the type and quantity of resources used for patients. This includes supplies, personnel, and time. Nurses need to know what costs are generated by their decisions and actions. Nurses also need to know what things cost and how they are paid for in an organization so that they can make cost-effective decisions. For example, nurses need to know per-item costs for supplies so that they can appropriately evaluate lower-cost substitutes.

In ambulatory and home health settings, nurses must be familiar with the various insurance plans that reimburse the organization. Each plan has different contract rules regarding preauthorization, types of services covered, required vendors, and so on. Although nurses must develop and implement their plans of care with full knowledge of these reimbursement practices, the payer does not totally drive the care. Nurses still advocate for patients in important ways while also working within the cost and contractual constraints. Moreover, when nurses understand the reimbursement practices, they can help patients maximize the resources available to them.

In hospitals, the cost of nursing care usually is not calculated or billed separately to patients but is part of the general per-diem charge. One major problem with this method is the assumption that all patients consume the same amount of nursing care. Another problem with bundling the charges for nursing care with the room rate is that nursing as a clinical service is not perceived by management as generating revenue for the hospital. Rather, nursing is perceived predominantly as an expense to the organization. Although this perception may not matter in a capitated setting where all provider services are considered a cost, accurate nursing care cost data are needed to negotiate managed care contracts. Additionally, patients do not see direct charges and so have no way to understand the monetary value of the services they receive.

Exercise 11-5

How was nursing care charged on the bill you obtained? What are the implications for nursing in being perceived as an expense rather than being associated with the revenue stream? Why will this perception be less important in a capitated environment?

Capturing All Charges in a Timely Fashion

Nurses also help contain costs by making sure that all possible charges are captured. Several large hospitals report more than $1 million a year lost from supplies that were not charged. In hospitals, nurses must know which supplies are charged to patients and which ones are charged to the unit. In addition, the procedures and equipment used need to be accurately documented. In ambulatory and community settings, nurses often need to keep abreast of the codes that are used to bill services. These codes change yearly, and sometimes items are bundled together under one charge, and sometimes they are broken down into different charges. Turning in charges in a timely manner is also important because delayed billing negatively affects cash flow by extending the time before an organization is paid for services provided. This is particularly considerable in smaller organizations.

In home health, hospice, and long-term care organizations, billing is closely integrated with the clinical information system. For example, to ensure reimbursement, the physician's plan of care and documentation that the patient meets the criteria for admission must be noted on the clinical record. Typically, nurses are responsible for documenting this information.

Exercise 11-6
You used three intravenous (IV) catheters to do a particularly difficult venipuncture. Do you charge the patient for all three catheters? What if you accidentally contaminated one by touching the sheet? How is the catheter paid for if not charged to the patient? Who benefits and who loses when patients are not charged for supplies?

Using Time Efficiently
The adage that time is money is fitting in health care and refers to both the nurse's time and the patient's time. When nurses are organized and efficient in their care delivery and in scheduling and coordinating patients' care, the organization will save money. With capitation, doing as much as possible during each episode of care is particularly important to decrease repeat visits and unnecessary service utilization. Because LOS is the most important predictor of hospital costs (Finkler & Kovner, 2000), patients who stay extra days cost the hospital a considerable amount. Decreasing LOS also makes room for other patients, thereby potentially increasing patient volume and hospital revenues. Nurses can become more efficient and effective by evaluating their major work processes and eliminating areas of redundancy and rework. Automated

clinical information systems that support integrated practice at the point of care will also increase efficiency and improve patient outcomes.

Exercise 11-7
The Visiting Nurse Association (VNA) cannot file for reimbursement until all documentation of each visit has been completed. Typically, the paperwork is submitted a week after the visit. When the number of home visits increases rapidly, the paperwork often is not turned in for 2 weeks or more. What are the implications of this routine practice for the agency? Why would the VNA be very vulnerable financially during periods of heavy workload? What are some options for the nurse manager to consider to expedite the paperwork?

Discussing the Cost of Care with Patients
Talking with patients about the cost of care is important, although it may be uncomfortable. Discovering during a clinic visit that a patient cannot afford a specific medication or intervention is preferable to finding out several days later in a follow-up call that the patient has not taken the medication. Such information compels the clinical management team to explore optional treatment plans or to find resources to cover the costs. Talking with patients about costs is important in other ways, too. It involves the patients in the decision-making process and increases the likelihood that treatment plans will be followed. Patients also can make informed choices and better use the resources available to them if they have appropriate information about costs.

Exercise 11-8
A new patient visits the clinic and is given prescriptions for three medications that will cost about $120 per month. You check her chart and discover that she has Medicare (but not Part D) and no supplemental insurance. How can you determine whether or not she has the resources to buy this medicine each month and if she is willing to buy it? If she cannot afford the medications, what are some options?

Meeting Patient Rather Than Provider Needs
Developing an awareness of how feelings about patients' needs influence decisions can help nurses better manage costs. A nurse administrator in a home health agency recently related the story of a nurse who continued to visit a patient for weeks after the patient's health problems had resolved. When questioned, the nurse said she was

uncomfortable terminating the visits because the patient continued to tell her he needed her help. Later, the patient revealed that he had not needed nursing care for some time, although he had continued telling the nurse he did because he thought she wanted to keep visiting him. This story illustrates how nurses need to verify whose needs are being met with nursing care.

Evaluating Cost-Effectiveness of New Technologies

The advent of new technologies is presenting dilemmas in managing costs. In the past, if a new piece of equipment was easier to use or benefited the patient in any way, nurses were apt to want to use it for everyone, no matter how much more it cost. Now they are forced to make decisions regarding which patients really need the new equipment and which ones will have good outcomes with the current equipment. Essentially, nurses are analyzing the cost-effectiveness of the new equipment with regard to different types of patients to allocate limited resources. This is a new and sometimes difficult way to think about patient care and at times may not feel like a caring way to make decisions regarding patient care. However, such decisions conserve resources without jeopardizing patients' health and thus create the possibility of providing additional healthcare services.

Exercise 11-9

Last year a new positive-pressure, needleless system for administering IV antibiotics was introduced. Because it was so easy and convenient for patients, the nurses in the home infusion company where you worked ordered them for everyone. Typically, patients get their IV antibiotics four times each day. The minibags and tubing for the regular procedure cost the agency $22 a day. The new system costs $24 per medication administration, or $96 a day. The agency receives the same per diem (daily) reimbursement for each patient. Discuss the financial implications for the agency if this practice is continued. Generate some optional courses of action for the nurses to consider. How should these options be evaluated? What secondary costs, such as the cost of treating fewer needlestick injuries, should be included?

Predicting and Using Nursing Resources Efficiently

Because healthcare organizations are service institutions, the largest part of their operating budget typically is for personnel. For hospitals, in particular, nurses are the largest group of employees and often account for most of the personnel budget. Staffing is the major area nurse managers can affect with respect to managing costs, and supply management is the second area. To understand why this is so, it is helpful to understand the concepts of fixed and variable costs.

The total **fixed costs** in a unit are those costs that do not change as the volume of patients changes. In other words, with either a high or low patient census, expenses related to rent, loan payments, administrative salaries, and salaries of the minimum amount of staff to keep a unit open must be paid. **Variable costs** are costs that vary in direct proportion to patient volume or acuity. Examples include nursing personnel, supplies, and medications. Break-even analysis is a tool that uses fixed and variable costs for determining the volume of patients needed to just break even (revenue = expenses) or to realize a profit or loss.

In hospitals and community health agencies, patient classification systems are used to help managers predict nursing care requirements (see Chapter 13). These systems differentiate patients according to acuity of illness, functional status, and resource needs. Some nurses do not like these systems because they believe the essence of nursing is not captured. However, we need to remember that these are tools to help managers predict resource needs. Describing all nursing activities and judgments is not necessary for a tool to be a good predictor. Misguided efforts to sabotage classification systems with the hope for better staffing work primarily to prevent the development of tools to better manage practice. Used appropriately, patient classification systems can help evaluate changing practice patterns and patient acuity levels as well as provide information for **budgeting processes.**

Exercise 11-10

Given the definitions for fixed and variable costs, why do you think nurse managers have the greatest influence over costs through management of staffing and supplies?

Managing staffing and decreasing LOS can achieve the most immediate reductions in costs. Hospitals strive to lower costs so that they will attract new contracts and be attractive as partners in provider networks. Therefore, staffing methods and patient care delivery models are being closely scrutinized. Work redesign, a process for changing the way to think about and structure the work of patient care, is the predominant strategy for developing systems that better utilize high-cost professionals and improve service quality. Increased staff retention, patient safety, and positive patient outcomes result from effective work redesign processes.

Using Research to Evaluate Standard Nursing Practices

Another way nurses are restructuring their work to make sure they add value for patients is through research. For example, in the internal medicine clinics at the University of Nebraska Medical Center, nurses and physicians developed a rule to predict which patients are at risk for orthostatic hypotension. This is significant because the mortality rates are high in patients who have orthostatic hypotension. Yet performing the sitting and standing blood pressure readings on all patients is costly in terms of nursing resources. Full implementation of the rule, which was developed and validated through research, results in nurses taking ortho-

static blood pressure readings on less than 25% of the clinic's patients. This chapter's Research Perspective illustrates cost savings from another practice alteration. Box 11-4 summarizes some cost-conscious strategies for nursing practice.

BOX 11-4

Strategies for Cost-Conscious Nursing Practice

1. Understanding what is required to remain financially sound
2. Knowing costs and reimbursement practices
3. Capturing all possible charges in a timely fashion
4. Using time efficiently
5. Discussing the costs of care with patients
6. Meeting patient, rather than provider, needs
7. Evaluating cost-effectiveness of new technologies
8. Predicting and using nursing resources efficiently
9. Using research to evaluate standard nursing practices

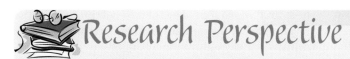

Research Perspective

Koelling, T. M., Johnson, M. L., Cody, R. J., & Aaronson, K. D. (2005). Discharge education improves clinical outcomes in patients with chronic heart failure. *Circulation, 111,* 179-185.

The purpose of this study was to isolate the effect that patient education by a nurse educator had on the clinical outcomes of heart failure patients. In this randomized, controlled trial of 223 heart failure patients, one group of patients ($n = 116$) received standard discharge information and the other group of patients ($n = 107$) received standard discharge information and 1 hour of one-on-one education from a nurse educator. All subjects were followed by telephone at 30, 90, and 180 days after discharge to collect data concerning post-hospitalization clinical events, symptoms, and self-care practices.

Patients who received the additional 1-hour teaching session with the nurse educator showed

improved clinical outcomes, increased adherence to self-care management, and reduced costs of care due to a reduction in rehospitalizations. The costs of care, including the costs associated with the additional education session, resulted in a savings of $2823 per patient in the education group as compared to the control group ($p = 0.035$).

IMPLICATIONS FOR PRACTICE
The findings from this economic evaluation support the implementation of nursing education programs for patients with chronic heart failure as evidenced by improved patient outcomes and reduced costs.

BUDGETS

The basic financial document in most healthcare organizations is the budget, a detailed financial plan for carrying out the activities an organization wants to accomplish for a certain period. An organizational budget is a formal plan that is stated in terms of dollars and includes proposed income and expenditures. The budgeting process is an ongoing activity in which plans are made and revenues and expenses are managed to meet or exceed the goals of the plan. The management functions of planning and control are tied together through the budgeting process.

A budget requires managers to plan ahead and to establish explicit program goals and expectations. Changes in medical practices, reimbursement methods, competition, technology, demographics, and regulatory factors must be forecast to anticipate their effects on the organization. Planning encourages evaluation of different options and assists in more cost-effective use of resources.

Exercise 11–11

A community nursing organization performs an average of 36 intermittent catheterizations each day. A prepackaged catheterization kit that costs the organization $17 is used. The four items in the kit, when purchased individually, cost the organization a total of $5. What factors should be considered in evaluating the cost-effectiveness of the two sources of supplies?

TYPES OF BUDGETS

Several types of interrelated budgets are used by well-managed organizations. Major budgets that are discussed in this chapter include the operating budget, the capital budget, and the **cash budget.** The way these budgets complement and support one another is depicted in Figure 11-2. Many organizations also use program, product line, or special purpose budgets. Long-range budgets are used to help managers plan for the future. Often, these are referred to as *strategic plans* (Finkler, 2001).

Operating Budget

The **operating budget** is the financial plan for the day-to-day activities of the organization. The expected revenues and expenses generated from daily operations, given a specified volume of

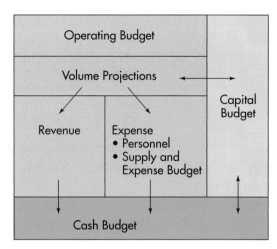

Figure 11-2   Interrelationships of the operating, capital, and cash budgets. (Modified from Ward, W. [1988]. *An introduction to health care financial management.* Ownings Mills, MD: National Health Publishing.)

patients, are stated. Preparing and monitoring the operating budget, particularly the expense portion, is often the most time-consuming financial function of nurse managers.

The expense part of the operating budget consists of a personnel budget and a supply and expense budget for each **cost center.** A cost center is an organizational unit for which costs can be identified and managed. The personnel budget is the largest part of the operating budget for most nursing units.

Before the personnel budget can be established, the volume of work predicted for the budget period must be calculated. A **unit of service** measure appropriate to the work of the unit is used. Units of service may be patient days, clinic or home visits, hours of service, admissions, deliveries, treatments, and so on. Another factor needed to calculate the workload is the patient acuity mix. The formula for calculating the workload or the required patient care hours for inpatient units is as follows: Workload volume = Hours of care per patient day × Number of patient days (Table 11-2).

In some organizations, the workload is established by the financial office and given to the nurse manager. In other organizations, nurse managers forecast the volume. In both situations, nurse managers should inform administration about any factors that might affect the accuracy of the forecast, such as changes in physician practice patterns,

Table 11-2 WORKLOAD CALCULATION (TOTAL REQUIRED PATIENT CARE HOURS)

Patient Acuity Level*	Hours of Care Per Patient Day (HPPD)†	×	Patient Days‡	=	Workload§
1	3.0		900		2,700
2	5.2		3,100		16,120
3	8.8		4,000		35,200
4	13.0		1,600		20,800
5	19.0		400		7,600
Total			10,000		82,420

*1, Low; 5, high.
†HPPD is the number of hours of care on average for a given acuity level.
‡1 patient per 1 day = 1 patient day.
§Total number of hours of care needed based on acuity levels and numbers of patient days.

new treatment modalities, or changes in inpatient versus outpatient treatment practices.

The next step in preparing the personnel budget is to determine how many staff members will be needed to provide the care. (This topic is discussed in more detail in Chapter 13.) Because some people work full-time and others work part-time, **full-time equivalents (FTEs)** are used in this step rather than positions. Generally, one FTE can be equated to working 40 hours per week, 52 weeks per year, for a total of 2080 hours of work paid per year. One half of an FTE (0.5 FTE) equates to 20 hours per week. The number of hours per FTE may vary within an organization in relation to staffing plans, so it is important to check.

The 2080 hours paid to an FTE in a year consist of both **productive** and **nonproductive hours.** Productive hours are paid time that is worked. Nonproductive hours are paid time that is not worked, such as vacation, holiday, orientation, education, and sick time. Before the number of FTEs needed for the workload can be calculated, the number of productive hours per FTE is determined by subtracting the total number of nonproductive hours per FTE from total paid hours. Alternatively, payroll reports can be reviewed to determine the percentage of paid hours that are productive for each FTE. Finally, the total number of FTEs needed to provide the care is calculated by dividing the total patient care hours required by the number of productive hours per FTE (Box 11-5).

The total number of FTEs calculated by this method represents the number needed to provide care each day of the year. It does not reflect the number of positions or the number of people

working each day. In fact, the number of positions may be much higher, particularly if many part-time nurses are employed. On any given day, some nurses will be off, on vacation, or ill. Also, some positions that do not provide direct patient care, such as nurse managers or unit secretaries, may not be replaced during nonproductive time. Only one FTE is budgeted for any position that is not covered with other staff when the employee is off.

Exercise 11–12

Change the number of patients at each acuity level listed in Table 11-2, but keep the total number of patients the same. Recalculate the required total workload. Discuss how changes in patient acuity affect nursing resource requirements.

The next step is to prepare a daily staffing plan and to establish positions (see Chapter 13). Once the positions are established, the labor costs that comprise the personnel budget can be calculated. Factors that must be addressed include straight-time hours, overtime hours, differentials and premium pay, raises, and benefits (Finkler, 2001). Differentials and premiums are extra pay for working specific times, such as evening or night shifts and holidays. Benefits usually include health and life insurance, Social Security payments, and retirement plans. Benefits often cost an additional 20% to 25% of a full-time employee's salary.

Exercise 11–13

If the percentage of productive hours per FTE is 80%, how many worked or productive hours are there per FTE? If total patient care hours are 82,420, how many FTEs will be needed?

BOX 11-5

Productive Hours Calculation

Method 1:   Add all nonproductive hours/FTE and subtract from paid hours/FTE

Example:	Vacation	15 days
	Holiday	7 days
	Average sick time	4 days
	TOTAL	26 days

26 × 8* hours = 208 nonproductive hours/FTE

2080 − 208 = 1872 productive hours/FTE

Method 2:   Multiply paid hours/FTE by percentage of productive hours/FTE

Example: productive hours = 90%/FTE

(1872 productive hours of total 2080 = 90%)

2080 × 0.90 = 1872 productive hours/FTE

Total FTE Calculation

Required Patient Care Hours	÷	Productive Hours Per FTE	=	Total FTEs Needed
82,420	÷	1872	=	44 FTEs

*Based on an 8-hour shift pattern.

The supply and expense budget is often called the *other-than-personnel services (OTPS) expense budget.* This budget includes a variety of items used in daily unit activities, such as medical and office supplies, minor equipment, books and journals, orientation and training, and travel. Although different methods are used to calculate the supply and expense budget, the previous year's expenses usually are used as a baseline. This baseline is adjusted for projected patient volume and specific circumstances known to affect expenses, such as predictable personnel turnover, which increases orientation and training expenses. A percentage factor is also added to adjust for inflation.

The final component of the operating budget is the revenue budget. The revenue budget projects the income that the organization will receive for providing patient care. Historically, nurses have not been directly involved with developing the revenue budget, although this is beginning to change. In most hospitals, the revenue budget is established by the financial office and given to nurse managers. The anticipated revenues are calculated according to the price per patient day. Data about the volume and types of patients and reimbursement sources, that is, the **case mix** and the **payer mix,** are necessary to project revenues in any healthcare organization. Even when nurse managers do not participate in developing the revenue budget, learning about the organization's revenue base is essential for good decision-making.

Capital Expenditure Budget

The **capital expenditure budget** reflects expenses related to the purchase of major capital items such as equipment and physical plant. A capital expenditure must have a useful life of more than 1 year and must exceed a cost level specified by the organization. The minimum cost requirement for capital items in healthcare organizations is usually from $300 to $1000, although some organizations have a much higher level. Anything below that minimum is considered a routine operating cost.

Capital expenses are kept separate from the operating budget because their high cost would make the costs of providing patient care appear too high during the year of purchase. To account for capital expenses, the costs of capital items are depreciated. This means that each year, over the useful life of the equipment, a portion of its cost is allocated to the operating budget as an expense. Therefore, capital expenditures get subtracted from revenues and in turn affect profits.

Organizations usually set aside a fixed amount of money for capital expenditures each year. Complete well-documented justifications are needed because the competition for limited resources is stiff. Justifications should include projected amount of use; services duplicated or replaced; safety considerations; need for space, personnel, or building renovation; effect on operational revenues and expenses; and contribution to the strategic plan.

Cash Budget

The cash budget is the operating plan for monthly cash receipts and disbursements. Organizational survival depends on paying bills on time. Organizations can be making a profit and still run out of cash. In fact, a profitable trend, such as a rapidly growing census, can induce a cash shortage because of increased expenses in the short run. Major capital expenditures can also cause a temporary cash crisis and so must be staggered in a strategic way. Because cash is the lifeblood of any organization, the cash budget is as important as the operating and capital budget (Finkler, 2001).

The financial officer prepares the cash budget in large organizations. Understanding the cash budget helps nurse managers discern when constraints on spending are necessary, even when the expenditures are budgeted, and the importance of carefully predicting when budgeted items will be needed.

THE BUDGETING PROCESS

The steps in the budgeting process are similar in most healthcare organizations, although the budgeting period, budget timetable, and level of manager and employee participation vary. Budgeting is done annually and in relation to the organization's fiscal year. A fiscal year exists for financial purposes and can begin at any point on the calendar. In the title of some financial reports, a phrase similar to "FYE June 30, 2005," appears and means that this report is for the fiscal year ending on the date stated.

Major steps in the budgeting process include gathering information and planning, developing unit budgets, developing the cash budget, negotiating and revising, and using feedback to control budget results and improve future plans (Finkler,

2001). A timetable with specific dates for implementing the budgeting process is developed by each organization. The timetable may be anywhere from 3 to 9 months. The widespread use of computers for budgeting is reducing the time span for budgeting in many organizations. Box 11-6 outlines the budgeting process.

The information-gathering and planning phase provides nurse managers with data essential for developing their individual budgets. This step begins with an environmental assessment that helps the organization understand its position in relation to the entire community. The assessment includes the changing healthcare needs of the population, influential economic factors such as inflation and unemployment, differences in reimbursement patterns, patient satisfaction, and so on.

Next, the organization's long-term goals and objectives are reassessed in light of the organization's mission and the environmental analysis. This helps all managers situate the budgeting process for their individual units in relation to the whole organization. At this point, programs are prioritized so that resources can be allocated to programs that best help the organization achieve its long-term goals.

BOX 11-6

Outline of Budgeting Process

1. Gathering information and planning
   - Environmental assessment
   - Mission, goals, and objectives
   - Program priorities
   - Financial objectives
   - Assumptions (employee raises, inflation, volume projections)
2. Developing unit and departmental budgets
   - Operating budgets
   - Capital budgets
3. Developing cash budgets
4. Negotiating and revising
5. Evaluating
   - Analysis of variance
   - Critical performance reports

Modified from Finkler, S., & Kovner, C. (2000). *Financial management for nurse managers and executives* (2nd ed.). Philadelphia: Saunders.

Specific, measurable objectives are then established, and the budgets must meet these objectives. The financial objectives might include limiting expenditure increases to 3% or making 4% reductions in personnel costs. Nurse managers also set operational objectives for their units that are in concert with the rest of the organization. This is where units or departments interpret what effect the changes in operational activities will have on them. For instance, how will using case managers and care maps for selected patients affect a particular unit? Establishing the unit-level objectives is also a good place for involving staff nurses in setting the future direction of the unit.

Along with the specific organization and unit-level operating objectives, managers need the organization-wide assumptions that underpin the budgeting process. Explicit assumptions regarding salary increases, inflation factors, and volume projections for the next fiscal year are essential. With this information in hand, nurse managers can develop the operating and capital budgets for their units. These are usually developed in tandem because each affects the other. For instance, purchasing a new monitoring system will have implications for the supplies used, staffing, and staff training.

The cash budget is developed after unit and department operating and capital budgets. Then the negotiation and revision process begins in earnest. This is a complex process because changes in one budget usually require changes in others. Learning to defend and negotiate budgets is an important skill for nurse managers. Nurse managers who successfully negotiate budgets know how costs are allocated and are comfortable speaking about what resources are contained in each budget category. They also can clearly and specifically depict what the effect of not having that resource will be on patient, nurse, or organizational outcomes.

Exercise 11–14

If you can interview a nurse manager, ask to review the budgeting process. Ask specifically about the budget timetable, operating objectives, and organizational assumptions. What was the level of involvement for nurse managers and nurses in each step of budget preparation? Is there a budget manual?

The final and ongoing phase of the budgeting process relates to the control function of management. Feedback is obtained regularly so that organizational activities can be adjusted to maintain efficient operations. **Variance analysis** is the major control process used. A **variance** is the difference between the projected budget and the actual performance for a particular account. For expenses, a favorable, or positive, variance means that the budgeted amount was greater than the actual amount spent. An unfavorable, or negative, variance means that the budgeted amount was less than the actual amount spent. Positive and negative variances cannot be interpreted as good or bad without further investigation. For example, if fewer supplies were used than were budgeted, this would appear as a positive variance and the unit would save money. This would be good news if it means that supplies were used more efficiently and patient outcomes remained the same or improved. A problem might be suggested, however, if using fewer or cheaper supplies led to poorer patient outcomes. Or it might mean that exactly the right amount of supplies was used but that the patient census was less than budgeted. To help managers interpret and use variance information better, some institutions use flexible budgets that automatically account for census variances.

Exercise 11–15

Examine Table 11-3 and identify major budget variances for the current month. Are they favorable or unfavorable? What additional information would help you explain the variances? What are some possible causes for each variance? Are the causes you identified controllable by the nurse manager? Why or why not? Is a favorable variance on expenses always desirable? Why or why not?

MANAGING THE UNIT-LEVEL BUDGET

How is a unit-based budget managed? At a minimum, nurse managers are responsible for meeting the fiscal goals related to the personnel and the supply and expense part of the operations budget. Typically, monthly reports of operations (see Table 11-3) are sent to nurse managers, who then investigate and explain the underlying cause of variances greater than 5%. Many factors can cause budget variances, including patient census, patient acuity, vacation and benefit time, illness, orientation, staff meetings, workshops, employee

Table 11-3 STATEMENT OF OPERATIONS SHOWING PROFIT AND LOSS FROM A NEIGHBORHOOD NURSING CENTER: MARCH 31, 2005

Current Month			REVENUES	Year-to-Date		
Budget	Actual	Variance		Budget	Actual	Variance
Patient Revenues						
11,500	12,050	550	Insurance payment	34,500	35,750	1,250
1,500	1,550	50	Donations	4,500	4,750	250
13,000	13,600	600	Net Patient Revenues	39,000	40,500	1,500
Nonpatient Revenues						
5,000	5,000	0	Grant income (#138-FG)	15,000	15,000	0
500	500	0	Rent income	1,500	1,500	0
5,500	5,500	0	Net Nonpatient Revenues	16,500	16,500	0
18,500	19,100	600	Net Revenues	55,500	57,000	1,500
Expenses						
			Personnel			
7,750	8,500	(750)	Managerial/professional	23,250	24,400	(1,150)
2,000	1,800	200	Clerical/technical	6,000	5,800	200
9,750	10,300	(550)	Net salaries and wages	29,250	30,200	(950)
1,200	1,400	(200)	Benefits	3,600	4,000	(400)
10,950	11,700	(750)	Net Personnel	32,850	34,200	(1,350)
			Nonpersonnel			
2,500	2,500	0	Office operating expenses	7,500	7,500	0
1,000	1,100	(100)	Supplies and materials	3,000	3,050	(50)
300	450	(150)	Travel expenses	900	450	450
3,800	4,050	(250)	Net Nonpersonnel	11,400	11,000	400
14,750	15,750	(1,000)	Net Expenses	44,250	45,200	(850)
3,750	3,350	(400)	Net Income	11,250	11,800	550
Revenues Over/Under Expenses						

mix, salaries, and staffing levels. To accurately interpret budget variances, nurse managers need reliable data about patient census, acuity, and LOS; payroll reports; and unit productivity reports.

Nurse managers can control *some* of the factors that cause variances, but not all. After the causes are determined, and if they are controllable by the nurse manager, steps are taken to prevent the variance from occurring in the future. However, even uncontrollable variances that increase expenses might require actions of nurse managers. For example, if supply costs rise drastically because a new technology is being used, the nurse manager might have to look for other areas where the budget can be cut. Information learned from analyzing variances also is used in future budget preparations and management activities.

In addition, nurse managers monitor the productivity of their units. Productivity is the ratio of outputs to inputs; that is, productivity equals output/input. In nursing, outputs are nursing services and are measured by hours of care, number of home visits, and so forth. The inputs are the resources used to provide the services such as personnel hours and supplies. Only decreasing the inputs or increasing the outputs can increase productivity. Hospitals often use hours per patient day (HPPD) as one measure of productivity. For example, if the standard of care in a critical care unit is 12 HPPD, then 360 hours of care are required for 30 patients for 1 day. When 320 hours of care are provided, the productivity rating is 113% (360/320 = 1.13), meaning productivity was increased or needed care was not delivered. One must consider the quality component into any productivity model related to care. In home health, the number of visits per day per registered nurse is one measure of productivity. If the standard is 5 visits per day but the weekly average was 4.8 visits per day, then productivity was decreased. Variances in productivity are not inherently favorable or unfavorable and thus require investigation and explanation before judgments can be made about them. For example, an explanation of the variance (4.8 visits per day) might include the fact that one visit took twice the amount of time normally spent on a home visit due to patient needs, thus preventing the nurse from making the standard 5 visits per day. The extra time spent on one patient was productive time but not adequately accounted for by this measure of productivity (visits per day).

Although they do not have a direct accountability for the budget, staff nurses play an important role in meeting budget expectations. Many nurse managers find that routinely sharing the budget and budget-monitoring activities with the staff fosters an appreciation of the relationship between cost and the mission to deliver high-quality patient care. Providing staff with access to cost and utilization data allows them to identify patterns and participate in selecting appropriate, cost-effective practice options that work for the staff and patients. Managers and staff who work in partnership to understand that cost versus care is a dilemma to manage rather than a problem to solve will develop innovative, cost-conscious nursing practices that produce good outcomes for patients, nurses, and the organization.

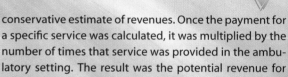

The Solution

I began by investigating the assumption that the IMC ambulatory clinic was losing money. Because expenses were reported as a whole for the IMC, they had to be broken down by section and by location where services were provided. A spreadsheet was used, and expenses were determined either by the hours of utilization or by the percentage of visit volume for that section. Once the expenses were calculated, the revenue needed to break even was determined for each section.

Next, revenues were predicted. This was challenging because of the complexity of the payer mix. The Medicare Resource-Based Relative Value Scale (RBRVS) was used to calculate all predicted payments. In this system, each physician service is assigned a "relative value" based on the time, skill, and intensity it takes to provide the service. Relative values are then adjusted for geographic variations and multiplied by a national conversion factor to determine the dollar amount of payment. This system was selected because it was the minimum payment expected for all categories of payers, including managed care contracts. Therefore, using this system provided a conservative estimate of revenues. Once the payment for a specific service was calculated, it was multiplied by the number of times that service was provided in the ambulatory setting. The result was the potential revenue for that service in that section. The potential revenues for each service were added to provide a total predicted revenue for the section.

Predicted revenue for each section was compared with the revenue required to break even. In every instance, the predicted revenue exceeded the break-even revenue. As a result of this work, the administrators changed their view of the IMC ambulatory service as a "loss leader," and staff reductions were not required. In addition, a performance strategy for physicians based on relative value units was developed, and some fees were increased because they were found to be lower than allowed by the RBRVS system.

— Robin Stoupa

 Would this be a suitable approach for you? Why?

CHAPTER CHECKLIST

Financial thinking skills are the cornerstone of cost-conscious nursing practice and are essential for all nurses. Nurses must also determine whether the services they provide add value for patients. Services that add value are of high quality, positively affect health outcomes, and minimize costs.

Understanding what constitutes profit and why organizations must make a profit to survive is basic to financial thinking. Knowing what is included in operating, capital, and cash budgets; how they interrelate; and how they are developed, monitored, and controlled is also important. Considering the ethical implications of financial decisions and collectively managing the cost-care dilemma is imperative for cost-conscious nursing practice.

- U.S. health indicators suggest that as a nation we are not getting a high value return on our healthcare dollar.
  - Infant mortality and breast cancer rates are two critical examples.
- Total healthcare costs are a function of price and utilization of services.
  - Administrative waste or inefficiency increases the price of healthcare services.
  - Our attitudes as consumers who want to be fixed, as well as healthcare insurance that buffers us from full healthcare costs, contribute to the high use of healthcare services.

- The government and insurance companies are the major payers for healthcare services. Individuals are the third major payer.
  - Payments may be based on cost reimbursement, flat rates, or capitated payments.
- Health care has moved toward managed care, organized delivery systems, and competition based on cost and quality outcomes.
- All private healthcare organizations must make a profit to survive.
- Nurses and nurse managers directly influence an organization's ability to make a profit.
- Cost-conscious nursing practices include the following:
  - Understanding what is required to remain financially sound
  - Knowing costs and reimbursement practices
  - Capturing all possible charges in a timely fashion
  - Using time efficiently
  - Discussing the costs of care with patients
  - Meeting patient, rather than provider, needs
  - Evaluating cost-effectiveness of new technologies
  - Predicting accurately and using nursing resources efficiently
  - Using research to evaluate standard nursing practices
- Nurse managers have the most influence on costs in relation to managing personnel and supplies.
- Variance analysis is the major control process in relation to budgeting.

TIPS ON MANAGING COSTS AND BUDGETS

- Know the cost and charges (if applicable) of the 20 most frequently used supplies on your unit.
- Evaluate what each of your patients would find most helpful during the time you will be caring for them.
- Decide which of your actions create costs for the patient or the organization.

- Be aware of how changes in patient acuity and patient census affect staffing requirements and the unit budget.
- Know how charges are generated and how the documentation systems relate to billing.
- Examine the upsides and downsides of the cost-care polarity thoughtfully.

TERMS TO KNOW

budget
budgeting process
capital expenditure budget
capitation
case mix
cash budget
contractual allowance
cost
cost-based reimbursement
cost center
fixed costs
full-time equivalent (FTE)
managed care
nonproductive hours

operating budget
organized delivery system (ODS)
payer mix
payers
productive hours
productivity
profit
prospective reimbursement
providers
revenue
unit of service
utilization
variable costs
variance
variance analysis

REFERENCES

Bodenheimer, T., & Grumbach, K. (2005). *Understanding health policy: A clinical approach* (4th ed.). New York: McGraw-Hill.

Finkler, S. A. (2001). *Budgeting concepts for nurse managers* (3rd, ed.). Philadelphia: Saunders.

Finkler, S., & Kovner, C. (2000). *Financial management for nurse managers and executives* (2nd ed.). Philadelphia: Saunders.

Healthy People 2010. Retrieved August 18, 2005, from www.health.gov/HEALTHYPEOPLE/document/.

Heffler, S., Smith, S., Keehan, S., Clemens, M. K., Zezza, M., & Truffer, C. (2004). Health spending projections through 2013. *Health Affairs*, suppl Web exclusives, W4, 79-93.

Medical Expenditure Panel Survey. Retrieved August 18, 2005, from www.meps.ahrq.gov/MEPSDATA/projected/mepsdata.htm.

Zelman, W., McCue, M. J., Millikan, A. R., & Glick, N. D. (2003). *Financial management of health care organizations: An introduction to fundamental tools, concepts, & applications.* Malden, MA: Blackwell.

SUGGESTED READINGS

Allen, V. M., O'Connell, C. M., Farrell, S. A., & Baskett, T. F. (2005). Economic implications of method of delivery. *American Journal of Obstetrics & Gynecology*, (193), 192-197.

Chang, C., Price, S., & Pfoutz, S. (2001). *Economics and nursing: Critical professional issues.* Philadelphia: F.A. Davis.

Chu, H., Liu, S., & Romeis, J. C. (2004). Does capitated contracting improve efficiency? Evidence from California hospitals. *Health Care Management Review*, 29(4), 344-352.

Contino, D. S. (2004). What's your project's ROI? *Nursing Management*, 35(2), 39-40.

Donaldson, N., Brown, D. S., Aydin, C. E., Bolton, M. L. B., & Rutledge, D. N. (2005). Leveraging nurse-related dashboard benchmarks to expedite performance improvement and document excellence. *Journal of Nursing Administration*, 35(4), 163-172.

Feldstein, P. (2004). *Health care economics* (6th ed.). Clifton Park, NY: Thomson Delmar Learning.

Finkler, S. A. & Ward, D. M. (1999). *Essential of cost accounting for health care organizations* (2nd ed.). New York: Aspen Publishers.

Haase-Herrick, K. S. (2005). The opportunities of stewardship. *Nursing Administration Quarterly*, 29(2), 115-118.

Huber, D. (2000). *Leadership & nursing care management.* Philadelphia: W.B. Saunders.

Inman, R. R., Blumenfeld, D. E., & Ko, A. (2005). Cross-training hospital nurses to reduce staffing costs. *Health Care Management Review*, 39(2), 116-125.

Johnson, B. (1996). *Polarity management: Identifying and managing unsolvable problems.* Amherst, MA: HRD Press.

Jones, D. (2003). Savings sharing: Rewarding staff for responsible decision-making. *Journal of Nursing Administration*, 35(4), 199-204.

Kirkby, M. P. (2003). Number crunching with variable budgets. *Nursing Management*, 34(3), 28-33.

Koelling, T. M., Johnson, M. L., Cody, R. J., & Aaronson, K. D. (2005). Discharge education improves clinical outcomes in patients with chronic heart failure. *Circulation*, 111, 179-185.

Kramer, M., & Schmalenberg, C. (2005). Revising the Essentials of Magnetism Tool: There is more to adequate staffing than numbers. *Journal of Nursing Administration*, 35(4), 188-198.

Lagoe, R. J., Westert, G. P., Kendrick, K., Morreale, G. & Mnich, S. (2005). Managing hospital length of stay reduction: A multihospital approach. *Health Care Management Review*, 30(2), 82-92.

Longest, Jr., B. B., & Lin, C. J. (2005). Can nonprofit hospitals do both well and good? *Health Care Management Review*, 30(1), 62-68.

Pilette, P. C. (2005). Presenteeism in nursing: A clear and present danger to productivity. *Journal of Nursing Administration*, 35(6), 300-303.

Revere, L., Large, J., & Langland-Orban, B. (2004). A comparison of inpatient severity, average length of stay, and cost for traditional fee-for-service Medicare and Medicare HMOs in Florida. *Health Care Management Review*, 29(4), 320-328.

Rosko, M. D., & Proenca, J. (2005). Impact of network and system use on hospital X-inefficiency. *Health Care Management Review*, 30(1), 69-79.

Shi, L., & Singh, D. (2004). Delivering health care in America: A systems approach (3rd ed.). Boston, MA: Jones & Bartlett Publishers.

Sultz, H., & Young, K. (2003). Health care USA: Understanding its organization (4th ed.). Boston, MA: Jones & Bartlett Publishers.

Vonderheid, S., Pohl, J., Schafer, P., Forrest, K., Poole, M., Barkauskas, V., & Mackey, T. A. (2004). Using FTE and RVU performance measures to assess financial viability of academic nurse-managed centers. *Nursing Economics*, 22(3), 124-134.

Ward, W. (1988). *An introduction to health care financial management*. Ownings, MD: National Health Publishing.

Wesorick, B., Shiparski, L., Troseth, M., & Wyngarden, K. (1997). *Partnership council field book: Strategies and tools for co-creating a healthy work place*. Grand Rapids, MI: Practice Field Publishing.

White, K. R., Bazzoli, G. J., Roggenkamp, S. D., & Gu, T. (2005). Does case management matter as a hospital cost-control strategy? *Health Care Management Review*, 30(1), 32-43.

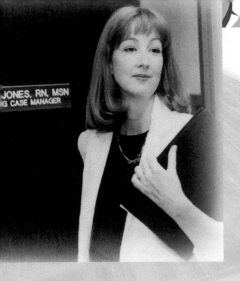

Chapter 12

Care Delivery Strategies

Karen A. Dadich

This chapter introduces models for nursing care delivery that are currently in use in healthcare agencies. The historical development of the case method, functional nursing, team nursing, primary nursing, and nurse case management is presented. Patient-focused care, disease management, and differentiated practice are also discussed. Each model is defined and discussed. The discussion summarizes the benefits and disadvantages of the model with an explanation of the nurse manager's and staff nurse's role.

Objectives

- Differentiate the characteristics of five care delivery models used in health care.
- Determine the role of the nurse manager and the staff nurse in each model.
- Describe the implementation of a disease-management program.
- Summarize the differentiated nursing practice model.

Questions to Consider

- *Which model of nursing care delivery would you select to implement? Why?*
- *How does your level of nursing education affect the care you provide?*
- *What are the satisfiers for the nurse manager in each care delivery model?*
- *How does the staff nurse influence the implementation of each care delivery model?*
- *How do reimbursement strategies impact the selection of a care-delivery model?*

The Challenge

Jacqueline Ward, RN, BSN
Assistant Director of Nursing, Texas Children's Hospital, Houston, Texas

As an Assistant Director of Nursing, on a newly designed 36-bed Hematology-Oncology Unit, I began to observe the Charge Nurses having increased difficulty in making patient assignments because of the layout and design of this new 36,000-square-foot unit. Other problems were also apparent. Throughout the shift, the nursing staff were having difficulty remaining engaged with the activities on the unit because of the distance between bedside stations. In addition, the layout of the unit made it difficult for a nurse to request help when needed.

After occupying the unit for several months and trying diverse methods to enhance teamwork and communication among the staff, it was apparent that there needed to be a more formal process in place to resolve these problems.

 What do you think you would do if you were this nurse?

INTRODUCTION

A **nursing care delivery model** is the method used to provide care to patients. Because nursing care is viewed by some as a cost rather than a source of revenue, it is logical for institutions to evaluate their method of providing patient care for the purpose of saving money while still providing quality care. In this chapter, five models of nursing care delivery are discussed: **case method, functional nursing, team nursing, primary nursing,** and nurse **case management.** The influence of **disease-management programs** and **patient-focused care** is introduced. The effect **differentiated practice** has on care delivery is described. Finally, emerging models of professional practice are presented.

Each nursing care delivery model has advantages and disadvantages, and none is ideal. Some methods are conducive to large institutions, whereas other systems may work best in smaller community settings. Managers in any organization must examine the organizational goals, the unit objectives, patient population, staff availability, and the budget when selecting a care-delivery model.

CASE METHOD

The case method, or **total patient care** method, of nursing-care delivery is the oldest method of providing care to a patient. This model should not be confused with nurse case management, which is introduced later in the chapter.

The premise of the case method is that one nurse provides total care for one patient during the entire work period. This method was used in the era of Florence Nightingale when patients received total care in the home. Care also included meeting the needs of the whole family, including cooking and cleaning (Nelson, 2000). Total patient care is used in critical care settings where one nurse provides total care to a small group of critically ill patients. Nurse educators often select this method of care when students are caring for patients.

Model Analysis

During an 8- or 12-hour shift, the patient receives consistent care from one nurse. The nurse, patient, and family share mutual trust and can work together toward specific goals. Usually, the care is patient-centered; comprehensive, continuous, and holistic. But the nurse may choose to deliver this care with a task orientation that negates the holistic perspective (Tiedeman & Lookinland, 2004). Changes in the patient's status are apparent to the nurse during the shift (Figure 12-1).

In today's costly healthcare economy, total patient care provided by a registered nurse (RN) is very expensive. The efficacy of this care delivery model is questionable. Is it realistic to use the highly skilled and extremely knowledgeable professional nurse to provide all the care required? Who over-

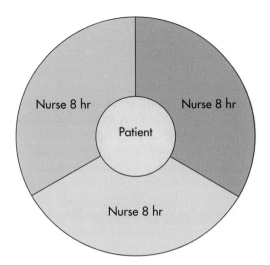

Figure 12-1 Case method of patient care for an 8-hour shift.

sees the care coordination in a 24-hour period (Tiedeman & Lookinland, 2004)? In times of managed care and nursing shortages, there may not be enough resources or nurses to use this model.

Total patient care is used in critical-care settings where one nurse provides total care to one or two critically ill patients. In the home setting, nursing care is supplemented by family members and home health aides in an effort to reduce the expense. In these settings, the RN becomes the coordinator of the care. Variations of the case method exist, and it is possible to identify similarities after reviewing other methods of patient-care delivery described later in this chapter.

Nurse Manager's Role

When using the case method of delivery, the manager must consider the expense of the system. The manager must weigh the expense of an RN versus the expense of licensed practical (vocational) nurses (LPNs/LVNs) and **unlicensed assistive (or nursing) personnel.** Unlicensed assistive personnel, as the name connotes, are not licensed as healthcare providers. They are technicians, nurse aides, and certified nursing assistants. The patient may require 24-hour care; however, the manager must decide whether the patient needs to have RN care or RN-supervised care provided by LPNs/LVNs or unlicensed personnel. To provide cost-effective care to patients, the staff must have adequate skills to provide total care.

The manager also needs to identify the level of education and communication skills of all staff. RNs must be educated in communicating and co-ordinating care, as well as supervising other staff members. LPNs/LVNs and unlicensed personnel also need continuing education to provide total care according to their level of practice.

Staff Nurse's Role

The staff nurse provides holistic care to a group of patients during a defined work time. The physical, emotional, and technical aspects of care are the responsibility of the assigned nurse. Some nurses thrive on this care delivery model, whereas others wish to delegate simpler, less complex aspects of care to assistive personnel. This care delivery model requires the total patient care nurse to complete the complex functions of care, such as assessment and teaching the patient and family, as well as the less complex functional aspects of care. Some nurses find satisfaction with this model of care because no aspect of nursing care is delegated to another, thus eliminating the need for supervision of others (Tiedeman & Lookinland, 2004). This model is especially useful in the care of complex patients who need active symptom management provided by an RN, such as the care of the client in a hospice setting.

Exercise 12-1

You have recently accepted a position at a home health agency that provides 24-hour care to qualified patients. You are assigned a patient who has 24-hour care provided by an RN during the day, an LPN/LVN in the evening, and a nursing assistant at night. You are concerned that the patient is not progressing well, and you suspect the evening and night shift personnel are not reporting changes in the patient's status. You want to change the situation. How would you justify any change in staffing? What recommendations would you make to the nurse manager, and why?

FUNCTIONAL NURSING

The functional model of nursing-care delivery became popular during World War II when there was a severe shortage of nurses in the United States. Many nurses entered the military to care for the soldiers. To provide care to patients at home, hospitals began to increase the number of LPNs/LVNs and unlicensed assistive personnel.

Functional nursing is a method of providing patient care by which each licensed and unlicensed staff member performs specific tasks for a large group of patients. For example, the RN may administer all intravenous (IV) medications and do admissions, one LPN/LVN may provide treatments, another LPN/LVN may give all oral medications, one assistant may do all hygiene tasks, and another assistant may take all vital signs (Figure 12-2). This division of aspects of care is similar to the assembly line system used by manufacturing industries. Just as an auto worker becomes an expert in attaching fenders to a new vehicle, the RN becomes expert in the tasks expected in functional nursing. A **charge nurse** coordinates care and assignments and may ultimately be the only person familiar with all the needs of any individual patient.

Model Analysis

There are several advantages to this model of patient-care delivery. First, each person becomes very efficient at specific tasks, and a great amount of work can be done in a short time. Another advantage is that unskilled workers can be trained to perform one or two specific tasks very well. The organization benefits financially from this model because care can be delivered to a large number of patients by mixing staff with a fixed number of RNs and a larger number of unlicensed assistive personnel. For example, a busy orthopedic unit may use the RN to do the patient assessments, the

LVN/LPN to do the dressing changes, nurse aides to complete the bed baths, and physical therapy aides to do the ambulation.

Although financial savings may be the impetus for organizations to choose the functional system of delivering care, the disadvantages may outweigh the savings (Figure 12-3). A major disadvantage is the fragmentation of care. The physical and technical aspects of care may be met, but the psychological and spiritual needs may be overlooked. Patients become confused with so many different care providers per shift. These different staff may be so busy with their assigned tasks that they do not have time to communicate with each other about the patient's progress. Because no one care provider sees patient care from beginning to end, evaluation of the patient's response to care is difficult to assess. Critical changes in patient status may go unnoticed. Fragmented care and ineffective communication can lead to patient and family dissatisfaction and frustration. Exercise 12-2 provides an opportunity to imagine how a patient would react to the functional method and also to imagine how the nurse may feel.

Exercise 12-2

Imagine your mother is a patient at a hospital that uses the functional model of patient-care delivery. She just had her knee replaced, and when you ask the nursing assistant for something for pain she says, "I'll tell the medication nurse." The medication nurse comes to your room and says that your mother's medication is to be administered intrave-

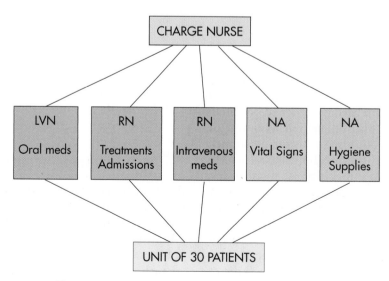

Figure 12-2 Functional method of nursing care delivery.

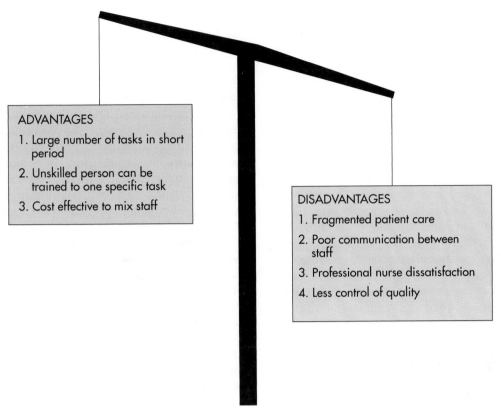

Figure 12-3   Advantages and disadvantages of functional nursing.

nously and the IV nurse will need to administer it. The IV nurse is busy starting an IV on another patient and will not be able to give your mother the medication for at least 10 minutes. This whole communication process has taken 40 minutes, and your mother is still in pain. Discuss your perception of the effectiveness of the functional method of patient care in this situation. How effective do you think communication among staff is when a patient has a problem? What could be done to improve this situation?

Nurse Manager's Role

In the functional nursing method, the nurse manager must be sensitive to the quality of patient care delivered and the institution's budgetary constraints. Because staff members are responsible only for their specific task, the role of achieving **patient outcomes** becomes the nurse manager's responsibility. Staff members can view this system as autocratic and may become discontented with the lack of opportunity for input.

By using effective management and leadership skills, the nurse manager can improve the staff's perception of their lack of independence. The manager can rotate assignments among staff within legal and organizational contexts to alleviate boredom with repetition. Staff meetings should be conducted frequently. This encourages staff to express concerns and empowers them with the ability to communicate about patient care and unit functions.

Staff Nurse's Role

The staff nurse becomes skilled at the tasks that are usually assigned by the charge nurse. Clearly defined policies and procedures are used to complete the physical aspects of care in an efficient and economical manner. However, the functional method leaves the professional nurse feeling frustrated because of the task-oriented role. Nurses are educated to care for the patient holistically, and providing only a fragment of care to a patient results in unmet personal and professional expectations of nurses.

■ *Exercise 12–3*

After 6 months of working on a unit that accommodates patients who have had general surgery, you realize that you are bored and frustrated with the functional model of care delivery. You have been doing all the IV medications and the administration of pain meds for your assigned patients. You have minimal opportunity to interact with the patients and learn about them, and you are unable to be innovative in your care. Discuss strategies you could use to resolve this dissatisfaction with functional nursing-care delivery.

The functional method of care delivery works well in emergency and disaster situations. Each care provider knows the expectations of the assigned role and completes the tasks in a quick and efficient style. Subacute care agencies, extended care facilities, and ambulatory clinics often use the functional model of care delivery. Severe budgetary cuts, reimbursement mechanisms, and nursing shortages have resulted in organizations changing the **staff mix** and increasing the proportion of unlicensed to licensed personnel. A modification of functional nursing is team nursing.

TEAM NURSING

After World War II, the nursing shortage continued. Many nurses who were in the military came home to marry and have children instead of returning to the workforce. Because the functional model received criticism, a new system of team nursing was devised to improve patient satisfaction. "Care through others" became the hallmark of team nursing.

In team nursing, a team leader is responsible for coordinating a group of licensed and unlicensed personnel to provide patient care to a small group of patients. The team leader is a highly skilled leader, manager, and practitioner, who assigns each member specific responsibilities according to role, licensure, education, ability, and the complexity of the care required.

The members of the team report directly to the team leader, who then reports to the charge nurse or unit manager (Figure 12-4). There are several teams per unit, and patient assignments are made by each team leader. Communication is enhanced through the use of written patient assignments, the development of nursing care plans, and the use of regularly scheduled team conferences to discuss patient status and formulate revisions to the plan of care.

Model Analysis

Some advantages of the team method are improved patient satisfaction, organizational decision-making

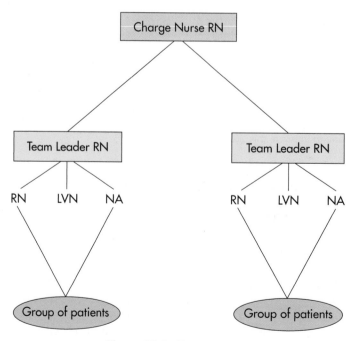

Figure 12-4　Team nursing.

occurring at lower levels, and cost effectiveness for the agency. Many institutions and community health agencies currently use the team nursing method.

Inpatient facilities may view team nursing as a cost-effective system because it works with an expected ratio of unlicensed to licensed personnel. Thus, the organization has greater numbers of personnel for a designated amount of money.

The team method of patient care delivery is a good system, if implemented properly; however, one major disadvantage arises if the team leader has poor leadership skills. The team leader must have excellent communication skills, delegation abilities, conflict resolution techniques, strong clinical skills, and effective decision-making abilities to provide a working "team" environment for the members. The team leader must be sensitive to the needs of the patient and at the same time, attentive to the needs of the staff providing the direct care (Moore, 2004). Often, the team leader is not prepared for this role, and the team method becomes a miniature version of the functional method, and the potential for fragmentation of care is high.

In times of nursing shortage, the lack of registered nurses (RNs) providing direct care impacts the quality of the care delivered (Aiken, Clarke, Sloane, Sochalski, & Silber, 2002). It is not uncommon to learn of the frustration nurses experience in this circumstance. Wishing to provide the care themselves is often an idea expressed by the RN in a short-staffed team setting (Moore, 2004). Instead, one must rely on those who are functioning with a task orientation to complete the essential elements of care.

■ *Exercise 12–4*

Think of a time when you worked with a group of four to six people to achieve a specific goal or accomplish a task (perhaps in school you were grouped together to complete a project). How did your group achieve the goal? Was one person the organizer or leader? How was the leader selected? Who assigned each member a component; or, did you each determine what skills you possessed that would most benefit the group? Did you experience any conflict while working on this project? How did the concepts of group dynamics and leadership skills affect how your group achieved its goal? What similarities do you see between the team nursing system of providing patient care and your group involvement to achieve a goal?

Nurse Manager's Role

The nurse manager, charge nurse, and team leaders must have management skills to effectively implement the team nursing method of patient-care delivery. The unit manager must determine which RNs are skilled and who is interested in becoming a charge nurse or team leader. Because the basic education of baccalaureate-prepared RNs emphasizes critical thinking and leadership concepts, they are likely candidates for such roles. The nurse manager should also provide an adequate staff mix and orient team members to the team nursing system by providing continuing education about leadership, management techniques, delegation, and team interaction (see Chapters 1, 2, 3, 17, and 23). By addressing these factors, the manager is aiding the teams to function optimally. Managing other staff members' care is viewed as a way of maintaining clinical competence (Nelson, 2000). Do you agree?

The charge nurse functions as a liaison between the team leaders and other healthcare providers. Some charge nurses have a difficult time relinquishing authority; however, the charge nurse needs to encourage each team to solve its problems independently.

The team leader plans the care, delegates the work, and follows up with members to evaluate the quality of care. In the ideal circumstance, the team leader updates the nursing care plans and facilitates patient care conferences. Time constraints during the shift may prevent scheduling daily patient care conferences or all team members may not be able to attend those that are held.

The team leader must also face the challenge of changing team membership. Diverse work schedules and nursing staff shortages may result in daily changes in the staff mix of a team and a daily assignment change for team members. The team leader assigns the professional, technical, and ancillary personnel to the type of patient care they are prepared to deliver. Therefore, the team leader must be knowledgeable about the legal and organizational limits of each role.

Staff Nurse's Role

Team nursing uses the strengths of each caregiver. The staff nurses, as members of the team, develop expertise in care delivery. Some members become known for their expertise in the psychomotor aspects of care. If one nurse is skilled at starting IVs, she will start all IVs for her team of patients. If a nurse is especially skillful in motivating postoperative patients to use the incentive spirometer and ambulate, he or she should be assigned to the surgical patients. The increasing complexity of the care of patients requires well-educated nurses who can critically solve complex and dynamic aspects of care. As a member of a group, each person strives to give the best care possible. Under the guidance and supervision of the team leader, the collective efforts of the team become greater than the functions of the individual caregiver.

Team Nursing Hybrid: Modular Nursing

A modification to team nursing is the modular method of patient-care delivery. The modular method focuses on the geographic location of patient rooms and assignment of staff members (Magargal, 1987). The unit is divided into modules, or districts, and the same team of staff is assigned consistently to the module. Each module has a modular, or team, leader RN who assigns the patients to module staff. Each module ideally consists of at least one RN, one LPN/LVN, and one nursing assistant. The charge nurse expects the module leaders to be accountable for patient care but assists in problem-solving when necessary.

Bennett and Hylton (1990) found increased continuity of care when staff was consistently assigned to the same module, and the geographic closeness of the modular system saved nursing time. The modular system can also cost money because it requires a redesign of the work environment to allow medication carts, supplies, and charts to be located in each module. Additionally, traditional long corridors are not conducive to **modular nursing.**

In the late 1960s, nursing care delivery methods were once again re-evaluated. Since RNs were educated to provide holistic care to patients, the primary nursing model evolved to provide increased autonomy for nurses.

▮ PRIMARY NURSING

A cultural revolution occurred in the United States during the 1960s. The revolution emphasized individual rights and independence from existing societal restrictions. This revolution also influenced the nursing profession because nurses were becoming dissatisfied with their lack of autonomy. In addition, the hierarchical nature of communication in team nursing caused further frustration. Institutions were also aware of the declining quality of patient care. The search for autonomy and quality care led to the primary nursing system of patient care delivery as a method to increase RN accountability for patient outcomes.

Primary nursing, an adaptation of the case method, was developed by Marie Manthey as a method for organizing patient care delivery in which one RN functions autonomously as the patient's **primary nurse** throughout the hospital stay (Manthey, Ciske, Robertson, & Harris, 1970).

Primary nursing brought the nurse back to direct patient care (Nelson, 2000). The primary nurse assumes 24-hour-a-day total patient care from admission through discharge. Conceptually, primary nursing care provides the patient and the family with coordinated, comprehensive, continuous care (Tiedeman & Lookinland, 2004). Care is organized to use the nursing process. The primary nurse collaborates, communicates, and coordinates all aspects of patient care with other nurses as well as other disciplines (Tiedeman & Lookinland, 2004). Advocacy and assertiveness are desirable leadership attributes for this care-delivery model.

The primary nurse, preferably baccalaureate-prepared, is held accountable for meeting **outcome criteria** and communicating with all other healthcare providers about the patient (Figure 12-5). For example, a patient is admitted to a medical unit with pulmonary edema. His primary nurse admits him and then provides a written plan of care. When his primary nurse is not working, an **associate nurse** implements the plan. The associate nurse is an RN who has been delegated to provide care to the patient according to the primary nurse's specification. If the patient develops additional complications, the associate nurse notifies the primary nurse, who has 24-hour accountability and responsibility. The associate nurse provides input to the patient's plan of care, and the primary nurse makes the appropriate alterations.

Model Analysis

Tiedeman and Lookinland (2004) cite numerous works that speak to the quality of care and patient satisfaction with primary care. Some studies cited

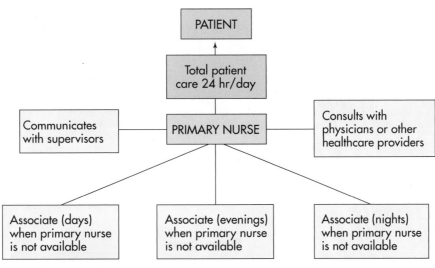

Figure 12-5 Primary nursing.

in their work speak to increased quality of care and patient satisfaction whereas others find no difference in these parameters when compared to team nursing.

Because of a decreased number of nonprofessional staff, healthcare agency costs are potentially reduced. Tiedeman and Lookinland (2004) state that lower costs for personnel are related to specific diagnosis-related groups.

RNs practicing primary nursing must possess a broad knowledge base and have highly developed nursing skills. In this system of care delivery, professionalism is promoted. Nurses experience job satisfaction because they are able to use their education to provide holistic and autonomous care for the patient. This high level of accountability for patient outcomes encourages RNs to further their knowledge and refine skills to provide optimal patient care. If the primary nurse is not motivated or feels unqualified to provide holistic care, job satisfaction may decrease.

In primary nursing, patients and families are satisfied with the care they receive because they establish a relationship with the primary nurse and identify the caregiver as "their nurse." Because the patient's primary nurse communicates the plan of care, the patient can move away from the sick role and begin to participate in his or her own recovery. By considering the sociocultural, psychological, and physical needs of the patient and family, the primary nurse can plan the most appropriate care with and for the patient and family.

A professional advantage to the primary nursing method is a decrease in the number of unlicensed personnel. The ideal primary nursing system requires an all-RN staff. The RN can provide total care to the patient, from bed baths to patient education, even both at the same time! Unlicensed personnel are not qualified to provide this level of inclusive care (Figure 12-6). The literature exposes the disagreements among authors about the appropriateness of LPN/LVNs as primary or associate nurses (Tiedeman & Lookinland, 2004).

A disadvantage of the primary nursing method is that the RN may not have the experience or educational background to provide total care. The agency needs to educate staff for an adequate transition from the previous role to the primary role. In addition, one has to ask whether the RN is ready and willing and capable of handling the 24-hour responsibility for patient care. In addition, the nursing practice acts must be evaluated to determine whether the primary nurse can be held accountable when she or he is off-duty.

In times of nursing shortage, primary nursing may not be the model of choice (Jonsdottir, 1999). This model will not be effective with a large number of part-time RNs who are not available to assume the primary nurse role.

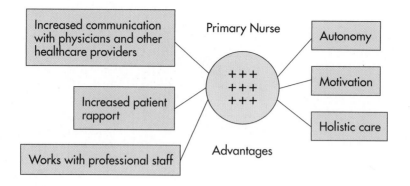

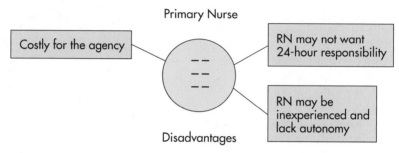

Figure 12-6   Advantages and disadvantages of primary nursing.

Exercise 12–5

Mr. Faulkner is admitted to the medical unit with exacerbated congestive heart failure. Mike Ross, RN, BSN, is Mr. Faulkner's primary nurse and will provide total care to Mr. Faulkner. Mike notes that this is Mr. Faulkner's third admission in 6 months for congestive heart failure–related symptoms. This is the first admission for which Mr. Faulkner has had a primary nurse. What do you think will be different about this admission with Mike providing primary nursing to Mr. Faulkner? Do you think there will be any difference in continuity of care? How involved do you think Mr. Faulkner will be with his own care in the primary nursing system?

With the arrival of managed care, patients' hospital stays are shorter than in the 1970s, when primary nursing became popular. Expedited stays make it challenging for primary nurses to adequately provide primary nursing. If the patient is admitted on Monday and discharged on Wednesday, the primary nurse has a difficult time meeting all patient needs before discharge if he or she is not working on Tuesday. The primary nurse must rely heavily on feedback from associates, which defeats the purpose of primary nursing.

Exercise 12–6

Imagine you are a primary nurse at an inpatient psychiatric facility. The patients you are assigned to are usually suicidal. How would you feel about the added responsibility for patients even when you were not at work? Is it realistic to expect the nurse to assume the role of the primary nurse with 24-hour responsibility? How would this responsibility affect your personal life? How would you make decisions about the patients and your home life?

Nurse Manager's Role

The primary nursing system can be modified to meet patient, nursing, and budgetary demands while maintaining the positive components that spawned its conception. The nurse manager needs to determine the desire of staff to become primary nurses and then educate them accordingly. The associate nurses and all other healthcare providers need clearly defined roles. They also need to be aware of the primary nurse's role and the importance of communicating concerns directly to that nurse.

The nurse manager who implements this care delivery model experiences some benefits. Primary nursing provides the nurse manager an opportunity to demonstrate leadership capabilities, clinical competencies, and teaching abilities to serve as a role model for professional practice. In addition, the role of budget controller and unit quality manager remain. The traditional roles of delegation and decision-making must be relinquished to the autonomous primary nurse. The nurse manager functions as a role model, advocate, coach, and consultant.

Staff Nurse's Role

The primary nurse uses many facets of the professional role—caregiver, advocate, decision-maker, teacher, collaborator, and manager. With 24-hour responsibility, the primary nurse has the autonomy and authority to deliver individualized, comprehensive, consistent care that is patient-focused (Johnson & Tahan, 1997). The associate nurse provides care using the plan of care developed by the primary nurse. Changes to the plan of care can be made by the associate nurse in collaboration with the primary nurse. This model provides consistency between nurses and shifts. To function effectively in this setting, staff nurses will need experience and opportunities to be mentored in this role.

Because it is not usually financially possible for an agency to employ only RNs, true primary nursing rarely exists. Some institutions have modified the primary nursing concept and implemented a **partnership model** to incorporate their current staff mix.

Primary Nursing Hybrid: Partnership Model

In the partnership model (or co-primary nursing model) of providing patient care, an RN is paired with a technical assistant. The partner works with the RN consistently. When the partner is unlicensed, the RN allows the assistant to perform basic nursing functions. This frees the RN to provide "semi-primary care" to assigned patients. Rehabilitative care settings may use the partnership model. A partnership between an RN and an LPN/ LVN is different. The RN's role is to encourage growth in the LPN/LVN partner, and the two share the patient assignments. In some settings, the partnership is legitimized with an official contract to formalize the relationship.

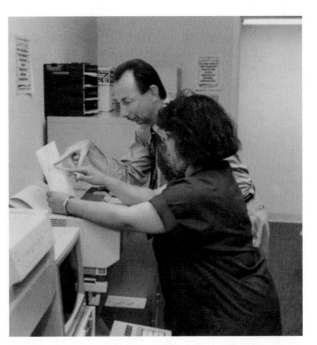

In the partnership model, the RN encourages the LPN/LVN partner's growth and the two share patient assignments.

Exercise 12–7

You are a primary nurse in a surgical intensive care unit of a small hospital. The unit you work on uses an RN-LPN/LVN partnership to decrease the number of RNs required per shift. You and your partner are assigned four surgical patients. Mr. Jones had a lobectomy 5 hours ago and is on a ventilator; Mrs. Martinez had a quadruple cardiac bypass 14 hours ago; Mr. Wong had a nephrectomy 2 days ago and is receiving continuous peritoneal dialysis; and Mr. Smith has a fractured pelvis and is comatose from a motor vehicle accident 24 hours ago. How would you distribute the staff to provide primary care to these four patients? Do you think it is possible to provide primary care in this situation? What responsibilities would you assume as the primary nurse, and what could you share with the LPN/LVN?

Primary Nursing Hybrid: Patient-Focused Care

Another view of primary care is the care delivered in a **patient-focused care** unit. The primary nurse in this model facilitates continuity of care; enhances collaboration with the patient, family, and interdisciplinary team; and controls practice through autonomous decisions (Johnson & Tahan, 1997). The multidisciplinary team formulates the plan of care after the primary nurse and the physician have assessed the patient.

Developed in the late 1980s, the patient-focused care model integrates principles from business and industry to decrease inefficiencies and create a plan that improves the quality of care, enhances patient and staff satisfaction, and reduces the cost of providing quality care. This model features decentralized, streamlined, and localized care (Graham, 2003).

Like modular nursing, discussed earlier, the patient-focused care unit requires a change in the physical environment. Services required by patients are decentralized. Satellite laboratories, radiology facilities, pharmacies, and supply rooms are geographically proximate to the patient rooms (Seago, 1999).

Original models of a patient-focused care unit included an RN paired with a cross-trained technician who provided patient-side care, including respiratory therapy, phlebotomy, and electrocardiographs. Modifications in this nurse-managed model include team members who provide direct care activities such as recording vital signs, drawing blood, and bathing patients.

In a patient-focused care unit, the role and scope of the nurse manager expand. No longer is the individual just a manager of nurses. Now the nurse manager assumes the accountability and responsibility to manage nurses and staff from other, traditionally centralized departments. Because the care is focused on the needs of the patient and not the needs of the department, the role of the manager becomes more sophisticated. The nurse manager orchestrates all the care activities required by the patient and family during the hospitalization. Implementing this philosophy and model of care requires new learning about one's beliefs, attitudes, and practices toward care (Graham, 2003). Another nursing-care delivery model that requires a complex set of expectations is the process of nursing case management.

NURSING CASE MANAGEMENT

Developed in 1985 as an outgrowth of primary care, **nursing case management** is a model used to coordinate care, maintain quality, and contain costs while focusing on the outcomes of care (Cohen & Cesta, 2001). Nursing case management is a collaborative activity that focuses on comprehensive assessment and intervention and holistic care planning with appropriate referrals to meet the healthcare needs of the patient and the family (Figure 12-7).

"Within the walls," or internal, nursing case management coordinates care in the acute care setting. "Beyond the walls," or external, case management, originally developed in the 1970s by insurance companies in an attempt to control extremely expensive claims, is used by community agencies, outpatient settings, and health maintenance organizations.

The success of nursing case management models has been demonstrated in all healthcare settings, including acute, subacute, and ambulatory settings; long-term care facilities; and health insurance companies and the community. Table 12-1 identifies

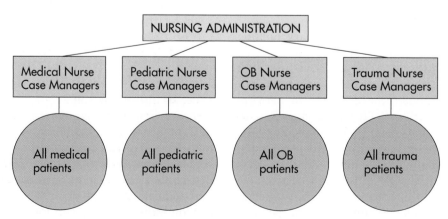

Figure 12-7   Nurse case management model in which all patients are assigned to a nurse case manager.

some of the service settings using this care-delivery model. The Research Perspective describes the process of implementing the case management model in a new setting.

The case management model of patient care delivery maintains quality care while streamlining costs and seeks the active involvement of the patient, the family, and diverse healthcare professionals. Healthcare organizations have tailored the case-management system to meet their specific needs. The elements of the **case-management model** are the **case manager** and the **critical pathway.**

Nurse Case Manager

Although there is inconsistency among professional standards about the education for case managers, many case-management services prefer master's-prepared clinical nurse specialists who have advanced preparation with the specific populations being served. The case manager is client-focused and outcome-oriented. The goal is to provide cost-effective care through integration of clinical services in combination with financial services. In addition, the nurse case manager (NCM) serves as an advocate for the patient and the family.

Depending on the facility, there may be several case managers to coordinate care for all patients, or a case manager may be assigned to a specific high-risk population (see Figure 12-7). The case manager may be responsible for coordinating care for 20 patients. It is essential that the case manager has frequent interaction with the patient and the healthcare provider to achieve and evaluate **expected outcomes.**

In organizations that use this process, the NCM is assigned a patient on admission (or pre-admission) based on the case manager's specialization. The NCM then coordinates patient care until discharge. The patient will have a specific **care MAP** (multidisciplinary action plan), or a critical path, based on an appropriate diagnosis-related group (DRG) category. The case manager will implement the plan and be responsible for monitoring patient progress toward the desired outcome criteria. This progress is communicated to the physicians, nurses, and other healthcare providers. All healthcare providers work together to decrease the patient's length of stay while addressing patient problems.

Example:
Imagine you are the NCM responsible for pediatric patients. Margo, age 3, is admitted to the emergency department (ED) with severe shortness of breath and a history of asthma. You introduce yourself to Margo and her mother as the case manager responsible for coordinating Margo's care throughout her hospital stay. You implement the care MAP used at your hospital and plan her care with the ED nurse and physician. After 2 hours, Margo is transferred to the pediatric intensive care unit (ICU). The ICU nurses follow the care MAP, identifying patient problems and the normal tests and treatments expected on day 1 (Box 12-1). On day 3, Margo is transferred to the pediatric floor, where you will coordinate her care with her mother, the nurse, and the physician. The nurses follow the care MAP you initiated and discuss any variations with you. When Margo is ready for discharge on day 4, you talk with her mother and arrange a follow-up phone call. You have been the pivotal person for Margo and her mother throughout this admission. Your main goal is to expedite Margo's hospitalization and prevent a readmission. If Margo is readmitted, you will be her NCM.

CRITICAL PATHWAYS AND CARE MAPS

The tool case managers use to achieve patient outcomes is a critical path. Critical paths are grids that outline the critical or key events expected to happen each day of a patient's hospitalization (Cohen & Cesta, 2001). The critical path component is based on the DRG services provided by all disciplines for the patient's particular DRG classification. Box 12-1 lists the various components of a critical path.

Care MAPs are a combination of the nursing care plan and the critical path. The care plan component is similar to the care plans typically used, except a time is indicated for each intervention of the nursing diagnosis. (See the example in Box 12-1.) The primary reason to implement a care MAP is to provide a written system for identifying patient and family needs. All healthcare providers follow the care MAP to improve the quality of care, decrease the length of stay, change practice patterns to increase efficiency, facilitate outcomes, and reduce costs.

Table 12-1   NURSE CASE MANAGEMENT SERVICE AREAS

Category	Service Setting
Acute	Orthopedics, cardiovascular, critical care, high-risk perinatal, oncology, emergency department
Subacute	Skilled nursing centers, rehabilitation units
Ambulatory	Physician's office, clinics
Long-term care	Nursing homes, group homes, assisted-living facilities
Insurance companies	Health maintenance organizations (HMOs), preferred provider organizations (PPOs), workers' compensation, Medicaid, Medicare
Community	Nurse-managed centers, home health agencies, urgent care centers, schools, rural settings

Modified from information presented in Cohen & Cesta (2001); Curtis, Lien, Grove, & Morris (2002); Huber (2000); Stanton & Packa (2001); and Tahan (1999).

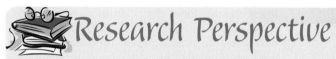

Research Perspective

Curtis, K., Lien, D., Grove, P., Morris, R. (2002). The impact of trauma case management on patient outcomes. *The Journal of Trauma, 53*(3), 477-482.

Trauma case management (TCM) was introduced to a 600-bed teaching hospital, a designated trauma center, in New South Wales, Australia. A pilot study was conducted over a 5-month period to determine the effectiveness of the care of the trauma case managers for those patients admitted to the hospital via the emergency department. In-hospital complications, missed injury rates, length of stay (LOS), staff satisfaction and use of allied health services were examined. Data from 148 patients with an Injury Severity Score less than 16 were compared with 327 patients from the previous year.

Study results revealed a 25% decrease in median LOS, from 4 days to 3. Patients with more severe injuries experienced a 2-day shorter LOS with TCM. Neither of these decreases was statistically significant. To reach a statistically significant 1-day reduction in LOS, each group in the study would have needed to enroll 1006 patients.

The complication rates did not change between the two groups. The authors indicate that this may have been due to small sample size and low complication rates. There was an increase in the detection of missed injuries during the study.

Physical and occupational therapists and social workers assist the trauma patient's return to activities of daily living. During the study, there was a 36% increase in the use of these allied health professionals.

Staff surveys indicated that trauma case management improved communication, coordination, and collaboration among staff ($P < 0.0001$). The authors also cite a clinical example demonstrating this improvement.

IMPLICATIONS FOR PRACTICE

Pilot projects can be conducted to improve patient care, reduce hospital and patient costs, and increase staff satisfaction.

BOX 12-1

Pediatric Asthma Care MAP (Example)

Critical Path

CARE CATEGORY	DAY 1	DAY 2	DAY 3	DAY 4
Consults	None	None	None	None
Tests	CBC, theophylline level, BMP, PPD, chest radiograph, ABGs, urine dipstick, and specific gravity × 1	Theophylline level, ABGs if indicated	Theophylline level, check PPD	Theophylline level
Treatments	Pulse oximetry, postural drainage, peak expiratory flow if cooperative every shift, O_2 therapy if indicated, IVs if indicated	Peak flow every shift, chest PT every shift	Peak flow bid, chest PT every shift	Peak flow q24h; consider discharge if increased peak flow
Medications	(Amount according to weight) Aminophylline and/or Proventil NEB/PO and/or steroids	Steroids may be discontinued within 48 hr or taper over 7-10 days; assess for change to PO medications	Assess change to PO medications	Consider discharge home within 24 hr of initiation of PO medications
Activity	As tolerated	As tolerated	As tolerated	As tolerated
Nutrition	As tolerated	As tolerated	As tolerated	As tolerated
Discharge plan	Inquire whether family used home care before admission; begin initial discharge plan	Initiate social work consult as indicated	Monitor progress on discharge plan, consult with physician, social worker, home health care; physician to give 24-hr notice to patient and write official discharge order	Before discharge, confirm home plan with parents, social worker, and home health care

Patient Variance (includes variances in response to treatment or special needs on admission; for example, the patient may also have an infection)

Patient Problems/Potential Problems

	DAY 1	DAY 2	DAY 3	DAY 4
Alteration in breathing patterns	a. Auscultate breath sounds for rales, wheezing, stridor, rhonchi	a. Auscultate breath sounds	a. Auscultate breath sounds, check color, retractions, nasal flaring q8h and prn	a. Auscultate breath sounds, check color, retractions, nasal flaring q8h and prn

Continued

BOX 12-1

Pediatric Asthma Care MAP (Example)—cont'd

	b. Assess skin and mucous membrane color and nasal flaring q4h	b. Assess color changes	b. Monitor and record vital signs q8h	b. Monitor and record vital signs q8h
	c. Note agitation, anxiety	c. Assess for retractions, nasal flaring q6h	c. Assess for retractions, O_2 saturation; determine discharge readiness	c. Assess for retractions, O_2 saturation; determine discharge readiness
	d. Note changes in vital signs or O_2 saturation	d. Note changes in vital signs and O_2 to discharge oximeter	d. Chest PT every shift unless contraindicated	d. Chest PT every shift unless contraindicated
	e. Monitor response to treatment (notify physician of headache, agitation, tachycardia, respiratory distress)	e. Chest PT every shift	e. Observe response to nebulizer treatment and check with physician	e. Observe response to nebulizer treatment and check with physician
	f. Chest PT every shift, position for chest expansion	f. Monitor response to treatment (report to physician changes, headache, increased respirations, distress, agitation, tachycardia)	f. Assess response to activity	f. Assess response to activity
	g. Encourage PO fluids, assess hydration status	g. Assess peak flow every shift	g. Assess clinical state, increased peak flow, tolerance of PO medications, theophylline level therapeutic	g. Assess clinical state, increased peak flow, tolerance of PO medications, theophylline level therapeutic
		h. Assess patient's response to activity		
		i. Encourage PO fluids		
Knowledge deficit	a. Orient to environment	a. Assess family and patient teaching needs	a. Continue discharge teaching	a. Discharge planning

BOX 12-1

Pediatric Asthma Care MAP (Example)—cont'd

		for disease process and begin discharge teaching	regarding medications, treatment, and importance of follow-up	
	b. Assess parent and child level of understanding	b. Assess need for visiting nurse, community referrals	b. Discharge plan with parents to minimize respiratory irritants at home and in the environment	b. Medication review
	c. Familiarize with hospital protocol (e.g., IV pump, medications, treatment)			c. Signs and symptoms of respiratory distress review
				d. Identify precipitating factors for asthma attack
				e. Exercise regimen
				f. Follow-up care
				g. When to call physician/ come to ED
Anxiety	a. Provide calm environment	a. Encourage family to state feelings, fears, and anxieties	a. Continue to encourage verbalization of concerns	a. Reevaluate level of anxiety and provide support
	b. Explore stressors and coping mechanisms	b. Evaluate anxiety level and provide supportive measures prn	b. Reevaluate level of anxiety	b. Reassure parents/child regarding knowledge of asthma
	c. Assess family dynamics			
	d. Encourage parent to stay with child			

Modified from Cohen, E. L., & Cesta, T. G. (1993). *Nursing case management: From concept to evaluation.* St. Louis: Mosby.
ABGs, Arterial blood gases; *BMP,* basic metabolic profile; *CBC,* complete blood count; *ED,* emergency department; *IV,* intravenous; *PPD,* purified protein derivative; *PT,* physiotherapy.

Development of critical paths and care MAPs can occur in various ways. Organizations can purchase paths for high-volume case types and individualize them according to the practice patterns within the organization, or the staff of a healthcare agency can develop its own care path/MAP. Accomplishing this process involves a number of steps.

Initially, the diagnosis for MAP development is determined. This decision is usually based on the volume of patients admitted with a particular diagnosis. For example, a patient with myocardial infarction, chronic obstructive pulmonary disease, or joint replacement might be a first choice. Evidence-based interventions for optimal care are assessed. (See Chapter 20 on evidence-based practices.) The clinical practice guidelines for the particular healthcare problem are reviewed. Retrospective chart review or concurrent chart review of patients currently receiving services for selected case types can identify patterns that can be incorporated into the path (Cardinal, Kraushar, & Wagie, 1994). This audit of charts can also identify costs associated with the treatment. Pathway/MAP development teams are organized to develop the tool. Membership on the team includes individuals from diverse departments involved in the care of the patient. For example, a team might include a physician, nurse manager, staff nurse, social worker, dietitian, occupational therapist, and pharmacist.

Following the audit, key patient care expectations and critical events are identified for incorporation into the path (Klenner, 2000). Small groups within the development team work to refine the elements of the path/MAP. Documentation strategies and discharge planning and instructions are affected by path/MAP development and may require revision. Newly developed tools can be tested on previously admitted patients. In essence, the patient's hospital stay is "redocumented" to identify usability of the tool (Klenner, 2000). Implementation of the tool can be enhanced through networking the development team members with their respective colleagues. Team cooperation and collaboration for path/MAP development improves utilization because all team members authored the tool and have a vested interest in the process (Berry, Cranston, & Fox, 2000).

If a patient's progress deviates from the normal path/MAP, a variance is indicated. A **variance** is anything that occurs to alter the patient's progress through the normal critical path. Analysis of variance is essential for effective utilization of a path/MAP. Circumstances that can cause a variance include operational, provider, patient, or clinical elements (Cohen & Cesta, 2001). Operational causes include broken equipment or interdepartmental delays. Changes in the practice pattern of the healthcare provider can affect the pathway and cause a variance. Complications in the patient's condition, such as a hemorrhage into the joint after total knee replacement, may increase total hospital days. A complication can inhibit the ability of the patient to meet the clinical indicator as described in the path/MAP. A patient or family's refusal of a specific component of care can create a variance.

Variances can be positive or negative. A negative variance is an undesired outcome, whereas a positive variance is an outcome that is achieved before it is expected (Cohen & Cesta, 2001). A patient undergoing a second hip replacement who attended preoperative classes and engaged in activities to "ready himself" for the surgery may actually leave the hospital sooner than predicted on the care MAP. The NCM on the orthopedic unit and the insurance company's case manager would view this as a positive variance.

Model Analysis

Nursing case management is a process for providing comprehensive care for those with complex health problems. Case management provides a well-coordinated care experience that can improve the care outcome, decrease the length of stay, and use multiple disciplines and services efficiently. Families and patients receive care across a continuum of settings, often from diverse institutions. NCMs can break down invisible institutional barriers for the client (Guttman, 1999). Nurses receive a sense of satisfaction knowing that the patient and family received coordinated, quality care in a cost-effective manner across the spectrum of the illness or injury.

Nursing leaders across the country and in diverse health settings identified major obstacles in the implementation of case-management services. Financial barriers, lack of administrative support, human resource inequities, turf battles, and the lack of information support systems have been identified as obstacles in the implementation of case management services (Rantz & Bopp, 1996). Case management is not a revenue-generating activity, but rather a "revenue-protecting" activity. It minimizes costs for those case types with the potential of high resource consumption (Rantz & Bopp, 1996). Consequently, case management may be seen as an expense.

The development of collaborative models of healthcare management incorporating nurses, social workers, and case managers have demonstrated significant cost savings. Some institutions have developed departments of healthcare case management. In this setting, the NCM works with the "medically complex," the social worker with the "socially complex," and utilization management for utilization review. This team of case managers, each with identified core functions, also has specialty functions based on the specific scope of responsibility (Cohen & Cesta, 2001). Collaboration among these case managers has positively affected health-delivery costs.

Education and preparation of case managers is a major human resource issue. The lack of nurses prepared at the BSN and MSN level, with the required clinical experience to be case managers has resulted in inadequately prepared staff being assigned to this role. The ideal case manager is the clinical nurse specialist. Another preparation for this role is that of the clinical nurse leader, which is discussed later in the chapter. Although this role, which is unit-based, is still evolving, it is designed to meet the clinical care needs of patients.

Performance appraisal of the case manager presents another human resource challenge. The case manager does not manage other employees; rather, the case manager manages patients and their care. How is this individual's performance evaluated? As with any other nursing position, performance appraisal criteria must be developed before the implementation of the process.

Who should be the case manager is a hotly contested question. Physicians see themselves as the managers of care. Social workers lay claim to this role. Nursing staff may see case management as utilization review. Nursing case management is a professionally autonomous role that requires expert clinical knowledge and decision-making skills.

Nurse Manager's Role

The nurse manager has increased demands when leading the case-management system. Quality improvement is constantly assessed to ensure the care MAP is DRG appropriate and that case managers are adequately managing their caseloads. Reimbursement for the care delivered is tied to effective planning and care delivery within the case-management process. Patient satisfaction is also pertinent to evaluate for quality. If patients are not satisfied with the system, the census may decline.

Communication among all systems must be coordinated. Because the NCM works with all departments, the nurse manager may need to facilitate interdepartmental communication. Educating the staff of other departments about the NCM's role and responsibilities will increase the effectiveness of the case-management process.

Staff Nurse's Role

The staff nurse provides patient care according to the case manager's specifications and must know the extent of the case manager's role. The case management system of patient care delivery is designed to move a patient from the illness state to optimal wellness as quickly as possible.

It is a concern that the art of nursing may vanish with an increased emphasis on moving patients quickly through the care delivery system to save money. The prospective payment system common in the managed-care environment dictates that nursing must develop new systems of care delivery to maintain quality care. One way to facilitate quality care is to consider the different abilities and education of the nurses caring for the patient. See the Literature Perspective for one organization's approach to creating a model of care to meet the needs of the increasing elderly population.

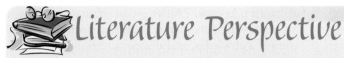

Literature Perspective

Clark, J. S. (2004). An aging population with chronic disease compels new delivery systems focused on new structures and practices. *Nursing Administration Quarterly, 22*(2), 105-115.

Managed care has impacted the delivery of health care. Hospital stays are shorter; patients are more acutely ill at the time of hospitalization and leave the hospital to recover at home or other extended care facilities. Shortages of nurses and other healthcare workers, and the diverse personnel from a wide array of disciplines, leave patients and their families coping with a disjointed and fragmented experience.

In an attempt to restore patient care to an integrated and holistic continuum, one hospital responded by developing a new model of care delivery. Baptist Hospital of Miami, a Magnet™ hospital recognized for nursing excellence, re-engineered its environment to create the "Twelve-Bed Hospital."

Initially, the design took a 51-bed cardiovascular telemetry and progressive care unit and broke it up into manageable segments of 12 to 16 beds with a Patient Care Facilitator (PCF) coordinating the care and advocating for the patient. The PCF is a clinical role; a liaison for physician and other team members to enhance the continuity of care. Strong teams develop within the 12-bed hospital because the PCF works with a consistent group of nursing staff to care for their assigned patients.

Ultimately, this pilot demonstration expanded to other areas of the hospital. Research is ongoing, but early findings indicate an improved hospital experience for patients with a PCF. This new model combines elements of traditional care models discussed in this chapter to create a new care-delivery model. Features of primary nursing, team nursing, case management, modular nursing, and patient-focused care are integrated into the design of the "Twelve-Bed Hospital" to improve the continuity of care, patient safety and satisfaction, and the overall effectiveness of the care.

IMPLICATIONS FOR PRACTICE

Nursing personnel from all levels and areas of practice can come together to alter care delivery to best meet the needs of the patient and their family. Seeking solutions to clinical challenges can be the first step in improving the patient-care experience. In addition, nursing staff satisfaction may improve as well.

DISEASE MANAGEMENT

Disease management has been in existence for many decades. Louis Pasteur's work focused on the containment and elimination of disease (Goldstein, 1998). **Disease management** is a model of care that coordinates healthcare interventions and communication for those individuals whose self-care needs are significant (Gorski, 2003). Those with chronic conditions who are high consumers of healthcare dollars are the recipients of disease-managed care. Chronic illnesses such as arthritis, asthma, cardiovascular disease, congestive heart disease, and diabetes are the prime focus of disease-management programs (Given, 2001). Disease-management programs for patients dealing with chronic illness build on the relationship with the healthcare team to prevent exacerbations and complications using evidence-based guidelines and patient empowerment techniques to improve the overall health and well-being of the client and family. Outcomes of this intervention are evaluated on an ongoing basis (Disease Management Association of America, 2006). This model of care has as its focus the concept of wellness; living well with a chronic disease. Determining the barriers to self care is an essential element of successful disease-management programs.

Disease-management programs consist of assessment to identify a specific population, comprehensive patient and family self-management education, use of evidence-based practice guidelines, medical management based on treatment algorithms, and focused visits with the healthcare team in an ambulatory setting to assist with adherence to the treatment protocol (Cohen & Cesta, 2001; Gorski, 2003). NCMs often decide whether a patient meets the specific criteria for a disease-managed program. Patients with complex healthcare needs and multiple diagnoses will continue to need extensive nursing case management and will not be eligible for a specific disease-management program (Goldstein, 1998).

DIFFERENTIATED NURSING PRACTICE

Differentiated nursing practice acknowledges the education, skill mix, and competency of each RN. Clearly defined competencies for the various levels of nurses are the foundation for differentiated practice (Foss & Koerner, 1997). Nurses prepared at the associate/diploma, baccalaureate, master's, and doctorate level are integrated in the differentiated practice model. Each defined role is different and complementary. Nurses choose the role based on their competency, skill, desire, and education (Foss & Koerner, 1997).

Refinements in differentiated practice have been in place in various clinical settings. Sioux Valley Hospital in Sioux Falls, South Dakota, has used a differentiated practice model in combination with a case-management model. Associate, primary, and advanced practice nurses were the cornerstone of the model. The associate nurse in the Sioux Valley Model was responsible for the assigned patient during a shift (Foss & Koerner, 1997). Critical paths guided the care delivered. The primary nurse coordinated care from admission to discharge for those with complex psychosocial, educational, or discharge planning needs (Foss & Koerner, 1997). Clinical nurse specialists and nurse practitioners were responsible for care throughout the illness episode. They interacted and collaborated with multiple disciplines to coordinate ongoing care across all healthcare settings (Foss & Koerner, 1997).

Incentives for implementing differentiated practice have been identified and include (1) the ability to identify the differences in preparation of nurses by level of education; (2) the ability to use different levels of nurses to meet the total needs of the patient; (3) improved clinical outcomes that are cost effective; (4) enhanced prestige of nursing through the identification of different levels of nursing to the public, the payers, and healthcare administration; (5) effective utilization of nursing resources to meet the diverse needs of managed care; and (6) career satisfaction with equitable compensation (Bellack & Loquist, 1999).

As the complexity of health care increases and the pressures of managed care exert their influence, areas such as communication and critical thinking will become more paramount. Differentiated practice in nursing can respond to these changing healthcare systems, payment strategies, and rising acuities and complex healthcare needs seen in patients and their families.

Nurse Manager's Role

Implementation of the differentiated practice model requires a shift in managerial style. Use of participatory managerial behaviors becomes essential. The nurse manager has the responsibility as a role model and mentor to encourage the professional growth of the staff. Collaborating with the staff to expand decision-making, problem-solving, and goal-setting becomes essential. The manager becomes a teacher, coach, and facilitator. Leadership behaviors of the manager in a differentiated practice setting become vital to the success of the organization. Successful managers demonstrate mutual trust, respect for ideas, and consideration of feelings. This leadership and management style expands the freedom of the nursing care delivered.

Staff Nurse's Role

Nursing staff practicing in the differentiated model find opportunities for more meaningful work. Increased autonomy, authority, and accountability provide opportunities to gain control over nursing practice. With greater control and responsibility comes a sense of empowerment.

Nursing competency and education can also determine advancement. Many organizations use clinical ladders for advancement. If a specific level is attainable with certain skills and education, a nurse can advance in position and salary according to the organization's structure. The differentiated model of care delivery describes a system of organizing nursing practice according to the education, clinical experience, competency, and decision-making required by the patient and family needs.

EVOLVING PROFESSIONAL PRACTICE MODELS/INFLUENCES

Magnet Recognition

Although no one model of care delivery is espoused by Magnet organizations, their use of models of care have led to new quality within health care. In 1982, a time of nursing shortage, the American Academy of Nursing recognized 41 hospitals that had a reputation for nursing excellence (Havens & Johnston, 2004).

These hospitals had a high level of nursing satisfaction characterized by high nurse retention, nurse autonomy, effective communication between nurses and physicians, organizational support for nursing, and nursing leadership that was strong, supportive, and visible (Havens & Johnston, 2004). These characteristics enabled the hospital to attract and retain nurses—thus the term *Magnet hospital.*

The Magnet Recognition Program, a program of the American Nurses Credentialing Center (ANCC), is designed for hospitals to achieve recognition of excellent nursing care through a self-nominating, self appraisal process to achieve **Magnet recognition.** The rigorous self-appraisal process is lengthy. The petitioning organization must assess its ability to meet the program standards and typically works for 2 years or more in the development of the application (Havens & Johnston, 2004). The hospital makes application for Magnet status, submits documentation to demonstrate its compliance with the Magnet standards and hosts a site visit by Magnet appraisers who assess and verify the presence of the "forces of Magnetism." For additional information on Magnet credentialing see: www.nursecredentialing.org/magnet/index.html. Magnet status is awarded for 4 years. Professional nursing practice at Magnet hospitals delivers quality patient care in excellent nurse work environments. In 2004, *U.S. News and World Report* added Magnet status to the criteria used in its judging of "best hospitals" (Trossman, 2004).

The Synergy Model

The American Association of Critical-Care Nurses (AACN) has adopted the **Synergy Model** as the framework for nursing practice as well as for the certification examination for the critical care nurse and the clinical nurse specialist (Kaplow, 2002). Predicated on the concept that the needs of the patient and their family influence the competencies of the nurse, the model outlines seven characteristics that patients exhibit during the course of their illness and eight nursing competencies that are essential for optimal patient outcomes.

The Synergy Model describes seven characteristics unique to every patient. These characteristics include stability, complexity, predictability, vulnerability, participation in decision-making and care, and resource availability (Edwards, 1999). The characteristics are further expanded with level descriptors. The patient characteristics drive the competencies of the nurse (Edwards, 1999).

Each of the nurse competencies (clinical judgment, advocacy and moral agency, caring practices, facilitation of learning, collaboration, systems thinking, response to diversity, and clinical inquiry) has levels of expertise, ranging from one through five (http://aacn.org/certcorp/certcorp.nsf/vwdoc/SynModel). Each of the competencies is essential in providing holistic care to the client. Depending on the acuity of the client, some competencies emerge as priorities whereas others are used to a lesser extent (Hardin & Hussey, 2003). When there is synergy between the patient characteristics and the competency of the nurse, patient care is optimized (Rohde & Moloney-Harmon, 2001).

The AACN website (www.aacn.org) provides information about the Synergy Model and its application in numerous and diverse care settings.

Clinical Nurse Leader

In this time of nursing shortage in a society with multitudinous healthcare needs, the American Association of Colleges of Nursing (AACN) has emerged with a document that describes a new role of the professional nurse—the **Clinical Nurse Leader** (CNL). The *Working Paper on the Role of the Clinical Nurse Leader* describes a professional nurse who is prepared for clinical leadership in all healthcare settings, who implements outcome-based practice and uses quality improvement strategies, and remains in and contributes to the profession of nursing. This individual will be able to create and manage responsive systems of care for patients and families (AACN, 2004).

As this role evolves and emerges, it is possible that the CNL will be integrated into models of care delivery discussed in this chapter or in new models yet to be developed. The AACN website (www. aacn.nche.edu) provides up-to-date developments of this attempt to influence the nursing profession and improve health care.

COMPARISONS OF CARE-DELIVERY MODELS

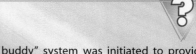

Each patient-care–delivery model has identified strengths and weaknesses. There is no perfect method for delivering nursing care to groups of patients and their families. No model is used in its "pure form." It is possible to see a variety of models used in an organization. Patient-care delivery must be individualized to the care setting. With modification, each model has the potential to be used effectively by hospitals, clinics, and home health and community agencies.

The Solution

As an Assistant Director of Nursing, I am responsible for ensuring the delivery of excellent patient care to patients accommodated on our Hematology-Oncology Unit. The nurses on the unit were committed to the same, but were faced with communication challenges. Collaborating with other members of the Leadership Team, receiving feedback from the staff nurses, and seeking out best practices from my peers in the healthcare community produced a solution. We initiated a sit-down report for all nurses called the "huddle" and established a "nurse buddy" system.

The "huddle" is conducted at the beginning of the shift after each nurse has obtained report from the nurse on the previous shift and has had the opportunity to review each patient's plan of care. The nurses are paged and notified that the "huddle" will occur. The "huddle" is facilitated by the Charge Nurse who surveys each nurse on his/her workload and the projected times he/she would need assistance with patient care.

The "nurse buddy" system was initiated to provide the patient-side nurse with an immediate resource—someone other than the Charge Nurse. These two nurses provide each other with assistance on an "as needed" basis. The "buddy" is assigned at the time all patient assignments are made and is in close proximity.

The feedback is very positive. The Charge Nurse has a clearer picture of the status of the patients, families, and staff. Because the staff nurses are more engaged, they state that they are involved with the unit's operational needs for the day. Planning patient care is done collaboratively so that each nurse is available to the "buddy" at times of need. Overall, teamwork and communication have been enhanced.

— Jacqueline Ward

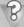 *Would this approach be suitable for you? Why?*

CHAPTER CHECKLIST

The roles of the nurse manager and staff nurse vary with each nursing-care delivery model. Regardless of the model, the nurse manager must have strong leadership and management skills for the model to be effective. Numerous issues must be considered when a care-delivery model is implemented. Without a competent manager, none of the discussed models would be effective.

- A care-delivery model is the method nurses use to provide care to patients.
- There are five models of patient-care delivery, each with its advantages and disadvantages:
  - The case method focuses on total patient care for a specific time period.
    - The nurse manager must consider the expense of this system and identify all staff members' level of education and communication skills.
  - The functional method emphasizes task-oriented care for a large group of patients.
    - The nurse manager is responsible for achieving patient outcomes, whereas staff members are responsible only for their specific tasks.
    - The functional method is most often used in subacute care facilities.
  - In the team method, a small team provides care to a small group of patients.
    - The nurse manager in this model needs strong management, critical thinking, and leadership skills.
    - The modular method is a modification of team nursing that focuses on the geographic location of patient rooms and assignments of staff members.
  - In the primary nursing method, a primary nurse provides total patient care and directs patient care from admission to discharge.
    - The nurse manager functions as role model, advocate, coach, consultant, budget controller, and unit quality manager.

  - The partnership model, or coprimary nursing model, pairs an RN with a technical assistant.
  - The patient-focused care unit employs a primary nurse and multiskilled team members.
- The nursing case management system is outcome-based and is facilitated by a case manager, who directs unit-based care using a critical path/care MAP.
  - The nurse manager in this care delivery system faces increased demands and pressure to move the patient through the system as quickly as possible.
  - Managed care is a way of organizing patient-care delivery with cost savings as the main goal.
- The nurse manager and charge nurse are responsible for directing patient care regardless of the delivery system. Key leadership and management concepts for directing patient care include the following:
  - Accountability
  - Delegation
  - Critical thinking
  - Communication
  - Promotion of autonomy
  - Collaboration
- Disease management programs assist those with chronic illness to manage their self-care to achieve their optimal health.
- The Nurse Case Manager plays a vital role in the management of care.
- The concept of differentiated practice emphasizes two levels of nursing practice: technical and professional.
- Each level has specific roles and responsibilities that depend on the nurse's educational preparation, experience, and clinical expertise.
- All the nursing roles complement each other.
- Emerging models of professional nursing practice continue to evolve.

TIPS FOR SELECTING A CARE DELIVERY MODEL

- Look at the organization and the population being served when selecting a care-delivery model.
- The mission and philosophy of an organization will affect the selection process.
- Evaluate staff mix trends to determine whether there is a potential impact on your care-delivery approach.
- There are advantages and disadvantages to any model; there is no ideal approach.
- Know that every model has specific expectations for both managers and staff.

TERMS TO KNOW

associate nurse
care MAP
case-management model
case manager
case method
charge nurse
Clinical Nurse Leader
critical path/critical pathway
differentiated nursing practice
disease management
expected outcomes
functional nursing
Magnet recognition
modular nursing
nursing care delivery model
nursing case management
outcome criteria
partnership model
patient-focused care
patient outcomes
primary nurse
primary nursing
staff mix
Synergy Model
team nursing
total patient care
unlicensed assistive (or nursing) personnel
variance

REFERENCES

Aiken, L. H., Clarke, S. P., Sloane, D. M., Sochalski, J., & Silber, J. H. (2002). Hospital nurse staffing and patient mortality, nurse burnout, and job dissatisfaction. *Journal of the American Medical Association, 88*(16), 1987-1993.

American Association of Colleges of Nursing. (2004). Working paper on the role of the clinical nurse leader. Retrieved July 3, 2005 from http://aacn.nche.edu/Publications/WhitePapers/ClinicalNurseeLeader.htm.

American Association of Critical Care Nurses. (2005). Retrieved July 3, 2005, from www.aacn.org.

American Nurses Credentialing Center. (2005). Retrieved July 3, 2005 from www.nursingworld.org/ancc/magnet.html.

Bellack, J. P., & Loquist, R. S. (1999). Employer responses to differentiated nursing education. *Journal of Nursing Administration, 29*(9), 4-8, 32.

Bennett, M., & Hylton, J. (1990). Modular nursing: Partners in professional practice. *Nursing Management, 21*(3), 20-24.

Berry, V., Cranston, B., & Fox, T. (2000). Caremapping: "What's in it for nurses?" *Nursing Case Management, 5*(2), 63-72.

Cardinal, J., Kraushar, V. K., & Wagie, T. (1994). Implementation of episodic case management in a managed care organization. In R. S. Howe (Ed.), *Case management for health care professionals.* Chicago: Precept Press.

Clark, J. S. (2004). An aging population with chronic disease compels new delivery systems focused on new structures and practices (electronic version). *Nursing Administration Quarterly, 28*(2), 105-115.

Cohen, E. L., & Cesta, T. G. (2001). *Nursing case management: From essentials to advanced practice applications* (3rd ed.). St. Louis: Mosby.

Curtis, K., Lien, D., Grove, P., & Morris, R. (2002). The impact of trauma case management on patient outcomes (electronic version). *The Journal of Trauma, 53*(3), 477-482.

Disease Management Association of America. (2006). Retrieved July 3, 2005, from www.dmaa.org.

Edwards, D. F. (1999). The Synergy Model: Linking patient needs to nurse competencies. *Critical Care Nurse, 19*(1). Retrieved July 3, 2005, from www.aacn.org/certcorp/certcorp.nsf/edcfc72ba47aaa708825666b0064bdcf/1e7a21e57.

Foss, N., & Koerner, J. (1997). The advanced practice nurse's role in differentiated practice: Martha's story. *AACN Clinical Issues, 8,* 262-270.

Given, B. A. (2001). Nurse practitioners: Issues within a managed care environment. In J. M. Dochterman & H. K. Grace (Eds.), *Current issues in nursing* (6th ed.). St. Louis: Mosby.

Goldstein, R. (1998). The disease management approach to cost containment. *Nursing Case Management, 3*(3), 99-103.

Gorski, L. (2003). A disease management program for heart failure: Collaboration between a home care agency and a care management organization [Electronic version]. *Lippincott's Case Management, 8*(6), 265-273.

Graham, I. (2003). Leading the development of nursing within a Nursing Development Unit: The perspectives of leadership by the team leader and professor of nursing (electronic version). *International Journal of Nursing Practice, 9*(4), 213-222.

Guttman, R. (1999). Case management of the frail elderly in the community. *Clinical Nurse Specialist, 13,* 174-178.

Hardin, S., & Hussey, L. (2003). AACN Synergy Model for patient care: Case study of a CHF patient (electronic version). *Critical Care Nurse, 23*(1), 73-76.

Havens, D. S., & Johnston, M. A. (2004). Achieving Magnet hospital recognition: Chief nurse executives and Magnet coordinators tell their stories (electronic version). *Journal of Nursing Administration, 34*(12), 579-588.

Huber, D. (2000). The diversity of case management models. *Lippincott's Case Management, 5,* 248-255.

Johnson, T., & Tahan, H. (1997). Care management: Outcomes-based practice for the primary nurse. *Journal of Nursing Care Quality, 11*(5), 55-68.

Jonsdottir, H. (1999). Outcomes of implementing primary nursing in the care of people with chronic lung diseases: The nurses' experience. *Journal of Nursing Management, 7,* 235-242.

Kaplow, R. (2002). The Synergy Model in practice: Applying the Synergy Model to nursing education (electronic version). *Critical Care Nurse, 22*(3), 77-81.

Klenner, S. (2000). Mapping out a clinical pathway. *RN, 63*(6), 33-36.

Magargal, P. (1987). Modular nursing: Nurses rediscover nursing. *Nursing Management, 18*(11), 98-104.

Manthey, M., Ciske, K., Robertson, P., & Harris, I. (1970). Primary nursing: A return to the concept of 'my nurse' and 'my patient.' *Nursing Forum, 9,* 65-83.

Moore, N. (2004) Notes from the floor (electronic version). *Nursing Administration Quarterly, 28*(4), 258-264.

Nelson, J. W. (2000). Models of nursing care: A century of vacillation (electronic version). *Journal of Nursing Administration, 30*(4), 156, 184.

Pontin, D. (1999). Primary nursing: A mode of care or a philosophy of nursing? *Journal of Advanced Nursing, 29,* 584-591.

Rantz, M. J., & Bopp, K. D. (1996). Issues of design and implementation from acute care, long term care and community based settings. In E. L. Cohen (Ed.), *Nurse case management in the 21st century.* St. Louis: Mosby.

Reisdorfer, J. T. (1996). Building a patient-focused care unit. *Nursing Management, 27*(10), 38, 40, 42, 44.

Rohde, D., & Moloney-Harmon, P. A. (2001). Pediatric critical care nursing: Annie's story. *Critical Care Nurse, 21*(5). Retrieved July 3, 2005 from http://www.aacn.org/certcorp/certcorp.nsf/e2adc54ac4b1fc078825692f006d1826/e10d46c9.

Seago, J. A. (1999). Evaluation of a hospital work redesign: Patient-focused care. *Journal of Nursing Administration, 29*(11), 31-38.

Stanton, M. P., & Packa, D. (2001). Nursing case management: A rural practice model (electronic version). *Lippincott's Case Management, 6*(3), 96-103.

Tahan, H. A. (1999). Clarifying case management: What is in a label? *Nursing Case Management, 4,* 268-278.

The AACN Synergy Model for patient care. (nd). Retrieved July 3, 2005 from http://www.aacn.org/certcorp/certcorp.nsf/vwdoc/SynModel.

Tiedeman, M., & Lookinland, S. (2004). Traditional models of care delivery: What have we learned (electronic version)? *Journal of Nursing Administration, 34*(6), 291-297.

Trossman, S. (2004). A magnetic force: ANCC program gains recognition in ensuring excellence in nursing services (electronic version). *American Journal of Nursing, 104*(12), 68-69.

SUGGESTED READINGS

Cox, K. (2003). The effects of intrapersonal, intragroup, and intergroup conflict on team performance effectiveness and work satisfaction. *Nursing Administration Quarterly, 27*(2), 153-163.

Felgen, J. (2004). A caring and healing environment. *Nursing Administration Quarterly, 28*(4), 288-301.

Heath, J., Johanson, W., & Blake, N. (2004). Healthy work environments: A validation of the literature. *Journal of Nursing Administration, 34*(11), 524-530.

Institute of Medicine. (2001). *Crossing the quality chasm: A new health system for the 21st Century.* Washington, DC: National Academy Press. Available at www.nap.edu.

Porter-O'Grady, T. (2001). Worker autonomy: The foundation of shared governance. *Journal of Nursing Administration, 31*(3), 100.

Upenieks, V. (2000). The relationship of nursing practice models and job satisfaction outcomes. *Journal of Nursing Administration, 30*(6), 330-335.

INTERNET RESOURCES

Agency for Health Care Research and Quality (AHRQ): www.ahrq.gov (provides clinical practice guidelines prior to 1996, as well as evidence reports).

Cochrane Collaboration: www.cochrane.org (Cochrane reviewers prepare, maintain, and promote the accessibility of systematic up-to-date reviews of healthcare interventions; a subscription is required; see your school librarian).

National Guideline Clearinghouse: www.guideline.gov (sponsored by AHRQ; provides clinical practice guidelines).

National Quality Measures: www.qualitymeasures.ahrq.gov (sponsored by AHRQ; public repository for evidence-based quality measures).

U.S. Preventive Services Task Force: http://ahrq.gov/clinic/uspstfix.htm (sponsored by AHRQ; premier source on effectiveness of clinical preventive health service).

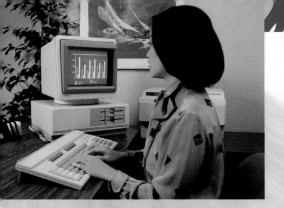

Chapter 13

Staffing and Scheduling

Mary Ellen Bonczek

This chapter explains key concepts related to staffing and scheduling. It defines and discusses the interrelationship between the personnel budget, the staffing plan, and patient outcomes. In this chapter, we also review measures for evaluating unit productivity and discuss the impact of various staffing and scheduling strategies on overall nursing satisfaction and continuity of patient care. These key points are critical to nurse managers' ability to deliver safe and effective care and service in their areas of responsibility while maintaining a high degree of employee satisfaction understanding the impact of nurse sensitive indicators on patient outcomes and controlling the unit's labor expenses. Nurse managers' ability to use this information and successfully communicate to staff is critical to their ability to lead productive services and be a valuable member of the leadership team.

Objectives

- Evaluate key external and internal organizational variables that affect staffing plans.
- Analyze activity reports to determine the effectiveness of a unit's productivity.
- Examine personal scheduling needs in relation to the patient's need for continuity of care and positive patient outcomes and the nurse manager's need to create a schedule that is balanced and fair for all team members.
- Relate floating, mandatory overtime, and the use of supplemental agency staff to staff satisfaction and patient-care outcomes.

Questions to Consider

- What activity measures can be used to assess unit workload levels?
- How do managers know that staffing on their units is adequate for the units' workload?
- What factors need to be considered by a manager to ensure that a schedule is both balanced and equitable?
- How do you engage staff in decisions about staffing plans and needed adjustments?

The Challenge

Mary Ellen Bonczek, BSN, RN, MPA, CNAA, BC
Senior Vice President, Chief Nurse Executive, New Hanover Regional Medical Center, Wilmington,
   North Carolina

The inpatient general surgical units at New Hanover Regional Medical Center total 54 beds, and our Surgical Trauma ICU (STICU) has 16 beds. Our organization was faced with severe capacity constraints as we prepared to begin a master site facility plan that would result in an additional 120 beds over the next 3 years. Our critical-care capacity was most challenged, and a void in service was a step-down unit for our surgical patients. The CCU, MICU, and CVICU all have step-down units to which they can transfer patients and free up beds for truly critical patients. A surgical step-down unit needed to be developed in beds that were already filled by the general surgery, postoperative patient. The challenge started with the need to identify the appropriate numbers of step-down beds needed. That assessment needed to meet two masters; one was the volume that was currently in STICU that could be transferred to the surgical step-down unit, and the second was what would be the best for a unit within a unit. Education plans needed to be developed, competencies identified, and a staffing plan developed. Admission and discharge criteria needed to be developed and approved by the medical staff. Communication to the nursing staff was critical—some feared that they would lose their positions and that critical-care staff would be substituted for their general surgical skills.

  What do you think you would do if you were this nurse?

Healthcare costs are escalating at a furious pace, and revenues continue to decelerate. Healthcare organizations have recognized that controlling labor costs is critical for overall cost reduction. Because nursing salaries constitute some of the major drivers of labor costs in a healthcare organization, nurse leaders are increasingly challenged to manage tightly both staffing and scheduling within their assigned cost centers. Nurse managers must make skilled staffing and scheduling decisions to ensure that safe and cost-effective care is provided by the appropriate level of caregiver. No matter what the practice setting—acute care, home care, or long-term care—there is an increased focus on manager accountability for establishing and monitoring effective and efficient staffing systems.

STAFFING

Nurse managers' roles are complex and demanding. They are the most essential positions to drive the successes of an organization. Of the many responsibilities and challenges the roles entail, staffing remains one of the most pivotal to daily unit operations, to patient safety, to patient and family satisfaction with care and services, to physician satisfaction and to employee satisfaction. Staffing issues often cause nurse managers great concern (and loss of sleep).

One solution may be to add more nurses. Mark, Harless, McCue, and Xu (2004) have shown that it is cost effective to increasing staffing levels. However, that is not always possible when the demand exceeds the supply. Therefore, staffing is always a driving issue in any organized nursing service.

Staffing is a function of planning for hiring and deploying qualified human resources to meet the needs of patients for care and services. Nurse managers have several opportunities to influence the use of staffing resources in the unit. First, nurse managers are responsible for their personal and professional knowledge of staffing benchmarks and productivity standards in their area of expertise. Second, during the preparation of a unit's personnel budget, nurse managers are accountable for projecting the staffing needs of a unit each year using established targets and projected volumes. Third, nurse managers are accountable for using the approved personnel budget to prepare a balanced staffing plan and schedule for a unit. Finally, nurse managers are responsible for monitoring, evaluating, and modifying the staffing plan over the course of the year based on a unit's volume, outcome measures, service needs, and acuity trends.

THE STAFFING PROCESS

Because the staffing process guides the development of a unit's staffing plan for the year, it is typically conducted in conjunction with the development of the personnel budget. Nurse managers must consider a number of variables that affect both the staffing process and the personnel budget. There must be routine assessments throughout the year to ensure acuity changes or service changes have not altered the required staffing.

External Variables That Affect Staffing Plans

Nurse managers must consider a number of external variables when preparing the personnel budget and projecting the unit's staffing needs. The external variables to be considered are highlighted in the following sections.

State Licensing Standards An important source for guidance in projecting staffing requirements is the licensing regulations of the state, typically through the department of health. **Staffing regulations** or recommendations can relate to the minimum number of professional nurses required on a unit at a given time or to the amount of minimum staffing in an extended-care facility or prison. Most states establish broad guidelines for minimum nurse staffing levels. However, a number of states, responding to the concerns of healthcare professionals and the public, have mandated or are attempting to mandate what the minimum nurse staffing level must be through the legislative process (www.nursingworld.org).

JCAHO and Other Regulatory Agency Standards There are a number of national organizations with missions related to continuous improvement of the safety and quality of health care provided to the public. The Joint Commission on Accreditation of Healthcare Organizations (JCAHO) is an example of this type of organization. JCAHO works to support performance improvement in healthcare organizations through establishing standards and survey accreditation processes. To comply with the

2005 JCAHO patient-care standards related to staffing, for example, an institution must provide an adequate number and mix of staff consistent with the hospital's staffing plan. The hospital needs to have an adequate number and mix of staff to meet the care, treatment, and service needs of the patients. JCAHO is not prescriptive as to what constitutes "adequate" staffing. However, in response to increasing public concerns about patient care safety and quality, JCAHO has initiated an effort to begin correlating an organization's clinical outcome data with its staffing ratios to determine the effectiveness of the overall staffing plan. Magnet™-designated hospitals have experienced the impact of this relationship (Kramer & Schmalenberg, 2005). Continuous reference to the website www.nursecredentialing.org is recommended to remain abreast of the research and standard recommendations.

The effectiveness of staffing is evaluated through the selection and correlation of data according to selected indicators. According to the 2005 JCAHO Hospital Accreditation Standards, "the hospital uses data on clinical/service screening indicators in combination with human resources screening indicators to assess staffing effectiveness." Two clinical or service indicators and two human resource indicators are to be selected according to the clinical focus of an area. The relationship between these indicators is the focus for assessing the effectiveness of staffing models and staffing mix ratios. These indicators appear in Box 13-1.

During the JCAHO accreditation process, the surveyor reviews the staffing plans developed by the nurse manager for any obvious staffing deficiencies—for example, a shift or series of shifts where the unit staffing plan is not met related to RN to patient ratios. The surveyor also interviews staff nurses outside of the presence of nurse managers to inquire about staff perceptions of the units' staffing adequacy. Surveyors may review the staffing effectiveness data for that unit as it compares to any variations from the staffing plan to identify quality of care concerns. Nurse managers are well advised to prepare a balanced staffing plan that supports a unit's unique patient care needs and the scrutiny of the JCAHO survey process. Nurse managers are also well advised to post this staffing plan and compliance reports for staff to visualize on a routine basis. In some states, this posting is required.

BOX 13-1

Assessment of Staffing Effectiveness Indicators

Clinical or Service Indicators
Family complaints
Patient complaints
Patient falls
Adverse drug events
Injuries to patients
Skin breakdown
Pneumonia
Postoperative infections
Urinary tract infections
Upper gastrointestinal bleeding
Shock/cardiac arrest
Length of stay

Human Resource Indicators
Overtime
Staff vacancy rate
Staff satisfaction
Staff turnover rate
Understaffing as compared to the hospital's staffing plan
Nursing care hours per patient day
Staff injuries on the job
On-call or per diem use
Sick time

Additional regulatory agencies that provide accreditation services similar to those provided by JCAHO include the American Osteopathic Association (AOA), the Center for Accreditation of Rehabilitation Facilities (CARF), the Accreditation Association for Ambulatory Health Care (AAAHC), the National Committee for Quality Assurance in Behavioral Health, and the Community Health Accreditation Program. Other groups are emerging.

American Nurses Association The American Nurses' Association (ANA) website, www.nursingworld.org, provides an abundance of resource information on staffing. One specific area of great interest is the American Nurses Association's National Center for Nursing Quality (NCNQ). This site contains information on a number of topics that address the safety and quality of nursing

care that patients receive and the quality of nurses' work lives. NCNQ is the overarching entity that includes a number of projects focused on patient safety, nursing care quality, nurse safety and quality of work life, and the factors that impact on these areas.

Three general approaches to ensure sufficient nurse staffing have been proposed. The first is to require and hold hospitals accountable for implementation of nurse staffing plans, with input from practicing nurses, to ensure that safe nurse-to-patient ratios are based on patient need and other criteria. The second approach is for legislators to mandate specific nurse-to-patient ratios in legislation or regulation. The third approach is a combination of nurse staffing plans and legislated nurse-to-patient ratios. Artz (2005) described the development of staffing systems through legislation as the politics of caring.

The debate over what constitutes minimum staffing is polarizing nurses and the organizations that employ them. The ANA speaks on behalf of professional nurses working in the United States. The ANA has established a number of standards for professional nursing practice, including principles for safe staffing that apply to all clinical care settings (Box 13-2). Nurse managers must consider the relationship between these standards of care and their staffing plans as they develop the unit budgets. Managers are as accountable for the safe provision of quality patient care as they are for fiscal management of the unit.

Although the ANA is not prescriptive relative to optimal staffing levels, they have supported research over the last decade to determine the effect of minimizing professional nursing positions in a staffing plan. Nursing researchers and others established a correlation between RN staffing levels and the quality of patient care outcomes, such as length of hospital stay, postoperative infection, and the development of hospital-acquired complications (e.g., pneumonia, urinary tract infections, pressure ulcers) (ANA, 2000b). Clarke (2005) identified policy implications of the research linking staffing and outcomes. Noting that these quality indicators show improvement with more RN involvement in patient care, professional nursing organizations such as the ANA are encouraging nurses to understand their clinical practice settings and ensure optimal RN-to-patient ratios (see the Research Perspective).

BOX 13-2

ANA Principles for Nurse Staffing

Principles

The nine principles identified by the expert panel for nurse staffing and adopted by the ANA Board of Directors on November 24, 1998, are listed below. A discussion of each of the three categories is available through ANA.

I. Patient Care Unit Related

a. Appropriate staffing levels for a patient care unit reflect analysis of individual and aggregate patient needs.

b. There is a critical need to either retire or seriously question the usefulness of the concept of nursing hours per patient day (HPPD).

c. Unit functions necessary to support delivery of quality patient care must also be considered in determining staffing levels.

II. Staff Related

a. The specific needs of various patient populations should determine the appropriate clinical competencies required of the nurse practicing in that area.

b. Registered nurses must have nursing management support and representation at both the operational level and the executive level.

c. Clinical support from experienced RNs should be readily available to those RNs with less proficiency.

III. Institution/Organization Related

a. Organizational policy should reflect an organizational climate that values registered nurses and other employees as strategic assets and exhibit a true commitment to filling budgeted positions in a timely manner.

b. All institutions should have documented competencies for nursing staff, including agency or supplemental and traveling RNs, for those activities that they have been authorized to perform.

c. Organizational policies should recognize the myriad needs of both patients and nursing staff.

From American Nurses Association. (2005). *Principles for nurse staffing.* Washington, DC: American Nurses Association.

In the 1990s, healthcare organizations focused efforts on reducing rising labor costs by undertaking major reengineering of traditional nursing staffing models and decreased the RN-to-patient ratios. As a result of these competing concerns, staff nurses and their professional nursing organizations found themselves in disagreement with the healthcare organizations regarding what constitutes a minimum safe staffing level. Nurse leaders learned from those experiences that our focus needs to be on retention of competent staff at the patient-side, as well as the outcomes of our patients.

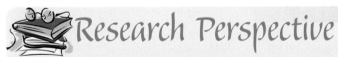

Research Perspective

Aiken, L., Clarke, S. P., Sloane, D.M., Scohalski, J., & Silber, J. H. (2002). Hospital nurse staffing and patient mortality, nurse burnout, and job dissatisfaction. *Journal of the American Medical Association, 288*(16), 1987-1993.

Responses from over 10,000 staff nurses were analyzed, along with information for more than 232,000 surgical patients and related administrative data. The key finding was that each additional patient per RN was associated with a 7% increase in likelihood of dying or failure to rescue.

IMPLICATIONS FOR PRACTICE

Correlation of human resource indicators such as nurse-to-patient ratios and RN turnover rates to patient outcomes such as patient mortality and failure-to-rescue should be incorporated into the performance improvement and planning initiatives for each hospital nursing department.

Consumer Expectations   Exceeding the expectations of consumers for care and services is a major strategy for maintaining and improving the long-term viability of the healthcare organization. Recognizing that the patient expects to receive high-quality nursing care, delivered promptly and efficiently by nurses who are satisfied with their workload, creates additional challenges that nurse managers must overcome as they prepare their budgets (Graf, Millar, Feilteau, Coakley, & Erickson, 2003). Organizational policies and clear expectations communicated to staff are essential to manage high and low volume as well as changes in acuity. Proposed personnel budgets and staffing plans that have no ability to flex up or down when patient acuity or volumes change put the nurse manager in a position in which the financial obligations of the position cannot be met. This poses a challenge to the provision of a professionally satisfying work environment. Patient, staff and physician satisfaction, service and care concerns, and improving patient safety are all outcomes of a solid staffing plan. Nurse managers are obligated to consider these variables when preparing the personnel budget.

Exercise 13-1

Review an organization's policies and procedures for assigning staff. Review a specific unit's staffing plan and current work schedule. Is the unit's actual schedule reflective of the organization's staffing policies? Is the unit's actual schedule consistent with the staffing plan? Review the nurse sensitive patient-care outcomes on the unit and assess for any trends in care concerns. Review the professional standards of care and practice. Interview two or three staff nurses on the unit as though you were a state or other regulatory surveyor, and ask them if they believe the unit usually has adequate staffing. What would these nurses' answers reveal to the surveyor?

Internal Organization Variables That Affect Staffing Plans

Nurse managers must also consider a number of internal organizational variables when preparing the personnel budget and projecting the unit's staffing needs. The internal organizational variables that are considered are highlighted in the following sections.

Organizational Staffing Policies   Nurse managers are guided in their development of unit personnel budgets by the organization's staffing policies. For example, the organization establishes the rate at which an employee earns overtime and what other benefit time will be paid for by the organization. Organizational staffing policies must comply with federal and state labor laws. Therefore, nurse managers will be in compliance with these laws if they adhere to their organizational staffing policies. An opportunity to apply qualitative judgment to policies was the basis of the article described in the Literature Perspective.

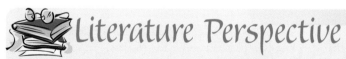

Literature Perspective

McCartney, P. (2005). Online bidding for open nursing shifts. *The American Journal of Maternal/Child Nursing,* *30*(5), 335.

Internet access and advancements in computer technology are now affording to staff nurses the opportunity to bid for shifts and self select opportunities for additional shifts. Managers spend an inordinate amount of time with increasing frustration calling off duty staff and begging for additional hours. In turn, staff are increasingly more devalued by the constant interruption of family life on days off.

IMPLICATIONS FOR PRACTICE
Filling vacant shifts with appropriately matched staff more efficiently reduces excess cost, as well as staff and manager frustration attempting to meet the unit staffing plans required.

Structure and Philosophy of the Nursing Services Department   A nursing philosophy statement outlines the vision, values, and beliefs about the practice of nursing and the provision of patient care within the organization. The philosophy statement is used to guide the practice of nursing in the various nursing units on a daily basis. Nurse managers must propose a staffing plan and a personnel budget that allow consistency between the written philosophy statement and the observable practice of nursing on their units. It is very demoralizing for nurses to feel that they cannot comply with their nursing philosophy statement or professional values because of problems associated with consistently inadequate staffing.

The philosophy statement also guides the establishment of the overall structure of the nursing service department and the staffing models that are used within the organization. The **staffing model** adopted by the organization plays a major role in determining the mix of professional and assistive staff needed to provide patient care.

Productivity targets such as nursing hours per patient day (NPPD) or hours per visit for emergency departments are referred to as Units of Service (UOS). These targets are used in staffing model forecasting for annual budgets. The UOS multiplied by the volume for a clinical area determine the number of staff needed. The formula can be adjusted for total paid staff or just for those required for the delivery of direct patient care. Determining the staffing skill mix that best meets the needs of the unit requires nurse managers to consider the intensity of nursing care generally required by unit patients. To determine the intensity of care, managers consider factors such as the severity of patient illnesses, the complexity of nursing care and procedures, the degree of patient dependency on the nursing staff, and the amount of time generally required to provide patient care. In the middle to late 1990s, reducing the complement of professional staff in the skill mix had become a major cost-saving strategy in many organizations. Focus on patient outcomes; service and operational excellence; and patient, staff, and physician satisfaction has drawn attention to these initiatives and refocused our attention.

Organizational Support Systems   Another critical variable that affects the development of the nursing personnel budget is the presence, or absence, of organizational systems that support the nurse in providing care. If the organization has recognized the need to keep the professional nurse at the bedside, support systems to allow that to happen will be evident. Examples of support systems that enhance the nurse's ability to remain on the unit and provide direct care to patients include transporter services, clerical support services, and hospitality services.

However, professional nurses often work in organizations that require them to function in the role of a multipurpose worker. Because nurses are generally scheduled in hospitals 24 hours a day, 7 days a week, they may be required to provide services for other professionals who provide more limited hours of care to patients. It is wise for nurse managers to identify what costs are being incurred in the unit as a result of the absence of adequate organizational support systems and to develop strategies to put those systems into place or justify the budget accordingly.

Changes in Services That Will Be Offered   Nurse managers must also consider organizational plans to expand existing clinical services or to develop new services or programs when preparing the personnel budget. For example, a manager of an inpatient surgical unit must consider the potential effect of offering a new surgical procedure to the community. What projections have been made for this market? What is the expected length of stay for patients undergoing this new procedure? What are the national standards for care for this type of patient? A nurse manager will use this information to project added staff to manage these changes in service.

A strategy to maximize capacity in constrained organizations may be to offer a complement of step-down critical care beds within the body of an existing inpatient surgical unit. Staffing plans need to be modified, and staff education and competencies need to be established and administered. A nurse manager is challenged with maintaining the appropriately competent staff to manage the internal flexing of patient acuity in the unit.

Conversely, nurse managers must also be aware of any organizational plans to delete an existing service that their new unit supports. For example, if a nurse manager in a home care setting knows that reimbursement for a certain procedure in the home has declined to the point that this service must be discontinued, allowances for fewer required staffing resources in the coming year must be made.

Projected Units of Service   The amount of work performed by a nursing unit, or **cost center,** is referred to as its **workload.** Workload is measured in terms of the **units of service** defined by the cost center. Nurse managers must understand the nature of the work in their area of responsibility to define the units of service that will be used as their workload statistic and to **forecast,** or project, the volume of work that will be performed by their cost center during the upcoming year (or validate the projection made by someone else) to propose an adequate personnel budget.

Productivity targets have been adopted by many organizations and, absent changes in scope of service or acuity, will drive the personnel budget calculations.

FORECASTING UNIT WORKLOAD

Nurse managers consider a number of factors besides projected units of service when beginning the process of forecasting the unit's workload for the upcoming year, including the following:

1. Historical staffing requirements
2. Effectiveness of the current staffing plan
3. Trends in acuity on the unit
4. Anticipated skill mix or other personnel changes
5. New physicians, programs, services, or technology anticipated to affect staffing
6. Patient outcomes; for example:
   a. Length of stay
   b. Urinary tract infections
   c. Patient falls

Nurse managers use this information and the information available in the unit's activity report to predict daily staffing needs for the upcoming budget period.

The Unit Activity/Productivity Report

Nurse managers rely on the unit's **activity or productivity report** for obtaining key statistics that can be used to project units of service for the upcoming

year. These statistics are also used to monitor the unit's current productivity performance. Institution-wide reports are generated that provide nurse managers with a variety of measures of unit workload. Although the format of these reports may vary, the kinds of information typically available to nurse managers in an activity report are included in Box 13-3.

In the inpatient setting, the **average daily census** (**ADC**) is one measure considered by nurse managers to project the potential workload of the unit. The ADC is a simple measure of the average number of patients being cared for in the available beds on the unit trended over a specific period. The formula for calculating the ADC is found in Box 13-4.

If a unit's ADC is trending upward, the nurse manager proposes additional personnel to manage this increase in patient volume. If the ADC is trending downward, the nurse manager proposes the need for fewer resources to manage this downward census trend. In the acute care setting, a unit's ADC can be extremely volatile based on the patterns of admissions, transfers, and discharges on the unit; in a long-term care setting, however, the unit's ADC may be very stable over prolonged periods. Nurse managers may note census trends based on a particular shift, the day of the week, or the season of the year. The addition of new physicians, the creation of new programs or services, and many other variables may also affect a unit's average daily census. The number of admissions and discharges per shift also increases staffing demands. Nurse managers must maintain a strong

---

BOX 13-3

Typical Report Indicators

- Volume statistic: number of units of service for the reporting period
- Capacity statistic: number of beds or blocks of time available for providing services
- Percentage of occupancy: number of occupied beds for the reporting period
- ADC (average daily census): average number of patients cared for per day for the reporting period
- ALOS (average length of stay): average number of days that a patient remained in an occupied bed

BOX 13-4

Formulas for Calculating Volume Statistics

- **ADC:** patient days for a given time period divided by the number of days in the time period
  566 patient days in June =
  566 patient days/30 days = ADC of 18.9
- **Percentage of Occupancy:** daily patient census divided by the number of beds in the unit
  18 patients in a 20-bed unit =
  18 patients/20 beds = 90% occupancy
- **ALOS:** the number of patient days for a specified period divided by the number of discharges for the same period
  There are 566 patient days and 98 discharges in June. 566 patient days divided by 98 discharges = 5.77 ALOS

grasp on these measures of workload to prepare an adequate staffing plan for their unit.

Another way of assessing a unit's activity level is to calculate the **percentage of occupancy.** The unit's occupancy rate can be calculated for a specific shift, on a daily basis, or as a monthly or annual statistic. The formula for calculating the percentage of occupancy is found in Box 13-4. Nurse managers use the percentage of occupancy to develop the unit's staffing plan. Optimal occupancy rates may vary by practice setting. In long-term care the organization would desire 100% occupancy rates. However, in acute care, 85% occupancy rates would ensure the best potential for patient throughput.

Another measure of unit activity that may be considered by nurse managers is the **average length of stay** (ALOS), or the number of days each patient stays in an occupied bed. As reimbursement dollars have decreased, so have lengths of stay. The cost of treating the patient has not decreased as dramatically because the patient's acuity is greater; essentially, hospitals need to provide more care in less time for fewer dollars with the same, if not better, outcomes. For this reason, as a unit's ALOS trends downward, the need for staffing resources may not

change substantially, or it may actually climb. The formula for calculating the average length of stay is also found in Box 13-4.

FORECASTING UNIT STAFFING REQUIREMENTS

Calculation of Full-Time Equivalents

Nurse managers use the unit's forecasted workload to calculate the number of **full-time equivalents** (FTEs) that will be needed to construct the unit's overall staffing plan. It is important to remember that there is a distinction between an employee in a position and an FTE. Chapter 11 describes FTEs and how they are calculated. To achieve a balanced staffing plan, nurse managers must determine the correct combination of full-time and part-time positions that will be needed.

Nurse managers must also consider the effect of productive and non-productive hours when projecting the FTE needs of the unit. **Productive time** is the paid hours that are actually worked on the unit. Productive hours can be further defined as direct or indirect. Direct care hours are used to pay for the care of patients. Indirect hours are used to pay for other required unit activities, such as staff meetings or continuing education attendance.

Nonproductive time (see Chapter 11) includes those hours of benefit time that are paid to an employee for vacation, holiday, personal, or sick time in some organizations, or for an employee attending orientation or continuing education activities. In most practice settings, nurses must be replaced when they are off duty and accessing their paid benefit time off. Managers must be aware of the average benefit hours required for their unit, or they will understate their FTE needs. This requires nurse managers to consider carefully how to allocate their budgeted FTEs into full-time and part-time positions to meet the staffing requirements for the unit when a portion of the staff is taking paid time off. In addition, looking at the number of employees being paid for any specific day may not reflect the number actually providing care. So, the nurse manager's role must include competencies in finances, information technology and automation of staffing and scheduling programs.

Exercise 13–2

Select a hospital-based department and determine the hours of operation for this organization. Assess the master scheduling plan and determine how many RNs are needed to ensure that each shift has one RN present. Assuming that a 36-hour work week (three 12-hour shifts) will equal one FTE; convert the required number of registered nurse positions to FTEs. Complete the exercise assuming a 40-hour work week (five 8-hour shifts) and compare the FTE variance.

Distribution of FTEs

Nurse managers must consider a number of variables when they begin the process of distributing FTEs into the **master staffing plan** for the unit. The master staffing plan, which is based on the unit's approved personnel budget, serves as a guide for creating the unit's schedules for the upcoming year. Variables that must be considered by managers when creating master staffing plans include the following:

1. The hours of operation of the unit
2. The basic shift length for the unit
3. Known activity patterns for the unit at various times of day
4. Maximum work stretch for each employee
5. Shift rotation requirements
6. Weekend requirements
7. Personal and professional requirements and requests for time off (e.g., school schedule, meetings for professional development and support for models of shared governance).

Each of these variables interrelates with the others, so few "absolutes" are possible. For example, initially one might think that a 24/7 unit might require more staff than a 7 AM to 6 PM area. If the first, however, is providing basic care all day and few activities at night (e.g., a long-term care facility), fewer staff might be needed than in the second if that were, for example, a day surgery unit.

The master staffing plan must consider the distribution of **fixed FTEs** in the plan. Fixed FTEs are held by those employees who will be scheduled to work, no matter what the volume of activity. These employees generally hold an exempt or salaried position, meaning their compensation does not depend on the unit's workload. Examples of employees who typically hold a fixed FTE include the nurse manager, the clinical nurse specialist, and the education staff.

The manager then distributes the **variable FTEs** into a master staffing plan. Variable FTEs are held by those employees who are scheduled to work based on the workload of the unit. These employees are considered nonexempt or hourly wage employees, meaning their compensation depends on the actual number of hours worked in a given pay period. Examples of employees who typically hold a variable FTE position include staff nurses, clerical staff, and other ancillary support staff assigned to the unit.

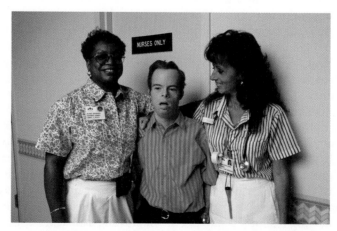

The purpose of the work about staffing and scheduling is to ensure safe patient care.

SCHEDULING

The Nursing Executive Center of the Advisory Board Company is a nationally recognized think-tank that studies complex or emerging issues confronting nursing administrators. Nursing retention and recruitment have been at the forefront of their research for the past several years. In studying the employment attributes most likely to result in nursing turnover in a hospital setting, the Nursing Executive Center found that having limited scheduling options was prominent as a factor in staff dissatisfaction.

Scheduling is a function of implementing the staffing plan by assigning unit personnel to work specific hours and specific days of the week. The nurse manager is greatly challenged to take the FTEs that are allotted through the personnel budget, distribute them appropriately, and create a master schedule for the unit that also meets each employee's personal and professional needs. Although completely satisfying each individual staff member is not always possible, a schedule can usually be created that is both fair and balanced from the employee's perspective while still meeting the patient care needs. Creating a flexible schedule with a variety of scheduling options that leads to work schedule stability for each employee is one mechanism for retaining staff within the control of nurse managers.

Self-scheduling or flexible scheduling needs to be properly managed. While personal needs of the staff are important to manage and meet, the patient care needs on the unit are the paramount focus for building a schedule. Unit standards for a staffing plan are established and then a negotiated schedule that results in meeting the needs of staff and patients is the expected and ultimate outcome.

Variables That Affect Staffing Schedules

Nurse managers must consider many variables to create a fair and balanced schedule. Examples of variables nurse managers can anticipate and must consider as they prepare the unit's schedule are found in Box 13-5.

Other unanticipated variables can complicate the best-prepared schedule. When faced with call-ins for illness, funeral leaves, jury duty, or an emergent need for a leave of absence (LOA), nurse managers must attempt to fill a shift vacancy on

BOX 13-5

Anticipated Scheduling Variables

Hours of operation
Shift rotations
Weekend rotations
Approved benefit time for the schedule period—vacations, holidays, and such
Approved leaves of absence/short-term disability
Approved seminar, orientation, or continuing education time
Scheduled meetings for the schedule period
Current filled positions and current staffing vacancies
Number of part-time employees

short notice. Requesting staff to add hours over their planned commitment, floating staff from another unit or securing someone from a staffing pool, contracting with agency nursing staff, or seeking overtime are examples of strategies that nurse managers may be compelled to use to ensure safe staffing of their units. However, many potential negative consequences are associated with using these strategies. For example, some states have passed legislation regarding mandatory overtime, which would eliminate the option of a manager telling another nurse to extend assigned hours. The strategies for adding supplemental staff to the unit are examined more carefully in the following sections.

Exercise 13-3

Assume you are going on a job interview. Considering your personal preferred work schedule, what scheduling practices would be most satisfying to you and might lead you to accept employment with the organization? What scheduling practices might cause you to look elsewhere for a job? Develop a list of questions to ask your potential employer regarding scheduling practices in their organization. What strategies do you have to offer as a team member in serving the organization's needs?

Increasing Staff FTEs   Upon being hired, employees create an implied contract with the organization for the FTEs they will work. Generally, full-time and part-time staff agree to work the FTEs that best meet their personal needs for income, benefits, time worked, and time off. When nurse managers are faced with an unanticipated staffing vacancy, the easiest remedy for fixing this problem may be to ask a staff member to work an additional shift or hours or to call an off-duty staff member and ask that person to come in on a scheduled day off. When nurse managers use this strategy often, they can potentially erode the professional environment and see an impact on retention. Although staff will be compensated for the inconvenience of adding hours above their FTE, and may even earn added bonus pay or overtime pay for the effort, an intrusion in their personal time and needed respite can take a toll on staff. Staff may ultimately become dissatisfied with this approach to managing staffing on the unit—especially if this is a recurring problem.

Exercise 13-4

Assume you are the senior staff leader working in the charge role of the shift. One of the staff assigned to work with you becomes ill and must go home suddenly, leaving his designated patient assignment to be resumed by someone else. As a unit leader, what factors would you consider as you determine how to reassign this work to other nurses? As a co-worker on the shift, what effective follower behaviors might you demonstrate to support the leader in this situation? Can you identify any behaviors that would complicate the staffing situation further?

Floating Staff   Another strategy that may be used to deal with unanticipated staff vacancies involves floating nurses from one clinical unit to another to fill the staffing vacancy. This can be an effective strategy if the nurses are being deployed from a centralized flexible staffing pool and they have the competencies to work on the unit to which they are assigned. Nurses working as float nurses are generally experienced nurses who maintain a broad range of clinical competencies. They usually receive added compensation for their willingness to be flexible and to float to a variety of units on short notice. Nurse managers are fortunate if they have a strong flexible staffing pool to draw upon when faced with unanticipated staffing vacancies.

When an organization does not have the flexibility of a staffing pool, nurses may be expected to float across clinical units to fill shift vacancies. There can be several areas of concern related to this strategy for meeting unanticipated staffing needs. The organization needs to protect the safe delivery of patient care and ensure a policy and prescribed practice is in place to reassign staff to the same or clinically similar areas. If a staff nurse is asked to

reassign to an area outside of his or her sphere of clinical competence, he or she should be utilized only to support the basic care needs and not assume a complete and independent assignment. Monitoring and evaluation of this practice is imperative to ensure safe and competent care delivery models. Specialized nursing competencies do not necessarily transfer across clinical practice settings. Floating a nurse should always raise the question about the practitioner's competence to provide safe care to patients in the unfamiliar unit.

Use of Agency Staff   Many nurses choose to work for staffing agencies. They may be hired by the nursing unit as independent contractors for a shift, a week, or a longer period. There are advantages to working for an agency, such as higher hourly rates of pay, diversity in work assignments, exposure to a variety of work teams, and the ability to travel. Use of agency nursing staff is a strategy used by an organization to fill temporary staff vacancies.

Despite advantages to using agency staff, nurse managers must consider the potential negative aspects of depending on supplemental staff to meet the unit's staffing plan. Patients should be unable to distinguish agency staff from unit staff. The professional behavior and clinical performance of the agency staff member needs to mirror those of the organization and therefore be seen as a reflection of the care provided on the unit. For this reason, nurse managers must expect agency staff to function as competent professionals in their unit following the organization's standards of behavior and/or performance.

It is difficult to monitor the performance of agency staff because they may work for only one shift in the unit before moving on to another unit or another facility. Managers may have difficulty documenting variations in performance or practice with agency staff members because of the sporadic nature of their assignment to a given unit.

Finally, if managers identify concerns about the competency of an agency employee, they may elect not to have that individual return to the unit in the future. However, if they do not communicate their performance concerns to that person's employer, the agency staff may not receive the necessary performance counseling. In that case, the agency employee may move from institution to institution perpetuating poor clinical performance practices until a serious patient outcome results. The use of agency personnel requires a high degree of supervision by nurse managers.

Overtime Requiring staff to stay on duty after their shift ends to fill staffing vacancies is called *mandatory overtime*. The issue of mandatory overtime is being discussed by professional nursing organizations and state boards of nursing across the country, and it has become a major negotiating point for nurses in unionized settings. Legislation prohibiting mandatory overtime has been adopted in some states and is pending in others. Mandatory overtime is a staffing strategy that is opposed by the ANA and many other professional nursing organizations because it is seen as a risk to both patients and nurses.

Asking staff to stay on duty after their shift ends to fill staffing vacancies is called overtime. This differs from mandatory overtime because there are no employment consequences based on the staff responses to the request. The nurse manager may be persuasive and the staff may be willing to accept this lengthened service. However, tired and overworked nurses are more likely to have compromised decision-making abilities and technical skills as a result of fatigue.

Once again, nurse managers may feel conflicted over this issue. Managers may feel compelled to require staff to work overtime out of a belief that a tired nurse is better than no nurse at all. When faced with an unsafe staffing situation, managers may believe no other options exist for providing care to the patients. Some organizations have policies regarding their right to mandate overtime. The policies may specify that refusing to work the required overtime has dire consequences and is punishable with corrective discipline. However, some states have made clear that refusing mandatory overtime does not constitute patient abandonment. Other organizations have taken a clear position on mandatory overtime and have not subscribed to that as a staffing strategy.

Exercise 13-5

Review a healthcare organization's policies on overtime. Is mandatory overtime covered in the policy? Are the consequences for failing to work mandatory overtime when requested to do so by a supervisor outlined in the policy? What does the state board of nursing allow regarding mandatory overtime? As a nurse manager, how would you respond to a staffing shortage without mandatory overtime as an option? How would you respond to a nurse manager who required you to stay on the job after your shift was over? Develop a list of questions you might ask on a job interview relating to use of overtime in the organization. Develop a list of strategies for eliminating mandatory overtime, if such exists.

Constructing the Schedule

Mechanisms are typically in place within an organization for staff to use in requesting days off and to know when the final schedule will be posted. In addition, most organizations have written policies and procedures that must be followed by nurse managers to ensure compliance with state and federal labor laws relative to scheduling. These policies also aid managers in making scheduling decisions that will be perceived as fair and equitable by all employees.

Schedules are usually constructed for a predetermined block of time based on organizational policy—for example, weekly, biweekly, or monthly. While the unit schedule may be prepared in a decentralized fashion by nurse managers or by unit staff through a self-scheduling method, the former may not support the clinical experience of staff or the autonomy that staff needs to fulfill their professional goals. In some organizations, centralized staffing coordinators may oversee all of the schedules prepared for the patient care units. Each method of schedule preparation has pros and cons.

Decentralized Scheduling—Nurse Manager One decentralized method for preparing the schedule involves nurse managers developing the schedule in isolation from all other units. In this model, nurse managers approve all schedule changes and actually spend time on a regular basis drafting the staff schedule considering only the staffing needs of the unit. In other decentralized models, managers do the preliminary work on schedules and then submit them to a centralized staffing office for review and for the addition of any needed supplemental staff. The advantage of this decentralized model is that the accountability for submitting a schedule in alignment with the established staffing plan rests with managers. These individuals are ultimately the ones accountable for maintaining unit productivity in line with the personnel budget, so the incentive to manage the schedule tightly is strong.

The negative aspect of this decentralized method relates to the inability of any individual nurse manager to know the "big picture" related to staffing across multiple patient care units. Requests for time off are approved in isolation from all other units, and there is a very real potential with this model that each manager will make a decision at the unit level that will be felt in aggregate as a "staffing shortage" across multiple units.

Staff Self-Scheduling   A self-scheduling process has the potential to promote staff autonomy and to increase staff accountability. In addition, team communication, problem-solving skills, and negotiating skills can be enhanced through the self-scheduling process. Successful self-scheduling is achieved when each individual's personal schedule is balanced with the unit's patient care needs.

Self-scheduling has become more complicated in the wake of care delivery changes and the decentralization of many activities to the individual patient care units. The professional nursing staff cannot work in isolation of other care members when creating a schedule. Assessing the readiness of support staff to participate in this type of initiative is critical as resource utilization and cost containment continue to be major focal points of concern.

Centralized Scheduling   One benefit to centralized scheduling is that the staffing coordinator is usually aware of the abilities, qualifications, and availability of supplemental personnel who may be needed to complete the schedule. In many organizations the centralized staffing coordinator is also aware of each unit's personnel budget and any constraints it may impose on the schedule. On the other hand, a disadvantage to centralized staffing is the limited knowledge the coordinator has relative to changing patient acuity needs or other patient-related activities on the unit. Developing a mechanism for the centralized staffing coordinator to share unit-specific knowledge with the respective nurse manager can resolve this disadvantage satisfactorily.

Many organizations have invested in computer software designed to create optimal schedules based on the approved staffing plans for individual units. The centralized staffing coordinator maintains the integrity of the computerized databank for each unit; enters schedule variances daily; generates planning sheets, drafts, and final schedules; and runs any specialized productivity reports requested by nurse managers. Nurse managers review the initial schedule created by the computer, make necessary modifications, and approve the final schedule.

The process for creating schedules selected by the organization depends on a large number of variables, including the size of the organization and the complexity of the staffing that must be produced.

Using Automation   There are various vendors available now that offer online scheduling or "bidding" for shifts. The concept is a win-win for staff and managers. Hospitals are using the concept for per diem scheduling, retention and recruitment of staff. In turn, this approach results in reducing the dependence on agency nurses and saving on nurse manager time (Trossman, 2004).

EVALUATING UNIT PRODUCTIVITY

Nurse managers are increasingly pressed to justify their staffing decisions. Managers have positions and subsequent budgeted nursing salary dollars in the personnel budget based on the estimated units of service that will be provided in the unit. If managers are able to provide more care to more patients while spending the same or fewer salary dollars, they have increased their unit productivity. Conversely, if the same or more salary dollars are spent to provide less care to fewer patients, managers have decreased their unit productivity.

Nursing productivity is a formula driven calculation. Unit of service (UOS) multiplied by the volume (patient days or Emergency Department visits) equals hours available to create direct productive staffing plans. Those hours multiplied by a non-productive factor (e.g., 1.12) to account for paid time off equals the total hours available for the staffing plan. A ratio of patients to RN is essential to set, apply to the total hours available and then build the support structure (nursing assistant or unit clerks) accordingly. Patient type, scope of service, acuity and/or classification of the patient are all factors correlated with patient outcomes that drive staffing decisions.

Calculating nursing productivity is challenging for nurse managers because it is difficult to quantify the efficiency and effectiveness of individual nurses providing care to patients. Individual nurses can vary greatly in their critical-thinking abilities, their skill levels, and their ability to make timely and accurate decisions that affect patient outcomes. Because patient care is an extremely dynamic process, patient acuity trending with a classification system is one method that can be used by nurse managers to project daily staffing needs and justify unit productivity.

Assessing and understanding staff competency is imperative. Dorothy Del Bueno's Performance Based Development System (PBDS) uses video simulations and written vignettes of patient care problems to assess selected competencies. PBDS is an extraordinary tool to understand the quality not just the quantity of an organization's nursing workforce.

Patient Classification Systems

One of the most commonly cited reasons for exceeding a unit's staffing plan is the increased acuity of the patients on that unit. However, the dynamic nature of patient care often makes it difficult to quantify and qualify the care needs of patients at any given time.

Patient classification systems have been developed in an effort to give nurse managers the tools and language for describing the acuity of patients on their unit. "Sicker" patients receive higher classification scores, indicating that more nursing resources are required to provide patient care. Nurse managers use the classification data to make adjustments to the unit's staffing plan for a given time or for quantifying acuity trends over longer periods as they forecast their staffing needs during the budget process.

Patient Classification Types

Two basic types of patient classification systems exist: prototype and factor. A **prototype evaluation system** is considered both subjective and descriptive. It classifies patients into broad categories and uses these categories to predict the patient care needs. The relative intensity measures (RIMs) system is a prototype system. This system classifies patient care needs based on their diagnosis related group (DRG). This system was first tried unsuccessfully in the early 1980s. Since then, Yale New

Haven Hospital in New Haven, Connecticut, has developed a RIMs system that is used to measure both workload and productivity. The data are then fed to a decision support system that integrates the clinical and financial information.

A **factor evaluation system** is considered more objective. It takes tasks, thought processes, and patient care activities and gives each one a time or rating. These associations are then summed to determine the hours of direct care required, or they are weighted for each individual patient. The Nursing Intervention Classification (NIC) system is a factor system that takes into consideration different interventions specific to each individual patient (McCloskey & Bulechek, 2000). Each intervention is given a name and a definition and is further specified to incorporate a list of all associated interventional activities. The list of interventions is comprehensive and applicable to inpatient, outpatient, home care, and long-term care patients.

Typically, organizations use a combination of systems. Some patient types with a single health care focus, such as maternal deliveries or outpatient surgical procedure patients, would be appropriately classified with a prototype system. Patients with more complex care needs and a less predictable disease course, such as those with pneumonia or stroke, are more appropriately evaluated with a factor system.

Advantages of Patient Classification Systems

On a broad scale, patient classification data can provide nurse managers with additional information that can be used when preparing the personnel budget. Acuity trending can help managers determine whether the unit's staffing model or skill mix should change. The system may also help managers determine the cost of care being provided to patients and may help justify changes in patient charges for services. On a daily basis, patient classification data can be used to fine-tune daily staffing requirements.

Disadvantages of Patient Classification Systems

Numerous potential problems exist with patient classification systems. The issue most often raised by the organization's administrators relates to the questionable reliability and validity of the data collected through a self-reporting mechanism. Nurses are often charged with the responsibility of classifying their patients.

Research compared actual time and motion studies, in which a single observer continuously timed the occurrences and duration of nursing activities, with self-reporting by nursing staff of the time and duration of each task performed. Biases of self-reporting were found to be no greater than observer-induced bias in time-and-motion measurement (Burke, McKee, Wilson, Donahue, Batenhorst, & Pathak, 2000).

Another concern with patient classification data relates to the inability of the organization to meet the prescribed staffing levels outlined by the patient classification system. Administrators worry that they risk potential liability if they do not follow the staffing recommendations of the patient classification system. If the classification data indicate that six caregivers are needed for the upcoming shift, but the organization can provide only five caregivers, what are the potential consequences for the organization if an untoward event occurs? Concern over the accuracy of biased data and the inability to meet predicted staffing levels outlined by the patient classification systems have caused many healthcare organizations to abandon patient classification as a mechanism for determining appropriate staffing levels. Staff morale is at risk when acuity models state one level and the organization cannot increase staffing to meet the unit's now defined needs. Likewise, staff morale is at risk without acuity models when it is clear to them that patient needs exceed care capacity. A truer approach is to measure and monitor patient outcomes and participate in national databases that monitor staffing effectiveness. For example the National Database for Nursing Quality Indicators (NDNQI) measures structure and outcome indicators and provides a comparative report comparing like organizations and units around the country.

Labor Cost Per Unit of Service

Organizations can use labor cost or a straight FTE model for comparison of actual to earned staff. **Labor cost per unit of service** is a simple measure that compares budgeted salary costs per budgeted volume of service (productivity target) with actual salary costs per actual volume of service (productivity performance). This measure requires managers to staff according to their staffing plan because

---

BOX 13-6

Analysis of Labor Costs per Unit of Service

1. A manager of a cardiac telemetry unit proposes the following in the personnel budget. These are the unit's productivity targets.
   Total patient days: 5840
   - ADC = 16
   - Staffing plan for ADC of 16:
     - Day shift: 3 RNs and 3 UAPs (50% RN skill mix)
     - Evening shift: 3 RNs and 3 UAPs (50% RN skill mix)
     - Night shift: 3 RNs and 1 UAP (75% skill mix)
   - Direct care labor costs are also projected by the manager based on the average RN and UAP salaries for this unit.
   - Target = $139.32 per patient, or $2229.12 per day
2. The manager actually staffs as follows:
   - ADC = 16
   - Actual staffing for ADC of 16:
     - Day shift: 4 RNs and 2 UAPs (66% RN skill mix)
     - Evening shift: 4 RNs and 2 UAPs (66% RN skill mix)
     - Night shift: 3 RNs (100% RN skill mix)
   - Direct labor costs for this day = $145.44 per patient, or $2327.04 per day.
3. The manager has incurred a variance:
   - Exceed target by $6.12 per patient, or $97.92 for the day.

ADC, Average daily census; *RN*, registered nurse; *UAP*, unlicensed assistive personnel.

---

the plan reflects the approved personnel budget. If managers compare their actual productivity performance to their productivity target and the two numbers match, managers know they have staffed productively. Box 13-6 provides an analysis of labor costs per unit of service.

If managers compare the two numbers and the actual productivity performance number is higher than the target, they have spent more money for care than they budgeted. Managers must explain change in productivity in a **variance report**. A number of variables may cause the labor costs to be higher than anticipated, such as increased overtime, paying bonus pay for regular staff, using costly agency resources, or a higher-than-anticipated amount of indirect educational or orientation time.

If managers compare the two numbers and the actual productivity performance number is lower than the target, they have spent less money for care than they budgeted. Managers must also explain this high degree of productivity. One variable that may cause the labor costs to be lower than anticipated is an increased nonprofessional skill mix. However, managers can also create lower labor costs by consistently understaffing their unit.

Impact of Leadership on Productivity

Nurse managers must possess staffing and scheduling skills to prepare a staffing plan that balances organizational directives with unit needs for care and services. They must spend time each month evaluating their unit's productivity performance. Yet recent research has shown that nurse managers can best improve unit productivity by spending more of their work time coaching and mentoring staff and providing them with clear information and direction related to meeting unit productivity goals. Nurse managers are the chief retention officers and need to perform their duties accordingly.

SUMMARY

Staffing is one of the greatest challenges a manager has. When performed well, it enhances satisfaction of the unit staff and contributes to positive patient outcomes. When not performed well, low morale and discontent result. The manager has various data available to help in planning the staffing patterns for the unit. Success, however, depends on the unit staff working collaboratively to meet the needs for care.

The Solution

Staff were convened to discuss the impact on the inpatient general surgery unit with a transition to a number of beds for surgical ICU step-down patients. Six beds were determined to be the initial number of step-down beds to be incorporated into the north side of the surgical inpatient unit. Staff were involved in the design of the space from the perspective of identifying which rooms were to be used and what in-room supplies and equipment would be necessary. Continuous pulse-oximetry and bedside computers were among the top needs identified. A staffing plan was established and staff on the unit were the first to be offered the positions. The unit's staffing plan was filled with staff from the general surgical unit on 9N and the related unit of 9S. Educational plans were developed and the STICU nursing staff were open and welcoming when the new step-down staff rotated and partnered with the STICU staff in the critical care environment. The staff completed didactic education and then those same STICU nurses provided back up for the new step-down staff when the unit opened. Continuous discussions were held with the medical staff involved through a champion who was identified within the Deptartment of General Surgery. Talking points were distributed to the medical staff and the other hospital staff to keep everyone current with the progress. Interdisciplinary teams were developed around the care models and are now engaged in daily patient care conferences to monitor progress of patients. The unit has been open for 6 months and is a great success. There are no vacant positions, critical care beds are more available, medical staff are very pleased with the care delivered, patient satisfaction for this unit is very good and the staff felt accomplished and proud of their contribution to the overall capacity challenge!

— Mary Ellen Bonczek

 Would this be a suitable approach for you? Why?

CHAPTER CHECKLIST

This chapter addresses the managerial functions of staffing and scheduling and asserts that skills in both functions are needed by the manager to maintain unit productivity and patient staff satisfaction.

- The nurse manager must consider the following external variables when developing the personnel budget and staffing plan:
  - State licensing regulations
  - JCAHO and other regulatory agency standards
  - ANA and other standards
  - Consumer expectations
- The nurse manager must also consider the following internal variables when preparing the budget and the unit staffing plan:
  - Organizational staffing policies
  - Structure and philosophy of the nursing services department
  - Organizational support services
  - Changes in services and programs
  - Projected units of service
- When forecasting the personnel needs for the unit, the nurse manager must consider the following:
  - The staffing model of the unit
  - The skill mix of the nursing staff
  - The number of positions and FTEs needed to meet the anticipated units of service
  - The amount of nonproductive paid-benefit time allotted to each staff member
  - Patient Outcomes
  - Availability of Resources
- When constructing the unit schedule, the nurse manager must consider the following:
  - Unit hours of operation
  - Shift or weekend rotations required in the unit
  - Approved paid time off for vacations, holidays, or other benefit hours
  - Staffing vacancies
  - Availability of automation
  - Organizational policies on overtime and use of agency personnel
- When evaluating unit productivity, the nurse manager should consider the following:
  - Acuity trends identified through patient classification systems
  - Labor cost per unit of service
  - Periodic unit activity reports

TIPS FOR STAFFING AND SCHEDULING

- Know state and federal laws regarding staffing and voluntary accreditation (professional society and institutional) standards for staffing.
- Understand current demands for staff and anticipate externally imposed changes, such as services offered, availability of registered nurses, and licensed practical/vocational nurses.
- Value the various responses to short staffing from the manager, staff, and patient perspectives.
- Understand the complexity of staffing issues and how they relate to staff satisfaction, community perception, budget, and accreditation standards.
  - Correlate structure and outcome indicators to assess effectiveness of staffing plans

TERMS TO KNOW

activity or productivity report
average daily census (ADC)
average length of stay
cost center
factor evaluation system
fixed FTEs
forecast
full-time equivalent (FTE)
labor cost per unit of service
master staffing plan
nonproductive time
percentage of occupancy
productive time
productivity report
prototype evaluation system
scheduling
staffing
staffing model
staffing regulations
units of service
variable FTEs
variance report
workload

REFERENCES

American Nurses Association. (2005). *Principles for nurse staffing.* Washington, DC: American Nurses Association.

American Nurses Association. (2000a, June 28). *ANA house of delegates sends strong message on mandatory overtime and nurse staffing* (press release). Washington, DC: American Nurses Association.

American Nurses Association. (2000b, May 2). *New ANA study provides more proof of link between RN staffing and quality patient care* (press release). Washington, DC: American Nurses Association.

Artz, M. (2005). The politics of caring: Setting nurse-patient ratios: ANA bill calls for development of staffing systems in hospitals. *American Journal of Nursing, 105*(5), 97.

Burke, T. A., McKee, J. R., Wilson, H. C., Donahue, R. M. J., Batenhorst, A. S., & Pathak, D. S. (2000). A comparison of time-and-motion and self-reporting methods of work measurement. *Journal of Nursing Administration, 30*(3), 118–125.

Clarke, S. P. (2005). The policy implications of staffing-outcomes research. *Journal of Nursing Administration, 35*(1), 17-19.

Graf, C. M., Millar, S., Feilteau, C., Coakley, P. J., & Erickson, J. I. (2003). Patients' needs for nursing care: Beyond staffing ratios. *Journal of Nursing Administration, 33*(2), 76-81.

Health Care Advisory Board. (1999). *Hardwiring for service excellence.* Washington, DC: Health Care Advisory Board.

Joint Commission on Accreditation of Health Care Organizations. (2001, January 11). *Joint commission to develop a new approach to assessing the effectiveness of staffing in health care organizations* (press release). Oakbrook Terrace, IL: Joint Commission on Accreditation of Health Care Organizations.

Joint Commission on Accreditation of Health Care Organizations, Section 2, Human Resources. (2005). *CAMH: Comprehensive accreditation manual for hospitals: The official handbook.* Oakbrook Terrace, IL: Joint Commission on Accreditation of Health Care Organizations.

Kramer, M., & Schmalenberg, C. (2005). Revising the Essentials of Magnetism Tool: There is more to adequate staffing than numbers. *Journal of Nursing Administration, 35*(4), 188-198.

Mark, B. A., Harless, D. W., McCue, M., & Xu, Y. (2004). A longitudinal examination of hospital registered nurse staffing and quality of care. *Health Services Research, 39*(2), 279-300.

McCloskey, J., & Bulechek, G. (2000). *Nursing interventions classification (NIC)* (3rd ed.). St. Louis: Mosby.

Trossman, S. (2004). Move over eBay? A potential trend involving bidding for shifts online. *American Nurse, 36*(3), 1, 8, 12.

SUGGESTED READINGS

Aiken, L. H., & Patrician, P. A. (2000). Measuring organizational traits of hospitals: The revised nursing work index. *Nursing Research, 49*(3), 146-153.

Bolton, L. B., Aydin, C. E., Donaldson, N., Brown, D. S., Nelson, M. S., & Harms, D. (2003). Nurse staffing and patient perceptions of nursing care. *Journal of Nursing Administration, 33*(11), 607-614.

Brooten, D., Youngblut, J., Blais, K., Donahue, D., Cruz, I., & Lightbourne, M. (2005). APN-physician collaboration in caring for women with high risk pregnancies. *Journal of Nursing Scholarship, 37*(2), 178-184.

Carter, M. R. (2004). Recruitment & retention report. The ABCs of staffing decisions. *Nursing Management, 35*(6), 16.

Connelly, L. M. (2005). Welcoming new employees. *Journal of Nursing Scholarship, 37*(2), 163-164.

Day, G. R. (2004). Is there a relationship between 12-hour shifts and job satisfaction in nurses? *Alabama Nurse, 31*(2), 11-12.

Hall, L. M., Doran, D., Baker, G. R., Pink, G. H., Sidani, S., O'Brien-Pallas, L., & Donner, J. (2003). Nurse staffing models as predictors of patient outcomes. *Medical Care, 41*(9), 1096-1109.

Hall, L. M., Doran, D., & Pink, G. H. (2004). Nurse staffing models, nursing hours, and patient safety outcomes. *Journal of Nursing Administration, 34*(1), 41-45.

Hart, S. E. (2005). Ethical climates and registered nurses' turnover intentions. *Journal of Nursing Scholarship, 37*(2), 173-177.

Hodge, M. B., Romano, P. S., Harvey, D., Samuels, S. J., Olson, V. A., Sauve, M. J., & Kravitz, R. L. (2004). Licensed caregiver characteristics and staffing in California acute care hospital units. *Journal of Nursing Administration, 34*(3), 125-133.

Hoffman, A. J., & Scott, L. D. (2003). Role stress and career satisfaction among registered nurses by work shift patterns. *Journal of Nursing Administration, 33*(6), 337-342.

Kaestner, R. (2005). An overview of public policy and the nursing shortage. *Journal of Nursing Administration, 35*(1), 8-9.

Lang, T. A., Hodge, M., Olson, V., Romano, P. S., & Kravitz, R. L. (2004). Nurse-patient ratios: a systematic review on the effects of nurse staffing on patient, nurse employee, and hospital outcomes. *Journal of Nursing Administration, 34*(7/8), 326-337.

Page, J. S. (2005). Nurse staffing and outcomes: Differentiating care delivery by education preparation. *Journal of Nursing Administration, 35*(1), 7.

Prater, M., & Getzoyan, T. (2005). Lessons learned: Safe scheduling practices for nursing staff. *Voice of Nursing Leadership, 3*(4), 4-5.

Rambur, B., McIntosh, B., Palumbo, M. V., & Reinier, K. (2005). Education as a determinant of career retention and job satisfaction among registered nurses. *Journal of Nursing Scholarship, 37*(2), 185-192.

Ray, C. E., Jagim, M., Agnew, J., McKay, J., & Sheehy, S. (2003). ENA's new guidelines for determining emergency department nurse staffing. *Journal of Emergency Nursing, 29*(3), 245-253.

Richie, K., & Peeler, C. (2005). R&R report. Plug into success with centralized flex staffing. *Nursing Management, 36*(2), 18.

Sadovich, J. M. (2005). Work excitement in nursing: An examination of the relationship between work excitement and burnout. *Nursing Economics, 23*(2), 91-96.

Sasichay-Akkadechanunt, T., Scalzi, C. C., & Jawad, A. F. (2003). The relationship between nurse staffing and patient outcomes. *Journal of Nursing Administration, 33*(9), 478-485.

Spetz, J. (2005). Public policy and nurse staffing: What approach is best? *Journal of Nursing Administration, 35*(1), 14-16.

Spetz, J. (2004). California's minimum nurse-to-patient ratios: The first few months. *Journal of Nursing Administration, 34*(12), 571-578.

Spetz, J. (2004). Hospital nurse wages and staffing, 1977 to 2002: Cycles of shortage and surplus. *Journal of Nursing Administration, 34*(9), 415-422.

Unruh, L. Y. (2005). Employment conditions at the bedside: A cause of and solution to the RN shortage. *Journal of Nursing Administration, 35*(1), 11-14.

Unruh, L. Y. (2003). The effect of LPN reductions on RN patient load. *Journal of Nursing Administration, 33*(4), 201-208.

Unruh, L. Y., Fottler, M. D., & Talbott, L. L. (2003). Improving nurse staffing measures: Discharge day measurement in "adjusted patient days of care." *Inquiry, 40*(3), 295-304.

Weinstein, S. M., & Antonova, S. (2003). International perspectives. Enhancing nurse-physician collaboration: A staffing innovation. *Journal of Nursing Administration, 33*(4), 193-195.

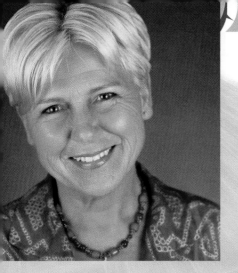

Chapter 14

Selecting, Developing, and Evaluating Staff

Diane M. Twedell

Individual employees need to understand clearly what is expected of them. Emphasis is placed on the selection interview and the importance of the orientation process for new staff. Role theory is a useful organizing framework for the manager and the employee to follow throughout all aspects of role performance. Effective communication of roles and role expectations among all members can facilitate improved performance, increased worker satisfaction, and most importantly, improved quality of care delivered. The role of the manager as a coach who empowers employees to grow as followers and develop their leadership skills in a learning environment is explored.

Objectives

- Relate concepts of role theory to position descriptions.
- Distinguish key points for the interview of a potential employee.
- Apply current philosophies of performance appraisal to a variety of situations.
- Differentiate five appraisal strategies.
- Examine specific guidelines for performance feedback.
- Evaluate components of the coaching process to develop followers.

Questions to Consider

- What is your role at work? at home? at school?
- How do you deal with conflict in these roles?
- How does a manager select and hire the right person for a position?
- How does a manager coach staff and create a learning environment?
- How does a manager empower staff members?
- What are some of your assumptions about performance appraisals?
- What type of appraisal methods are you familiar with?
- How would you improve performance appraisals?
- What do you believe empowers you to improve your performance?

The Challenge

Linda Gates, RN, BSN
Clinical Nurse Manager, Memorial Hospital, Colorado Springs, Colorado

The nursing units were tasked with improving evaluations for all nurses. The staff wanted more specific guidelines that validated competencies that were unique to their units. They also wanted professional recognition of their work on various committees with the hospital and activities within local, state, and national organizations. The managers were challenged to develop an improved and more comprehensive evaluation method that would incorporate the overall goals of the organization, evaluate the competencies critical to each specific nursing unit, and serve to develop the professionalism of the staff.

 What do you think you would do if you were this nurse?

INTRODUCTION

Healthcare delivery systems are businesses that are economically driven. Whether the setting is inpatient or outpatient, the emphasis is on providing the highest quality care at an affordable price. The nurse manager is a key individual whose leadership can directly influence many environmental functions. Kleinman (2004) indicates that effective leadership styles of nurse managers enhance staff nurse retention. Other functions begin with the selection of the right person for the right position and having the manager function in the role of coach. As a coach, the nurse manager can assist and encourage employees to perform at their highest levels in an empowered and self-directed manner. The nurse manager also functions to clarify the organization's mission and expectations.

The role of follower cannot be overrated! A strong patient-care unit has both effective leadership and team members who understand their role in meeting the goals for quality patient care. Professional healthcare providers must clearly understand what is expected of their performance, including the ramifications of not meeting those expectations. This performance can be achieved only when all members of the organization have clearly defined roles and overall objectives. Ambiguous roles are more detrimental to role performance and employee work satisfaction than conflict within the role.

ROLE CONCEPTS AND THE POSITION DESCRIPTION

The acquisition of a role requires an individual to assume the personal, as well as the formal, expectations of a specified role or position. Many individuals function within multiple roles. As discussed in the Theory box, **role theory** provides an appreciable framework for the development and evaluation of staff. Today's professional nurse is often a parent, spouse, and community volunteer and maintains full-time employment outside the home. Many skills are necessary for each role. In addition, the role-taker (i.e., the individual actually performing the role) has specified performance objectives within the social context in which the role is enacted. The social context includes the physical and social environment. Acquisition of the role is time-dependent; individuals apply their life experiences.

Role ambiguity in the workplace creates an environment for misunderstanding and hinders effective communication. In this situation, individuals do not have a clear understanding of what is expected of their performance or how they will be evaluated. In contrast, **role conflict** is easier to recognize. Employees know what is expected of them, but they are either unwilling or unable to meet the requirements.

Employees must have clear role expectations and perceive that their contributions are valued. Empowerment and control for certain aspects of

Theory Box

ROLE THEORY

THEORY/CONTRIBUTOR	KEY IDEAS	APPLICATION TO PRACTICE
Role Theory and Role Dynamics in Organizations Kahn et al. (1964) developed this theory.	Roles within organizations affect an individual's interactions with others. Acquisition of these roles is time-dependent and varies based on individual experiences and value systems. For effective communication to take place, role expectations for performance must be understood by all individuals involved.	The role of the professional nurse is complex. Role acquisition, role clarity, and role performance are enhanced by the use of clear position descriptions and evaluation standards.

the environment have been linked to increased personal health, job satisfaction, and individual performance. They are then more likely to be committed to the organization and to provide a higher level of patient care. These principles are applicable to both managers and staff members. A consistent focus on developing staff creates a learning environment directed toward excellence.

Acquisition of the role is time-dependent; individuals apply their life experiences to each role and interpret the role within their own value system. As roles become more complex, the individual may take longer to assimilate the components of each particular role. Nursing graduates enter the profession with various levels of educational and life experiences. The nurse manager plays an integral role in assisting these individuals in the development and acquisition of the complex role of the professional nurse. The important thing to remember is that role-development evolves over time and with consideration to individual needs. Coaching is a technique that the manager can use to facilitate individual development; this technique is discussed later in this chapter within the context of performance appraisal.

The position description provides written guidelines detailing the roles and responsibilities of a specific position within the organizational context. The position description reflects functions and obligations of a specific work position. It is a contract for the individual that describes responsibilities of the work assignment, as well as to whom the individual reports.

The position description should reflect current practice guidelines for individuals and may have competency-based requirements. As paradigms of nursing delivery systems shift to the home and community, professional nurses must have a clear understanding of the performance that is expected. The nurse is also responsible for clearly understanding the position descriptions of the paraprofessionals to whom care is delegated. Clear and concise position descriptions for all employees are extremely important because they provide the basis for roles within the organization. Example statements from a position description for a staff nurse in the emergency room appear in Box 14-1.

Exercise 14-1

Obtain a position description for a registered nurse from a community nursing service and a hospital. Compare them. Analyze the general categories (e.g., communication, and responsibilities) and the specific behaviors. What competencies do you already have? How will you develop other competencies? What are common competencies for registered nurses?

BOX 14-1

Excerpts From a Position Description

- Responsible for the provision of direct patient care to all age groups
- Must have current certification in advanced cardiac life support (ACLS) and pediatric advanced life support (PALS)
- Required to accurately assess and prioritize patient-care needs and delegate care appropriately to paraprofessionals, including LPNs/LVNs (licensed practical nurses/licensed vocational nurses) and EMTs (emergency medical technicians)
- Responsible for therapeutic communication to patients, families, and staff

SELECTING STAFF

The selection of staff would seem to be a relatively simple process. The manager wants the most qualified individual for the position. Choosing the right individual is the challenge! Clinical skills are important; however, a manager needs to hire individuals who "make good nurses, not just good clinicians" (Nelson, 2004, p. 36). Health care is centered on caring for people, and nurses with appropriate people skills are essential for producing satisfied patients and families. Kelly (2004, p. 6) states "during the interview process, nurse managers must identify those candidates who possess the professional and personal values that are compatible with the organization's values." For example, if an applicant values that the needs of the patient come first and this value is also articulated via the organization, they have similar values related to the work of the organization. The applicant and the manager must agree on what defines quality care and the manner in which it should be delivered. The manager must also decide whether members of the existing staff are to be included in the screening and interview process for new employees. The following guidelines are suggestions for the manager and staff, as well as for the prospective employee.

The manager's focus before and during the interview is to be prepared and have well-thought-out questions. The environment should be comfortable and provide privacy without interruptions. The interview questions can be related to the applicant's previous experience or be directed to evaluate values and critical-thinking skills. This may be accomplished by asking the applicant to describe his or her reactions to challenging situations previously experienced. Questions may link to behavioral competencies that lead to a successful nurse including: judgment, sensitivity, teamwork, quality-orientation, critical-thinking, and communication (Nelson, 2004). A question related to teamwork in an interview could be, "Tell me about a time when you were working in a group and there were problems with other individuals who were not pulling their weight. What did you do to maintain a team environment?"

Technical skills, such as specific certifications, are also important for the work environment and, therefore, also must be discussed or validated. The applicant may be given a case study to read and discuss with the interviewer. The case study could describe a situation for the unit in which the applicant is being interviewed; it could also contain content that would require the applicant to prioritize the care of one patient or a group of patients. Nelson indicates that the case study simulation can assist managers in assessing the candidate for both behavioral and clinical competencies (2004).

Questions from the applicant should be answered honestly. Kelly (2004, p. 6) notes that "it is essential that during the interviewing process the interviewer give the potential candidates a clear picture of what will be expected of them." A tour of the unit and a review of the position description are helpful to give the applicant information about the expectations of the role. Staff members also may be included in the interview and can provide information to the applicant as appropriate. The Research Perspective points out that recruitment of nurses is related to positive work experiences; that is what the applicant is looking for. At the conclusion of the interview, it is important for the nurse manager to clarify concrete issues. Offering details regarding who will contact the applicant with the decision and whether it will be via personal phone call or written letter is important (Iacono, 2004). Thank the applicant for the interview, and end the interview on a positive note.

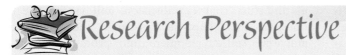

Research Perspective

Cameron, S., Armstrong-Stassen, M., Bergeron, S., & Out, J. (2004). Recruitment and retention of nurses: Challenges facing hospital and community employees. *Nursing Leadership, 17*(3), 79-92.

This exploratory study examined nurses' perceptions of their work experiences in both hospitals and community settings using selected Magnet™ characteristics. Mail surveys were completed by 1248 nurses in Canada. Multiple research-proven scales were used to measure organizational factors, participation in decision-making, nurse–physician relationships, support from co-workers, autonomy and control, job challenge, work demands, fair treatment, work schedule, and satisfaction with career. Nurses working in community settings were more satisfied with their workplaces than hospital nurses. Lack of perceived organizational support was noted in both community and hospital nursing settings.

IMPLICATIONS FOR PRACTICE

It is essential to address nurses' concerns about their work environments. Nurse managers and their staff need to work continuously toward creating a more positive work experience. Shared decision-making and being respected for nursing's contribution is vital to recruitment and retention of nursing staff.

The applicant also has responsibilities in preparation for the employment interview. It is important to be on time and appropriately dressed. Conservative dress is always acceptable. A uniform is not necessary and usually not even preferable. First impressions may be lasting impressions. Previous review of the organization's goals and mission statement, as well as a review of the **position description** for which the interview is being conducted, is also appropriate. The applicant should be prepared to answer each question honestly and thoughtfully. It is equally important to the prospective employee to make the right decisions as it is to the employer. The manager and the applicant must have a clear understanding of the values and organizational goals for nursing care for a good fit within the role to occur. The applicant should focus on the topic and avoid irrelevant conversations. The individual must prepare in advance for any questions that might be discussed. In addition to describing previous situations and how they were handled, the applicant may be asked to describe personal strengths and weaknesses. At the end of the interview, the applicant should thank the manager for his or her time and verify when the selection will be made and how it will be communicated. It is also appropriate to send the manager a brief note of appreciation for the interview. Preparing for and participating in interviews appear in Chapter 27.

Developing Staff

Once the interview and offer are completed and an applicant has accepted the position, orientation should be planned. Orientation to the organization usually is a structured program that is generally applicable to all new employees. It may include outlining the mission, benefits, safety programs, and other specific topics. Orientation to the work area usually depends on the specialty area involved, the skills that need to be verified, and the environment itself. Every individual brings various experiences and skills to a new position. A nurse manager will assist new employees by advising them about educational programs and experiences that will aid in their entry to the organization. It is imperative that the orientation period be used efficiently for both the employee and the organization. Orientation is a very expensive endeavor for the organization. Baggot, Hensinger, Parry, Valdes, and Zaim (2005, p. 139) note that RN turnover is costly and that "this includes $15,000 in direct costs for hiring and orientation based on an 8 week orientation."

Orientation can accomplish a variety of things. It is a time for new employees to learn the work environment and the staff. Many institutions provide preceptors, who are considered to be expert clinicians and resources. Hensinger, Minerath, Parry, and Robertson (2004, p. 268) stated that "nurse preceptors add significant value to the health care community." Preceptors teach newly hired nurses in the clinical setting. In some settings, the Kolb (1985) Learning Style Inventory (LSI) may be administered to new employees and the information then shared with the preceptors and the new employees. When preceptors understand the learning styles of new employees, a better focus for implementation of the orientation goals is provided. After learning styles have been identified, new employees work with preceptors who understand specifically how to address the individualized learning needs of new employees in a manner that enhances learning.

Continued development of the staff is a unique role for the nurse manager. It is a challenge to merge a group of individuals with varying levels of expertise and experience. If the focus is centered on professional socialization and development, a common thread will "weave" itself throughout all employees. That common thread may be a particular philosophy of care delivery, further development of critical-thinking skills for a specific specialty, or political activities in which members are involved. Some units encourage a monthly journal club or a brief presentation by employees to summarize information learned from a conference. One nursing unit could send a staff member to monthly open meetings of the state board of nursing. This staff member then could give a summary of the report of the meeting to the rest of the staff—an exciting way to keep informed of the role of professional nursing.

Empowerment strategies are useful for individual professional development, as well as overall staff development. Empowerment is a process that acknowledges the values and judgment of individu-

als and trusts that their decisions will be the correct ones. In this chapter's Challenge and Solution, employee self-development and professional empowerment were the results of intervention.

For an individual to feel empowered, the environment must be open and individuals must feel safe to explore and develop their own potential. O'Connor (2004, p. 3) states that "keeping the door open to new learning, attending to self, family, and friends and finding occasions to teach or mentor new nurses and leaders are at the core of professional and personal life." The organizational environment must allow individuals the freedom of making decisions while retaining the accountability for the consequences of those decisions. Management must release control to followers so that they might perform work more effectively, individually, and as a team. Specific environmental challenges and situations can influence employee attitudes, feelings of empowerment, and performance within roles. These challenges can affect commitment to the organization and individual work satisfaction. Positive feedback or coaching, achievement recognition, and support for new ideas may enhance employee feelings of empowerment and their ability to perform effectively.

One strategy for staff empowerment includes providing timely feedback for performance contributions, not simply during the annual **performance appraisal.** Supporting the implementation of innovative ideas and providing opportunities for mentoring relationships are also valuable approaches for the manager and staff. Many organizations use shared governance as a guide for accountability. A premise of shared governance is that power, control, and decision-making can empower staff and enhance individual and group accountability.

PERFORMANCE APPRAISALS

Providing feedback to employees regarding their performance is one of the strongest rewards an organization can provide. Performance appraisals are individual evaluations of work performance. Ideally, evaluations are conducted on an ongoing basis, not at the conclusion of a predetermined period. Evaluations, however, are usually done annually and also may be required after a scheduled orientation period for new employees. Chandra and Frank (2004) note that performance appraisals can serve to motivate employees and improve their performance.

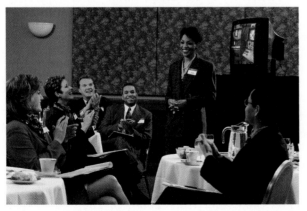

Providing off-site learning opportunities can help staff know they are valued.

The process of providing feedback, for either above-average or below-average performance, is best received at a time closest to the incidents being evaluated. The actual appraisal is sometimes viewed as a negative experience. Many nurse managers perceive the appraisal as a time-consuming process of endless paperwork. Instead, nurse managers should embrace the appraisal process as a key time for assisting with staff development. The performance appraisal process can assist in correcting current performance and stimulate improvement, be used for wage/salary and personnel issues, and promote improved career planning (Chandra & Frank, 2004). Appraisals should be designed so that they can be supported in court, should the need arise. Court decisions can be made based on the evidence, or lack of evidence, presented in the evaluation instrument. Consider, for example, the individual who has been fired for reasons of poor work performance. The employee must be provided written notice that performance is unsatisfactory, and that notice must specify what the employee must accomplish for satisfactory performance. This simple condition can make the difference for either the employee or the employer to justify the fairness for termination. Performance appraisals can be either formal or informal. Performance appraisals may also include personal and peer evaluations as well as managerial components.

An informal appraisal might be as simple as immediately praising the individual for performance recognized. A compliment from a family member or patient might be conveyed. Some units have a specific bulletin board for thank-you notes from patients and their families. Sometimes a simple "Thank you for all your hard work today!" can be extended from the manager to the staff. In addition, staff members have a responsibility to show the manager their appreciation and give positive and negative feedback.

The formal performance appraisal involves written documentation according to specific organization guidelines. Whether the evaluation is informal or formal, it does not preclude interim evaluations. The primary reason for an interim evaluation is so that praise or corrections are made as close to an episode as possible.

Brief anecdotal notes entered into the employee's file on a regular basis are important. These anecdotal notes, when accumulated over time, provide a more accurate cumulative appraisal. The anecdotal note describes an occurrence, either favorable or unfavorable, in a brief and concise manner. The purpose is to assist the manager with information throughout an entire rating period.

These notes, combined with variance reporting, are another means of documenting employee performance and provide a more conclusive appraisal that reflects the entire rating period. Variance reporting identifies specific occurrences, based on benchmarks or specific standards. As an example, "The employee will have CPR certification by January 1." If the employee does not meet this deadline, a variance is recorded along with the specific circumstances or discipline planned.

Example of an Anecdotal Note: Nurse "Smith"

2/14/03: Patient (Samuel Karruthers) and family stated how much they appreciated Ms. Smith's nursing care during this hospitalization. Her coordination of rehabilitation services in a competent and caring manner decreased their anxiety and assisted them in learning what they needed to know for care in the home. Ms. Smith had the family demonstrate dressing changes and transfer techniques under her supervision to establish their confidence and competence in being able to care for the patient in their home. She made the patient feel "special," not like just another number. Compliment relayed to employee. [Note in employee's anecdotal record with a signature and date by nurse manager.]

Additional methods may also be incorporated into the performance appraisal in the form of competency assessment tools. These may include observation of daily work, case studies, exemplars, self assessment, mock events, presentations, return demonstrations, and quality improvement monitors (Wright, 1998). Integration of competency assessment data into the evaluation process further enhances the individual employee's sense of empowerment, as well as accountability for the evaluation process.

Coaching

The overall evaluative process can be enhanced if the manager employs the technique of coaching. **Coaching** is a process that involves the development of individuals within an organization. This coaching process is a personal approach in which the manager and the employee interact on a frequent and regular basis with the ultimate outcome that the employee performs at an optimum level. Coaching can be individual or may involve a team approach; when implemented in a planned and organized manner, it can promote team building and optimal performance of the employees. Coaching is a learned behavior for the nurse manager and takes time and effort to be developed. The rewards for both the employee and the nurse manager are significant; communication is enhanced, and the performance appraisal process is an active one between the employee and the manager.

Exercise 14-2

Select a partner. Observe some behavior and prepare an anecdotal note. Ask your partner for feedback about the content.

The formal performance appraisal usually involves some type of predetermined evaluation tool or instrument. The tool may be a simple one or may involve the integration of a variety of measuring methods. The instruments should reflect the philosophy of the organization and be as objective and specific regarding the employee's performance as possible. Numerous instruments and a variety of simple to complex scoring methods for each exist. The new employee must have a clear understanding of timing and the content of the appraisal tool at the onset of employment. The example in Box 14-2 illustrates a type of peer appraisal method in which a staff nurse could evaluate another staff nurse within the area-specific context of assessment documentation.

Exercise 14-3

Think back to your last performance appraisal, either in the clinical situation as a professional nurse or in the role of nursing student. Did you feel you were fairly and adequately evaluated? Were the comments reflective of your current practice and made by someone who had directly observed the care that you provided? What was the environment like for the interview? Were you comfortable with the evaluator? Was feedback given, both positive and negative? How did you feel at the conclusion of the interview? Taking the time to think about the answers to these questions might provide you insight and direction before your next performance appraisal interview.

The scoring procedures for evaluations can be as simple as satisfactory/unsatisfactory. A more complex scoring system that includes a numerical rating scheme (using a range of 1 to 4, with 1 meaning "rarely meets standards," to 4 meaning "always exceeds standards") also appears in Box 14-2. The results from the peer-review process are then summarized and incorporated into the manager's formal performance appraisal.

PERFORMANCE APPRAISAL TOOLS

The type of appraisal tool used is not as important as how it is used. A formal written tool may have specific guidelines or a more open-ended format. General topics may be addressed in an anecdotal or "incident" type of format. The tool or evaluation form should facilitate accurate appraisal of the

---

BOX 14-2

Peer Performance Appraisal, Staff Nurse

Area of Responsibility
Assessment/Diagnosis: Provides continuous holistic assessment to include physical, psychosocial, spiritual, and educational needs. Directs outcome criteria so that discharge plans are timely and optimum quality care is delivered.

a. Completes database (history/physical assessment) within 12 hours of admission   (Score 4)

b. Illustrates documentation reflective of continuous assessment per unit guidelines (e.g., neurovascular assessment of extremity following cardiac catheterization)   (Score 3)

c. Initiates plan of care according to critical path guidelines within 12 hours of admission   (Score 4)

d. Provides for safe environment   (Score 4) individual's performance and provide an opportunity to identify personal goals of the individual and goals of the organization.

There are primarily two categories of performance appraisal tools: structured and flexible. Table 14-1 summarizes examples of structured and flexible tools.

Structured Performance Appraisal Tools

Forced Distribution Scale   The forced distribution scale is a norm-referenced tool that prevents the evaluator from rating all individuals in the same manner. The evaluator is provided a schematic diagram and asked to rate the individual according to all individuals the manager evaluates. As depicted in Figure 14-1, the evaluator has indicated that the individual rated is in the top 10% of employees but is not the best employee. This scale also provides the employee with a brief visual picture of how this evaluator has ranked the individual's performance in reference to others. It further illustrates that this particular evaluator has an even distribution of

scores for the evaluation summary of all employees. This type of scale can undermine group cohesion and communication effectiveness by its very nature of rank-ordering individual performance. This employee should feel positive about the evaluation. In reality, however, the employee is likely to feel just the opposite. The employee can see how many other employees, above him or her on the scale, are perceived as being better. The forced distribution scale can also undermine morale and group cohesion, as well as stifle creativity or the uniqueness of the individual employee.

Graphic Rating Scales   Graphic rating scales are another example of a structured approach to evaluation. They comprise a numbering system that indicates high and low values for evaluating performance. The rating scale is popular because it is easy to construct and easy to use. Problems with this type of scale are that it lacks specificity and may promote a **halo or recent behavior bias effect**. Arnold and Pulich (2004, p. 228) describe the halo effect as "when a manager perceives one positive characteristic about an employee on his or her performance and generalizes it into an overall high rating." The same, but opposite, effect is known as the **horn effect**. The total person is seen as negative based on a negative characteristic or effect. The recent behavior bias occurs when "the rater remembers behavior primarily from the most recent event of the employee's performance period as opposed to the entire time period" (Arnold & Pulich, 2004, p. 268). For example, the employee performs in a satisfactory or less than satisfactory manner up until the month before the evaluation is due and then becomes "superemployee." If most of the information used for an evaluation is collected during the last month of the rating period, it may

Table 14-1 EXAMPLES OF STRUCTURED AND FLEXIBLE PERFORMANCE APPRAISAL TOOLS

Structured (Traditional Method)	Flexible (Collaborative Method)
Forced distribution	Behaviorally anchored scale rating scales (BARS)
Graphic rating scale	Management by objectives (MBO)
Rating scales	Peer review

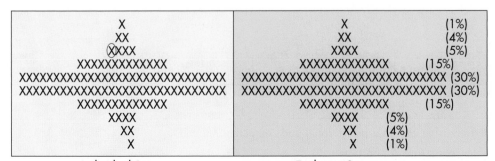

Figure 14-1   Forced distribution scale. X, Employee; ⊗, individual whom the employer is rating (evaluation history).

not accurately reflect the total performance. The evaluation then reflects the "best" behavior rather than behavior that occurred during the majority of time in the rating period. Supervisors tend to rate people the same from one rating period to the next. Thus, there is the potential for overinflation of the evaluation if the recent performance is all that is included.

Anecdotal notes compiled consistently over the entire rating period are a much more equitable method for providing an accurate summary of the employee's performance. Some managers use small notes with adhesive backs to place inside an employee's informal file to document behaviors quickly as situations warrant. A sheet of paper for notes placed in the front of each file would also serve the same purpose. The manager might also keep secured electronic data files for the same purpose. Security of the files, electronic or paper, is important to maintain confidentiality.

Rating Scales   Rating scales are relatively easy to construct and easy to complete (Table 14-2). On the downside, they usually consist of generalizations, not specific behaviors, and the rating is relatively subjective in nature. Some managers never give a "5," with the rationale that no employee always exceeds expectations.

Flexible Performance Appraisal Tools

The evaluation focus can also be conducted with a collaborative approach. How can the manager assist the individual to develop professionally?

Behaviorally Anchored Rating Scales   Behaviorally anchored rating scales (BARS) can be implemented as a collaborative or flexible approach. The focus is on behavior and should include

employees in the development. BARS combine ratings with critical incidents (specific examples that have occurred) or criterion references (examples usually based on standards of practice or competency-based standards). The criteria used for this scale are specific to the specialty of nursing delivered and preestablished outcomes. This scale is also considered more advantageous in terms of litigation. BARS describes the employee's performance both quantitatively and qualitatively. Staff who are involved in the development of these instruments are more likely to understand the importance of evaluation for each criterion selected and to have an understanding of their performance expectations. This is another example of clarification of roles and role expectations within the organization. The primary drawback of this scale is that it is expensive to develop and time consuming to implement; it must be designed for each specific position description or standard of practice. However, it provides the manager with concrete information regarding an employee's performance, with minimal subjective interference. Box 14-3 provides an example of how established nursing standards of practice, or protocols for practice, can be incorporated into the appraisal process using peer review. The data might also be used in an outcome review process as a component of a continuous quality-improvement program. The final result would be summarized by the manager and incorporated into the employee's performance appraisal.

Management by Objectives   One method that has been used for many years is management by objectives (MBO). Arnold and Pulich (2004, p. 229) state MBO "involves establishing performance goals jointly between the manager and the employee

Table 14-2   EXAMPLE OF A RATING SCALE

Criteria	Almost Never				Always Exceeds
1. Completes nursing care in a professional and competent manner	1	2	3	4	5
2. Is reliable; comes to work on time	1	2	3	4	5
3. Provides patient teaching as appropriate	1	2	3	4	5

BOX 14-3

Example of a Behaviorally Anchored Rating Scale

Emergency room (ER) staff nurse responsibilities for patient admitted with chest pain: (ER records evaluated per protocol; minimum 10/rating period). Met/Unmet
1. Vital signs recorded within 5 min of admission _____
2. Cardiac monitor, IV, lab tests, and ECG done within 15 min _____

3. If sublingual nitroglycerin given, vital signs recorded every 5 min for 30 min _____
   a. Chest pain changes evaluated per protocol _____
   b. Post–chest pain 12-lead ECG documented _____

for the upcoming appraisal period." Progress regarding the accomplishment of these goals is documented throughout the rating period. An MBO approach requires that the employee establishes clear and measurable objectives at the beginning of each rating period. Then, during the performance appraisal evaluation, both the employee and the manager address these objectives individually and in writing. In effect, the employee has created a "performance contract," as well as having defined goals for future professional performance. Box 14-4 illustrates goals and accomplishments.

Peer Review Peer review is also a flexible or contemporary strategy. If the guidelines are developed collaboratively, peer review may also be considered a developmental method of evaluation. That is, employees are involved in the development and implementation process. Nurses tend to function in their normal patterns in the presence of peers, and this can be a very solid rating method. However, it is important to obtain objective ratings based on performance, not subjective ratings based on personal friendships. This method should not be used if the manager is attempting to institute team-building strategies or if the unit is unstable and employees do not like each other. The employees must trust and respect each other to participate willingly in the peer appraisal process. Arnold and Pulich (2004, p. 231) state that, "Objectivity may suffer as some employees seek to sabotage the ratings of those they dislike or view as rivals for a future promotion."

Summary of Appraisal Instruments

Which instrument/method of appraisal is best? The missions and goals of the organization determine

BOX 14-4

Learning Goals and Accomplishments

Learning Goals
1. Prepare for and take advanced cardiac life support (ACLS) certification examination
2. Participate in shared governance committee as unit representative

Accomplishments (12 Months Later—Summary)
1. Successfully passed certification examination
2. Participated in monthly meetings; chaired task force for development and implementation of new delivery system; presented in-service class to staff on several units

the tools used. A combination of several tools is most likely superior to any one method. The primary success of any performance appraisal lies in the skills and communication abilities of the manager. It is also the manager's responsibility to educate employees about the process and tools for performance appraisals. Role ambiguity and uncertainty of standards of practice and methods for evaluation are significant contributors to decreased work satisfaction. The best-designed instrument will fail if the manager is ineffective and unable to communicate with the employee.

Exercise 14-4

Obtain a performance appraisal tool from the local healthcare organization from which you obtained a position description. Based on the descriptions provided, how would you characterize it? Is it structured or flexible? Is it quantitatively based, qualitatively based, or both? How does the tool reflect the position description?

Appraisal Interview Environment

The appraisal instrument is not the only factor in the evaluation process. Scheduling the appraisal in advance and allowing both parties to prepare for the appraisal is important (Feuer, 2003). The interview should be conducted professionally and in a positive manner. It is an ideal time for communication between the employee and the manager. There should be no interruptions, if possible. This time is important for clarification of employee and organizational goals. Evaluation of employee performance should be objective and nonemotional. The evaluation instruments should be clearly completed, and time should be allowed for discussion. Goals may be established. The manager and the employee should sign the appraisal forms, and each should be provided a copy. The effectiveness of the entire appraisal method relies on the manner in which the manager uses the tools and the feedback that the employee receives. Effective communication between the manager and employees can prevent potential performance problems on a unit. Specific behaviors by the manager enhance the actual appraisal process (Box 14-5).

Exercise 14-5

Find a partner. Using an audiotape recorder or a videotape recorder (preferred), conduct a performance appraisal. Seek feedback using the key behaviors in Box 14-5.

BOX 14-5

Key Behaviors for the Performance Appraisal Session

- Provide a quiet, controlled environment, without interruptions.
- Maintain a relaxed but professional atmosphere.
- Put the employee at ease; the overall objective is for the best job to be done.
- Review specific examples for both positive and negative behavior (keep an anecdotal file for each employee).
- Allow the employee to express opinions, verbally and in writing.

- Write future plans and goals, training needs, and such (a "performance contract" for the future).
- Set follow-up date as necessary to monitor improvements, if cited.
- Show the employee confidence in his or her performance.
- Be sincere and constructive in both praise and criticism.

The Solution

The managers decided to apply the performance appraisal principles and develop guidelines for comprehensive portfolio development. The clinical portfolio represents a strategy to manage and achieve quality outcomes. The planning and implementation of the portfolio included (1) analysis of existing evaluation components; (2) current institutional requirements (e.g., fire, safety, immunizations, certifications); (3) collaboration of the nurse manager committee and professional development committee; (4) integration of previous department-specific competency components; (5) evidence of continuing education; (6) peer-review evaluations; (7) personal notes from patients, families, and staff; and (8) a personal reflective self-evaluation.

The managers and staff believe that this comprehensive approach provides a more complete picture of the employee's performance for the entire rating period. Portfolio development is the responsibility of each employee and thus mandates employee accountability and responsibility for the inclusion of the information as listed above.

— Linda Gates

 Would this be a suitable approach for you? Why?

CHAPTER CHECKLIST

The manager plays a key role in the selection and development of staff. As a role model, the manager is also key in the establishment of the type of work environment that exists. Managers must be supportive and develop their staff to their highest potential. They must have accurate position descriptions and tools for evaluation of employee performance. These are integral to role development and professional socialization. Managers must also use various communication methods to empower their employees. Coaching and implementation of empowerment strategies positively contribute to overall staff performance as well.

- The interviewer should do the following:
  - Prescreen the applicants.
  - Prepare questions in advance.
  - Control the environment.
  - Provide role clarification.
  - Be a good listener.
  - Give honest answers to questions.
  - Provide closure.
  - Inform the applicant when he or she will be notified.
- The applicant should do the following:
  - Be on time and dressed appropriately.
  - Review the organization's mission and goals.
  - Prepare questions in advance.
  - Answer questions honestly and completely.
  - Note appreciation for the interview.
- Development of the staff includes the following:
  - Organized and efficient orientation
  - Plans for education, team building, and professional socialization

- Active coaching
- Implementation of empowerment strategies
- Development of accurate position descriptions and tools for evaluation of employees is integral to role development and professional socialization. Nurse managers should use various communication methods, including coaching techniques.
- Role theory describes how individuals perceive their position in an organization.
- Distinction and clarity among the various positions are imperative if partnerships in quality patient care are to exist.
  - The position description serves several purposes:
    - Provides written guidelines that describe roles and responsibilities
    - Reflects the position's overall function and obligations
    - Serves as a contract between manager and employee
    - Reflects current practice guidelines for the position
- Performance appraisals are a method of providing feedback to the employee in relation to individual performance.
  - Types of structured (traditional) performance appraisals include the following:
    - Forced distribution method
    - Graphic rating scales
    - Rating scale
  - Types of flexible (collaborative) performance appraisals include the following:
    - Behaviorally anchored rating scales (BARS)
    - Management by objective (MBO)
    - Peer review

TIPS FOR CONDUCTING AN INTERVIEW

- Prescreen the applicant and schedule a time for the interview.
- Prepare questions in advance. Be concise but thorough.
- Control the environment for noise and interruptions.
- Explain and clarify the role for which the applicant is interviewing.
- Be a good listener.
- Answer questions honestly.

- Inform the applicant when he or she will be informed of the decision.

TERMS TO KNOW

coaching
empowerment
halo or recent behavior bias effect
horn effect
performance appraisal
position description
role ambiguity
role conflict
role theory

REFERENCES

Arnold, E., & Pulich, M. (2003). Personality conflicts and objectivity in appraising performance. *Health Care Manager, 22*(3), 227-232.

Baggot, D., Hensinger, B., Parry, J., Valdes, M., & Zaim, S. (2005). The new hire/preceptor experience: Cost benefit analysis on one retention strategy. *Journal of Nursing Administration, 33*(9), 468-477.

Cameron, S., Armstrong-Stassen, M., Bergeron, S., & Out, J. (2004). Recruitment and retention of nurses: Challenges facing hospital and community employers. *Nursing Economics, 22*(5), 231-239.

Chandra, A., & Frank, Z. (2004). Utilization of performance appraisal systems in health care organizations and improvement strategies for supervisors. *The Health Care Manager, 23*(1), 25-39.

Feuer, L. (2003). The management challenge: Making the best of your next performance appraisal. *Case Manager, 14*(5), 22-24.

Heinsinger, B., Minerath, S., Parry, J., & Robertson, K. (2004). Asset protection: Maintaining and retaining your workforce. *Journal of Nursing Administration, 34*(6), 268-272.

Iacono, M. (2004). The selection process: Interview tips for nurse managers. *Journal of PeriAnesthesia Nursing, 19*(5), 345-347.

Kahn, R. L., Wolfe, D. M., Quinn, R. P., Snoek, J. D., & Rosenthal, R. A. (1964). *Occupational stress: Studies in role conflict and ambiguity.* New York: Wiley.

Kelly, D. (2004). Improving nurse managers' interviewing skills. *Journal of Nursing Administration, 34*(1), 6-8.

Kleinman, C. S. (2004). Leadership: A key strategy in staff nurse retention. *The Journal of Continuing Education in Nursing, 35*(3), 128-132.

Kolb, D. A. (1985). *Learning-style inventory.* Boston: McBer.

McGillis Hall, L., Waddell, J., Donner, G., & Wheeler, M. M. (2004). Outcomes of a career planning and development program for registered nurses. *Nursing Economics, 22*(3), 227-232.

Nelson, G. (2004). Hiring the complete nurse: Selecting the right nurses means looking beyond clinical skills. *Nurse Leader, August,* 36-39.

O'Connor, M. (2004). Strategic planning for career development. *Journal of Nursing Administration, 34*(1), 1-3.

Wright, D. (1998). *The ultimate guide to competency assessment in health care* (2nd ed.). Eau Claire, WI: PESI Health Care.

SUGGESTED READINGS

Kalisch, K. (2003). Recruiting nurses: The problem is the process. *Journal of Nursing Administration, 33*(9), 468-477.

Lauer, C. S. (2004). How to land the best. *Modern Health Care, 34*(3), 26.

Maxwell, M. (2004). Recruitment realities: Building a HR/nursing partnership. *Nursing Economics, 22*(2), 86-87.

Part 3

Changing the Status Quo

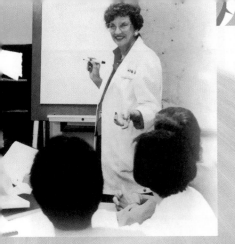

Chapter

15

Strategic Planning, Goal-Setting, and Marketing

Darlene Steven

This chapter discusses the application of several organizational elements of planning for the future, such as the strategic planning process, goal-setting, management by objectives, and marketing. Examples of planning and marketing strategies used in the healthcare field are presented when appropriate.

Objectives

- Value the importance of environmental assessment.
- Explain the planning process.
- Inter-relate the purpose of a mission statement, a philosophy, goals, and objectives.
- Describe goal-setting and strategic planning.

- Describe the process of strategic planning in establishing an entrepreneurial business in the healthcare field.

- Value the importance of marketing plans in the healthcare field.

Questions to Consider

- How is the strategic plan used to implement change in an organization?
- How do the mission statement, philosophy, goals, and objectives merge with the strategic plan of the facility?
- How can you influence the direction of your organization by effective planning?
- If you had a "vision" of where your facility should be directed in the future, how would you go about making your vision a reality?

The Challenge

Tim Porter-O'Grady, RN, PhD, FAAN
Senior Partner, Tim Porter-O'Grady Associates, Inc., and Associate Professor, Emory University,
   Atlanta, Georgia

As the nurse manager on the medical surgical unit, I was dealing with an unmotivated and "burned out" staff. They could only complain about the workload and the increasing demands that the organization was placing on their shoulders. They felt no one cared and that things were out of control. The staff believed that management was making decisions about their work and lives and they had no role to play in it. I had done everything I could to motivate them but found they still complained and exhibited no accountability for what was happening. I sensed the staff felt impotent and passive.

 What do you think you would do if you were this nurse?

The current healthcare system is in a state of change. The pressure to contain costs in health care has resulted in major reforms. Restructuring of our healthcare system includes patient empowerment; comprehensive and coordinated service delivery; efficient and effective use of resources, manpower, and technology; and emphasis on health promotion and prevention. The demographics of our society are also in a state of change and include a dramatic increase in the elderly population.

Nurses have the opportunity to make a difference by planning new strategies for the future and by influencing the direction of health care. As nurses, our new paradigm shift is about embracing technology. We must be proactive in our use of it so that we may become active in its development. Only by fearlessly adopting and using new technologies can we garner the expertise and earn the credibility to serve as advisors, directors, and influencers of technology. Only by influencing technology can we ensure that it will be used to meet nursing's information needs, to advance nursing practice, and to ensure nursing's continued viability. In short, where twenty-first century technology is concerned, it is embraced or replaced (Redd & Kongstevedt, 2004).

Proactive simply means "aggressive planning," which provides direction for one's efforts and toward which others must then react. Thus, greater control is possible so that the preferred future becomes a probability, not just a possibility. The importance of proactive, thoughtful, deliberate planning in the face of uncertainties cannot be overstated. Proactive means that every person in the organization must manage their work and their professional lives and how they relate to the organization's goals and missions.

In this chapter, the strategic planning process takes on significance. Planning is followed by an introduction to goal-setting and management by objectives. The key concepts of marketing as it relates to the healthcare industry are discussed. When appropriate and feasible, examples of planning and marketing strategies used in the healthcare field are presented as case studies.

STRATEGIC PLANNING

Definition

Strategic planning is a process that is designed to encompass the organization's emphasis on mission statements, strategic action plans, changes in policies and procedures, environmental factors affecting the organization, and the development of new services.

The strategic planning process shown in Figure 15-1 consists of the following series of steps:

- Search of the environment to determine those forces or changes that may affect the work of the organization or that may be crucial to its survival
- Appraisal of the organization's strengths and weaknesses and its potential for dealing with change
- Appraisal of major environmental opportunities and threats in light of the organization's capacity

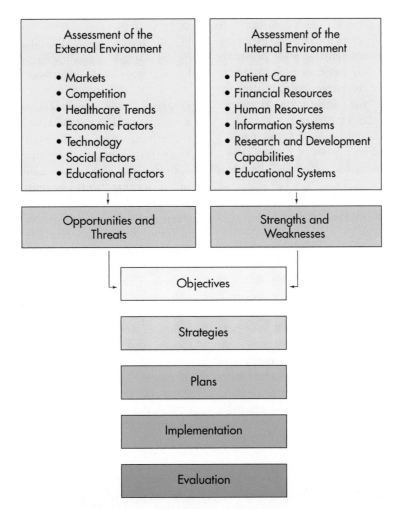

Figure 15-1   Key steps in strategic planning.

- Identification and evaluation of the various strategies available to the organization to meet these opportunities and threats
- Selection of the best option that balances the organization's potential with the challenges of changing conditions, taking into account the values of its management and its social responsibilities
- Preparation of the strategy
- Implementation and evaluation of the strategy

Reasons for Planning

To survive the ongoing change and restructuring of the healthcare system, thoughtful and deliberate planning becomes a necessity. This process leads to success in the achievement of goals and objectives, gives meaning to work life, and provides direction for operational activities of the organization. Furthermore, planning may result in efficient and effective use of resources and may assist in the formulation of visionary activities and the future direction of the agency. There are numerous reasons why nursing administrators should plan in a systematic manner: Knowledge regarding philosophy, goals, and external and internal operations of the organization are necessary; an understanding of the planning process is essential; and time must be divided based on day-to-day operations rather than on short- and long-range plans.

Phases of the Strategic Planning Process

The strategic planning process is proactive, vision-directed, action-oriented, creative, innovative, and oriented toward change. "Health care providers increasingly are relying on strategic planning to guide the allocation of capital and other resources. Strategic planning helps identify and prioritize opportunities for financial improvement, particularly revenue-generating initiatives, which offer the greatest opportunities for significant long-term benefits" (Zuckerman, 2000, p. 54).

The term *strategic planning process* usually entails the development of a plan of action covering 3 to 5 years. The initial phase is the most difficult.

Phase 1: Assessment of the External and Internal Environment

External Environmental Assessment   Assessment of the external environment is the initial phase in the strategic-planning process. The economic, demographic, technologic, social, educational, and political factors are assessed in terms of their impact on opportunities and threats within the environment. Healthcare managers can assess the effect of competitors on their environment and thus plan and monitor their own operations and develop other creative and visionary programs. An example appears in Box 15-1.

Exercise 15-1

What is your opinion about the economic situation in the city in which you live? What are the demographics of the area? What are the educational resources?

Internal Environmental Assessment   The internal assessment of the environment includes a review of the effectiveness of the structure, size, programs, financial resources, human resources, information systems, and research and development capabilities of the organization. The management team involves all levels of staff in this process and focuses on the purpose of the organization; the mission; the capabilities, skills, and relationships of various professional and related staff; and the weaknesses and strengths of staff in such areas as leadership, planning, coordination, research, and staff development.

Phase 2: Review of Mission Statement, Philosophy, Goals, and Objectives

Mission Statement   A mission statement reflects the purpose and direction of the healthcare agency or a department within it. A statement of philosophy provides direction for the agency and/or depart-

---

BOX 15-1

An Example of Environmental Assessment

A rural northern community is undertaking a study to examine accessibility, availability, quality, and effectiveness of primary, secondary, and tertiary cardiac and cancer services provided to patients. One of the initial steps is to conduct an environmental scan. The factors taken into consideration include the following:

- Economic forces and the escalating rates of healthcare costs
- The numbers and types of health professionals, including shortages of adequately trained cardiologists, radiologists, physicists, internists, and family physicians
- Shortages of nurse practitioners, nurses, radiation therapists, and technicians
- The social, political, and regulatory forces, including strategic priorities of the government in health promotion and disease prevention
- The diagnostic services available, including magnetic

resonance imaging (MRI) and nuclear diagnostic imaging
- Therapeutic capabilities (gene therapy, chemotherapy, radiation therapy, chelation, and laser therapy)

Patient Trends
- Demographic and population trends (population, employment, socioeconomic indicators, education, ethnicity, and lifestyle issues, with particular emphasis on minority groups)
- Trends in health care (increased emphasis on wellness programs and enhanced technologies)
- Through a process of participatory research, the investigators plan to undertake "town hall" meetings so that residents can give thoughtful deliberation to the services that exist and provide visionary ideas for services in the future.

ment within it. The content usually specifies beliefs regarding the rights of individuals, beliefs regarding health and nursing, expectations of practitioners, and commitment of the organization to professionalism, education, evaluation, and research. The importance of the mission statement cannot be overstated, yet it is questionable how many individuals in an organization, when questioned directly, could enunciate the key points in the mission statement or the philosophy of a healthcare setting.

Covey (1990), in his classic book, related that the mission statement is vital to the success of an organization. He believes that everyone should participate in the development of the mission statement: "The involvement process is as important as the written product and is the key to its use" (p. 139).

Covey related the belief system of IBM: the dignity of the individual, excellence, and service. Everyone in IBM is committed to these values. This illustration of a mission statement is worthy of further consideration by healthcare agencies. "An organizational mission statement, one that truly reflects the deep shared vision and values of everyone within that organization, creates a unity and tremendous commitment" (p. 143).

Exercise 15–2

Select a clinical organization with which you have been affiliated. How effective is the structure? (Does the organization operate effectively and efficiently?) What overall human resources are present (e.g., various titles and numbers of people)? What information systems are used? Apply these questions to the nursing component only.

An example of a mission statement of a newly developed community congestive heart failure program is to provide quality, patient-centered, and integrated care, using the primary healthcare model.

Goal-Setting Goal-setting is the process of developing, negotiating, and formalizing the targets or objectives of an organization.

The community congestive heart failure program has six goals:

1. Provide comprehensive patient/family education through inpatient and outpatient programs.

2. Develop protocols for standardized patient care programs in terms of diet, exercise, smoking cessation, and other aspects of prevention and control.
3. Provide a multidisciplinary approach to patient care through the use of physicians, nurse practitioners, nurses, social workers, psychologists, physical and occupational therapists, dietitians, home care personnel, and pastoral care.
4. Enhance community support programs.
5. Develop telemetry and telemedicine programs in northern and remote communities.
6. Ensure that current information and services are available to patients on websites.

Exercise 15–3

Review a healthcare organization's mission statement. Tell a colleague in your own words what the statement means in general; give specific examples of how it translates to nursing.

Practical insights from these studies that are important to nurse administrators are that specific goals are more likely to lead to higher performance than are vague or very general goals, such as "do your best." Feedback, or knowledge of results, is likely to motivate individuals toward higher performance levels and commitment to the achievement of goals.

Three key steps in implementing a goal-setting program are as follows:

1. Set goals that are specific and adhere to a deadline.
2. Promote goal commitment by providing instructions and support to employees and managers.
3. Support the achievement of goals with appropriate feedback as soon as possible.

Objectives The ability to write clear and concise objectives is an important aspect of nursing administration. Characteristics of well-written objectives include the following:

1. The objective statement is properly constructed.
   - It begins with the word to, followed by an action verb.
   - It specifies a single result to be achieved.
   - It specifies a target date for its attainment.

2. The objective is measurable.
3. The objective can be easily understood by those required to attain it.
4. The objective conforms to SMART criteria: *S*pecific, *M*easurable, *A*chievable, *R*esult-oriented, and *T*ime bound.

Phase 3: Identification of Strategies   The third phase of the strategic planning process involves identifying major issues, establishing goals, and developing strategies to meet the goals. Strategy "is a broad plan of action by which an organization intends to reach its objectives" (Sommers & Barnes, 2001, p. 59). All departmental managers are involved in this process and are responsible for preparing a detailed plan of action, which may include the following: development of short- and long-term objectives, formulation of annual department objectives, resource allocation, and preparation of the budget.

Phase 4: Implementation   In the fourth phase of the strategic plan, the specific plans for action are implemented in order of priority. This entails open communication with staff in regard to the priorities for the next year and subsequent periods; formulation of revised policies and procedures in regard to the changes; and formulation of area and individual objectives related to the plan. The specific plans to be focused on include market plans, program plans, operating plans and budget, and human resource plans.

Phase 5: Evaluation   At regular intervals, the strategic plan is reviewed at all levels to determine whether the goals, objectives, and activities are on target. As stated previously, it is important to consider that objectives may change as a result of legislation, budget cutbacks, and change in structure or other environmental factors. Therefore, optional activities may need to be adapted to the situation. For example, one agency was informed that there had to be a decrease in the budget of $500,000 over the next 6 months. The staff were involved in the development of creative methods for ensuring that the necessary changes occurred. Savings were realized with organizational restructuring, the elimination of nursing supervisor positions, and changes in medication administration to a unit dose system.

Exercise 15–4

You are a staff nurse at a public health department in a small rural town. The director of nursing has assigned you to work on a planning committee. The purpose of the committee is to devise long- and short-term departmental goals.

The population of the town is 25,000, and the chief industry is agriculture. It is estimated that 8000 more people will move there in the next 5 years; most will be immigrants from Asia and Mexico.

The health department currently has four full-time baccalaureate nurses, and the state has not approved additional funding for this year.

Considering the concepts of strategic planning you have just read, in what direction should this department consider moving during the next 5 years? Does the department have an adequate number and mix of staff to accommodate this growth? How will you determine between long-term and short-term plans? What additional information will your committee need to plan realistically for the next 5 months and the next 5 years?

An example of a strategic plan of action for the development of a community congestive heart failure program is available at the website for this text.

MARKETING

Marketing may be defined as the "activities designed to generate and facilitate exchanges intended to satisfy human wants and needs" (Sommers & Barnes, 2001, p. 4). Social marketing emphasizes ideas, attitudes, and lifestyle changes. Social marketing is used in a number of health-promotion activities undertaken by nurses. The benefits of marketing include increased consumer satisfaction, improved resource attraction, and improved organizational efficiency. The underlying assumption is that marketing helps manage the exchange of goods and services in a more efficient manner. Marketing principles have been used successfully in a number of community programs designed to decrease the risks of heart disease (diet, exercise, antismoking campaigns; alcohol and drug use awareness; and sexual assault services). One particular program that has generated a great deal of interest is the social marketing approach to advertise Sexual Assault Nurse Examination (SANE) services to college students. The researchers planned an advertising campaign to reach university students. Posters were placed in several strategic points, including hallways and bathrooms. A survey of 1051 sociology students was then conducted, with the result that posters placed in private viewing spaces as opposed to public spaces were found to be more effective (Konradi & DeBruin, 2003).

An example of a survey designed to assess the knowledge, attitudes, and beliefs and practices regarding breast and cervical cancer screening of selected ethnocultural groups is presented in the Research Perspective box.

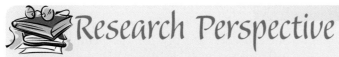 *Research Perspective*

Steven, D., Fitch, M., Dahliwal, H., Kirk-Gardner, R., Sevean, P., Jamieson, J., Stafford, J., & Woodbeck, H. (2004). Knowledge, attitudes, beliefs and practices regarding breast and cervical cancer screening in selected ethnocultural groups in northwestern Ontario. *Oncology Nursing Forum, 31*(2), 305-311.

THE CONCEPTS OF RESEARCH

The objective of the project was to examine the knowledge, attitudes, beliefs, and practices regarding breast and cervical cancer screening of selected ethnocultural groups in a northern region.

SAMPLE SIZE

A convenience sample of 125 women aged 40 years and older who were of Italian, Ukrainian, Finnish, Ojibwa, and Oji-Cree descent was selected.

METHODOLOGY

An interview guide was designed specifically for this study. The interview guide contained information related to knowledge, attitudes, beliefs, and practices about breast self-examination (BSE), clinical breast examination (CBE), mammography, and cervical cancer screening procedures. A demographic data sheet was used to assess age, marital status, educational level, number of dependent children, and town of residence. A pilot study consisting of 25 women was conducted to determine the appropriateness of the tool.

FINDINGS

A comparison of groups regarding health-related behaviors was conducted. Aboriginal women were more likely to have ever smoked (77% compared with 40% or less in other groups). Most women exercised twice a week, and the exercise of choice was walking. The aboriginal women related that they consumed foods higher in fat

and were more likely to add salt to food and had more than four drinks per day. First Nations Women (aboriginal women in northwest Ontario, including those who live on and off reserves) were more likely than any other group to have not performed a BSE, have refused a BSE or mammogram, have not been told how to do a breast examination, have not received written information about BSE, and state they were uncomfortable and fearful about cervical cancer screening procedures (33% refused an internal examination compared with 0% to 8% in other ethnic groups).

IMPLICATIONS FOR PRACTICE

This study has tremendous implications for designing marketing strategies that are culturally sensitive and that take into consideration the literacy level of participants in any screening program. The researchers offer the following recommendations regarding education.

- Develop culturally sensitive health education programs and resources (pamphlets, videos, television, and media programs).
- Develop culturally appropriate written materials with consideration for literacy and visual appeal.
- Develop educational programs in the school system regarding the importance of screening, prevention, and early detection of breast and cervical cancer.
- Develop educational programs for health-care professionals on cultural sensitivity regarding breast and cervical cancer screening for specific populations.

Strategic Marketing Planning Process

The strategic marketing planning process is similar in nature to the strategic planning process and the nursing process. Figure 15-2 offers a comparative chart outlining the steps in the process.

The steps of the strategic marketing planning are as follows:

- Analyze the organization-wide mission, objectives, goals, and culture to which the marketing strategy must contribute.
- Assess organizational strengths and weaknesses to respond to threats and challenges presented by the external environment.
- Analyze the future environment the marketer is likely to face with respect to the public served; competition; and the social, political, technologic, and economic environment.

- Determine the marketing mission, objectives, and specific goals for the relevant planning period.
- Formulate the core marketing strategy to achieve the specified goals.
- Implement the necessary organizational structure and the systems within the marketing function to ensure proper follow-through of the designed strategy.
- Establish detailed programs and tactics to carry out the core strategy for the planning period, including a timetable of activities and the assignment of specific responsibilities.
- Establish benchmarks to measure interim and final achievements of the program.
- Implement the planned program.
- Measure performance, and adjust the core strategy, tactical details, or both as needed.

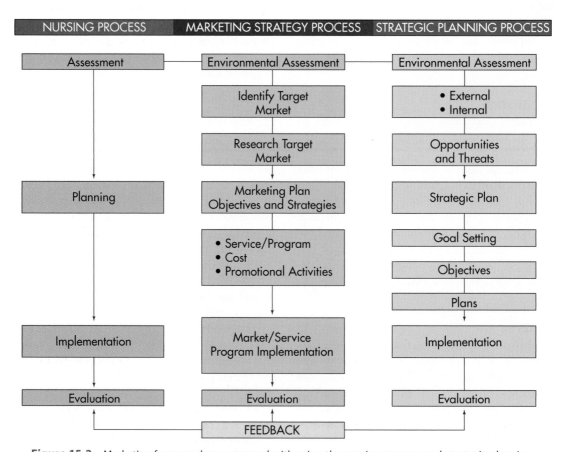

Figure 15-2   Marketing framework as compared with using the nursing process and strategic planning.

Assessment

Determining Organization-Level Missions, Objectives, and Goals A marketing plan is developed by the top-level managers and advisory board to do the following:

1. Determine the organization-level long-term culture, mission, objectives, and goals.
2. Assess the organization's likely future external environment.
3. Assess the organization's current and potential strengths and weaknesses.

Analyzing Organizational Strengths and Weakness During the marketing process, an environmental assessment is conducted to identify and research the target market. An example of this is conducting a needs assessment of the services currently provided by an agency to develop new services or promotional activities to meet the needs of the population being served.

An audit may consist of interviews with key staff; review of documents; observation of staff; visits to competitors; and overview of advertisements, brochures, and other documents as deemed appropriate.

Analyzing External Threats and Opportunities The three components of the external environment are (1) the public environment, which consists of groups and organizations that affect the organization (e.g., public, media, regulatory agencies), (2) the competitive environment, which consists of other organizations that vie for the attention and loyalty of clientele, and (3) the macroenvironment, consisting of demographic, economic, technologic, political, and social forces to which the organization must adapt. Pamphlets and brochures are promotional materials that inform clients about the benefits of a healthcare agency's programs and services.

Setting Marketing Mission, Objectives, and Goals The marketing mission, objectives, and goals must be aligned with the organizational mission, objectives, and goals. The marketing focus is geared to changing market conditions, much as a financial advisor evaluates changing investment market conditions. The market, comprised of both external and internal markets, influences the way an organization moves toward its vision.

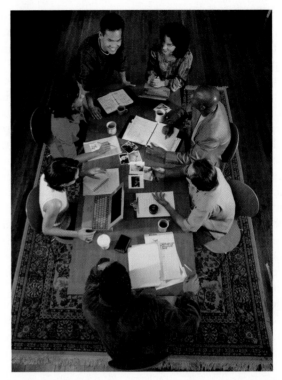

Strategic planning requires open, honest communication about the current view of the organization, its strengths and limitations, and its future.

Planning

The environmental assessment is followed by the development of a marketing plan. This plan outlines the service or program to be provided, includes a detailed budget-cost analysis, and describes the promotional activities designed to promote the program. "Predicting the future" is difficult in turbulent times. Forecasting involves considering multiple factors that could happen to anticipate problems and plan for the future. The process requires several components:

- Assessment of the current situation
- Identification of strengths and weaknesses
- Outline of the driving forces in the environment
- Development of optional scenarios
- Identification of the preferred action
- Development of a plan of action
- Implementation of the plan of action
- Evaluation

Forecasts should be estimates of how accurately a situation can be predicted, provide optional futures, be considered for their influence in convincing managers of the need for change, be a learning experience, be cost effective, and be used for their ritualistic purpose. Rather than using the "shooting at a target" metaphor, it may be more appropriate to think of forecasters as art teachers, helping line (and clinical) managers to paint updated pictures of their future. For example, in forecasting the number of patients who will need cardiac services in a community, a manager needs to consider an environmental scan, including factors related to mortality and morbidity; the fact that individuals are living longer as a result of medical, technologic, and pharmaceutical interventions; and the effect of lifestyle and co-morbidity. In the rural community described in the Research Perspective, diabetes is becoming more common among aboriginal people because of hereditary and lifestyle changes; these changes could lead to an increased incidence of heart disease in the future. The community is developing culturally sensitive preventive programs for this population.

Implementation

The implementation phase includes the establishment of the program and promotional activities designed to communicate benefits of the service or program to patients. Forms of promotion may include media releases, brochures, pamphlets, newsletters, and "word-of-mouth" advertising.

Evaluation

The evaluation may incorporate satisfaction surveys, interviews with clients, and further research studies designed to assess reasons that clients are using or not using the service, program, or product. Feedback is an essential component of the marketing process.

Box 15-2 and Table 15-1 present steps in the strategic marketing planning process in relation to the

---

BOX 15-2

Mission Statement, Goals, and Objectives of the Northwestern Ontario Breast Cancer Screening Program

Mission Statement

To reduce the leading cause of cancer deaths in women by delivering a comprehensive, organized, and evaluated breast cancer screening program for women between the ages of 50 and 69 years. In accordance with Ontario's health goals, the Cancer Care Ontario is committed to deliver a program that is sensitive to women's needs, builds on health-promoting behaviors, and fosters partnerships with interest groups in the community.

Overall Goal

To integrate health promotion strategies and medical practice to reduce mortality from breast cancer by 40% using breast screening of women aged 50 to 69 years.

Objectives

- To detect breast cancer earlier than would occur if organized screening were not available
- To develop and implement a community mobilization plan for the program
- To develop and implement a social marketing plan, including a health education component for the program

- To establish protocols and standards for healthcare professionals associated with the program
- To establish protocols for the interaction of the target population with the program
- To develop and implement training and technical assistance for those associated with the delivery of the program
- To develop a partnership with healthcare professionals that will facilitate program delivery
- To establish a regional breast screening service so that all women in the target population have equal access to breast screening
- To ensure that a minimum of 70% of women in the target population participate in screening every 2 years
- To document the follow-up of all women in whom an abnormality has been detected
- To provide screening that is sensitive and acceptable to the target population
- To evaluate the program on a continual basis, including needs assessment and measurement of process, economic, and outcome variables

Table 15-1 STRATEGIC PLAN OF ACTION FOR THE DEVELOPMENT, IMPLEMENTATION, AND EVALUATION OF A WOMAN'S HEALTH CENTER

Objective	Activities	Responsible Council	Time Frame
1. To develop a women's health center in a remote rural community	1.1 To conduct a needs assessment	Nurse practitioners	January 2007
	1.2 To conduct a literature review related to each of these topics: • Women's health • Entrepreneurship • Programs related to women's health	Nurse practitioners and students	January 2007
	1.3 To form an advisory committee comprising community representatives to oversee the development and implementation of the center	Nurse practitioners	February 2007
	1.4 To develop the organizational structure, mission statement, philosophy, and objectives, and revise accordingly	Nurse practitioners and advisory committee	February 2007
	1.5 To develop policy and procedure manuals for staff	Nurse practitioners	Ongoing
	1.6 To determine the business structure of the organization (i.e., legalities regarding partnerships, corporations, and proprietorship)	Nurse practitioners	Ongoing
	1.7 To develop a budget	Nurse practitioners	January 2007 Ongoing
	1.8 To develop a business site for the organization: • All renovations • Office equipment • Supplies • Special healthcare equipment • Filing and billing systems	Consultants and nurse practitioners	February 2007

Continued

Table 15-1 STRATEGIC PLAN OF ACTION FOR THE DEVELOPMENT, IMPLEMENTATION, AND EVALUATION OF A WOMAN'S HEALTH CENTER—cont'd

Objective	Activities	Responsible Council	Time Frame
	1.9 To develop a marketing program (newspapers, telephone, radio messages, signs, and direct mailings)	Nurse practitioners	February 2007 Ongoing
2. To implement and evaluate the effectiveness and efficiency of these programs	2.1 To develop patient questionnaires related to satisfaction regarding care provided	Nurse practitioners	March 2007 Ongoing
	2.2 To develop cost-effective analysis studies to evaluate each of the programs being provided	Nurse practitioners	Ongoing
	2.3 To collect and collate data related to utilization of services by clientele	Nurse practitioners	Ongoing

delivery of breast cancer screening services to women in a widespread rural area of Ontario, Canada.

Nurses in all roles have rights and responsibilities relating to planning, goal-setting, and marketing. Each of us has some sense of what is important today and sustainable for tomorrow in the context of our cultural perspective. Most of us sense the difference between fads and trends and how each affects us personally and professionally. Leaders are accountable for setting goals, including followers in those activities, and aligning tasks with the goals. Additionally, all of us, as we represent our profession, organization, or community, are marketing each of those elements. We can contribute to formal marketing strategies through activities such as focus groups, or we can evaluate responses to marketing materials. Always, however, the focus should be on how what we are doing contributes to future quality.

The Solution

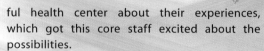

I had read an article by a staff nurse from a large health center about forming a unit staff council that would be empowered to make decisions and solve problems. This council was totally led by the staff and its consultant/advisor. What are the lines below?

I decided to get something like this started on my unit and undertook the following plan:

1. I copied the article for the staff, and I talked to the informal leaders about their interest in it. I had my staff talk with the staff at the success-

ful health center about their experiences, which got this core staff excited about the possibilities.

2. I talked with the staff about what decisions they wanted to control and found that they were interested in self-scheduling, time and job sharing, clinical problem-solving, and better time management. I set up a charter of authority with them and a process for getting together regularly to deal with their issues.

The Solution—cont'd

3. The staff set up a mechanism for getting everyone involved by rotating their tasks, processes, and decision-making responsibilities among the staff members. They determined that everyone on the staff would have to participate or move to another unit. They decided that this was the way they intended to "do their business."

4. I made sure that beginning issues were easy and resolvable, with measures of success built in. I celebrated the staff's successes with them, no matter how small. As the staff got more confident and proficient, I introduced them to issues with more critical value and supported them with information, skill development, and good process.

5. As the staff became stronger and felt a higher level of ownership, I backed off and let them take more control and authority, and the council became an integral part of the unit's way of working. The staff

had more authority, felt more autonomy, and had more control.

The result of this approach was a stronger investment of the staff in their own issues, a mechanism for managing their own issues, and a way to directly address problems they previously thought they had no control over. Energy and enthusiasm returned; a growing sense of maturity and accountability emerged; and other units and staff became intrigued enough with what was happening that they, too, wanted to establish similar approaches on their units. In many cases, the staff became mentors and consultants to the efforts of other units in the system.

— Tim Porter-O'Grady

 Would this be a suitable approach for you? Why?

CHAPTER CHECKLIST

The effectiveness of any organization depends on its strategic planning. Nurse leaders/managers must be aware of the critical elements to facilitate the process. Setting goals and defining marketing strategies for product lines are part of the role professional nurses must perform to achieve effective organizational results in creating a niche in healthcare services.

- The planning process leads to success in the achievement of goals and objectives, gives meaning to work life, and provides direction for the organizational activities of the organization.
- Strategic planning is similar in nature to the nursing process and involves the following:
  - Assessment of the environment (internal and external)
  - Appraisal of the organization's strengths and weaknesses

- Identification of the major opportunities and threats
- Development of strategies to meet these opportunities
- Implementation and evaluation of the strategy
- Marketing strategies will continue to play a vital role in healthcare settings as competition increases to provide services and programs to the public. Steps in the strategic marketing planning process are as follows:
  - Assessment
  - Planning
  - Implementation
  - Evaluation
- Nurses can play a pivotal role in the development of visionary programs and services that meet the needs of the population.

TIPS FOR PLANNING, GOAL SETTING, AND MARKETING

- Be clear about the organization's mission and vision.
- Read and listen to wide sources of data to determine what is happening and what trends could affect you and your organization.

- Be clear about your role in the organization and its success.
- Think about what messages others need to hear about you and your services.

TERMS TO KNOW

marketing
strategic planning

REFERENCES

Covey, S. (1990). *The seven habits of highly effective people.* Toronto: Simon & Schuster.

Konradi, A., & DeBruin, P. (2003). Using a social marketing approach to advertise Sexual Assault Nurse Examination (SANE) services to college students. *Journal of American College Health, 52*(1), 33-39.

Redd, L., & Kongstevedt, P. (2004). Are you ready for 2004 challenges? *Health Care Financial Management, 58*(2), 36-39.

Sommers, M., & Barnes, J. (2001). *Fundamentals of marketing.* Boston: McGraw-Hill Ryerson.

Steven, D., Fitch, M., Dahliwal, H., Kirk-Gardner, Sevean, P., Jamieson, J., & Woodbeck, H. (2004). Knowledge, attitudes, beliefs and practices regarding breast and cervical cancer screening in selected ethnocultural groups in Northwestern Ontario. *Oncology Nursing Forum, 31*(2), 305-311.

Zuckerman, A. (2000). Leveraging strategic planning for improved financial performance. *Healthcare Financial Management, 54*(12), 54-57.

SUGGESTED READINGS

Beyerlein, M. M., Freedman, S., McGee, C., & Moran, L. (2003). The 10 principles of collaborative organizations. *Journal of Organizational Excellence, 22*(2), 51-63.

Bhuian, S. N., Mengue, B., & Bell, S. J. (2005). Just entrepreneurial enough: The moderating effect of entrepreneurship on the relationship between market orientation and performance (electronic version). *Journal of Business Research, 58*, 9-17. Retrieved February 14, 2005, from www.sciencedirect.com/science?_ob=MImg&_imagekey=B6V7S-48R1YNM-1-3&_cdi=5850&_user=10&_orig=browse&_coverDate=01%2F31%2F2005&_sk=999419998&view=c&wchp=dGLbVzb- zSkzS&md5=1424463e0b457a66b3f4d5931ed8fe06&ie=/sdarticle.pdf.

Florida Centre for Nursing. (2004). Statewide strategic plan for nursing workforce in Florida. Orlando, FL: Florida Centre for Nursing.

Higgins, J. M., & Mcallaster, C. (2004). If you want strategic change, don't forget to change your cultural artifacts. *Journal of Change Management, 4*(1), 63-73.

Hooley, G. J., & Greenley, G. E. (2005). The performance impact of marketing resources (electronic version). *Journal of Business Research, 58*, 18-27. Retrieved February 14, 2005, from www.sciencedirect.com/science?_ob=MImg&_imagekey=B6V7S-494HRY8-2-5&_cdi=5850&_user=10&_orig=browse&_coverDate=01%2F31%2F2005&_sk=999419998&view=c&wchp=dGLbVzb-zSkzS&md5=db5af3df5a591557163e60011c65576d&ie=/sdarticle.pdf.

Kim, W. C., & Mauborgne, R. (2004). Blue ocean strategy. *Harvard Business Review, 82*(10), 76-84.

Lee, L., & Jones, L. (2004). Developing a strategic plan for a neonatal practitioner service. *Advances in Neonatal Care, 4*(5), 292-305

Lowry, R., Hardy, S., Jordan, C., & Wayman, G. (2004). Using social marketing to increase recruitment of pregnant smokers to smoking cessation service: A success story. *Public Health, 18*, 239-243.

Parnell, J. A., & Lester, D. L. (2003). Towards a philosophy of strategy: Reassessing the five critical dilemmas in strategy formulation and change. *Strategic Change, 12*(6), 291-303.

Phillips, K., Haas, J., Liang, S., Baker, L., Tye, S., Kerlikowske, K. et al. (2004). Are gatekeeper requirements associated with cancer screening utilization. *Health Services Research, 39*(1), 153-178.

Philpott, E., Hamblin, D. J., Bains, T., & Kay, G. (2004). The use of models and methods for strategic planning: Towards an holistic view of strategy. *International Transactions in Operational Research, 11*(2), 203-216.

Pool, S. W. (2004). Prepared minds: Developing executives for success in the strategic planning process. *Developing and Learning in Organizations: An International Journal, 18*(5), 14-16.

Roland, T. R., Ambler, T., Carpenter, G. S., & Kumar, V. (2004). Measuring marketing productivity: Current knowledge and directions. *Journal of Marketing, 68*(4), 76-89.

Saxe, J., Burgel, B., Collins-Bride, G., Stringar-Murray, S., Dennehy, P., & Holzemer, W. (2004). Strategic planning for UCSF's community health nursing faculty practices. *Nursing Outlook, 52*(4), 179-188.

Sehwail, L., & DeYong, C. (2003). Six sigma in health care. *Leadership in Health Services, 16*(4), 1-5.

Zwick, D., & Dholakia, N. (2004). Whose identity is it anyway? Consumer representation in the age of database marketing [Electronic Version]. *Journal of Macro-marketing, 24*(1), 31-43. Retrieved February 16, 2004 from http://jmk.sagepub.com/cgi/reprint/24/1/31.

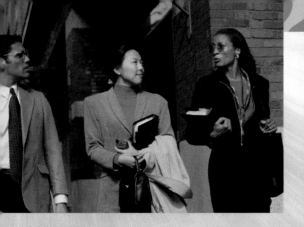

Chapter

16

Leading Change

Patricia S. Yoder–Wise
Kristi Menix

This chapter describes the general nature of change in healthcare organizations. The theories and models, processes, responses, principles, and strategies typically involved in creating and leading change are discussed. The manager's primary role is that of change agent. This role includes responsibilities to anticipate, create, and manage the dynamic forces of change for desired outcomes and goal achievement. How to react to imposed change is part of that responsibility, but leading proactively to create change offers opportunities to better control outcomes. The followership role change is critical to effectiveness and efficiency in transitioning to the new. The effective change agent ensures staff empowerment to achieve change outcomes. The term change agent is used in this chapter to describe the nurse responsible and accountable for achieving a defined set of work outcomes through the efforts of an employee group. Change refers to an alteration in the work environment that is new or different from what existed previously. Change management refers to the overall processes and strategies used to moderate and manage the preparation for, effect of, responses to, and outcomes for conditions that are new and different from those that existed previously.

Objectives

- Analyze the general characteristics of change in open-system organizations.
- Relate the models of planned change to the process of low-level change.
- Evaluate nonlinear theories for managing high-level change.
- Evaluate the use of select functions, principles, and strategies for initiating and managing change.
- Formulate desirable qualities of effective change agents.

Questions to Consider

- What are your beliefs about the benefits and disadvantages of change?
- What is your usual response to unexpected change? To deliberate, planned change? To sustained ambiguity in a change situation?
- Do you actively seek change to improve practice and management outcomes?
- What kinds of expertise and values do you possess that could facilitate change in a work setting?
- What strategies do you propose to support continuous learning?

The Challenge

Joel Graeter, RN, BSN
Clinical Manager, East Texas Medical Center Specialty Hospital, Tyler, Texas

As a specialty hospital clinical manager accountable for the safe, quality care of acutely ill patients with multiple, complex, and long-term care needs and average lengths of stay of 30 to 32 days, I must simultaneously respond to constant administrative pressures to reduce operational costs. Recently, pay schedules for nurses changed hospital-wide. New pay incentives made it more appealing for nurses to work as much or as little (prn) as they wish with no benefits but at a higher hourly wage or as nurses contracted to the hospital through an agency at a high hourly wage. Full-time nurses, employees of the hospital, have benefits, but

they earn less per hour than agency and prn nurses. Their services are available and more cost effective, and, therefore, they are asked to work overtime and engage in other unit responsibilities. The challenge is to maintain appropriate staffing levels and mixes, as well as continuity of care, in the face of managing the dynamics of a nursing staff with varying commitment, values, and aptitudes. How could I manage this change and its forces effectively?

 What do you think you would do if you were this nurse?

INTRODUCTION

Change is a natural social process of individuals, groups, organizations, and society. The forces of change originate inside and outside healthcare organizations. Change today is constant, inevitable, pervasive, and unpredictable and varies in rate and intensity, which unavoidably influences individuals, technology, and systems at all levels of the organization. Even if we did not want to change, the rapidity of change and the volume of changes affecting health care dictate that we must embrace change or face inevitable frustration.

Because most healthcare organizations operate as open systems, they are receptive to external and internal influences originating from a rapidly changing healthcare delivery system. Organization-wide change depends on the organization's stage of development, degree of flexibility, and history of response to change, as well as the maturity of its systems. The role of **change agents** is to lead change efforts through thinking that is systems- and theory-based, tolerant of ambiguity, and mindful of the whole picture. Therefore, the management of change in organizations requires moving from an emphasis on long-range planning and established goals to a greater focus on managing the dynamic forces in the **change situations** while moving toward a set of achievable outcomes.

Balancing change in the long and short view is a key challenge today.

CONTEXT OF THE CHANGE ENVIRONMENT

The transformation of healthcare delivery is occurring rapidly, creating contextual alterations in change situations in such factors as time, information, decision-making, and planning (Begun & White, 1995). Increased uncertainty challenges change agents to communicate differently and more extensively than is required, with less complex change (Freeman, 1999; Geddes, Salyer, & Mark, 1999). Nursing entities, as open systems, need to begin viewing their work in less bureaucratic, inflexible ways and open themselves up to responding with flexibility and creativity to today's dynamic environment (Begun & White, 1995). Using planned linear change was useful when society and health care were somewhat stable (low-complexity change). The highly complex, accelerated, and unpredictable change situations of today still require planning, but on a constantly changing basis.

Nurses are key players in healthcare delivery. They are partners with multiple-care providers, and pivotal players in open-systems organizations.

In the classic work, Begun and White (1995) said, "In order for the nursing profession to strategically adapt in a rapidly changing environment, it is important to consider its current dominant logic; as a source of structural inertia. A system's dominant logic is a screen that filters information deemed relevant by historical antecedents and by those analyzing the data" Using **chaos theory** components, Begun and White (1995) suggested that nursing in various areas is too stable and thus too unresponsive and unable to adapt to the influences of rapid change. Today, nursing organizations that achieve Magnet™ status, the designation for healthcare facilities that indicates excellence in nursing care, are typically ones that are flexible, adaptive, and innovative; they capitalize on rapid change to improve patient safety, work conditions, and quality. Box 16-1 shows guidelines for altering the dominant logic. Forecasting for shorter terms (no more than 3 to 5 years) and using scenario planning to answer multiple "what if" questions are examples of the needed flexibility and creativity in nursing today.

Planned change models, or linear approaches, can guide directional, more incremental, low-level, less complex changes, such as those needed to be systematic in reorganizing the storage of unit supplies or to recommend a series of staff-development offerings for nursing staff. High-level change, on the other hand, is characteristically more fluid and complex because of the interactions and activities of multiple players and influences across the organization. **Nonlinear change** approaches are found in complexity/chaos and **learning organization** theories. They offer helpful approaches for understanding dynamic, open-system healthcare organizations and for guiding change agents in managing accelerated, increasingly uncertain change environments (Menix, 2000, 2001). Change agents in planned changes focus on specific goals and the incremental steps to attain that goal. Change agents in nonlinear, complex changes serve as monitors of the environment, negotiators of influences on a change, and forecasters of various scenarios and possible outcomes.

PLANNED CHANGE USING LINEAR APPROACHES

Most **planned change** models—linear models—advocate that change can occur in a sequential and directional fashion when guided by effective change agents. Planned change models, such as those of Lewin (1947); Lippitt, Watson, and Westley (1958); and Havelock (1973), explain the nature of **change processes** and offer systematic problem-solving methods designed to achieve change. The use of

BOX 16-1

Guidelines for Altering the Dominant Logic

Decrease	Increase
Long-term forecasting	Short-term forecasting
Preplanned strategies	Emergent strategies
Emphasis on past successes	Search for new opportunities
One future vision	Multiple scenarios
Rigid, permanent structures	Self-organizing, temporary structures
Structural isolation in the workplace	Structural interdependence in the workplace
Stability of leadership	Leadership turnover
Standardization	Innovation, experimentation, diversity
Insulation from other professions and marketplace	Cooperation and competition
Marketplace "passivity"	Marketplace "aggression"
Expectation of job security	Self-learning

From Begun, J. W., & White, K. R. (1995). Altering nursing's dominant logic: Guidelines from complex adaptive systems theory. *Complexity and Chaos in Nursing, 2*(1), 10.

planned change can be useful for low-level change in more stable environments. Flexibility in implementing the plan and moderating the situational factors, as is advocated by nonlinear approaches, can improve the overall outcomes. However, to make change happen, the group has to move through it. The group cannot let only a few make the change. Sticking with and advancing the change is daily work that requires the attention of all involved.

Lewin (1947) suggested that an analysis of change situations, which he called *force field analysis*, includes early and ongoing assessment of **barriers** and **facilitators**. Barriers in change situations are factors that can hinder the change process; facilitators are factors that can expedite the process. These elements may originate with people, technology, structure, or values. For change to be effective, the force of facilitators must exceed the force of barriers; thus, the work of change agents is to reduce the barriers in the situation and support or enhance the facilitators. Figure 16-1 illustrates an example of how to diagram forces so that a visual portrays the strengths and barriers of any change. In this case, the strengths outweigh the barriers.

Lewin (1947) describes change as having three stages:

- Unfreezing
- Experiencing the change
- Refreezing

Unfreezing refers to the awareness of an opportunity, need, or problem for which some action is necessary; it also requires subsequent mental readiness to approach the issue. This phase may occur naturally as a progressive development, or it may result from a deliberate activity as a first step in planning a change. For example, when the current way of giving shift reports is ineffective, as evidenced by errors occurring in care delivery, the staff become aware of a problem and the need for change. As in The Challenge presented earlier, changes in nurses' pay schedules and their effects on staffing and scheduling brought about unfreezing for hospital leadership and all staff.

Exercise 16-1

Identify the facilitators and barriers in the following situation. Rate the potential strength of each in hindering or expediting attainment of the change. Use +5 for the highest positive strength toward change occurring and −5 for the greatest negative strength against the change:

Nursing administration wants the pediatric neurology unit to merge with the pediatric cardiac unit for improved care delivery and cost-effectiveness. Staff nurses and managers from both units—some enthusiastic, some reluctant—participate on the merger planning committee. The appointed chair is the organization's powerful personnel director. Administration wants a new facility to house the merged unit.

"Experiencing" the change or solution leads to incorporation of what is new or different into work and interpersonal processes (Lewin, 1947). Deciding to begin to use the change or being thrust into the change can result in potential integration of the new way of thinking or doing.

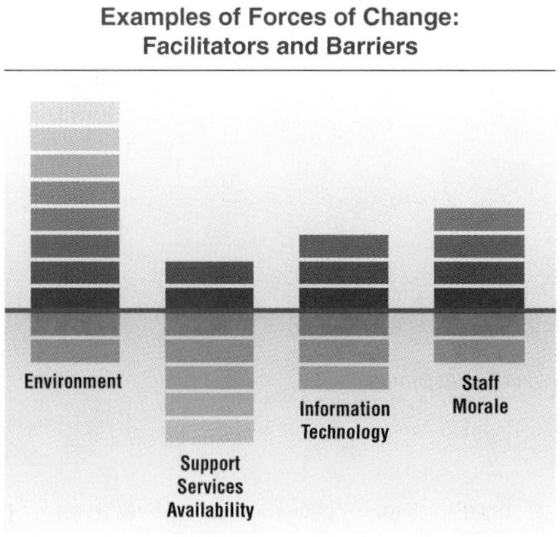

**Examples of Forces of Change:
Facilitators and Barriers**

Figure 16-1   Examples of forces of change: facilitator and barriers.

"Refreezing" occurs when the participants in the change situation accept and use the new attitude or behavior (Lewin, 1947). Acceptance is assumed once most staff integrate the change into their work processes. Surveys, structured or unstructured observations, or other data-collection methods can be conducted at various points after the implementation of a designated change. Analysis of these data can help evaluate the degree of implementation and identify additional alterations needed to ensure an effective **change outcome**.

Although Havelock's (1973) six-stage model for planning change had particular application to educational entities (see Theory box), it shows similarities in the elements of the directional phases recommended by other planned-change models. Two adjuncts to Havelock's model advocate development of the effective change agent and use of his model as a rational problem-solving process. The rational problem-solving process is "how change agents can organize their work so that successful innovation will take place" (p. 3).

Lippitt, Watson, and Westley's (1958) model suggests seven sequential phases to use to plan change (see Theory box). Inherent in this model is the change agent's appraisal of the "change and resistance forces which are present in the client system at the beginning of the change process as well as others which may be revealed as the process advances. Being continuously sensitive to the constellation of change forces and resistance forces is one of the most creative parts of the change agent's job" (p. 92).

The innovation-decision process (Rogers, 1995) describes the choice of an individual, over time, to accept or reject a new idea for use in practice (see Theory box). According to Rogers' work, the individual's decision-making actions pass through five sequential stages. The decision to not accept the new idea may occur at any stage. However, the change agent can facilitate movement by others through these stages by encouraging the use of the idea and providing information about its benefits and disadvantages.

Theory Box

THEORIES FOR PLANNED CHANGE

KEY CONTRIBUTORS	KEY IDEA	APPLICATION TO PRACTICE
Six Phases of Planned Change* Havelock (1973) is credited with this planned change model.	Change can be planned, implemented, and evaluated in six sequential stages. The model is advocated for the development of effective change agents and used as a rational problem-solving process. The six stages are as follows: 1. Building a relationship 2. Diagnosing the problem 3. Acquiring relevant resources 4. Choosing the solution 5. Gaining acceptance 6. Stabilizing the innovation and generating self-renewal	Useful for low-level, low-complexity change.
Seven Phases of Planned Change† Lippitt, Watson, and Westley (1958) are credited with this planned change model.	Change can be planned, implemented, and evaluated in seven sequential phases. Ongoing sensitivity to forces in the change	Useful for low-level, low-complexity change.

Continued

Theory Box—cont'd

THEORIES FOR PLANNED CHANGE

KEY CONTRIBUTORS	KEY IDEA	APPLICATION TO PRACTICE
	process is essential. The seven phases are as follows: 1. The client system becomes aware of the need for change. 2. The relationship is developed between the client system and change agent. 3. The change problem is defined. 4. The change goals are set and options for achievement are explored. 5. The plan for change is implemented. 6. The change is accepted and stabilized. 7. The change entities redefine their relationships.	
Innovation-Decision Process‡ Rogers (1995) is credited with formulating this process.	Change for an individual occurs over five phases when choosing to accept or reject an innovation/idea. Decisions to not accept the new idea may occur at any of the five stages. The change agent can promote acceptance by providing information about benefits and disadvantages and encouragement. The five stages are as follows: 1. Knowledge 2. Persuasion 3. Decision 4. Implementation 5. Confirmation	Useful for individual change.

*Modified from Havelock, R. G. (1973). *The change agent's guide to innovation in education.* Englewood Cliffs, NJ: Educational Technology Publications.

†Modified from Lippitt, R., Watson, J., & Westley, B. (1958). *The dynamics of planned change.* New York: Harcourt Brace.

‡Modified from Rogers, E. M. (1995). *Diffusion of innovations* (4th ed.). New York: The Free Press.

NONLINEAR CHANGE: CHAOS AND LEARNING ORGANIZATION THEORIES

Chaos Theory

Organizations can no longer rely on rules, policies, and hierarchies to get work accomplished in inflexible ways. According to chaos theory perspectives, the rapidly changing nature of human and world factors suggest that emphasizing rules and policies is short-sighted and wastes time. Organizations are open systems operating in complex, fast-changing environments. The term, open, by itself suggests that such systems (organizations/services) are affected by and simultaneously affect the environment in which they exist. These systems are like semipermeable membranes, allowing some exchanges between the internal and external environments. Non–human-induced responses are characterized by random-appearing yet self-organizing patterns. This constant adaptation and anticipation forces organizations to remain relevant in their environment. Typically, organizations experience periods of stability interrupted with periods of intense transformation, thus demonstrating "spurts" of change rather than smooth, incremental change. Although not predictable in the long run, small changes in the internal or external environment can result in significant consequences to organizational work processes and outcomes. Chaos theory further explains that the conditions present in a particular organizational change will not occur again in the same form (Vicenzi, White, & Begun, 1997). Figure 16-2 illustrates the contrasting patterns.

Organizations have always been self-organizing systems with the potential for self-renewal. Magnet hospitals, as a key example, illustrate how organizations dedicated to excellence capitalize on a vision of quality to create shared values and beliefs. Furthermore, the focus on interrelationships (CNO to and from staff, nurses with physicians, and employees with patients) creates new camaraderies for change. Their use of evidenced-based outcomes research has been exemplary. Continuous learning by personnel as a matter of organizational philosophy further promotes adaptation to accelerated change.

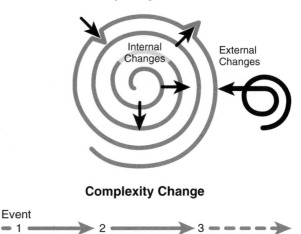

Figure 16-2   Contrasting patterns of linear and complexity theories.

Learning Organization Theory

Learning organizations are organizations that place emphasis on flexibility and responsiveness (Senge, 1990). Specifically, complex organizations that are responsive to internal and external influences are trying to survive in an unpredictable healthcare environment. They can best respond and adapt when members of the organization complete their work with others using a learning approach. Enactment of Senge's five disciplines is essential to achieving learning organization status. *Disciplines* refers to the critical and interrelated elements that comprise a grouping that can function effectively only when all elements are present, linked, and interacting. For example, a car with a working engine and other essential operational features but no tires could not be driven as designed. Without the knowledge of the interrelatedness of the car's operational features, one might not be able to take the right action to use this form of transportation.

Senge's (1990) five disciplines of learning organizations are the following:

1. Systems thinking
2. Personal mastery

3. Mental models
4. Shared vision
5. Team learning

Dialogue (two-way discussion) promotes the individual, group, and organizational learning process. *Systems thinking* refers to the need for the organization to view the world as a set of multiple visible and invisible parts that interact constantly. When the organization values and facilitates development of the deeper aspirations of its members in addition to professional proficiency, it successfully matches organizational learning and personal growth or *personal mastery*. Each individual and each organization bases its activities on a set of assumptions, beliefs, and mental pictures about the way the world should work. When these invisible *mental models* are uncovered and consciously evaluated, it is possible to begin to determine, in a "learningful" (Senge, 1990, p. 9) way, their influence on work accomplishment. *Building shared vision* occurs when leaders involve all members in moving personal visions of the future into a consolidated yet ongoing vision common to members and leaders. *Team learning* refers to the need for a cohesive group to learn together to benefit from the abilities of each member, thereby enhancing the overall outcomes of the team's efforts. Organizations value employees who can learn continuously, interact and communicate effectively as team members, and seek to meet their potential as team members.

An example of the application of chaos and learning organization theories is a community hospital that has been sensitive to and has adapted to external and internal environmental influences, such as the need to make changes in reimbursement and accreditation policies. The process of adaptation involves times of fluctuation interrupted with times of stability. The implications of managed care induced by major insurance players may not be predictable, but they have significant consequences for the financial survival of the community hospital. New reimbursement strategies have forced community hospitals and other area hospitals to interact to seek consolidation for all to survive. Accelerated change of such magnitude has created change that appears chaotic. However, all hospitals are becoming transformed, and some order exists in the middle of perceived general chaos. It is likely that these exact conditions will not occur again for these hospitals. Hospital administrators and other personnel have shown resilience and assumed a "learning" philosophy to seek overall organizational adaptation.

MAJOR CHANGE MANAGEMENT FUNCTIONS

Change agents selectively use **change management** functions and activities to assist in the creation and management of change to reach specific outcomes. They may or may not be used sequentially; they may be applied simultaneously, based on the nature of the change process. Flexibility and appropriateness of use are essential. The five functions are as follows:

1. Planning (includes assessment)
2. Organizing
3. Implementing
4. Evaluating
5. Seeking feedback

Feedback functions in conjunction with the first four management functions as a way to assess the ongoing status of the change process and movement toward desired change outcomes.

Planning is simply the activity of looking ahead to decide how to achieve some result, goal, or outcome. For any plan to be effective, both those who will implement the plan and those who will be affected by the changes must participate in the change-planning process from the beginning. Planning ideally occurs before implementation. Part of the initial and ongoing planning activity includes assessing the who, what, when, where, how, and why of the situation needing change and the factors desired to achieve the change. It is important to carefully assess factors in the change situation that will predictably support or interfere with the progress of a change (Lewin, 1947). This information clarifies the conditions and direction of the advancing plan. Putting general plans for change in writing can establish a visual method to communicate ideas, decisions, and responsibilities to others.

Organizing entails making decisions about reaching outcomes in terms of time, personnel, materials, communication, or other activities and resources. For reasons of efficiency, it is important to weigh the costs and benefits of options to reach several possible change outcomes. Organizing builds clarity into the plan by formalizing the desired sequence and means of accomplishing the change.

Exercise 16-2

From the perspective of a manager applying these functions to a change process, consider the manager's responsibility to orient a new staffing coordinator for a large surgicenter, and identify the appropriate management function for each member. Ideally, the manager, the new staffing coordinator, and the assistant nurse manager will map out in writing (1) the goals of the orientation, (2) the activities for meeting goals, and (3) a schedule for accomplishing them. The assistant nurse manager and staffing coordinator agree to meet as needed, as well as to meet weekly to review progress and to address informational or confidence needs. Part of this plan includes the option to alter the plan based on unexpected changes. The staffing coordinator will begin the position in 2 weeks and put the prearranged outline of activities into action. The assistant nurse manager's responsibility will be to guide and support the education of the new staffing coordinator. Unexpected occurrences, such as the staff coordinator being absent for a few days, will create the need to modify the goal, activities, or time frame of the orientation plan (dynamic quality of process). New information (feedback) guides the overall process.

Implementing ideally occurs after a plan is established. However, unexpected change may sometimes require immediate action. Plans made quickly after the change can facilitate handling the effects of the change. Successful implementation, or putting the plan into action, depends on the appropriateness of the change and the involvement of those involved in the change. An important aspect of change is that change in one part of a system can affect the function in other, related systems.

Evaluating entails continually judging the degree to which the change process is moving acceptably toward desired outcomes or goals and whether or when outcomes are met. Monitoring, or ongoing data collection, assists the change agent to recognize and correct process problems early. Judging whether or not an outcome has been fully or partially met occurs in the final stage of the change process.

Effective change agents obtain feedback by continuously gathering accurate, comprehensive, timely information about the progress of the change process through a variety of sources. Classic references (Ashby, 1957; Cadwallader, 1959) describe that **cybernetic theory** purports that access to what the theory calls **negative feedback** can be accomplished by establishing communication networks that act as monitors of specific types of information. Analysis of this negative feedback, or information indicating a correction is needed in the system, informs the change agent where problems exist: whether the course of the accelerated change process has veered away from its progress toward desired outcomes or some action is needed to facilitate continued progress. Although some typical organizational feedback mechanisms include computerized data findings, staff meeting discussions, and informal or formal observations, negative feedback sources are found specifically in the reports of exceptions, such as incident reports, variances in budget expenditures, or new reimbursement policies. Multiple sources of unexceptional feedback produce information to build a picture of success for the change process.

Another way to view the approach to change is described by Hirschhorn (2002). He suggests that there are three aspects to effecting a change, and each aspect is equally important to the success of a change. Described as campaigns, these three aspects are political, marketing, and military. Table 16-1 illustrates the key concepts of each of the campaigns and provides an example of each. The key, however, is that these are three interrelated efforts that must be addressed for change to be effective.

Furthermore, it is critical to use emotional intelligence rather than knowledge intelligence. What this means is that a change agent has to have the knowledge of both the nature of the change and the nature of the people with whom he or she is working to effect the change. Lakoff (2004) suggests that we think in frames, and if the knowledge we are given does not fit our frame about a topic or event, we dismiss the information. It is a challenge when working with another to help that other person adjust the frames. Think what it is like when working with a group of people with multiple frames and helping them to exchange a well-entrenched frame for something new. The critical issues are to help people change their behavior and to realize that communication more likely involves people's emotions and feelings rather than their intellect. Therefore, to bring about change, a leader

Table 16-1 EXAMPLES OF THE THREE CAMPAIGNS FOR CHANGE

Type of Change	Description	Example
Political	Coalition-building to create more influence. Changes in structures.	Working with pharmacy to effect a change in the delivery of medications to patients. Creating new communication approaches to enhance patient-safety outcomes.
Marketing	Listening to what is important to team members. Working with key groups such as physicians who typically admit to a given unit. Creating a theme.	Describing to patient families why certain approaches are taken. Determining what motivates others to change. Creating huddles to map out the plan for the day. Using messages to convey a full set of values around a change (for example, nothing about me without me . . . a theme for patient safety).
Military	Engaging with resistance by providing attention, testing beachheads, and creating a war room.	Paying attention (asking questions about, seeking reports about) to the change outcomes. Determining the tough choices that need to be made and going after them strategically. Creating a space for resources and meetings about the change that symbolizes to others that the change is moving ahead.

Based on Hirschhorn, L. (July, 2002). Campaigning for change. *Harvard Business Review, 80*(7), 98-104.

of change must be equally skilled at knowing the various elements of the change and how to affect them and at knowing how to "read" people and their relationships with the change at hand.

RESPONSES TO CHANGE

Change, whether proactively initiated at the point of change or imposed from external sources, affects people, technology, and systems. Change can be mandated by higher administration, or it can originate within any department or unit or at the level of care delivery. Often, higher administration creates a change for managerial staff to integrate into their work areas. Therefore, it follows that the responses that arise across the organization will depend on how change is perceived. Effective change agents anticipate possible responses and apply strategies to deal with them for the best possible change outcomes.

Organizational culture and staff readiness influence responses to change. Knowing values and beliefs of work groups (staff and their managers

and administrators—all part of organizational culture) is critical to identifying responses to change. Readiness can be viewed as individuals' current attitudes or willingness, as well as their nursing abilities. Assessment of organizational culture and the readiness of staff and others to engage in making or participating in a change, whether minor or extensive, sets the stage for the selection and use of strategies. For example, in Exercise 16-2, the willingness of the nursing and administrative managerial staff to merge successfully is interdependent with the different nursing and organizational skills required by the new unit. Answering the self-assessment questions in Table 16-2 can help determine how receptive one is to change and innovation.

Human Side of Change

The *human side* of managing change refers to staff responses to change that either facilitate or interfere with change processes. Responses to all or part of the change process by individuals and groups may vary from full acceptance and willing participation to open rejection. Some nurses may manifest

Table 16-2 SELF-ASSESSMENT: HOW RECEPTIVE ARE YOU TO CHANGE AND INNOVATION?

Read the following items. Circle the answer that most closely matches your attitude toward creating and accepting new or different ways.

1. I enjoy learning about new ideas and approaches.	Yes	Depends	No
2. Once I learn about a new idea or approach, I begin to try it right away.	Yes	Depends	No
3. I like to discuss different ways of accomplishing a goal or end result.	Yes	Depends	No
4. I continually seek better ways to improve what I do.	Yes	Depends	No
5. I commonly recognize improved ways of doing things.	Yes	Depends	No
6. I talk over my ideas for change with my peers.	Yes	Depends	No
7. I communicate my ideas for change with my manager.	Yes	Depends	No
8. I discuss my ideas for change with my family.	Yes	Depends	No
9. I volunteer to be at meetings when changes are being discussed.	Yes	Depends	No
10. I encourage others to try new ideas and approaches.	Yes	Depends	No

If you answered "yes" to 8 to 10 of the items, you are probably receptive to creating and experiencing new and different ways of doing things. If you answered "depends" to 5 to 10 of the items, you are probably receptive to change conditionally based on the fit of the change with your preferred ways of doing things. If you answered "no" to 4 to 10 of the items, you are probably not receptive, at least initially, to new ways of doing things. If you answered "yes," "no," and "depends" an approximately equal number of times, you are probably mixed in your receptivity to change based on individual situations.

their dissatisfactions visibly; others may quietly accommodate the change. Some individuals consistently reject any new thinking or ways of doing things.

The initial responses to change may be, but are not always, reluctance and resistance. Resistance and reluctance are common when the change threatens personal security. For example, changes in the structure of an agency can result in changes of position for personnel. Changing the position of a nurse from critical care nurse to home health nurse can result in the nurse feeling temporarily incompetent and isolated.

The change agent's recognition of the ideal and common patterns of individuals' behavioral responses to change can facilitate an effective change (Rogers, 1995). These responses and brief descriptions are as follows:

- *Innovators* thrive on change, which may be disruptive to the unit stability.

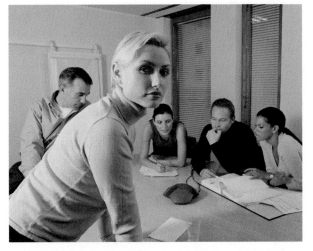

In system organizations, remote-site staff need to participate in making changes to feel a part of the process and have the same understanding as those within the primary site.

- *Early adopters* are respected by their peers and thus are sought out for advice and information about innovations/changes.
- *Early majority* prefer doing what has been done in the past but eventually will accept new ideas.
- *Late majority* are openly negative and agree to the change only after most others have accepted the change.
- *Laggards* prefer keeping traditions and openly express their resistance to new ideas.
- *Rejectors* oppose change actively, even use sabotage, which can interfere with the overall success of a change process.

The change agent's challenge is to deal with these behavioral patterns of individuals by providing opportunities to channel their responses into those supportive of the change process. Helping innovators "test" new ideas might be accomplished in a contained manner so that they are not disruptive, yet they feel supported. In one sense, the work of the Institute for Healthcare Improvement (IHI) uses this approach. The focus of the Institute is to accelerate change. Unit-based decision-making to change processes and policies is built around the microcosm of the unit and the ongoing adaptation to evolving realities. The more rapidly change can be incorporated, the more effective the organization is at remaining relevant. Connecting early adopters to new ideas and to innovators keeps them at the cutting edge. When these two groups are supported, an early majority can occur. The challenge of working with the late majority and the laggards is making them feel comfortable to transition to new practices. Thus, the equal challenge is to help them feel sufficiently uncomfortable that remaining where they are is no longer the place of comfort. Finally, the goal of working with the rejectors is to minimize their effects and to encourage them to find work that is more satisfying. The change agent's challenges are to be sensitive to employees' stages of loss and to promote transition by responding with appropriate interventions.

Jost (2000) reported her development of an assessment tool using concepts from Levine's conservation model. The tool's purpose was to assess and address staff members' issues systematically. Discovering the nature of their concerns, the nurse manager intervened appropriately to support staff during times of change and transition, which ulti-

mately had positive outcomes for productivity, job satisfaction, and employment longevity.

Systems and Technologic Side of Change

The *systems and technologic side of managing change* refers to responses that influence the efficiency and effectiveness of work processes and outcomes. The change agent's challenge is to monitor, recognize, and apply appropriate strategies to minimize responses that are destructive and maximize those that support the dynamics of an ongoing change.

Organizational systems and technology can both influence and be influenced by change. System responses to change may emerge as signs of more or less efficiency or effectiveness. Changes in the type of staff or technology used to deliver care may lead to initial responses of confusion, then to a period of adaptation by the staff and other systems. The quality of care and the morale of staff may change. Productivity and safety outcomes may be different. Reparation of the breakdowns in the affected work processes can restore efficient and effective functioning. Managing uncertainty is critical.

STRATEGIES

The change agent uses various strategies to facilitate both planned and nonlinear change processes (Figure 16-3). **Strategies** are approaches designed to achieve a particular purpose based on anticipation and consideration of myriad human, technologic, and system responses. The intent of the change agent and those supporting the change is to promote the continued movement toward integrating the change and achieving outcomes and to decrease and eliminate, if possible, any harmful resistance to the change (Wheeler, 1995). The key to using the various strategies effectively is to learn to match the appropriate strategies with the demonstrated response as it relates to the change situation.

Strategies, such as education and communication; participation and involvement; facilitation and support; negotiation and agreement; and manipulation and cooptation, or coercion, can be used individually or in combination with each other (Kotter & Schlesinger, 1979). As supported by chaos and learning organization theory, the change agent also uses vision development, rela-

MATCHING STRATEGIES TO SITUATIONS

Situation	Education	Support	Facilitation	Communication	Participation	Negotiation	Manipulation	Cooptation	Coercion	Learning	Visioning	Relationships	Information
Staff not sure of next best step in change process	√	√	√	√						√	√	√	√
Two staff members reluctantly try change	√	√	√	√	√	√				√		√	√
Staff has heard rumors about new program	√			√						√	√		√
Several staff members propose a different method		√	√		√					√	√	√	√
One nurse consistently lags behind in accepting a change	√		√		√					√	√	√	√
A group of staff expresses loss of previous roles		√	√	√						√		√	√
Three staff members challenge the need for a change	√		√	√	√	√				√	√		√
Staff member avoids change task force membership				√		√			√	√		√	√
Four staff members have become change agents with manager	√	√	√	√	√					√	√		√
A group of staff verbalizes satisfaction with status quo	√			√	√	√	√	√		√	√	√	√
One nurse disrupts the change process with other ideas	√			√	√	√	√	√		√	√	√	√
Two nurses try to get others to oppose change	√			√		√	√	√	√				

Figure 16-3 Matching strategies to situations.

tionship building, and information management strategies.

Communication and *education* refer to interchanges among the change agent, the change participants, and others for the purpose of integrating the elements of the change process. Staff meetings, focus groups (Carney, 2000), and informal discussions inform staff and clarify change activities. Active and empathetic listening is essential. Early explanation and education, especially of informal leaders, can facilitate change.

Empowerment of staff through *participation* and *involvement* promotes ownership of both the process and the decisions made during the process. It is important to incorporate staff at all levels at the beginning or as early as possible and then throughout the change process.

Facilitation and *support* strategies typically are used to reassure and assist those in the change situation who do not accept a change because of anxiety and fear. When personal security is threatened or when loss and grief are experienced, people tend to want to continue doing what they have always done. A staff member with financial problems may believe that a new benefit plan or implementation of no mandatory overtime policy will result in less take-home pay. The change agent can reassure that person by providing the actual calculation to show that the fear is unfounded.

Individuals or groups in the change situation may have the power or resources to adversely affect the success of a particular change. *Negotiation* and agreement strategies can revise these terms of the change to accommodate the involved parties.

Cooptation usually entails manipulated involvement through an appointed or assigned role. An example of this strategy is appointing a highly resistant individual to a change task force that necessitates more active involvement in the change process. *Manipulation* appeals to the motivational needs of others and influences them to participate in change when they might not do so on their own initiative. Expecting staff to be cooperative by participating in a pilot project of the proposed change on a 3-month basis can reduce barriers.

Coercion involves the use of power to force others to make a change, particularly when time is critical to implementation. An example of coercion would be offering to retain a staff member's position during staff reductions if that individual accepts certain conditions.

The ongoing creation of goals and visions *(visioning)* by all the change participants or change teams shows overt responsiveness to the dynamic nature of change (Senge, 1990). This required dialogue continually redefines the future, whether for the organization or for a project. Development of a set of possible outcomes rather than rigid pursuit of one outcome opens the possibilities to respond to unpredictable environmental influences (Begun & White, 1995). Change agents build work environments that support the time needed to create a shared vision and accept varied beliefs of staff (Senge, 1990).

Information management by the change agent focuses on delivery of the right information to the right place at the right time. Information may produce decisions that are relevant and flexible!

Managing *relationships* involves how individual capabilities and potential can facilitate creative solutions to projected organizational outcomes and is essential to change management. Formal position titles become irrelevant. Matching a staff member who has the needed abilities and attitudes with the demands of an appropriate project, for example, can lead to more creative outcomes. Peers can become coaches and teachers to help develop others' competencies.

The strategies discussed are useful when used appropriately. It is important to recognize cognitive responses or concerns, for example, that can be met with education, information, or other forms of communication. Participation, facilitation, and support can be choices to address the emotional components of accepting change, such as fear, anxiety, or grief. When the issue is sustained lack of motivation or unwillingness to cooperate, the more effective strategies may be manipulation, cooptation, or coercion. Effective change agents develop work environments that support continuous individual and group learning. Because of the dynamic nature of accelerated change environments, effective change agents stay focused on the dynamics of change by consistently managing information, relationships, and vision.

Typically, combinations of strategies are applied simultaneously, rather than one at a time. Figure 16-3 captures the deliberate selection of appropriate strategies to fit the ongoing needs and responses associated with leading change.

ROLES AND FUNCTIONS OF CHANGE AGENTS AND FOLLOWERS

Initiating change and managing its dynamics using linear and nonlinear approaches are key roles of change agents, with shared responsibilities by followers. Appropriate application of related functions, principles, and strategies can assist in meeting the challenges of any kind of change on the change continuum from **low-complexity change** to **high-complexity change**. The ultimate goal is a unified movement toward the adoption of something new or different. For example, in nursing homes, reducing turnover is a reflection of a change in the industry (see the Research Perspective). Anthony and colleagues (2005) indicate that retention is a key element of the professional role of nurse managers.

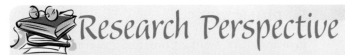

Research Perspective

Anderson, R. A., Corazzini, K. N., & McDaniel Jr., R. R. (2004). Complexity science and the dynamics of climate and communication: Reducing nursing home turnover. *Gerontologist, 44,* 378-388.

Using complexity theory, these researchers analyzed the effects of administrative climate, communication patterns, and the interaction of both on turnover. Using a hierarchical regression to test the hypotheses, the researchers collected data from 3449 employees in 164 randomly sampled nursing homes. The lowest turnover of licensed practical nurses and certified nurse assistants (the most frequently employed staff in nursing homes) occurred when the two factors of climate and communication interacted in the analysis. Open communication was a key factor as was a reward-based climate. Additionally, key predictors of lower turnover related to higher staffing levels and longer tenure of the nursing director.

IMPLICATIONS FOR PRACTICE

Creating climates that are rewarding and that support open communication is possible in any setting and leads to lower turnover rates. Stabilizing staff, especially at the leadership level, can also contribute to the intents of licensed practical nurses and certified nurse assistants to turnover.

Effective followership requires that followers communicate constructively with the formal or **informal change agent** to offer information, suggestions, or concerns. Followers also benefit by actively seeking participation in change, staying flexible, tolerating ambiguity, and thoughtfully supporting change efforts (Menix, 2001). Lencioni (2002) suggests that the key dysfunction of a team is lack of trust. Building trust, therefore, is critical for both leaders and followers.

Change agents use their personal, professional, and managerial knowledge and skills to lead or influence change and to build trust in the team. Staff members who are not officially in charge—possessing only informal power—can also play important change agent functions. Through their early interest and expertise (early majority), informal leaders can model the new way of doing or thinking for others to simulate. Their positive attitudes toward integrating the change can positively influence staff participation and unity. The informal leader's close interaction with the formal change agent can lead to reinforcement with other staff members about changes in direction.

Knowing how to build relationships, interact with others, and empower change participants is also critical to the achievement of change outcomes (Menix, 2001). Staff who share the creation of change that affects them directly and who trust the change agent usually are more receptive to change and integrate change more willingly. Giving and receiving information that includes clear explanations also encourages receptivity. Assertive communication projects self-confidence. Persistence and persuasion can communicate the change agent's commitment to the change outcome.

Because the human, systems, and technologic responses to change are unpredictable, flexibility, timing, and conflict management by the change agent can keep the change on course (Menix, 2001). It is important to deal with potential or real conflict in effective ways. Understanding the interrelatedness of change and group dynamics assists the change agent in selecting appropriate strategies. Change participants are members of unique work cultures, and, therefore, the change agent's selection of strategies to manage responses should take the culture's dominant values and beliefs into consideration. Creating change that is viewed as culturally appropriate is more valued than change that is imposed on people.

Having credibility, often as a result of their expertise and legitimate power, allows change agents to sometimes make independent decisions without negative responses. Change agents can role model the change by actively participating in the change situation, which can translate into expectations for others to follow. For example, a manager who uses the new computerized medication dispenser may be more likely to earn the respect of the change participants.

Exercise 16–3

Recall a work or personal situation in which a particular individual tried to get you or a group to do something. What rationale supported the decision to cooperate or not? Was the idea worthwhile from your perception? Was the person making the suggestions known, understood, and trusted? Was the person making the suggestions aware of the real situation, an essential part of carrying out the idea, or had he or she not received official sanctioning to influence activities? Can you see that change agents need specific qualities and abilities to be trusted by others?

PRINCIPLES

Principles are assumptions and general rules that guide behavior and processes. Principles are useful for creating and leading change. Classic principles that characterize effective change implementation are provided in Box 16-2 (Harper, 1993).

Exercise 16–4

Prepare an actual or hypothetical change that is meaningful to you in your personal, work, or school life. Select a change that provides an opportunity to apply the linear (planned) and nonlinear principles of change. Draft a hypothetical or actual plan for change, drawing on the chapter content and paying particular attention to the array of change principles discussed. Share your plan and the rationale used with peers or a small group of other healthcare providers. Ask for their comments and suggestions. (If you need a hypothetical change to work with, consider this one: You are the assistant manager for a home health agency. The agency administrator just informed you by memorandum that in 1 month, because of new reimbursement rules, the agency will begin caring for patients receiving chemotherapy. How will you prepare for this change?)

BOX 16-2

Classic Principles Characterizing Effective-Change Implementation

- Change agents within healthcare organizations use personal, professional, and managerial knowledge and skills to lead change.
- The recipients of change believe they own the change.
- Administrators and other key personnel support the proposed change.
- The recipients of change anticipate benefit from the change.
- The recipients of change participate in identifying the problem warranting a change.

- The change holds interest for the change recipients and other participants.
- Agreement exists within the work group about the benefit of the change.
- The change agents and recipients of change perceive a compatibility of values.
- Trust and empathy exist among the participants of the change process.
- Revision of the change goal and process is negotiable.
- The change process is designed to provide regular feedback to its participants.

Modified from Harper, C. L. (1993). *Exploring social change* (2nd ed.). Englewood Cliffs, NJ: Prentice Hall.

The Solution

The changes in nurses' pay schedules essentially rearranged both the tangible and less tangible incentives of employment. Some nurses decided to stay in full-time positions; some became prn nurses. I continue to use prn and agency nurses, despite their higher costs. My goal in managing this change was to maintain the standards and continuity of care by providing the right number and type of competent staff around the clock. The hospital has clinical coordinators, too, who offer the added expertise and support for all staff and patients, regardless of their pay schedule classification. Most of my change management strategies had to do with keeping frequent contact with staff, being approachable, and addressing individual issues of concern before they became unit issues. Building trust, keeping their confidence, and always seeking to know their opinions and needs work toward retention of full-time nurses and hopefully making this place a quality place to work for all. My phi-losophy is to keep employees happy, not to just keep them! Besides staying informed about what is going on in this hospital and outside about the supply of nurses and other related issues, I do a variety of things to attract and interest future nursing staff. I talk with nursing students and serve as a preceptor for them. I talk to high school students as well. I support the informal learning and continuing education of my current staff. I try to help them meet their goals and the unit's needs. I observe for tiredness and burnout and try to act in their interest. I never discourage staff from leaving the unit; many times they return because they had positive experiences.

— Joel Graeter

 Would this be a suitable approach for you? Why?

CHAPTER CHECKLIST

Change is an unavoidable constant in the rapidly transforming healthcare delivery system. As a result, uncertainty is an element in most healthcare institutions. Creating and leading change rather than merely reacting can promote overall organizational effectiveness.

The nature of accelerated change demands flexibility and prompt response to sometimes unpredictable environmental pressures as opposed to inflexible thinking and acting. Planned change as a linear approach to managing change can be useful for dealing with low-level, less complex change. Nonlinear approaches offered by chaos and learning organization theories focus more on managing the dynamic elements of more complex, high-level change situations.

- Characteristics of change include the following:
  - Is a natural social process
  - Involves individuals, groups, organizations, and society
  - Is constant and accelerates at various rates and intensities
  - Is inevitable and unpredictable
  - Varies from high complexity to low complexity
- Planned change occurs in sequential stages, according to planned change theorists:
  - Lewin:
    - Awareness of need for change
    - Experience of change
    - Integration of change
  - Havelock:
    - Building a relationship
    - Diagnosing the problem
    - Acquiring relevant resources
    - Choosing the solution
    - Gaining acceptance
    - Stabilizing the innovation and generating self-renewal
  - Lippitt, Watson, and Westley:
    - Client system becomes aware of need for change
    - Relationship between client system and change agent
    - Change problem defined
    - Change goals set and options for achievement explored
    - Plan for change implemented

- – Change accepted and stabilized
- – Change entities redefine relationship
- Rogers:
  - – Knowledge
  - – Persuasion
  - – Decision
  - – Implementation
  - – Confirmation
- Nonlinear change occurs in a different manner according to nonlinear change theorists:
  - Chaos theory:
    - – Organizations as open systems
    - – Non–human-induced self-organizing patterns
    - – Periods of stability interrupted with intense transformation
    - – Small changes resulting in significant consequences
    - – Conditions in one situation not recurring in the same pattern
  - Learning organization theory:
    - – Emphasis on flexibility, responsiveness, and learning
    - – Five disciplines interrelated by dialogue
  - Systems thinking:
    - – Personal mastery
    - – Mental models
    - – Shared vision
    - – Team learning
  - Major change management functions:
    - – Planning
    - – Organizing
    - – Implementing
    - – Evaluating
    - – Providing feedback/cybernetic theory
- The human responses to change manifest in various behavioral patterns that may help or hinder movement toward achievement of the change outcome:
  - Innovators
  - Early adopters
  - Early majority
  - Late majority
  - Laggards
  - Rejectors
- Multiple strategies are used selectively to promote involvement by the participants of change and to facilitate the overall change process:
  - Education and communication
  - Participation and involvement
  - Facilitation and support
  - Negotiation and agreement
  - Manipulation and cooptation
  - Coercion
  - Information management
  - Relationship facilitation
  - Ongoing vision development
  - Continuous learning
- Effective change agents, both formal and informal (those not in charge), exhibit the following characteristics in the change situation:
  - Display leadership
  - Possess excellent communication skills
  - Use observation skills
  - Know how groups work
  - Are perceptive about political issues
  - Are trusted by others
  - Establish positive relationships
  - Empower others
  - Are flexible
  - Manage conflict
  - Participate actively in change
  - Are respected, credible members of organization or community
  - Possess expert and legitimate power
  - Understand change process
  - Display appropriate timing
- Principles guide change:
  - Ownership of change
  - Anticipated benefits as change consequence
  - Negotiability between change agent and participants
  - Benefits of feedback to change process

TIPS IN LEADING CHANGE

- Whether involved in planned (low-complexity) or nonlinear (high-complexity) change, create a group of outcome/goal scenarios with prospective actions to achieve.
- Expect people to respond differently to change, which may either keep movement toward the outcome on course or slow it down.
- People cope and adapt better when they assume the role of continuous learner during accelerated change.
- People involved in change may assume the roles of followers or leaders and may emerge from both informal and formal, or internal and external sources.
- Creating a detailed plan and rigidly adhering to it reduces opportunities to moderate the inevitable and changing aspects of a change process, especially in an accelerated change environment. Building ambiguity and flexibility into a plan and how it is managed promotes responsiveness and movement toward desired outcomes.

TERMS TO KNOW

barriers
change agents
change management
change outcome
change process
change situations
chaos theory
cybernetic theory
facilitators
high-complexity change
informal change agent
learning organization
low-complexity change
negative feedback
nonlinear change
planned change
strategies

REFERENCES

Anderson, R. A., Corazzini, K. N., & McDaniel Jr., R. R. (2004). Complexity science and the dynamics of climate and communication: Reducing nursing home turnover. *Gerontologist, 44,* 378-388.

Anthony, M. K., Standing, T. S., Glick, J., Duffy, M., Paschall, F., Sauer, M. R., Sweeney, D. K., Modic, M. B., & Dumpe, M. L. (2005). Leadership and nurse retention: The pivotal role of nurse managers. *Journal of Nursing Administration, 35,* 146-155.

Ashby, W. R. (1957). *An introduction to cybernetics.* New York: John Wiley & Sons.

Begun, J. W., & White, K. R. (1995). Altering nursing's dominant logic: Guidelines from complex adaptive systems theory. *Complexity and Chaos in Nursing, 2*(1), 5-15.

Cadwallader, M. L. (1959). The cybernetic analysis of change in complex social organizations. *The American Journal of Sociology, 65,* 154-157.

Carney, M. (2000). The development of a model to manage change: Reflection on a critical incident in a focus group setting. An innovative approach. *Journal of Nursing Management, 8,* 265-272.

Freeman, S. J. (1999). The Gestalt of organizational downsizing: Downsizing strategies as packages of change. *Human Relations, 52*(12), 1505-1541.

Geddes, N., Salyer, J., & Mark, B. M. (1999). Nursing in the Nineties: Managing the uncertainty. *Journal of Nursing Administration, 29*(5), 40-48.

Harper, C. L. (1993). *Exploring social change* (2nd ed.). Englewood Cliffs, NJ: Prentice Hall.

Havelock, R. G. (1973). *The change agent's guide to innovation in education.* Englewood Cliffs, NJ: Educational Technology Publications.

Hirschhorn, L. (July, 2002). Campaigning for change. *Harvard Business Review, 80*(7), 98-104.

Jost, S. J. (2000). An assessment and intervention strategy for managing staff needs during change. *The Journal of Nursing Administration, 30*(1), 34-40.

Kotter, J., & Schlesinger, L. (1979, March/April). Choosing strategies for change. *Harvard Business Review, 57,* 106-114.

Lakoff, G. (2004). *Don't think of an elephant! Know your values and frame the debate.* White River Junction, Vermont: Chelsea Green Publishing.

Lencioni, P. (2002). The five dysfunctions of a team: A leadership fable. San Francisco: Jossey-Bass.

Lewin, K. (1947). Frontiers in group dynamics: Concept, method, and reality in social science, social equilibria and social change. *Human Relations, 1*(1), 5-41.

Lippitt, R., Watson, J., & Westley, B. (1958). *The dynamics of planned change.* New York: Harcourt Brace.

Menix, K. D. (2000). Educating to manage the accelerated change environment. Part 1. *Journal for Nurses in Staff Development, 16,* 282-288.

Menix, K. D. (2001). Educating to manage the accelerated change environment. Part 2. *Journal For Nurses in Staff Development, 17,* 44-53.

Porter-O'Grady, T. (1997). Quantum mechanics and the future of health care leadership. *The Journal of Nursing Administration, 27*(1), 15-20.

Porter-O'Grady, T. (2002). *Quantum Leadership: A Textbook of New Leadership.* Gaithersburg MD: Aspen.

Rogers, E. M. (1995). *Diffusion of innovations* (4th ed.). New York: The Free Press.

Senge, P. M. (1990). *The fifth discipline.* New York: Doubleday.

Vicenzi, A. E., White, K. R., & Begun, J. W. (1997). Chaos in nursing: Make it work for you. *American Journal of Nursing, 97*(10), 26-31.

Wheeler, M. M. (1995, January/February). The human side of change. *Canadian Journal of Nursing Administration, 8*(1), 26-32.

SUGGESTED READINGS

Asselin, M. (2001). Time to wear a third hat? *Nursing Management, 32*(3), 25-28.

Bennis, W. G., Benne, K. D., & Chin, R. (1984). *The planning of change* (4th ed.). Fort Worth: Holt, Rinehart & Winston.

Buonocore, D. (2004). Leadership in action: Creating a change in practice. *AACN Clinical Issues, 15,* 170-181.

Hawkins, A.L. & Kratsch, L.S. (2004). Troubled units: Creating change. *AACN Clinical Issues, 15,* 215-221.

Perra, B. M. (2000). Leadership: The key to quality outcomes. *Nurse Administrator Quarterly, 24*(2), 56-61.

Rycroft-Malone, J. (2004). The PARIHS framework—A framework for guiding the implementation of evidence-based practice. *Journal of Nursing Care Quality, 19,* 297-304.

West, B., Lyon, M. H., McBain, M., & Gass, J. (2004). Evaluation of a clinical leadership initiative. *Nursing Standard, 19,* 33-41.

Witkin, B. R., & Altschuld, J. W. (2000). *From needs assessments to action.* Thousand Oaks, CA: Sage Publications.

Wolf, F., Bradle, J., & Nelson, G. (2005). Bridging the strategic leadership gap: A model profram for transformational change. *Journal of Nursing Administration, 35*(2), 54-60.

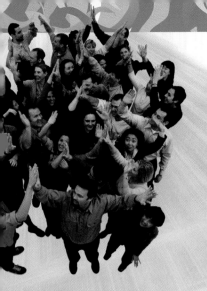

17

Building Teams Through Communication and Partnerships

Karren Kowalski

T his chapter explains major concepts and presents tools with which to create and maintain a smoothly functioning team. Life requires that we work together in a smooth and efficient manner, communicate effectively, and develop relationships that produce partnerships. Many important team efforts occur in the work setting. Such teams often include members with various backgrounds and educational preparation (e.g., physicians, nurses, administrators, allied health professionals, and support staff such as housekeeping and dietary staff members). Each team member has something valuable to contribute and deserves to be treated honorably and with respect. When teams are not working effectively, all team members must change how they communicate and interact within the team.

Objectives

- Evaluate the differences between a group and a team.
- Value four key concepts of teams.
- Demonstrate an effective communication interaction.
- Identify at least five communication pitfalls.
- Apply the guidelines for acknowledgment to a situation in your clinical setting.
- Compare a setting that uses the "rules of the game" with your current clinical setting.
- Develop an example of a team that functions synergistically, including the results such a team would produce.

Questions to Consider

- *What differentiates a team from a group? How is a team created?*
- *What are the most common communication breakdowns?*
- *What are key aspects of a well-functioning team?*
- *What are the key issues team members face or questions team members want to know?*
- *How are communication and self-worth connected?*
- *What role do agreements or guidelines play in a team?*
- *What are the behaviors and attitudes that destroy teams?*
- *Do teams go through stages of development?*

The Challenge

Diane Gallagher, RN, MS
Director, Women's and Children's Services, Rush-Presbyterian-St. Luke's Medical Center,
  Chicago, Illinois

An extensive "team" of people works together to care for the neonate in a neonatal intensive care unit (NICU). They include physicians, registered nurses, respiratory therapists, physical therapists, social workers, neonatal nurse practitioners, and ancillary staff. Occasionally, specialists are consulted for specific cardiac, neurologic, or gastrointestinal problems. These are intermittent "team" members who play a crucial role in the baby's care.

Recently, a new group of specialists joined our team. They were identified as a top-notch group who would, by virtue of their expertise and reputation, increase the census and revenues for the hospital. Our team was excited to have this opportunity to grow in an area where we had infrequent experience. However, things did not go smoothly. There were clinical disagreements, communication breakdowns, and interpersonal conflicts. The experience evolved into mutual distrust and control issues.

As disagreements, insults, and complaints escalated on both sides, the situation came to a defining moment when the director of the specialty group said, "I'm never bringing any of our patients here. I'm sending them to the PICU." The response from the NICU team was, "Fine with us; we don't need you, your patients, or the hassle." It seemed reasonable to not work together because in fact, functionally, we were already not working together. This response was in direct conflict with our belief that we could provide a valuable service and make a difference for both the patients and their families. This posed a dilemma for the staff, but everyone felt the situation was hopeless.

No one believed we could function as a team, and, therefore, further efforts to work together were futile. We had tried and failed. Let's just cut our losses and move on. How does one create a team when no one believes it is possible and some believe it is not even necessary?

 What do you think you would do if you were this nurse?

INTRODUCTION

As we experience changes such as cost-cutting and downsizing in health care, teamwork becomes critical. The adage "If we do not all hang together we will all hang separately" was never more true than now as we move through an era in which health care is rapidly changing. To create finely tuned teams, communication skills must improve. Each team member must focus on improving his or her own skills, as well as supporting other team members, to grow in **effective communication.**

In our society, where so much emphasis is placed on the individual and individual achievement, teamwork is the quintessential contradiction. In other words, with all the focus on individuals, we still need individuals to work together in groups to accomplish goals. Everybody knows and understands this, particularly individuals who spend their Sundays watching football or basketball. These team sports are premier models of cooperation and competition. They are the model for teamwork for business today, and they represent a group following their respective leader or "coach" (Parcells, 2000).

GROUPS AND TEAMS

The definition of **group** is a number of individuals assembled together or having some unifying relationship. Groups could be all the parents in an elementary school, all the members of a specific church, or all the students in a school of nursing, because the members of these various groups are related in some way to one another by definition of their involvement in a certain endeavor. A **team,** on the other hand, is a number of persons associated together in specific work or activity. Not every group is a team, and not every team is effective.

A group of people does not constitute a team. From Parker's (1990) perspective, a team is a group of people with a high degree of interdependence geared toward the achievement of a goal or a task. Often, we can recognize intuitively when the so-called team is not functioning effectively. We say things such as, "We need to be more like a team" or "I'd like to see more team players around here." Consequently, in the process of defining *team,* effective versus ineffective teams should be considered. Teams are groups that have defined objectives, ongoing positive relationships, and a supportive environment and that are focused on accomplishing a specific task. Teams are essential in providing cost-effective, high-quality health care. As resources are expended more prudently, patient-care teams must develop clearly defined goals, use creative problem-solving, and demonstrate mutual respect and support. Facilities with ineffective teams will find themselves out of business.

Exercise 17–1

Think of the last team or group of which you were a part. Think about what went on in that team or group. Specifically think about what worked for you and what did not work. Use the "Team Assessment Questionnaire" in Table 17-1 to evaluate these aspects more specifically. When you have finished answering the questions, use the scoring mechanism at the bottom to discover how well your team or group functioned in terms of roles, activities, relationships, and general environment.

When a team functions effectively, a significant difference is evident in the entire work atmosphere, the way in which discussions progress, the level of understanding of the team-specific goals and tasks, the willingness of members to listen, the manner in which disagreements are handled, the use of consensus, and the way in which feedback is given and received. The original work done by McGregor (1960) sheds light on some of these significant differences, which are summarized in Table 17-2.

Ineffective teams are often dominated by a few members, leaving others bored, resentful, or uninvolved. Leadership tends to be autocratic and rigid, and the team's communication style may be overly stiff and formal. Members tend to be uncomfortable with conflict or disagreement, avoiding and suppressing it rather than using it as a catalyst for change. When criticism is offered, it may be destructive, personal, and hurtful rather than constructive and problem-centered. Team members may begin to "stuff" their feelings of resentment or disagreement inside, sensing that they are "dangerous." This creates the potential for later eruptions and discord. Similarly, the team avoids examining its own inner workings, or members may wait until after meetings to voice their thoughts and feelings about what went wrong and why.

In contrast, the effective team is characterized by its clarity of purpose, informality and congeniality, **commitment,** and high level of participation. The members' ability to listen respectfully to each other and communicate openly helps them handle disagreements in a civilized manner and work through them rather than suppress them. Through ample discussion of issues, they reach decisions by consensus. Roles and work assignments are clear, but members share the leadership role, recognizing that each person brings his or her own unique strengths to the group effort. This diversity of styles helps the team adapt to changes and challenges, as does the team's ability and willingness to assess its own strengths and weaknesses and respond to them appropriately.

The challenges encountered in today's health-care systems are prodigious. Ongoing rounds of downsizing budget cuts, declining patient days, reduced payments, and staff layoffs abound. Effective teams participate in effective problem-solving, increased creativity, and improved health care. While this challenge to be clear in communications may seem daunting, there are many tools to help leaders develop teams. One source is described in the Literature Perspective.

Table 17-1 TEAM ASSESSMENT QUESTIONNAIRE

Circle the appropriate number using the following scale. (1, Not at all; 2, limited extent; 3, some extent; 4, considerable extent.)

1. People are clear about goals for the group.	1 2 3 4
2. Unnecessary procedures, policies, and formality are minimized.	1 2 3 4
3. Team members feel free to develop and experiment with new ideas and approaches.	1 2 3 4
4. The allocation of rewards is perceived to be based on excellent performance.	1 2 3 4
5. Recognition and praise outweigh threats and criticism.	1 2 3 4
6. Calculated risk-taking is encouraged.	1 2 3 4
7. People are clear about their responsibilities and expectations for performance.	1 2 3 4
8. People are clear about how their roles and responsibilities interrelate with those of others.	1 2 3 4
9. People perceive others in the work group to be high performers.	1 2 3 4
10. People are clear about what personal characteristics/competencies are necessary for superior performance in their jobs.	1 2 3 4
11. The team produces high-quality decisions, products, and/or services.	1 2 3 4
12. The team is able to conduct effective meetings.	1 2 3 4
13. The team achieves its goals.	1 2 3 4
14. The team and its individual members are able to interact effectively with others outside the team.	1 2 3 4
15. The team makes decisions and produces output in a timely fashion.	1 2 3 4
16. The team members truly support each other in carrying out their respective responsibilities.	1 2 3 4
17. Team members are open in their communications with each other.	1 2 3 4
18. Team members follow through on commitments.	1 2 3 4
19. Team members trust each other.	1 2 3 4
20. All team members are equal contributors to the team process.	1 2 3 4
21. The group often evaluates how effectively it is functioning.	1 2 3 4
22. Individual members feel committed to the team.	1 2 3 4

If you would like to score your team assessment questionnaire, enter the score you selected for each question. Next, take the scores for each area; then calculate the average score.

Roles Item/Score	Activities Item/Score	Relationships Item/Score	Environment Item/Score
7 _____	2 _____	5 _____	1 _____
8 _____	3 _____	14 _____	2 _____
9 _____	11 _____	16 _____	3 _____
10 _____	12 _____	17 _____	4 _____
18 _____	13 _____	19 _____	5 _____
20 _____	15 _____	22 _____	6 _____
21 _____			
Total Score _____	Total Score _____	Total Score _____	Total Score _____
Average Score = _____	Average Score = _____	Average Score = _____	Average Score = _____
(Total Score ÷ by 7)	(Total Score ÷ by 6)	(Total Score ÷ by 6)	(Total Score ÷ by 6)

If the average for a column (e.g., Activities) was 3.5, it means the group is fairly productive in its activity, falling halfway between "some extent" and "considerable extent." If the average for the relationships column was 1.5, it indicates that the respondent believes that team members have not been effective in developing relationships with one another that are clearly defined, effective, or respectful of one another.

From Dubnicki, C. (1991, May-June). Building high-performance management teams. *Healthcare Forum Journal, 34*, 19-24.

Table 17-2 ATTRIBUTES OF EFFECTIVE AND INEFFECTIVE TEAMS

Attribute	Effective Team	Ineffective Team
Working environment	• Informal, comfortable, relaxed	• Indifferent, bored; tense, stiff
Discussion	• Focused • Shared by almost everyone	• Frequently unfocused • Dominated by a few
Objectives	• Well understood and accepted	• Unclear, or many personal agendas
Listening	• Respectful—encourages participation	• Judgmental—much interruption and "grandstanding"
Ability to handle conflict	• Comfortable with disagreement • Open discussion of conflicts	• Uncomfortable with disagreement • Disagreement usually suppressed, or one group aggressively dominates
Decision-making	• Usually reached by consensus • Formal voting kept to a minimum • General agreement is necessary for action; dissenters are free to voice	• Often occurs prematurely • Formal voting occurs frequently • Simple majority is sufficient for action; minority is expected to go along with opinion
Criticism	• Frequent, frank, relatively comfortable, constructive • Directed toward removing obstacle	• Embarrassing and tension-producing; destructive • Directed personally at others
Leadership	• Shared; shifts from time to time	• Autocratic; remains clearly with committee chairperson
Assignments	• Clearly stated • Accepted by all despite disagreements	• Unclear • Resented by dissenting members
Feelings	• Freely expressed, open for discussion	• Hidden, considered "explosive" and inappropriate for discussion
Self-regulation	• Frequent and ongoing, focused on solutions	• Infrequent, or occurs outside meetings

Modified from McGregor, D. (1960). *The human side of enterprise.* New York: McGraw-Hill.

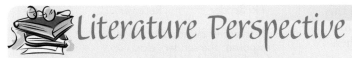 Literature Perspective

Davis, H., & Sharon, B. (2002). *Teambuilding: High-performance team models and strategies.* Malvern, PA: Indaba Press.

This is a workbook that will guide the reader through the team-building process. It provides specific models and guidelines for team development. There are tools and skill sets supplied that enable you to achieve results in team situations. Some of these include team commitment contracts, stages of team development, a formula for stress control and stress relief, tools for giving feedback and for coaching, brainstorming, tools for evaluating team effectiveness, and ideas about negotiation and influencing. Criteria are described for achieving peak performance for both individuals and teams. Team goal development including vision, mission, and purpose are reviewed. Theories of team behavior are identified. There are tools that look at the development of each individual team member and the importance of effective communication within the team. If readers work through the exercises in the book, they will have a much better perception of how to participate on a team.

COMMUNICATING EFFECTIVELY

Communication in the work environment is not only important to good working conditions that retain nurses but also critical to reduction of medical errors (American Association of Critical-Care Nurses [AACN] & VitalSmarts, 2005; Arford, 2005). Due to such issues, new graduates go through a facility orientation, which emphasizes communication skills. Many nurses view this as a waste of time that could be used to further technical skills; however, at evaluation time, communication skills are often seen as an area for improvement (Buckman, Korsch, Baile, & Jason, 2000; Weiner, Barnet, Cheng, & Daaleman, 2005). The only thing human beings do more often than communicate is breathe. It is the most important component of daily activities. It is essential to clinical practice, to building teams, and to leadership. A person cannot *not* communicate. Because communication consists of both verbal and nonverbal signals, humans are continuously communicating not just thoughts, ideas, and opinions but also feelings and emotions (Morreale, Spitzberg, & Barge, 2001). Once the message is sent, it cannot be retracted; it can be amended, but the first impression of the communication usually is lasting. However, as important as this initial impression is, it is often an unconscious response or reaction.

How we communicate is also a reflection of self-worth: Once a human being has arrived on this earth, communication is the largest single factor determining what kinds of relationships she or he makes with others and what happens to each in the world (Satir, 1988, p. 51). Self-worth is a major influence in all communication. Stress results whenever self-worth is threatened.

Communication is learned from watching others. A host of poor examples can be seen in movies and television. Poor communication leads to relationship breakdowns, misunderstandings, high levels of emotion, judgment, and an excess of drama. Nursing programs teach therapeutic communications with patients and their families. However, little focus is placed on effective communication in the workplace, although communication is essential to building and maintaining smoothly functioning teams.

A basic model of communication patterns between the sender and the receiver is found in Figure 17-1. Effective communication develops a rhythm in which messages are sent and received in a productive, respectful, and supportive manner (Wilson, 1999). Communication begins to break down as the rhythm is disrupted. The **sender-receiver** pattern disintegrates into a nonrhythmic event, as described in Figure 17-1. When nonrhythmic patterns develop, the participants may feel disrespected, upset, and even fearful.

Stress

In her classic work, Satir (1988) identified the connection between stress and self-worth that can evolve as a result of a breakdown in communication. She defined stress as a threat to positive self-

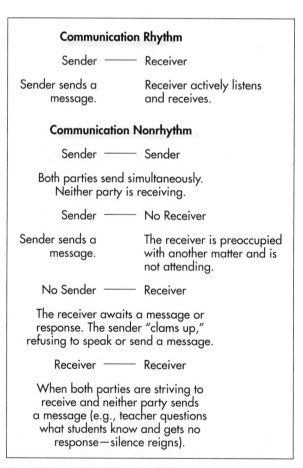

Communication Rhythm

Sender ——— Receiver

Sender sends a message.   Receiver actively listens and receives.

Communication Nonrhythm

Sender ——— Sender

Both parties send simultaneously. Neither party is receiving.

Sender ——— No Receiver

Sender sends a message.   The receiver is preoccupied with another matter and is not attending.

No Sender ——— Receiver

The receiver awaits a message or response. The sender "clams up," refusing to speak or send a message.

Receiver ——— Receiver

When both parties are striving to receive and neither party sends a message (e.g., teacher questions what students know and gets no response—silence reigns).

Figure 17-1 Potential communication rhythms. (Modified from Satir, V. [1988]. *The new peoplemaking.* Mountain View, CA. Science & Behavior Books; and Olen, D. [1993]. *Communicating speaking & listening to end misunderstanding and promote friendship.* Germantown, WI: JODA Communications.)

worth. Human beings tend to feel stress or anxiety whenever there is an unconscious linking of feelings, behaviors, or comments from others to a lowering of self-esteem or an attack on self-worth. A conscious effort should be made to relieve stress through activities such as ensuring specific/scheduled quiet time, requesting peer support, keeping a journal, treating yourself to something special, or going for a walk (Weiss, 2001).

Stress Response Model

When this threat is identified, the receiver often reacts using one of the five communication patterns: attribution of blame, placation, constrained cool headedness, immaterial irrelevance, or congruence (Bradley & Edinberg, 1990; Satir, 1988). Each pattern interaction and the source of the interaction is described with examples of each pattern in Table 17-3. The pattern that produces effective communication, the one to strive for, is congruence. Congruent communication occurs when both the verbal and nonverbal actions fit the inner feel-

ings of the sender and are appropriate to the context of the message. This communication pattern creates the kind of connection between the sender and the receiver that fosters respect, support, and the creation of relationship.

Communication Barriers

In today's busy world, many interruptions and interferences to clear, focused, effective communication create breakdowns. According to Ceccio and Ceccio (1982), to be aware of these potential problems allows both sender and receiver to be prepared to minimize such barriers.

Distractions: Distractions most commonly come through sensory perceptions, such as poor lighting or background noise, including music, talking, ringing phones, and interruptions by others. Papers, reports, and heavy workloads can also be distracting.

Inadequate knowledge: The sender and receiver may be at different levels of knowledge, particularly in this time of highly specialized and technical

Table 17-3 COMMUNICATION PATTERNS

Pattern	Interaction	Source	Example
Attribution of blame	Sender blames receiver	Fault-finder dictator acts superior as camouflage for fear and low self-esteem	Mostly "you" messages; for example, "You really blew it!"
Placation	Sender placates receiver	Sender's low self-worth: puts herself/himself down	"I was wrong. I'm sorry. It's all my fault."
Constrained cool headedness	Sender is correct and very reasonable without feeling or emotion	Feelings of vulnerability covered by cool analytical thinking	"Studies have shown that in 75% of cases the patient is correct. I decided to use research data in coming to a solution."
Irrelevant	Sender is avoiding the issue, ignoring own feelings and feelings of the receiver	Fear, loneliness, and purposelessness	"Wait a minute. Let me tell you about . . ." (changes the subject)
Congruence	Sender's words and actions are congruent; inner feelings match the message	Any tension is decreased and self-worth is at a high level	"For now, I feel concerned about the anger and hostility exhibited by Dr. X. I'm wondering what approach would de-escalate him?"

Modified from Satir, V. (1988). *The new peoplemaking.* Mountain View, CA: Science & Behavior Books; and Bradley, J., & Edinberg, M. (1990). *Communication in the nursing context* (3rd ed.). Norwalk, CT: Appleton & Lange.

knowledge bases. For multiple reasons, one person may not seek clarity from the other.

Poor planning: The process of organizing, planning, and clearly thinking through what needs to be communicated is very helpful. If the interaction is more spontaneous, it can more easily fall into a nonrhythmic pattern.

Differences in perception: Both the sender and the receiver have their individual mental filters—the way in which they see the world. Because of this individuality, no two filters are the same. Thus, the same message is interpreted differently. Add to this sociocultural, ethnic, and educational differences, to name a few, and it is easy to see how these differences can occur.

Emotions and personality: Someone who is experiencing distress may not be able to receive another message or may have difficulty keeping his or her emotions out of an unrelated message. Most humans, at some point, bring distress or problems from home to the workplace. If these remain unconscious, they can influence the work setting in a negative or nonproductive way.

Communication Pitfalls

Effective communication suggests that the interaction is a rhythmic pattern that is respectful and clear, promotes trust, and encourages the expression of feelings and viewpoints. On the other hand, pitfalls in communication comprise actions, behaviors, and words that create distrust, are dishonoring, and decrease the feelings of self-worth in the receiver. Box 17-1 lists the major pitfalls of communication. These pitfalls lead to communication breakdowns that affect not only the team but also the quality of care to patients (Jason, 2000).

Communication Guidelines

There are effective guidelines that can be used when communicating. These are used mostly to facilitate a positive outcome and to create an environment in which the communicator can achieve the desired outcome. Unconscious use of any of the pitfalls will most likely result in thwarting the desired outcome. Box 17-2 lists effective guidelines for communication.

Exercise 17–2

In pairs or small groups, compare the effective guidelines for communication with the communication pitfalls. Give examples of each from your own recent personal experience. Hypothesize how you could have changed the pitfalls into a positive interaction.

KEY CONCEPTS OF TEAMS

In rare instances, a team may produce teamwork spontaneously, like kids in a schoolyard at recess. However, most management teams learn about teamwork because they need and want to work together. This kind of working together requires that they observe how they are together in a group and that they unlearn ingrained self-limiting assumptions about the glory of individual effort and authority that are contrary to cooperation and teamwork. Keys to the concept of team include the following:

- Conflict resolution
- Singleness of mission
- Willingness to cooperate
- Commitment

Conflict Resolution

When thinking about conflict, it is helpful to realize that conflict is fundamental to the human experience and is an integral part of all human interaction (Porter-O'Grady, 2004a). Therefore, the challenge is to recognize the breakdown in the communication process and to deal appropriately with it (Porter-O'Grady, 2004b). Conflicts are usually based on attempts to protect a person's self-esteem or to alter perceived inequities in power because most human beings believe that other people have greater power, and thus, most human beings are unlikely to achieve their objectives (Sportsman, 2005). For example, when a nurse recognizes upset and reaction between two nursing assistants with whom he or she is working, the following steps can be helpful: identify the triggering event; discover the historical context for each person; assess how interdependent they are on each other; identify the issues, goals, and resources involved in the situation; and uncover any previously considered solutions (Sportsman, 2005). Assessing the level of working relationship between the conflicted parties is essential, particularly if they work together on a regular basis.

The word *team* is usually reserved for a very special type of working together. This working together requires communication in which the members understand how to conduct interpersonal relationships with their peers in thoughtful, supportive, and meaningful ways. It requires that team members be able to resolve conflicts among

BOX 17-1

Communication Pitfalls

1. Giving Advice

It is so tempting to give advice when a co-worker comes with an issue or problem. *Don't!* Most often what the person wants is to work through the issue by talking out loud. Just listen.

2. Making Others Wrong

When telling others "our" story of distress, the adversary is always "wrong." The telling of the story to a third party only reinforces how right "I" am and how wrong, bad, or terrible the other person is. If you have an issue or problem, take the problem to the person with whom you are upset. "Take the mail to the correct address." Don't gossip!

3. Defensiveness

Defensiveness occurs when you do not listen, are hostile or aggressive, or respond as if attacked when there was no attack. Look for a physiologic signal in your body so that you can identify your own distress. Stop. Breathe. Acknowledge that the message did not come out the way you intended and begin again.

Also, defensiveness can occur when met with hostile, aggressive behavior from another. Rather than choose an emotional response or react to the attack, know that the other person's behavior has nothing to do with you personally but is the response chosen by that person in a moment of stress. Any one of a dozen other responses could have been chosen. Understand the person is motivated by fear or hurt.

4. Judging the Other Person

Evaluating another person as "good" or "bad," as someone you like or do not like, or judging their actions or behavior as "stupid" or "crazy" or "inappropriate" is a reflection of how you judge yourself. Who is the hardest person on you? Of course, you are. Know that you can have feelings about situations or behaviors without judging the other person in a negative way. Rather, you can feel compassion for their stress and fear, which often drives behavior. This is true particularly when a supervisor or physician is reprimanding you.

5. Patronizing

Speaking to others as though they are less than human or in need of custodial care fails to honor them as human beings. You do not have to be condescending or seek to humiliate in an overly sweet voice. These are merely other versions of judging or making the person wrong. Another approach is to question what is at issue for them in the moment.

6. Giving False Reassurance

One of the great temptations of nurses is to "fix" things and make them better, to rescue the situation or the person involved. To accomplish this goal, sometimes we reassure inappropriately. Know that you do not have to fix every situation. You can support people to work through situations themselves.

7. Asking Why Questions

When working in the team, refrain from asking why questions. These tend to create a defensive response in the other person. Instead, ask "What makes you think . . ."

8. Blaming Others

Saying things such as "You make me so angry" is blaming the other person for your feelings, which you choose at any given time. In nearly every situation, the responsibility for communication breakdown is a joint responsibility. You can always choose your response, even if that response is to say, "I can't discuss this with you now. I would like to talk about this later when I am more calm."

themselves and to do so in ways that enhance rather than inhibit their working together. In addition, team members must be able to trust that they will receive what they need while being able to count on one another to complete tasks related to team functioning and outcomes. To communicate effectively, people must be willing to confront issues and to express openly their ideas and feelings—to use interactive skills to accomplish tasks. In nursing, constructive confrontation has not been a well-used skill. Consequently, if communication patterns are to improve, the onus is on each of us as individuals to change communication patterns. In essence, for things to change, each of us must change.

Singleness of Mission

Each and every team must have a purpose—that is, a plan, aim, or intention. However, the most successful teams have a mission—some special work

BOX 17-2

Guidelines for Communication

- Approach each interaction as though the other person has no knowledge of effective communication. Assume responsibility for creating the sender-receiver rhythm.
- Share your thoughts and feelings. Be self-revealing.
- Use casual conversation or "small talk"; it can be important to relationships, particularly when it is light and humorous. It balances the deep meaningful talk.
- Acknowledge, praise, and encourage the other person; doing so is supportive and brings life and energy to the relationship.
- Present messages in a way that the other person can receive them.
- Take responsibility for any problem or issue you have with another and speak about it as your problem or issue also.
- Use language of equality even when position titles are not of the same level.

Modified from Olen, D. (1993). *Communicating speaking & listening to end misunderstanding and promote friendship.* Germantown, WI: JODA Communications.

or service to which the team is 100% committed. The sense of mission and purpose must be clearly understood and agreed to by all (Fisher & Thomas, 1996). The more powerful and visionary the mission is, the more energizing it will be to the team. The more energy and excitement are engendered, the more motivated all members will be to do the necessary work.

Willingness to Cooperate

Just because a group of people has a regular reporting relationship within an organizational chart does not mean the members are a team. Boxes and arrows are not in any way related to the technical and interpersonal coordination or the emotional investment required of a true team. In effective teams, members are required to work together in a respectful, civil manner. Most of us have been involved in organizations in which people could accomplish assigned tasks but were not successful in their interpersonal relationships. In essence, these employees received a salary for not getting along with a certain person or persons. Some of these employees have not worked cooperatively for years! Organizations can no longer afford to pay people to not work together. Personal friendship or socialization is not required, but cooperation is a necessity. Traditionally, these interpersonal skills were considered "soft" skills and difficult to coach people or hold them accountable. That is no longer the case. In most organizations employees can now be terminated for a lack of willingness to work cooperatively with team members.

Commitment

Commitment is a state of being emotionally impelled and is demonstrated when there is a sense of passion and dedication to a project or event—a mission. Often, this passion looks a little crazy. In other words, people go the extra mile because of their commitment. They do whatever it takes to accomplish the goals or see the project through to completion. An example of commitment is discussed by Charles Garfield when he talks about being a part of the team that created the lunar landing module for the first man to walk on the moon. People did all kinds of things that looked crazy, including working extended hours and shifts, calling in to see how the project was progressing, and sleeping over at their work station so as not to be separated from the project—all because everybody knew they were a part of something that was much bigger than themselves. They were a part of sending a man to the moon, something that human beings had been dreaming about for thousands of years. It was a historical moment, and people were intensely committed to making it happen.

Many people go through their entire lives hating every single day of work. Needless to say, most of them are not committed. Because we spend an extensive amount of time in the work setting, it is critically important to both physical and mental well-being that people enjoy what they do. If this is not the case for you, then try to find a different job or profession—one you might love. Life is too short to do something that you hate doing every day. While you are moving into whatever you decide you love doing, commit to yourself to do your best at whatever you are now doing. Be 100% present wherever you are. Do the best work you are capable of doing. This honors you as a human being, and it honors your co-workers and patients.

■ Exercise 17–3

Box 17-3 contains eight questions. Spend at least 20 minutes in a quiet place thinking about and writing answers to these eight questions. Pay particular notice to question 7.

There are many examples of commitment, such as that of Jan Skaggs, the Vietnam veteran who was the driving force behind the building of the Vietnam War Memorial. He was a clerk in the Washington, DC, bureaucracy who attended a veterans' meeting and decided there needed to be a memorial to those who lost their lives in Vietnam, a memorial that had all 58,000 names inscribed on it. He had only a high school diploma and did not even own a suit, but 5 years and $7 million later, the wall was dedicated (Lopes, 1987). This is a demonstration that one does not have to have a college degree to be committed. Sometimes a college degree can inhibit people from accomplishing their goals because they become diverted from a purpose, from a mission, or from life goals by things such as good grades. Rather than understanding grades as a tool of measurement, they see them as an end in themselves.

Almost anyone can be taught the technical aspects of what needs to be done in most patient-care settings. Teaching people to love what they do or to care about patients and their families—even the most difficult and unique patients and families—is far more difficult.

TOOLS AND ISSUES THAT SUPPORT TEAMS

When individuals come together in a group, they spend considerable time in group process or social dynamics, which allows the group to advance toward becoming a team and completing a goal. Each person within the group struggles with three key questions that must continually be reevaluated and renegotiated. These three questions, according to Weisburg's classic work (1988), are as follows:

1. Am I in or out?
2. Do I have any power or control?
3. Can I use, develop, and be appreciated for my skills and resources?

"In" Groups and "Out" Groups

Most of us want to be valued and recognized by others as a part of the group, one who "knows" or understands. Most people want to be at the core of

BOX 17-3

Exploring Commitment

The key to finding your compelling mission/passion that will lead you to success and peak performance is to ask yourself the right questions. Your answers to these questions will help you understand what you need to know about yourself. Read each question, then think carefully for a few minutes and answer each question honestly. Do not censor or edit out anything, even if it seems impossible or unrealistic—allow yourself to be surprised. Let your imagination soar.

1. Am I deriving any satisfaction out of the work I am now doing?
2. If they did not reward (praise or pay) me to do what I now do, would I still do it?
3. What is it that I really love to do?
4. What do I want to pursue with my time and energy that is worthwhile?
5. What motivates me to reach out and do my very best to excel?
6. What is it that only I can say to the world? What needs to be done that can best be done only by me?
7. If I won $10 million in the lottery tomorrow, how would I live? What would I do each day and for the rest of my life?
8. If I were to write my own obituary right now, what would be my most significant accomplishment? Is that enough?

Repeating this exercise often will give you additional insights and information about what you really want and love to do. If taken seriously, the exercise should help you to have an understanding of why you selected this profession and whether or not you have the stamina to do whatever it takes to make a contribution and to make a difference in the practice of nursing.

decision-making, power, and influence. In other words, they want to be part of the "in" group, and researchers have demonstrated that those who feel "in" cooperate more, work harder and more effectively, and bring enthusiasm to the group. The more we feel we are not a part of the key group, the more "out" we feel, and the more we withdraw, work alone, daydream, and engage in self-defeating behaviors. Often, intergroup conflict results when individuals who feel they are "out" and want to be "in" create a schism or a division that prohibits the team from accomplishing its goals.

Power and Control

Everybody wants at least some power, and everybody wants to feel they are in control. When faced with changes that we are unable to influence, we feel impotent and experience a loss of self-esteem. Consequently, all of us want to feel we are in control of our immediate environment and that we have enough power and influence to get our needs met. When a situation or an event arises that we are unable to handle, we attempt to compensate for it in some way; most of these ways are not productive to smoothly functioning teams.

Exercise 17-4

Think about a time when you and a small group of classmates or co-workers wanted to change something, such as a scheduled time (a class or meeting), an assignment, or an outcome measure (grading curve of a test or a performance evaluation criterion), and the faculty or administration adamantly refused. How did you feel? What was the response? Did you engage in gossip to make others appear wrong? You may have been "right," but the sense of a loss of control or power is very uncomfortable, sometimes resulting in stress and fear. Very mature behavior is required to maintain a positive, problem-solving approach.

POSITIVE COMMUNICATION MODEL

Whenever human beings are in distress or are having an emotional reaction to a situation or the actions of another, a conditioned response is to move into one or all of the following: *blame, judgment,* or *demand.* These are depicted in the awareness model found in Figure 17-2. With effort and practice, it is possible to create a communication interaction that produces a significantly improved outcome.

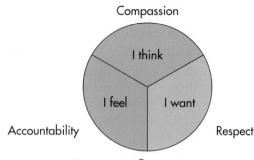

Awareness Model

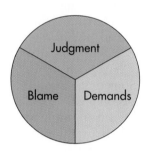

Figure 17-2 Awareness model: differentiating between conscious and unconscious responses. (Modified from St. Charles Medical Center. [1993]. *People centered teams.* Bend, OR: SCMC.)

When an individual is reacting at the feeling level, he or she tends to move unconsciously to blame. By taking accountability for these feelings, one can move out of blame and own one's feelings by stating, "I feel . . ."

Likewise, when an individual is trapped in distress or reaction at the thinking level, he or she most often turns to judgment. By thinking compassionately, one can dismantle the judgment and state what one thinks in a compassionate way: "I think . . ."

Finally, when in distress, we make demands that are often unreasonable. By calming oneself, one can find respect for the other human being and make a request: "I want . . ."

Most broken relationships are stuck in blame, judgment, and demand. Being accountable, compassionate, and respectful helps clarify what goes on inside each of us.

Everyone needs to feel as though his or her skills, tools, and contributions are needed and valued and that he or she is respected for what personal contributions are offered to the workplace, team, or group. Everyone has weaknesses, and there is no need to emphasize these or to spend time in ongoing correction. Rather, focus should be placed on people's strengths, specifically, acknowledging and emphasizing what people do well.

Part of focusing on people's strengths is being willing to acknowledge peers, faculty, and the other significant people in one's life (Roman, 2001). In contrast, many role models focus on correction. Consequently, many of us spend a large portion of our time correcting others rather than appreciating people for all the wonderful things they are. We seem to believe a finite number of available **acknowledgments** exists, and we must not give out too many of them because they must be held in reserve for very important events. In addition, we do not always give acknowledgments in a way they can be received and valued. Box 17-4 can serve as a guide for giving acknowledgment.

To deal with the three personal issues discussed in this section, team members must learn how to state openly what is on their minds and be responsive and respectful as other members of the team do the same. In other words, team members must give and receive feedback constructively. These are essential elements that must be in place for people to be able to give and receive feedback in constructive ways.

Exercise 17–5

Within the next 3 days, find three opportunities to acknowledge a peer or acquaintance using the five guidelines for acknowledgment shown in Box 17-4. In addition, use the guidelines to accept at least one self-acknowledgment.

Group Agreements

One of the most helpful tools available is to have the team members come to an agreement about the ground rules concerning their relationships with one another (Mears, 1997). This can take place in various ways. There are even multiple kinds of guidelines or rules that can be used to set the context for how people relate. One example of a set of guidelines can be found in Box 17-5. These are called "The Rules of the Game." They have gone through multiple transitions and redesign, but the basic tenets are essentially the same. People must agree on the goals and mission with which they are involved. They have to reach some understanding of how they will exist together. Tenets or rules such as "We will speak supportively" go a long way to avoid gossiping, backbiting, bickering, and misinterpreting others. As you review these group agreements, keep in mind that a part of this process is the willingness of members of the team to be accountable for upholding the agreements and to give feedback when the agreements have been violated. Without rules, people have implicit

---

BOX 17-4

Guidelines for Acknowledgment

1. Acknowledgments must be specific. The specific behavior or action that is appreciated must be identified in the acknowledgment; for example, "Thank you for taking notes for me when I had to go to the dentist. You identified three key points that appeared on the test."
2. Acknowledgments must be "eye to eye," or personal. Look the person in the eye when you thank them. Do not run down the hall and say "Thanks" over your shoulder. Written appreciation also qualifies as "eye to eye."
3. Acknowledgments must be sincere, that is, from the heart. Each of us recognizes insincerity. If you do not truly appreciate a behavior or action, do not say anything. Insincerity often makes people angry or upset, thus defeating the goal.

4. Acknowledgments are more powerful when they are given in public. Most people receive pleasure from public acknowledgment and remember these occasions for a long time. For people who are shy and may prefer no public acknowledgment, this is an opportunity to work on a personal growth issue with them. Public acknowledgment is an opportunity to communicate what is valued.
5. Acknowledgments need to be timely. The less time that elapses between the event and the acknowledgment, the more powerful and effective it is and the more the acknowledgment is appreciated by the recipient.

BOX 17-5

"Rules of the Game" for Women's and Children's Hospital, Rush-Presbyterian–St. Luke's Medical Center

These "Rules of the Game" were adapted from a San Francisco real estate broker who was the founder and president of Hawthorn-Stone. Dr. Karren Kowalski proposes that we use them not only among ourselves but with each new person who joins the organization, asking if we/they are willing and able to do the very best we/they can to support the rules.

1. Be willing to support Rush's purpose, games, rules, and goals

By first asking if people will support the rules, we have their agreement that they can be held accountable for times when they violate the "rules of the game."

2. Speak supportively

This means no swearing; if it does not serve, do not say it; if it does not support, do not say it; do not make other people wrong; you may choose not to say negative things. Language either empowers or limits people in terms of achieving their potential. How we speak about a colleague, the institution, our job, the workplace, and so forth, does make a difference.

3. Correct supportively

Dr. Kowalski says, "Make corrections without invalidation or correct without crucifixion."

4. Acknowledge that whatever is being communicated is true for the speaker at that moment

Most of the time, people make comments because they truly believe them. Therefore, it is important not to judge what is being said and misinterpret it, but to listen so that we can understand what is being said. Emphasis is on active listening.

5. Complete your agreement

Only make agreements that you intend to and are willing to keep. This is especially important for those who (1) procrastinate and (2) say "yes" to everything. If you must break an agreement, communicate this information as soon as possible.

6. If a problem arises, first use the system for corrections, then communicate the problem with optional solutions to the person who can do something about the problem

This is another way to eliminate gossip, judgment, and self-righteousness.

7. Be effective and efficient

8. Optimize every event—create more with less

Items 7 and 8 go together. Look for value in every event. Focus on what can be learned or done; use "lateral thinking" to create effective options.

9. Have the willingness to win and to allow others to win

"Win/lose" is a "zero sum game." Effective problem-solving allows everyone to win—to get their needs met.

10. Focus on what works

The corollary is, get beyond what's not working. Be willing to try something new. When it's broke, fix it!

11. When in doubt, check out feelings

When there seem to be blocks to communication or progress, it is often related to how people are feeling. Check this out, ask the person/people in question. Get the feelings out in the open where they can be checked out, tested, responded to.

12. Agree to disagree until reaching consensus

Commit to working together toward mutually agreeable solutions. This keeps things in a forward motion without judgment. It keeps things hopeful.

13. Tell the truth from the point of view of personal responsibility

Always begin with the pretense that you are willing to assume 50% of the responsibility. This eliminates "you, you, you" messages and allows you to work with others toward a solution, not toward blame.

Modified from Thurber, M. (1973). *Rules of the game.* San Francisco: Hawthorne-Stone Real Estate.

permission to behave in any manner they choose toward one another, including angry, hurtful acting-out behavior.

Trust

Trust is the basis by which leaders/managers facilitate the activities and the progress of the team. Hogan defines *leadership* as "the ability to persuade a group to set aside individual preoccupations in order to pursue a common goal, and leadership should be evaluated in terms of how a group performs vis-à-vis the other groups with which it competes" (1997, p. 1). Hogan concludes that the essential task of leadership is to build high-performance teams. Thus, the key sign that leaders/ managers are performing poorly is the degree to which their team members do not trust them.

Trust is also a major issue among group members, and one of the first questions to come up in the group concerns whom one can trust or not trust. In the early days of organizational development, McGregor (1967) defined *trust* in the following way:

Trust means: "I know that you will not—deliberately or accidentally, consciously or unconsciously—take unfair advantage of me." It means, "I can put my situation at the moment, my status and self esteem in this group, relationship, my job, my career, even my life, in your hands with complete confidence" (p. 163).

One can see from this description how critical trust is within a team (Druskat & Wolff, 2001). The leader models trust through behaviors such as setting the ground rules by which the team will function and holding team members accountable for adhering to the rules. Trust is probably the most delicate aspect within relationships and is influenced far more by actions than by words. In other words, what people do is more powerful than what they say. Trust is a fragile thread that can be severed by one act. Once destroyed, trust is more difficult to reestablish than its initial creation.

QUALITIES OF A TEAM PLAYER

For students, it soon becomes clear that working in teams is important. Understanding what is required of a strong team mate becomes clear as students are assigned teams for various projects. Most people have participated in teams that did not work

and in those that worked very well. Maxwell (2002) identified 17 characteristics that make a good team player.

1. Adaptability—Inflexibility does not work in teams. Being rigid in thinking or behavior is destructive to both the individual and to the team.
2. Collaboration—Collaboration is more than cooperation. It means each person brings something to the project that adds value to the team and supports the creation of synergy.
3. Commitment—It is a passion in the face of adversity to take action and make things happen. It is the passion to do whatever it takes to accomplish the team objectives.
4. Communicate—Communication should happen early and often. Frequency of interaction with other team members, talking with them and sharing thoughts, ideas, and experiences—these are the activities that support teamwork.
5. Competence—Competence translates as someone who is quite capable, highly qualified, and does the job well.
6. Dependable—Team members who are dependable follow through and do what they have agreed to do well, without prodding or delay.
7. Disciplined—Discipline is doing what you really do not want to do so you can accomplish the goals you really want and includes paying attention to the details in thinking, in emotions, and in the actions they take.
8. Adding Value—Helping a teammate advance or grow into a better person or team player; helping teammates advance the team; believing in your teammates before they believe in themselves are examples of value-added.
9. Enthusiastic—Enthusiasm focuses on becoming a highly energetic team member who has a positive attitude and believes that the team, together, can be better than anyone dreamed they could.
10. Intentional—The team and its members have a purpose for themselves and for the team. Every action counts and is meaningful. Focusing on doing the right things in each moment and following through with these actions to their logical conclusion.
11. Awareness of the Mission—Each team member has a sense of purpose and mission that drives

all thoughts, ideas, and actions to do what is best for their team and their cause.

12. Prepared—Being prepared translates as preparation for every meeting and event and begins with a thorough assessment of what is needed, aligning the appropriate work with the appropriate effort, addressing the mental aspects of the right attitude, and being ready to take action.

13. Relationship-oriented—The ability to be connected to other members of the team, to be in a relationship with them is the core of being relationship-oriented. These relationships and the mutual respect upon which they are built create cohesiveness on the team.

14. Improve Yourself—As a team member, you strive to continually grow and reflect, both routinely and periodically, on how well each venture of assignment went and what you could have done better. This is a process of self-reflection.

15. Selflessness—Putting others on the team ahead of yourself through being generous to team members, avoid "playing politics," show loyalty toward team members, and value interdependence among team members over the American value of being independent are all examples of selflessness.

16. Solution-Focused—Do not be consumed with all of the problems associated with the endeavor; rather, focus on finding the solutions; think about what is possible.

17. Tenacious—Being tenacious means giving your all, with determination, and refusing to stop until the goal has been accomplished.

Exercise 17-6

Think about the last team project in which you participated. What worked about the team? What did not work about the team? Was there a member who did not carry his/her share of the work? Was there a team member who was a "know it all"? How did you handle the situation? Was there a person on the team who took the lead? How many of the qualities of a good team player do you possess? Be honest. What are areas in which you could improve? What are your strengths; that is, where do you shine?

CREATING SYNERGY

Teams function with varying levels of effectiveness. The interesting part of this is that effectiveness can be created systematically. Truly effective teams are ones in which people work together to produce extraordinary results that could not have been achieved by any one individual (Mears, 1997). This phenomenon is often described as **synergy**. In the physical sciences, synergy is found in metal alloys. Bronze, the first alloy, was a combination of copper and tin and was found to be much harder and stronger than either copper or tin separately; the tensile strength of bronze can be predicted by merely adding the tensile strength of tin and of copper.

We see the same properties of synergy in human endeavors; for example, in the 1980 U.S. Olympic hockey team. Many people remember this hockey game, in which the Americans defeated the Russians. The team consisted of a group of college kids, none of whom could establish a successful career in the National Hockey League. However, for 2 weeks they were the best hockey team in the world—and they were the best because they knew how to work together to produce extraordinary results. Working cooperatively, an effective team produces extraordinary results that no one team member could have achieved alone To create synergy consistently, certain basic rules must be followed:

- Establish a clear purpose.
- Listen actively.
- Be compassionate.
- Tell the truth.
- Be flexible.
- Commit to resolution.

Establish a Clear Purpose

Creative synergy requires a clear purpose. Each member of the team must understand the reason the team is together, determine what he or she wishes to accomplish (as delineated by defined goals and objectives), and express his or her belief in both the value and feasibility of the goals and tasks. Teams function best when the members can not only tell others about their purpose but also define and operationalize succinctly the meaning and value of this purpose.

Listen Actively

Listening actively means that you are completely focused and tuned in to the individual who is speaking. It means listening without judgment. It means listening to the essence of the conversation so that you can actually repeat to the speaker most of the speaker's intended meaning. It means being 100% present in the communication. (For guidelines for active listening, see Box 17-6.)

It does not mean developing a defensive response or argument in your head while the other person is still speaking. To listen actively, a person must be absolutely focused on the speaker, absorbing words, posture, tone of voice, and all the clues accompanying the message, so that the intent of the communication can be received. Specific purposes used in **active listening,** including examples, are found in Table 17-4.

BOX 17-6

Guidelines for Active Listening

1. Slow down your internal processes and seek data. Do not interrupt the speaker.
2. The more information you acquire through listening, the less interpretation you do (making up the missing pieces or motivations). The less information you have, the more interpretation you do.
3. Realize that the first words from the other person are not necessarily representative of inner thoughts and feelings. Be patient.
4. When listening, suspend your own beliefs and views and judgments, at least temporarily. Attempt to understand the perspective of the other person, particularly if it is different from yours.
5. Realize that any judgments or "labels" strongly influence the manner in which you listen to the other person.
6. Appreciate the difference between understanding other people's perspective and agreeing with them. First strive to understand. Then you may agree or disagree.
7. Effective listening is based on an inner desire to learn about another's unique experience of the world.

Modified from Olen, D. (1993). *Communicating speaking & listening to end misunderstanding and promote friendship.* Germantown, WI: JODA Communications.

Table 17-4 ACTIVE LISTENING

Use of Active Listening	Examples
To convey interest in what the other person is saying	I see! I get it. I hear what you're saying.
To encourage the individual to expand further on his or her thinking	Yes, go on. Tell us more.
To help the individual clarify the problem in his or her own thinking	Then the problem as you see it is . . .
To get the individual to hear what he or she has said in the way it sounded to others	This is your decision, then, and the reasons are . . . If I understand you correctly, you are saying that we should . . .
To pull out the key ideas from a long statement or discussion	Your major point is . . . You feel that we should . . .
To respond to a person's feelings more than to his or her words	You feel strongly that . . . You do not believe that . . .
To summarize specific points of agreement and disagreement as a basis for further discussion	We seem to be agreed on the following points . . . But we seem to need further clarification on these points . . .
To express a consensus of group feeling	As a result of this discussion, we as a group seem to feel that . . .

Be Compassionate

To be compassionate means to have a sympathetic consciousness of another's distress and a desire to alleviate the distress. Consequently, it is inappropriate to focus time and energy on making the other person wrong, especially when your perspective differs from his or hers. It means listening from a caring perspective—one that is focused on understanding the viewpoint of the other person rather than insisting on the "rightness" of one's own point of view.

Tell the Truth

To tell the truth means to speak clearly to personal points and perspectives while acknowledging that they are, merely, personal perspectives. If an observation is made about the tone or behavior of a speaker that affects the ability of others to hear the message, feedback can be provided in a way that does not make the speaker wrong. This is accomplished in an objective rather than subjective manner using neither a cynical nor a critical tone of voice. To be effective, one must own—be responsible for—personal opinions and attitudes.

Be Flexible

Flexibility and openness to another person's viewpoint are critical for a team to work well together.

No single person has all the right answers. Therefore, acknowledging that each person has something to contribute and must be heard is important. Flexibility reflects a willingness to hear another team member's point of view rather than being committed to the "rightness" of a personal point of view.

Commit to Resolution

To commit to resolution means that one can agree to disagree with someone even when that perspective is different. Rather than assuming the person is wrong, this is a commitment to hear his or her perspective, listen to the real message, identify differences, and creatively seek solutions to resolve the areas of differences so that there can be a common understanding and shared commitment to the issue. Both parties need to then agree that they feel heard and agree to the resolution. This differs greatly from compromise and majority vote seen in the democratic process. When compromise exists, there is acquiescence or relinquishing of a significant portion of what was desired. This generally leaves both parties feeling negative about themselves or the agreement. Consequently, most compromises must be reworked at some future date. Working on conflict and its resolution (Table 17-5) is time-consuming but essential to effectively functioning teams (Eisenhardt, Kahwajy, & Bourgeois, 1997).

Table 17-5   ASPECTS OF CONFLICT

Destructive	Constructive
Diverts energy from more important activities and issues	Opens up issues of importance, resulting in their clarification
Destroys the morale of people or reinforces poor self concepts	Results in the solution of problems
Polarizes groups so they increase internal cohesiveness and reduce intergroup cooperation	Increases the involvement of individuals in issues of importance to them
Deepens differences in values	Causes authentic communication to occur
Produces irresponsible and regrettable behavior such as name-calling and fighting	Serves as a release for pent-up emotion, anxiety, and stress
	Helps build cohesiveness among people sharing the conflict, celebrating in its settlement, and learning more about each other
	Helps individuals grow personally and apply what they learn to future situations

Modified from Hart, L. B. (1980). *Learning from conflict*. Reading, MA: Addison-Wesley.

Commitment to resolution is integral to the needs of the team. One team member may be in disagreement with another team member, but the successful work of the team is what is at stake in this conflict. Without commitment to resolution for the sake of the team, individuals often have less impetus to seek a common ground or to agree to disagree.

Synergy cannot occur when one team member becomes a self-proclaimed expert who has the "right" answer. Nor can synergy occur when people refuse to speak. Each team member has good ideas, and these need to be shared. They are not shared, however, when someone feels uncomfortable in the team. It is difficult to speak up and appear wrong or inadequate. The challenge each person faces is to push through discomfort and become a full participant in problem identification and resolution for the overall benefit of the team.

Our society tends to be dualistic in nature. **Dualism** means that most situations are viewed as right or wrong, black or white. Answers to questions are often reduced to yes or no. As a result, we sometimes forget there is a broad spectrum of possibilities. Exercising creativity and exploring numerous possibilities are important. This allows the team to operate at its optimal level.

We have all known people who were self-proclaimed experts, to whom it was critically important that they be right and acknowledged as right, who become judgmental of others whose perspectives and opinions differ from theirs. Consequently, being able to tell the truth to one's synergistic team and to encourage team members to stretch and look at different ways of functioning is vital. This requires strong skills in good negotiation and conflict resolution, something for which few of us have been trained. If self-proclaimed experts think we are judging them, they will not hear the questions, the observations, or the "truth" because the message seems to be making them wrong rather than originating from compassion. The most valuable contribution an individual can make to an organization is a passionate commitment to the creation of synergistic teams.

INTERDISCIPLINARY TEAMS

Interdisciplinary teams are essential to quality patient care. Nurses, physicians, dietitians, social workers, case managers, pharmacists, and physical therapists, to name but a few, must work together to achieve cost-effective care while achieving the highest quality of care in the healthcare setting. This means there must be efforts to understand the various roles and backgrounds of each discipline. At the same time, nurses are frequently leading teams comprising licensed practical/vocational nurses and technicians or assistants of various kinds. Here again, it is critical to understand everyone's role and job description as well as their backgrounds and who they are as individuals and human beings. In addition, the collaboration needed in interdisciplinary teams cannot be created without mutual trust and respect between the members (Brown, Ohlinger, Rusk, Delmore, & Ittmann, 2003).

Several additional aspects of interdisciplinary work are crucial to creating and maintaining these teams. Coyne (2005) emphasizes *the importance of understanding each situation*, which includes clarifying misperceptions and inaccurate information about others within the team including any assumptions that one professional group is favored over another. *Noticing professional expectations and unwritten processes* and cultures of the various professions within the team are also critical to working together seamlessly. It is helpful for nurses to note how other groups talk and behave and to note the special language they use. *Encourage the different disciplines to learn* from each other. For example, in comparing the different codes of ethics, it is quite amazing to discover similarities as opposed to the differences. Most are focused on the patient. The team leader must *set a positive tone*. If the leadership expects interdisciplinary teamwork and verbalizes and models positive and upbeat attitudes, the various disciplines will work together smoothly.

Frequency of interaction of the team members can create ongoing interactions and familiarity with one another. Team members who are in a professional relationship with one another are more apt to work together smoothly. There may be a weekly patient-care meeting in which patients with significant needs or problems are reviewed and each profession addresses issues from the specific area of expertise. *Keep communication open* includes telling the truth in a way that it can be heard and understood. If an aspect of care is governed by regulations, it is helpful when a knowledgeable member of the team speaks to the issue or regulation, always remembering to phrase the information in a way that facilitates hearing and understanding. At all times the interdisciplinary team must *focus on the patient.* When the deliberations are focused on the delivery of best patient care for the specific patient, mutual respect can be developed, and open sharing of ideas and problem-solving occurs.

THE VALUE OF TEAM-BUILDING

The value of team-building is to enhance functioning in any one or all of the following processes (Herman & Reichelt, 1998; Coyne, 2005):

- The establishment of goals and objectives
- The allocation of the work to be performed
- The manner in which a group works: its processes, norms, decision-making processes, and communication patterns
- The relationships among the people doing the work

When things are not going well in an organization and there are problems that need to be resolved, the first intervention people think of is "team-building." Naturally, for teams (a collection of people relying on each other) to be effective, they must function smoothly and communicate effectively to create the best possible work environment (Amos, Hu, & Herrick, 2005). The difficulty is that when organizations are feeling stress and facing difficulties, they generally do not have teams whose members function well together. Team-building can address any one of the aforementioned activities, depending on the available time and other resources. A team-building consultant can teach a team how to set goals and priorities; help a team analyze the distribution of the workload using various team members' strengths; examine a team's process, norms, decision-making processes, and communication patterns; and promote resolution of interpersonal conflicts or problems within the team.

Regardless of which areas are problematic, appropriate assessment of the team is essential. The problems may be in priority or goal setting, allocation of the work, team decision-making, or interpersonal relationships among the members. The success of the team depends on its members and its leadership.

Team-building has grown out of an area of social psychology that focused on group dynamics. In the late 1950s and early 1960s, group dynamics centered on an entity called *training groups,* or "T" groups. As is often the case with new technology, some people did not have positive experiences with T groups, and as a result, such groups acquired a questionable reputation. The notoriety focused on the confrontational style and lack of sensitivity in sharing observations and information. People within the groups felt they were considered to be wrong about various behaviors, attitudes, and activities. As a result, distrust often predominated.

Druskat and Wolff (2001) build a strong case for dealing constructively with building an underlying foundation for teams. They believe that three major components of smoothly functioning teams must be created:

- Mutual trust among the members
- A strong sense of team identity (that the team is unique and worthwhile)
- A sense of team efficacy (that the team performs well and its members are synergistic in their manner of working together)

At the heart of these components are the emotions we often work so hard to keep out of the workplace. However, as human beings we function in the same way in both work and personal lives. Mutual trust can be developed only when each team member tells the truth about feelings, thoughts, and wants *and* listens and supports other members of the team to do likewise. Every person yearns to be a part of something bigger than himself or herself to do something important that makes a difference. Well-functioning teams allow this to happen. Developing such teams can increase nursing job satisfaction and group cohesiveness, as well as decrease nurse turnover rates (DiMeglio et al., 2005).

Understandable anxiety exists concerning the safety of being vulnerable and exposed if personal issues are revealed. That is why it is helpful for the team-building facilitator to make a thorough assessment of major issues and the willingness on the part of members to work on issues. One approach is to interview members of the team individually to discover what the critical issues are. The kinds of

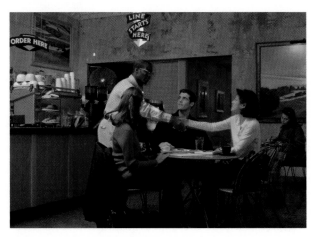

Teams can form strong relationships external to the work environment.

questions that might be asked are found in Box 17-7.

The kind of tool presented in Box 17-7 enables the leader of the team to understand what the issues are before going into the team-building exercise so that he or she is not surprised and does not become defensive. This kind of tool also gives the facilitator some sense of what the major issues are within the group so that he or she has a better understanding of how to work with the group.

MANAGING EMOTIONS

Probably one of the greatest fears in team-building exercises is that people will become emotional, that they will lose control of themselves or the environment, or that they will appear weakened or vulnerable. Men have a particularly difficult time with this fear, but many women also want to appear strong and are hesitant to be open and vulnerable. Although many people acknowledge that we are all thinking and feeling persons, management/leadership is usually more willing to deal with the "thinking" side than the "feeling" side of individuals within the team.

Because people spend such a large percentage of their time in the work setting, it would be unrealistic to believe that they always and continually appear in an unemotional and controlled state. Human beings simply do not function that way. What is observed is people's aspirations, their achievements, their hopes, and their social

consciousness; they are observed falling in love; falling in hate and anger; winning and losing; and being excited, sad, fearful, anxious, and jealous. Consequently, these "feelings" are important components of organizational life and do much to undermine work effectiveness. Most of us know of situations in which, because of an emotional disagreement, two individuals have avoided each other for years. Because of the power of emotions and the inevitability of their presence, their effect on interpersonal relationships, and their influence on productivity and the quality of work, emotions should be a high priority when examining the functioning of the team. Fortunately, research is now appearing that addresses the importance of emphasizing the "emotional intelligence" of individuals and teams when working in teams (Druskat & Wolff, 2001). Those teams that address these issues are much more successful and create a positive work environment.

According to Bocialetti (1988), people are sensitive to what happens when emotions are revealed. When people yell or get angry or upset, and when goals, objectives, and tasks are disputed, employees see the following:

- A member intimidating and frightening others within the group
- Embarrassment
- A member overstating or exaggerating another's view to appear right

- Provocation of defensive and hostile responses
- Overconcern with oneself—self-absorption
- Gossip
- Loss of control
- A member distracting others from "real work"
- Disruption or termination of relationships within a group

These are behaviors that destroy any hope of creating a smoothly functioning team, one that supports its members to grow and learn and provide quality patient care. On the other hand, the cost of suppressing emotions or "feelings" includes the following:

- Physical and psychological stress
- Withdrawal from participation
- Loss of energy and depression
- Reduction of learning
- Hiding of important data because of fear
- Festering problems and emotions
- Prevention of others from being acknowledged
- Decreased motivation
- Weakening of the ability to receive constructive feedback
- The loss of one's influence

These kinds of outcomes lead to the conclusion that suppressing emotions at work is neither healthy nor constructive for team members.

When emotions are handled appropriately within the team, there are several positive outcomes for the work setting. One creates a sense of internal comfort with the workings of the team and the organization. When stress is lowered and kept at lower levels on average, problems are much more easily resolved. This phenomenon is similar to releasing steam slowly with a steam valve rather than having the gasket blow. Interpersonal relationships on the team are more stable, and people have a sense of closer ties and collegiality when emotions are addressed. Fewer negative relationships or interactions develop, which results in more effective and pleasant working relationships all around.

Work group effectiveness improves when the team is functioning smoothly and emotions and "feelings" are being addressed on a routine basis rather than waiting for a volcanic eruption. Problems of withdrawal, boredom, and frustration are much less likely to overwhelm the team and

lead to its breakdown (Turpin, 2000). The skills and tools previously discussed (e.g., speaking supportively) are the basic tools one needs to handle the emotional aspects of the team. Choosing to cope with emotional upset must be a conscious choice, one that requires practice to improve the skill.

THE ROLE OF LEADERSHIP

Teams usually have a leader. In addition, teams function within large organizations that have leaders. Without the approval and the support of the leader, team-building, which can be a costly endeavor in terms of consultation fees as well as work time and resources of the team, is difficult to undertake and of questionable effectiveness. Although very strong teams may be able to educate themselves regarding some of the issues, such as establishing goals and priorities or clarifying their own team process, addressing any kind of relationship issue among team members without a more objective outside party facilitating the process is exceedingly difficult.

Because leadership is such a pivotal part of smoothly functioning teams, it is illuminating to examine leaders more carefully. Truly progressive leaders understand that leadership and followership are not necessarily a set of skills; rather, these are qualities of character, a manifestation of a person's own being (Tracey & Hinkin, 1998). On speaking specifically to leadership, we are not talking about "putting on a role." In actuality, leaders realize their capacity for influence, risk taking, and decision making more fully. Leadership, and to some degree followership, is as much about character and development as it is about education. According to Peter Vaill (1989), leadership is concerned with bringing out the very best in people. For a leader who truly believes this, team-building is a natural outgrowth. This type of leader understands that the very best in a person is tied intimately to the individual's deepest sense of himself or herself—to one's spirit. The efforts of leaders must touch the spiritual aspect in themselves and others. Warren Bennis (1989) once said that leaders simply care about more people. Consequently, this caring manifests itself in doing whatever it takes to improve team functioning. This may imply involving oneself in team-building with the team. The

BOX 17-8

The "Can Do" Brigade: An Army Nurse's Study in Character Development

As life events are reviewed, important or pivotal learning can be identified. One life event that significantly affected me was the year I spent as an Army Nurse Corps officer in South Vietnam. This was the first time I remember an awareness and understanding of confidence in the face of incredible obstacles. I had spent the first 10 months of my nursing career in labor and delivery at Indiana University before volunteering for a guaranteed assignment to Vietnam. I went to Fort Sam Houston for 6 weeks of basic training, where they taught me really important things like how to salute, how to march, and how many men are in a battalion. No one ever asked me if I could start an IV or draw a tube of blood. This was important because Indiana University had the largest medical school class in the United States at that time and nurses did nothing that interfered with medical education. Therefore, I had never started an IV or drawn blood. When I arrived in Saigon, they put me in a sedan with another nurse and sent me up to the Third Surgical Hospital, one not unlike the one in MASH. We even had a Major Burns—that was not his name but it was his function. Surgical hospitals receive only battle casualties; their purpose is to stabilize and to transport.

The Third Surgical Hospital was located in the middle of the 173rd Airborne Brigade, whose job it was to defend the Bein Hoi Air Base, where all the sorties in the south were flown during the war. We were stopped at the gate by an MP who stepped up and saluted very snappily. He knew that a staff car must contain either a very-high-ranking officer or, if it was his lucky day, females.

When I was in Vietnam, 500 American women and 500,000 American men were there. The MP looked in the window, saluted snappily, and said "Afternoon, ma'am!" He wanted to know where we were going; he talked to us for a few minutes and assured us if there was anything he could do for us we should just give him a call. He saluted us and said, "CAN DO." I didn't understand because I did not know that there are units with very high esprit de corps who attach snappy little sayings at the end of things like salutes, phone conversations, memos, and so forth.

The 173rd was the "CAN DO" brigade. When we got to the hospital and met the chief nurse, she took us down to the mess hall and introduced us to all the doctors and nurses. We were sitting and having coffee when the field phone rang in the kitchen and the mess sergeant yelled out, "Incoming wounded." Everybody got up and started to leave for the preop area. I just sat there until the chief nurse said, "Come on." I said, "You don't understand, I deliver babies." She was not impressed! She took me by the arm and led me to preop.

When we got there, we discovered there were not just a few incoming wounded, there were more than 30, and some were very seriously injured. She immediately told the sergeant to call headquarters battalion of the 173rd Airborne and tell them that the Third Surg needed blood. She turned to me and said, "Lieutenant, you are responsible for drawing 50 units of fresh whole blood." I was shocked! I had never drawn a tube of blood, but I found in the back section of preop a Specialist 4th class who was already setting up "saw horses" and stretchers, putting up IV poles, and hanging plastic blood sets. I started to help, and soon I heard trucks out back. I opened the door and looked outside. There were two huge Army trucks, and kids—17, 18, 19, and 20 years old—were jumping out. They were covered with red mud from the bottom of their boots to the tops of their helmets. I looked at them, and I looked at the clean cement floor, and in an instant my mother came to me. I put my hand on my hip and said, "Where have you boys been?" One PFC stepped forward and saluted me very snappily and said, "Ma'am, we just came in this afternoon from 30 days in the field, we have been out in the rice paddies chasing the Viet Cong, we have not had a hot meal, and we've not had a shower but Sergeant Major said the Third Surg needs blood!" He saluted smartly and said, "CAN DO!" They were very clear. After 30 days of chasing and being chased by the Viet Cong, giving a unit of blood was easy. "CAN DO!" They were confident. They were kids who had looked into the face of death. At that moment, I knew if they CAN DO, I Can Do! Life requires confidence. With confidence, you can make your dreams come true!

risk in such an endeavor is that the team leader is open to being vulnerable, to being judged by others, and to being wrong. However, if the leader has modeled the "rules of the game" and has held people to these rules, as well as holding himself or herself to them, the team-building exercise will not degenerate into judging and placing blame.

If true leadership is about character development as much as anything, then character development is also beneficial for followers—that is, members of the team. The areas of character development often addressed include communication, particularly those aspects of speaking supportively that avoid placing blame and justifying and enhance understanding the other person's message. Box 17-8 highlights an example of character development from personal experience.

Leaders understand the multiple aspects of the issue of control. They take control of their lives rather than being at the mercy of others—rather than being victims. They have clarity regarding their own control issues. They focus time and energy primarily and almost exclusively on those issues, events, and behaviors over which they have control. Their activities are thus primarily focused on areas relating directly to them—not on world events or other happenings over which they have neither influence nor control.

Confidence, which loosely translates as faith or belief that one will act in a correct and effective way, is a key aspect of character. Thus, it follows that confidence in oneself can be closely tied to self-esteem, which is satisfaction with oneself. The greatest deterrent to self-esteem and self-confidence is fear. Fear is described by some as "false evidence appearing real." Susan Jeffers (1987) believes the core fear—the one that rules our lives—is one of "I can't handle it." So, the core of our fears is "I can't handle it," and it is exactly the opposite of being confident or holding oneself in high esteem. Working on self-confidence requires an attitude of belief, of confidence, of I "CAN DO" whatever is required (see Box 17-8) (Fisher & Thomas, 1996).

False
Evidence
Appearing
Real

Simply caring about more people translates into a willingness to focus time and energy on members of the team. From one perspective, caring is risking being with someone and sharing both suffering and joy. Healing often emerges from caring. Behaviors that demonstrate caring include giving of oneself in terms of warmth and love and particularly giving one's time. The second aspect of caring is truly listening to team members and hearing and understanding them. The third aspect includes being 100% present for them. The fourth is to honor the other person—to see their wholeness, their possibilities, their hopes, and their dreams.

Leading the team is clearly not the easiest thing to do, but neither is being an active, fully participating member of the team. Both require taking risks, including being in a relationship. Being in a team-building experience and hearing those things that have not worked for people in their interactions with peers and the leader can be scary but worthwhile. It requires a focus on personal and professional growth. It requires building character.

Exercise 17-7

The "Gordian Knot": A Team-Building Game

Gordian knot is a term sometimes used to describe a problem that cannot be solved. However, teamwork can sometimes solve seemingly impossible problems, as this game will illustrate.

In a group of 8 to 10 people, form a tight circle facing inward with your shoulders touching and your hands placed in the center. Take the hand of two other people across the circle from you. The goal is to unwind the knot until the entire circle is holding hands side by side. You may not let go of hands to unwind the knot unless your facilitator gives you special permission to do so!

After your group has unwound its knot, together choose one or two categories of questions from Part I of the "Team-Building Discussion" outline that follows. Discuss these questions, writing down your answers as you go so that you can report to the class later. Be sure to support your answers with examples from your group's experience with the game. Then, complete all questions in Part II.

GORDIAN KNOT ANALYSIS

PART I

LEADERSHIP AND BUILDING TEAMWORK

What did it feel like not to have a designated leader?

_____

Who became the leader?

_____

How?

_____

Did the leadership process work?

_____

How did you feel about it?

_____

Who came up with new ideas?

_____

Did the team support this process?

_____

How were conflicts resolved and problems solved?

_____

How did you build a sense of teamwork?

_____

TEAM MEMBERSHIP

Did you feel like a part of the team?

_____

Why or why not?

_____

Did your team have a good mix of skills and abilities?

_____

Did you adapt to the needs of others or to the needs of the team?

_____

Did you meet your objectives without wasting time and energy?

_____

What role did you play as a team member?

_____

TRUST AND OPENNESS

What was the team's level of trust and open communication?

_____

Great Deal = 10, Much = 7, Some = 5, Little = 3, None = 0

What contributed to this level of trust?

_____

Did you deal with issues candidly and honestly?

_____

What was your level of trust?

_____

What would have increased the team's level of trust and openness?

_____

CONTRIBUTION TO THE TEAM-DEVELOPING RELATIONSHIPS

Did you all know and agree to the mission of the team?

_____

How were decisions made?

_____

Who participated in making them?

_____

When did you need to make decisions?

_____

Were they primarily about what to do (tasks) or how to do it (process)?

_____

Did you use each other as resources?

_____

Did you work well together?

_____

How did your relationships develop and strengthen?

_____

How do you feel about each other now?

_____

CULTIVATING A FEELING OF SATISFACTION ABOUT YOUR TEAM

Do you feel proud of your team?

_____

How do/did you feel rewarded by being a member of this team?

_____

Did you have fun?

_____

Did the challenge cease to be fun?

_____

How did the team handle this?

_____

Are you satisfied with your results?

_____

DEVELOPING THE TEAM THROUGH RISK-TAKING

Did you, individually or as a team, try out any new or uncomfortable communications or behavior? Give examples. _____

Did that feel safe?

_____

Did you support each other in your risk taking?

_____

PART II

EVALUATE AND SHARE WITH THE REST OF THE TEAM HOW YOU FEEL YOU DID AS A PARTICIPANT

Consider the following:

Was I active or passive?

_____

Did I communicate clearly?

_____

Did I take risks?

_____

Did I support others?

_____

Did I ask for help or support from others?

_____

Was my behavior typical for me?

_____

How would I do it differently?

_____

Give each other honest and helpful feedback on the congruency of self-perception versus the perception of other team members.

Debriefing exercise courtesy of Walter Kowalski, BreakThroughs, Inc., Englewood, Colorado.

The Solution

The first question that needed to be asked was, "Were we committed to providing the most optimal care for the neonate?" In other words, why would teamwork be important in this situation? What's the vision or mission? After achieving agreement among the NICU team, we strategized on how to create a "team" with the specialists. Making our intent clear was very important. A meeting with the director of the specialty team, the NICU medical director, and nursing leadership was arranged. We discovered that we shared a common goal: to provide the best care possible for the baby. Keeping that goal as the focus, we then identified areas of mutual respect. From there, both sides were willing to listen to each other's concerns. Care guidelines could be identified, as well as areas of responsibility. Ideas on how to improve the communication process were also discussed. A plan based on patient needs, complete with agreements, was implemented.

Were we a team yet? The answer is no. There was still a little skepticism and reserve. Everyone seemed to have a "wait-and-see" attitude. The first big chance was identified when the specialty group insisted a patient of theirs be admitted to the NICU because they believed it was the best place for the baby to be. Another measurable outcome was having the agreements honored. This reinforced to everyone that his or her concerns had been heard and respected. Mutual trust was building, and a collegial relationship began. A year later, it is hard to imagine that this situation ever occurred. There is enthusiasm for this specialty's physicians and their patients. It is certainly a change in attitude.

There are many components to team-building, but the most important component is to be clear about your mission and intentions when working with potential team members. The intention to provide the best care possible assisted each one of us to be more open, creative, and trusting. These are all necessary components of team-building. Remember, teams are made up of individuals. Ask yourself if you are willing to accept responsibility for your response and actions. Be the change that you want to see.

— Diane Gallagher

 Would this be a suitable approach for you? Why?

CHAPTER CHECKLIST

Nurse managers must help build teams. Although the manager does not have to lead the team, the manager must ensure that the group can function effectively as a team. The team members must be able to communicate with each other effectively, share a single mission, be willing to cooperate with each other, and be committed to achieving their objectives. Successful teamwork requires leadership, trust, and willingness to take risks.

- A team is a highly interdependent group of people that has the following characteristics:
  - Has defined goals and objectives
  - Communicates effectively with one another
  - Has an ongoing relationship
  - Is focused on accomplishing a task

- Attributes of effective teams include the following:
  - Clarity of purpose
  - Informality
  - Effective communication
  - Participation
  - Listening
  - Civilized disagreement
  - Consensus decisions
  - Clear roles and work assignments
  - Shared leadership
  - Diversity of styles
  - Self-assessment and self-regulation
- Each team member deals continually with three questions:
  - Am I in the "in" group or the "out" group?
  - Do I have any power or control?
  - Can I use, develop, and be appreciated for my skills and resources?

- Focusing on team members' strengths and acknowledging what they do well are two of the keys to team-building.
  - To be effective, acknowledgments must be the following:
    - Specific
    - Personal
    - Sincere
    - Timely
    - Public
- One of the most helpful tools for teams is a set of ground rules that govern how members will interact with each other.
- Trust is essential for successful teamwork.
- Synergy allows a team to produce results that could not have been achieved by any one individual. Creating it requires the following:
  - Active listening
  - Compassion
  - Honesty
  - Flexibility
  - Commitment to resolution of conflicts
- Managing emotions is a key strategy in team-building.
- Leadership is a pivotal part of a smoothly functioning team.
  - Leadership relies on personal character development as much as on education.
  - Confidence is a key aspect of the leader's character.
    - A "can do" attitude is one of the most important confidence-building strategies a leader can adopt.
- Taking a risk and experimenting with a new behavior is the most effective way to change behavior.

TIPS FOR TEAM-BUILDING

- Commit to the purpose of the team.
- Develop team relationships of mutual respect.
- Communicate effectively and actively listen.
- Create and adhere to team agreements concerning function and process.
- Build trust.

TERMS TO KNOW

acknowledgment
active listening
commitment
dualism
effective communication
group
sender-receiver
synergy
team

REFERENCES

American Association of Critical-Care Nurses (AACN) & VitalSmarts. (2005). *Silence kills: The seven crucial conversations for healthcare.* San Francisco: The Association.

Amos, M., Hu, J., & Herrick, C. (2005). The impact of team building on communication and job satisfaction of nursing staff. *Journal for Nurses in Staff Development, 21*(1), 10–16.

Arford, P. (2005). Nurse-physician communication: An organizational accountability. *Nursing Economics, 23*(2), 72–77.

Bennis, W. (1989). *On becoming a leader.* Reading, MA: Addison-Wesley.

Bocialetti, G. (1988). Teams and management of emotion. In W. B. Reddy & K. Jamison (Eds.), *Team building blueprints for productivity and satisfaction* (pp. 62–71). Alexandria, VA: NTL Institute for Applied Behavioral Sciences; and San Diego: University Associates.

Bradley, J., & Edinberg, M. (1990). *Communication in the nursing context* (3rd ed.). Norwalk, CT: Appleton & Lange.

Brown, M., Ohlinger, J., Rusk, C., Delmore, P., & Ittmann, P. (2003). Implementing potentially better practices for multidisciplinary team building: Creating a neonatal intensive care unit culture of collaboration. *Pediatrics, 111*(4), 482–488.

Buckman, R., Korsch, B., Baile, W., & Jason, H. (2000). Review and commentary: A practical guide to communication skills in clinical practice. *Education for Health, 13*(2), 221–227.

Ceccio, J., & Ceccio, C. (1982). *Effective communication in nursing: Theory and practice.* New York: John Wiley & Sons.

Coyne, C. (2005). Strength in numbers: How team building is improving care in a variety of practice settings. *PT—Magazine of Physical Therapy, 13*(6), 40–51.

Davis, H., & Sharon, B. (2002). *Teambuilding: High-performance team models and strategies.* Malvern, PA: Indaba Press.

DiMeglio, K., Padula, C., Piatek, C., Korber, J., Barrett, A., Ducharme, M., Lucas, S., Piermont. N., Joyal, E., DeNicola, V., & Corry, K. (2005). Group cohesion and nurse satisfaction: Examination of a team-building approach. *The Journal of Nursing Administration, 35*(3), 110–120.

Druskat, V., & Wolff, S. (2001). Building the emotional intelligence of groups. *Harvard Business Review, 79*(3), 81–91.

Dubnicki, C. (1991, May–June). Building high-performance management teams. *Healthcare Forum Journal, 34,* 19–24.

Eisenhardt, K., Kahwajy, J., & Bourgeois, L. (1997, July–August). How management teams can have a good fight. *Harvard Business Review, 75,* 77–85.

Fisher, B., & Thomas, B. (1996). *Real dream teams: Seven practices used by world class team leaders to achieve extraordinary results.* Delray Beach, FL: St. Lucia Press.

Hart, L. B. (1980). *Learning from conflict.* Reading, MA: Addison-Wesley.

Herman, J., & Reichelt, P. (1998). Are first line nurse managers prepared for team building? *Nursing Management, 29*(10), 68–72.

Hogan, R. (1997). What we know about leadership. *Academic Leader, 13*(12), 1.

Jason, H. (2000). Communication skills are vital in all we do as educators and clinicians. *Education for Health, 13*(2), 157–161.

Jeffers, S. (1987). *Feel the FEAR and DO IT anyway.* Columbia, NY: Fawcett.

Lopes, S. (1987). *The wall.* New York: Collins.

Maxwell, J. (2002). *The 17 essential qualities of a team player.* Nashville, TN: Thomas Nelson Publishers.

McGregor, D. (1960). *The human side of enterprise.* New York: McGraw-Hill.

McGregor, D. (1967). *The professional manager.* New York: McGraw-Hill.

Mears, P. (1997). *Health care teams: Building continuous quality improvement.* Boca Raton, FL: St. Lucia Press.

Morreale, S., Spitzberg, B., & Barge, K. (2001). *Human communication: Motivation, knowledge, & skills.* Belmont, CA: Wadsworth.

Olen, D. (1993). *Communicating speaking & listening to end misunderstanding and promote friendship.* Germantown, WI: JODA Communications.

Parcells, B. (2000). The tough work of turning around a team. *Harvard Business Review, 78*(6), 179–184.

Parker, G. M. (1990). *Team players and teamwork.* San Francisco: Jossey-Bass.

Porter-O'Grady, T. (2004a). Constructing a conflict resolution program for health care. *Health Care Management Review, 29*(4), 278–283.

Porter-O'Grady, T. (2004b). Embracing conflict: Building a healthy community. *Health Care Management Review, 29*(3), 181–187.

Roman, M. (2001). Teams, teammates, and team building. *MedSurg Nursing, 10*(4), 161–165.

Rosenstein, A., & O'Daniel, M. (2005). Disruptive behavior and clinical outcomes: Perceptions of nurses and physicians. *American Journal of Nursing, 105*(1), 54–64.

Satir, V. (1988). *The new peoplemaking.* Mountain View, CA: Science & Behavior Books.

Sportsman, S. (2005). Build a framework for conflict assessment. *Nursing Management, 36*(4), 12–40.

Thurber, M. (1973). *Rules of the game.* San Francisco: Hawthorne-Stone Real Estate.

Tracey, J., & Hinkin, T. (1998). Transformational leadership or effective managerial practices? *Group & Organizational Management, 23*(3), 220–237.

Turpin, C. (2000). Creating winning teams. *Nephrology Nursing Journal, 27*(2), 171.

Vaill, P. (1989). *Managing as a performing art.* San Francisco: Jossey-Bass.

Weiner, S., Barnet, B., Cheng, T., & Daaleman, T. (2005). Processes for effective communication in primary care. *Annals of Internal Medicine, 142*(8), 709–714.

Weisburg, M. (1988). Team work: Building productive relationships. In W. B. Reddy, & K. Jamison (Eds.), *Team building blueprints for productivity and satisfaction.* Alexandria, VA: NTL Institute for Applied Behavioral Sciences; and San Diego: University Associates.

Weiss, W. (2001). Attitude: A major managerial challenge. *Supervision, 62*(6), 3–7.

Wilson, J. (1999). Improving communication skills. *Management Accounting, 77*(3), 88.

SUGGESTED READINGS

Dubnicki, C. (1991, May-June). Tuning up your team. *Healthcare Forum Journal, 34,* 25–28.

Dyer, W. (1987). *Team building issues and alternatives.* Reading, MA: Addison-Wesley.

Francis, D., & Young, D. (1979). *Improving work groups: A practical manual for team building.* San Diego: University Associates.

Jeffers, S. (1992). *Dare to connect: Reaching out in romance, friendship and the workplace.* Columbia, NY: Fawcett.

Nanus, B. (1992). *Visionary leadership.* San Francisco: Jossey-Bass.

Schmieding, N. J. (1993). Nurse empowerment through context structure and process. *Journal of Professional Nursing, 9,* 239–245.

Sibbet, D., & O'Hara-Devereaux, M. (1991). The language of teamwork. *Healthcare Forum Journal, 34,* 27–30.

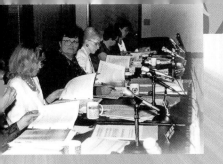

Collective Action

Fran Hicks

T oday's employees in many fields expect, and in some situations, demand a greater voice in decisions involving their work life. These decisions involve both the context and the content of their work. Policy, education, and experience influence healthcare professionals to engage the consumer in healthcare decisions. These professionals see merit in being part of decision-making processes about their work lives. Specifically, participation in decisions regarding practice is an appropriate expectation of a professional nurse. Collective action is one mechanism available to achieve that participation. The manager can capitalize on this strategy to accomplish positive outcomes.

Objectives

- Evaluate how participation of staff nurses in decision-making relate to job satisfaction.
- Analyze the influence of culture on the selection of a governance model.
- Evaluate how key characteristics of selected collective action strategies apply in the workplace: shared governance, workplace advocacy, and collective bargaining.
- Distinguish between the rights of individuals included in collective bargaining contracts and the rights of at-will employees.
- Compare the factors that contribute to nurses' decisions to be represented for the purpose of collective bargaining and the decision for no representation.

- Evaluate decision-making strategies for their effectiveness within diverse workplace environments.

Questions to Consider

- *How does nurse participation in decision-making influence job satisfaction?*
- *What strategies can you use to participate in decision-making?*
- *How can you transfer your knowledge of advocacy to the workplace?*
- *What would influence you to make the decision to practice in an organization in which nurses are organized for the purpose of collective bargaining?*
- *Within the context of labor law, how do the responsibilities of nurses who are considered supervisors differ from the responsibilities of nurses who are considered nonsupervisory?*

The Challenge

Peggy Reiley, RN, MSN, ScM
Vice President, Scottsdale Memorial Hospital—Osborn, Scottsdale, Arizona

I was a new vice president for patient services. After several months of assessing the new organization, I determined that I would like to redesign how care was delivered on the patient care unit. Specifically, I wanted to reevaluate various roles and possibly redesign certain roles to better meet the need of patients and their families.

 What do you think you would do if you were this nurse?

INTRODUCTION

The excitement of beginning a career in nursing or assuming the position of a manager is balanced by events taking place in health care and the effect of these events on nursing, nurses, and health care. The knowledge gained about health care provides a background for considering issues within health care and factors that promote or inhibit the achievement of professional nursing practice.

Nurses are deeply involved in the complex clinical problems of individuals, families, and communities because nursing practice requires the acquisition, synthesis, and retrieval of knowledge to provide competent nursing care. Having the time and resources to engage in high-level preparation for each situation may be viewed as unattainable, especially in some situations in which nurses are concerned about providing basic safe care.

COLLECTIVE ACTION

Collective action is a benign phrase; it refers to many aspects of daily life, including work. When parishioners make a contribution to a mission that is the result of collective action; when nurses work to achieve Magnet™ status, that is the result of collective action; when patient care is delivered in hospitals 24 hours per day, that is the result of the collective action of shifts of nurses. The collective action of nurses requires a level of independence during the shift and interdependence between shifts and with other healthcare professionals. Nurses learn quickly to rely on their colleagues. Nurses have been less comfortable with formal collectives than some other occupational groups. Several

factors may contribute to this discomfort. Chief among those factors are gender, career focus, and view of power. Women have had less experience in working and playing within a team structure than men. As a female-dominated profession, nursing has manifested this lack of experience. Before Title IX (prior to 1972), few girls participated in competitive team sports. Additionally, many women, including nurses, view employment as a job rather than a career. For these individuals, the time to work with others to achieve common goals deprived them of personal time. Women have not perceived themselves to be powerful. Nursing has been characterized as an "oppressed group" (Roberts, 2000). The "good" nurse was considered obedient. The Nightingale Pledge reinforced obedience: "With loyalty will I endeavor to aid the physician in his work . . ." (Dock & Stewart, 1920). This obedience or acquiescence to authority appears to have been transferred to other authority figures, including but not limited to, hospital administrators.

Minarik and Catramabone (1998) described four main purposes of collective participation for nurses: (1) to promote the practice of professional nursing, (2) to establish and maintain standards of care, (3) to allocate resources effectively and efficiently, and (4) to create satisfaction and support in the practice environment. Collective action helps define and sustain individuals in achieving their purposes. In the absence of collective action, the average individual has limited influence in achieving his or her purpose. Many children learned the strength and value of collective action early in life as siblings banded together to make a request to their parents. The same strategy has probably served in an organization when, together, a group of peers makes a point or pleads a case. Nurses have identified practice concerns and have joined together to bring about change in numerous practice settings.

Exercise 18-1

Identify three collectives to which you belong. List the purposes of each. How do you feel as a member of these groups?

The strategies for developing networks, developing a collective voice, and cultivating a collective require strong leaders and a broad **followership.** Leaders and followers have separate and distinct roles. Those roles are complementary—each requires the other. The relationship is interdependent. Followers and leaders also share many characteristics. Successful people move easily between the roles of follower and leader. The knowledge and skills of followers may differ from those of the leader; they are not less. Leaders and followers are knowledgeable of the context and content of their practice. Followers are active, involved participants committed to an agreed-upon agenda. They are loyal and supportive to the individual who is setting the pace and the agenda. The nurse who becomes a leader finds that the absence of followers is personally painful.

Changes in an initiative or an agenda may result in today's leader being tomorrow's follower. The opposite may be applicable: Today's follower may be tomorrow's leader. The change may result from the context of the situation. In the operating room, the surgeon is the acknowledged leader, and the anesthesiologist follows that lead with respect to the extent of the anesthesia. If the patient's condition changes, the anesthesiologist becomes the leader, and the surgeon may simply step away from the table, an overt act that demonstrates a change in leadership. As healthcare consumers and participants, we salute the clarity.

 Exercise 18-2

Identify two groups in which you have been a leader (e.g., school, church, sports, and clubs). Was your specific role the result of a group decision? How did your role as a leader differ from your role as a follower? List the skills you used in each role.

Informed followers are not submissive partisans blindly following a cultist personality. They are effective group members, not "groupies." They are skilled in group dynamics and accountable for their actions. They are willing and able to question, debate, compromise, collaborate, and act. Consider potential differences between being a subordinate in a hierarchical organization and being a follower committed to one's practice.

Collective action provides a mechanism for achieving professional practice through greater participation in decision-making. The governance structure provides the framework for participation. Participation in decision-making regarding one's practice is an appropriate expectation for professionals, provides for greater autonomy and authority over practice decisions, contributes to supporting the professional nurse, and is a major component of job satisfaction. The privilege and the obligation to participate are inherent in the discipline of nursing. Consistent with the *Code of Ethics for Nurses* (ANA, 2001), members of the discipline participate based on their competence. Although nurses are expected to be informed, active participants, not all nurses wish to participate in decisions. For these nurses, going to work and doing their assigned job may fulfill their expectations. They may not perceive themselves as being in a subordinate position, or if they do, it is not a concern for them. Their orientation is to serve the care recipient and to be loyal to the organization. For these individuals, asserting the right and responsibility to participate in decisions may be considered disrespectful to the organization's policies and to the physician, or they may be energy-draining. For the professional nurse, participation in practice-related decisions is critical to quality patient care, expected by society, and essential to autonomy for nursing. Today's healthcare environment demands that nurses exercise the four key historical concepts identified by Lewis and Batey (1982): responsibility, authority, autonomy, and accountability.

Responsibility

The history of nursing provides evidence of nurses accepting responsibility or the "charge to act." Historically, this charge took the form of unquestioningly and meticulously following the "physician's orders" and "hospital procedures." The "good" nurse rendered disclosure at the convenience of the physician and management. Today, healthcare organizations achieving Magnet recognition are characterized by the control of nursing practice by nurses (Kramer & Schmalenberg, 2004). Nursing and individual nurses must have the power to control practice. The recognition of credentialing, especially certification, has contributed to the exercise of expert power by nurses.

Authority

Authority based on preparation and experience suggests a departure from the tradition of delegating authority to individual nurses based on the physician's or nurse manager's knowledge of the nurse—knowledge that too often was based on personal characteristics, not clinical competence. That statement does not denigrate the collegial relationship between and among nurses and physicians, relationships that are based on mutual respect and trust. There is evidence that patient care improves when these relationships exist. Authority suggests that nurses use the power of their professional status to act in behalf of the best interest of patients.

Autonomy

Autonomy, the freedom to make independent decisions exceeding the standard nursing practice and that are in the best interest of the patient (Kramer & Schmalenberg, 2004), is critical to the control of nursing practice. Aiken, Clarke, and Sloane (2000) demonstrated ". . . that nurse control over the practice setting explains almost all of the variation in patient satisfaction that is associated with different organizational forms of AIDS care" (p. 462). To maximize the clinical effectiveness of registered nurses (RNs), they must have autonomy consistent with their scope of practice. Multiple studies demonstrate that a healthcare organization that provides a climate in which nurses have authority and autonomy has better patient outcomes, retains nurses at a higher rate, is more cost effective, and has evidence of greater patient satisfaction than an organization in which such a climate does not exist (Kramer & Schmalenberg, 2004). According to Kennerly (2000), the future depends on designing and implementing freedom in decision-making to create and sustain positive work environments in nursing. Nurse involvement in decision-making contributes to higher levels of job satisfaction for

the nurse and higher levels of satisfaction with care for the patient and positively influences health outcomes.

Autonomy encourages innovation and increases productivity. A lack of autonomy and advocacy for standards frequently results in organizational silence and marginalization of nurses (Hascup, 2003; Duchscher & Cowin, 2004). Nurse managers have influence in this area of working with staff. Mrayyan (2004) found that nurses in an international study reported that the three most important variables in increasing nurse autonomy were supportive management, education, and experience. Specific managerial actions were defined as elements of interactions with others, especially when conflict was involved. Helping nurses communicate and supporting them in dealing with conflict helps nurses describe themselves as having more autonomy. The Research Perspective defines further outcomes of this study.

The "failure on the part of healthcare delivery organizations, physicians, and policy-making bodies to fully recognize the decision-making abilities of RNs has contributed to problems in recruiting and retaining nurses, hindered the development of a career orientation in professional nursing, and limited the efficiency and effectiveness of patient care delivery" (U.S. Department of Health and Human Services, 1988, p. vii). This statement was accurate when written and has become more important as the delivery of and payment for health care evolve.

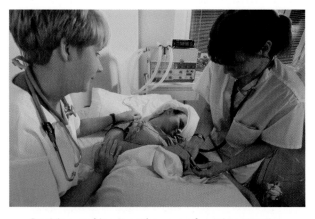

Decision-making is at the core of nursing practice.

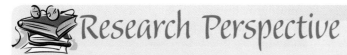
Research Perspective

Mrayyan, M. T. (2004), Nurses' autonomy: Influence of nurse managers' actions. *Journal of Advanced Nursing*, 45(3), 326-336.

This international study (Canada, United Kingdom, and United States), using a convenience sample, represented 317 hospital nurses. Listservs were used to solicit participants. Specifically, this study looked at how nurse managers can enhance staff nurses' autonomy. Nurse managers had major influence on patient care. Autocratic management, physicians, and workloads were most commonly associated with a decreased sense of autonomy. Respondents reported the greatest autonomy as serving as patient advocates, questioning physician orders, teaching about patient medication, consulting with medical doctors and other professionals, and preventing skin breakdown. The greatest unit operation-related decisions had to do with scheduling, patient assignments, service on committees, and unit-based educational offerings. Nurse managers greatly influence the staff nurses' perceptions of their autonomy.

IMPLICATIONS FOR PRACTICE

Nurse managers can influence staff nurses' perceptions of their autonomy through supportive management, education, and experience. Using a participative method of management and leadership can enhance the view of staff nurses in terms of their satisfaction with their autonomy.

Although automobile manufacturing is a highly mechanized process, management has learned that it is cost effective to give the employee on the shop floor the autonomy to "stop the line" when the potential for error is detected. Stopping errors before they occur is more efficient than recalling items and retrofitting and is more humane than causing injury and perhaps death. In health care, "failure to rescue" is a recognized indicator of patient safety (Agency for Healthcare Research and Quality, 2003). Unlocking minds by providing greater autonomy and diversifying tasks decreases fear, specifically fear of ridicule, fear of punishment, fear of loss of job, and even fear of favors. The Institute for HealthCare Improvement (IHI) takes the concept of change as events unfold to the unit level with its 100,000 Lives Campaign. By supporting unit-level change without complex organizational structure approvals, change occurs in real time, and patients benefit.

Accountability

Accountability focuses the organization and all its members on the purposes and the outcomes of their collective activities. Accountability requires ownership. Porter-O'Grady and Malloch (2002) assert, "Accountability is always internally generated. It rests first and foremost within" (p. 261). Although they make many points about accountability, the following are five critical considerations: (1) accountability is about outcomes, not processes, (2) accountability is individually defined, (3) accountability is inherent in the role—it is not delegated, (4) accountability must be clear to all those in related roles, and (5) accountability is the foundation for evaluation.

The value of process is determined by the extent to which individuals observe a particular protocol while accomplishing a goal. Accountability focuses on the achievement of the specified outcome. This shift in thinking has had a tremendous effect on healthcare reimbursement. An example of the shift is evident in patient education. Initialing a form to indicate that patient teaching has occurred is no longer acceptable. The criteria now expect that the patient's behavior has changed. Porter-O'Grady and Malloch (2002) call this the Age of Accountability; work is viewed in terms of outcomes. To achieve positive outcomes within an organization, shared accountability is critical. "When responsible adults refuse to share accountability, it poisons human relationships, corrupts professions, and makes self-esteem impossible" (Kupperschmidt, 2004, p. 115).

GOVERNANCE

Nursing **governance** is the methodology or system by which a department of nursing controls and directs the formulation and the administration of nursing policy. Organizational structure provides a framework for fulfilling the organization's mission. Organizational charts show the relationship among and between roles. The structure of the organization and the relationship among the components of the structure are influenced by the individuals selected to interpret and implement the organization's philosophy. A particular form of governance evolves from the mission and values of the organization and the relationships among and between its components. Thus, managers and leaders who enact the mission and values on a daily basis support nursing more openly. To paraphrase an adage, behavior speaks louder and has more clout than organizational charts.

Nurses have multiple strategies to achieve collective action at their disposal; three prevalent ones are **shared governance, workplace advocacy,** and **collective bargaining.** These strategies are not mutually exclusive. As noted, governance is influenced by the context within which the organizational culture is embedded. Often the culture itself dictates the avenue of collective action.

The **culture** of the geographic area influences the organizational culture and the selected governance structure. For example, in right-to-work states, collective bargaining may be tolerated more than supported by nurses and administration. Box 18-1 summarizes some key factors about these states. Although mobility and the mass media have diluted the "purity" of geographic cultures, it is prudent to acknowledge how deeply embedded these cultural influences are within the fabric of American society.

When a **subculture** is clearly rooted in the mission of the organization (delivery of quality care in a cost-effective environment), the possibility of genuine negotiation or problem solving is enhanced. A subculture has its own unique and distinctive features, even as other features overlap with those of the larger culture. Members may adhere to values that are specific to their group, while at the same time espousing values of the larger society. The presence of congruent subcultures supports healthy relationships. Healthy relationships are an impor-

BOX 18-1

Right-to-Work Legislation

Right-to-work legislation prevents unions from mandating membership by workers in a given organization. In states with right-to-work laws, unions are not allowed to mandate membership of employees in a bargaining unit. Therefore, unionization is less prevalent. Nurses working in these states are less likely to choose unionization as a strategy to achieve collective action in part because they may see fewer examples in society at large.

tant variable in the development of a strong internal governance structure capable of supporting a professional practice environment that works well for everyone involved.

Exercise 18-3

Is your state a right-to-work state? If it is not, what is the nearest state that is a right-to-work state? Are any workers in the right-to-work state organized for the purpose of collective bargaining? How would you describe these workers (e.g., laborer, professional)?

Nurses and administrators are often members of separate subcultures. This phenomenon should not be given a negative connotation. Several factors may increase the distinct ideologies of the two groups, including the existence of a distant corporate structure and the presence of a union. Both factors may be considered external tensions. By tradition, decision-making in the United States has been centralized at the top administrative level. There is a tendency to increase the concentration of decision-making during economic downturns and the pressures inherent in maintaining a healthy "bottom-line." Actions are taken to avoid risk. However, history shows that broader input, not less, is important during these times.

When efforts have been made to address nurses' perceptions about job satisfaction, there has been a resulting effect on the relationship between nursing and the top administration of a hospital. Job satisfaction and the perceived level of care are greater when organizations provide for interaction between staff and management and when decision-making is at the point of service (Parker & Gadbois,

2000). The relationship is damaged when organizations do not address job satisfaction.

Exercise 18-4

Identify four factors in your practice (experience) that contribute to job satisfaction. Compare your responses to those of three practicing nurses who are not supervisors and three practicing nurses who are supervisors. Are your factors similar to the responses of others? Are you surprised by the responses?

In the past, nurses experienced practice environments and working conditions controlled by the medical profession and hospital administration. Increasingly, nurses expect a motivating, satisfying work environment that includes a role in decision-making. Many nurses today are unwilling to remain outside of the decision-making loop. Work redesign efforts to increase productivity and lower costs have contributed to increased tension regarding the role of nursing and nurses in decision-making. Evolving or creating a system that incorporates others in the decision-making process may be difficult for many individuals in upper management positions. High-performing organizations that provide quality health care create climates that provide for participation by all stakeholders. Each

stakeholder shares responsibility and risk; and that requires optimism and trust.

Contractual models allow nurses to form an organization and contract with the healthcare organization to provide nursing services. A contractual model can be characterized as a self-governance model as opposed to shared governance. Nurses become contract providers instead of employees. Historically, nurses were direct contractors as private-duty nurses prior to becoming hospital employees. Free agency may be the contractual model for the 2000s and beyond (Manion, 2000).

Shared Governance

Shared governance is described as a democratic, egalitarian concept; it is a dynamic process resulting from shared decision-making and accountability (Porter-O'Grady, 2001). According to Porter-O'Grady, Hawkins, and Parker (1997), basic principles of shared governance include partnerships, equity, accountability, and ownership. It is more accurate to say that shared governance demands participation in decision-making rather than provides for participation. The Literature Perspective describes one organization's implementation in an integrated healthcare network through its use of a shared governance model.

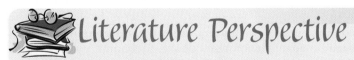

Literature Perspective

Batson, V. (2004). Shared governance in an integrated healthcare network. *AORN Online, 80*(3), 493-496.

Seton Healthcare Network, a network of more than 20 hospitals across central Texas, created an implementation team to create a shared governance model when the network agreed to assume operation of other hospitals in Austin. Nursing created a four-part model: a nurse executive council, a nursing practice congress, nursing specialty councils, and support councils. Each had distinct roles. One of the early tasks of the nurse executive council was to evaluate nursing positions and position descriptions to redesign and align them to fit the new network approach. This group subsequently evolved into the group addressing working conditions and salaries and benefits. The practice congress deals with the

broad issues of practice; specialty councils focus on areas of common practice or types of settings. The support councils focus on providing consultation about important aspects of the nursing role, educational development, issues of patient safety, and information systems issues.

IMPLICATIONS FOR PRACTICE

Shared governance is a complex, time-consuming process that can provide depth and breadth to the implementation of the mission and values of the organization. Nurse managers have specific roles to fulfill in supporting others' involvement in the process.

Through numerous reports and stories about organizations that have experienced the Magnet journey, staff nurses have praised the quality of their direct involvement through shared governance. Additionally, they favor work and learning (consistent with the Institute of Medicine [IOM] report, 2003) that is interdisciplinary and patient focused.

Some organizations mislabel their governance structures. Although structures may be labeled "shared governance," they possess few of the characteristics outlined by those who are recognized as experts on the topic. In addition, many organizations have developed thinly veiled mechanisms designed to preclude nurses from participating in collective action. In today's competitive environment, it is critical that nurses are informed of potential implications of various approaches. Professional-practice climates recognize individual and team performance. Increasingly nurses are seeking organizations that provide professional-practice climates, ones that have effective activities, not just effective documents. Thus, when considering any new position, planning to interview nurses within the organization before finalizing employment decisions is a wise strategy.

Workplace Advocacy

Workplace advocacy is an umbrella term encompassing activities within the practice setting. The choice of advocacy to reflect the framework in which nurses control the practice of nursing is consistent with the goals of the profession. Workplace advocacy includes an array of activities undertaken to address the challenges faced by nurses in their practice settings. The focus of these activities is on career development, employment opportunities, terms and conditions of employment, employment rights and protections, control of practice, labor-management relations, occupational health and safety, and employee assistance. The objective of workplace advocacy is to equip nurses to practice in a rapidly changing environment. Advocacy occurs within a framework of mutuality, facilitation, protection, and coordination.

Gadow's (1990) historic discussion of the manifestations of advocacy is relevant to a discussion of today's workplace advocacy. These manifestations include (1) ensuring relevant information, (2) enabling the selection of information, (3) disclosing a personal view, (4) providing support for making and implementing decisions, and (5) helping determine personal values.

Exercise 18-5

Contact nurses who are not represented by contract. Discuss the strategies they use to influence practice decisions (e.g., staffing, skill mix, responsibilities) and economic decisions (e.g., wages, benefits, time off, retirement).

Ensuring Relevant Information   Nurses must have relevant information to support their practice. Access to information is the basis for initiatives, full participation, and sharing information. Clinical nursing practice demands that nurses begin with patient information. The use of clinical data is necessary for patient well-being. However, patient information is the beginning of data gathering, not the end. It is equally important for nurses to have information related to how decisions are made for determining nurse staffing, occupational health and safety issues, equal employment opportunity information, professional liability, and **labor law.**

Enabling the Selection of Information   Just as healthcare patients must have relevant information to make good decisions; nurses must be able to select information that is relevant to their practice. Nurses have an obligation to know about a workplace. A good way to begin is by learning the mission of the organization and becoming knowledgeable of the culture. Acquaint yourself with nurses who practice in the organization. The time and effort devoted to this activity will be well spent. Many nurses and other individuals spend more time making decisions about the cars that they drive than a potential employment site. Think about a time when you were deciding about a car. You probably checked various makes and models and determined price; you may have visited a website or visited the dealership; you may have visited the service department and talked with those who had purchased a car from the dealership; you may have, literally or figuratively, kicked the tires. A similar process is appropriate in selecting a place of employment. Data regarding the workplace inform nurses of the history of the workplace. These data are available through the organization's Occupational Safety and Health Administration (**OSHA**) 200 Logs (www.OSHA.gov).

Disclosing a Personal View   Nurses and managers disclose their views on issues related to the work environment. Disclosure of management's perspective is important. The failure to build a trusting relationship jeopardizes the achievement of outcomes. Similarly, when nurses do not disclose their perspective, the relationship is at risk.

Risk takes many forms. Healthcare organizations constitute one of the most unsafe work environments in the United States. This environment is characterized by "speed-ups," fewer personnel, fewer full-time personnel, and a propensity to underemploy. An increasingly cynical public holds the "face" of the organization accountable for their pain and frustration. Often, a nurse is that organizational face. Violence toward healthcare personnel continues to increase. Risk is greater in emergency departments and psychiatric settings. Evidence reveals that many incidents are not reported. The identified toxins in the workplace are also a factor. Latex is a particular problem. Disinfectants, sterilants, antineoplastic agents, radiation, and noise are constants. The organization has a responsibility to ensure a safe environment for staff and patients. Obviously, nurses need to be involved in addressing workplace safety. Occupational health nurses provide expert consultation in the identification of potential hazards and suggestions for change, yet many healthcare organizations do not seek such experts. Box 18-2 describes two key sources of environmental support.

Providing Support for Making and Implementing Decisions   The support needed to make and implement decisions is achieved through **role models, mentors,** and **empowerment.** Role models may include the nurse who has exquisite clinical skills in assessment. Perhaps you have had the opportunity to observe nurses who seem to "absorb" information when they enter a patient's environment. Gladwell (2005) calls this thin slicing. This is a rare and coveted skill. Similarly, observing someone who is skillful in assertive communication transforming an explosive situation into a positive interaction is impressive. The implementation of a primary mentorship program may contribute to the development of these and other skills. A brief program with an external expert will not achieve the goal. A mentoring relationship is an ongoing, "hands-on" process. Individuals who have experi-

BOX 18-2

Safety in the Workplace

The **Occupational Safety and Health Act** of 1970 requires employers to provide a safe and healthy environment. Fire protection, construction and maintenance of equipment, worker training, machine guarding, and protective equipment are specified. Employers are required to familiarize themselves with applicable standards.

The **Centers for Disease Control and Prevention (CDC)** guidelines assume that all patients are infectious for HIV and other bloodborne pathogens. Although the CDC is not an enforcement agency, its guidelines are adopted as professional practice standards.

enced a successful mentorship have identified positive, frequently occurring behaviors that characterized their mentor. These behaviors include trust and the opportunity to make decisions that derive from that trust. The value to the individual is professional growth (Restifo & Yoder, 2004). The value to the organization is in the outcome: The individual will make better decisions.

Exercise 18-6

List the characteristics that you would want a mentor to possess. If you have identified a person you would want as a mentor, ask if he or she is willing to mentor you. Identify factors that are contributors and barriers to your seeking a mentorship relationship with the individual. Consider ways that you can address these factors.

Empowerment, or supporting other nurses, is a complex process. It can be demonstrated in repetitive assertive behaviors, such as requiring an accuser to confront the accused directly. That action supports the accused and eliminates a third-party translator. A more complex example involves the act of documenting an unsafe assignment. Accepting an unsafe assignment or refusing an assignment is difficult for nurses—both those at the beginning of their careers and those who are experienced. Critical elements to note are date, unit, assignment, staff available, rationale for objections, and documentation of notification of supervisor. Accurate, concise, and clear documentation can assist the nurse manager by providing a source of data necessary to support the preparation of their budgets and to support the documenters of such occurrences. Many assignments are classified as unsafe because of a lack of personnel and a lack of training of the existing personnel; therefore, nurses need to be prepared to respond when an assignment is inappropriate. Consider the consequences of accepting an assignment that is beyond your scope of practice and skills. These consequences have the potential to affect a patient, the organization, your colleagues, and yourself. One consequence may be conflict, and intense conflict may require a formal resolution. The Alternative Dispute Resolution (ADR) model provides assistance to nurses and is particularly useful in noncontract facilities. ADR uses techniques other than litigation. These techniques include negotiation, facilitation, mediation, and arbitration (Bachman, 2001). Gerardi (2004) defined direct costs of conflict (obvious) as such factors as turnover, management productivity, disability claims, and litigation. Indirect costs of unresolved conflict include team morale, loss of reputation, and thus market, and delay in patient services. Gerardi also defined four elements in mediation. Listening for understanding is important to clarify the specific conflict. Reframing allows progress in conversation as a result of neutralizing language. Elevating the definition of the problem is designed to incorporate all of the elements of the conflict so that common ground can be established. Finally, clear agreements are used to define future behavior. Thus, when a nurse complains about the way in which a physician interacts, a nurse manager could use these steps to attempt to resolve the issue. In some cases, it clearly would be wiser to use an external mediator who could be seen as totally neutral. The federal Office of Personnel Management provides a useful guide (www.opm.gov/er/adrguide/toc.asp).

Helping Determine Personal Values Professional values evolve through education in classroom settings, clinical assignments, and interactions with other nurses. "Professional values are beliefs and ideologies that are generally held in common by members of the profession and are used to guide professional practice" (Chinn & Kramer, 1999, p. 42). You will have an opportunity to solidify your own values as skillful mentors guide your practice and assist you to engage in value clarification. Inherent in professional values are ethical codes, standards of practice, standards for protect-

ing participants, willingness to challenge social traditions, priorities for allocating resources, cultural mores, and priorities for allocating resources (Chinn & Kramer, 1999).

Determining personal values increases an individual's value to an organization because the individual is empowered to make decisions within his or her scope of practice. This situation is both that simple and that complex. Empowerment requires redefining the managerial role and a change in behavior by nurses and administrators. The behavior change is one in which trust replaces distrust and respect replaces disrespect. How will the beginning nurse determine individual values within various types of decisions if there are inadequate, guided opportunities to practice decision-making?

Organizational patterns may segment the responsibility for the provision of care and the management of resources for that care. It is in the best interest of healthcare consumers for nurses to participate in decisions regarding the provision of care and resources. The involvement of nurses can vary from none whatsoever to a high degree of input by nurses in virtually every decision affecting the conditions of employment and their practice. Nurses must be prepared and willing to participate.

Exercise 18-7

Identify three factors that you consider most empowering in a governance model. Would the presence of one or more of these factors influence you to practice in such an environment? Identify three factors that you would consider least empowering in a governance model. Would the presence of one or more of these factors influence you to avoid practicing in this environment?

Collective Bargaining

Collective bargaining is the performance of the mutual obligation of the employer and representatives of the employees to meet at reasonable times and confer in good faith with respect to wages, hours, and other terms and conditions of employment or the negotiation of any agreement or any question arising from those terms and conditions. The purpose of collective bargaining by nurses (Box 18-3) is to secure reasonable and satisfactory conditions of employment, including the right to participate in decisions regarding their practice.

BOX 18-3

Unionization

In non-healthcare industries, unionization is acknowledged as a usual and expected business practice. Improved communication and good will cannot eliminate the gap between labor and management. Cooperation between management and labor will remain an illusion unless or until there is sharing of responsibility, power, and profits (Levitan & Johnson, 1983). If cooperation and trust exist between the union and the company, the members of the union will understand when the company is experiencing financial difficulties, and management will understand when members of the union experience difficulties. In 1996, the Malden Mills continued to assist employees from company funds when the company was unable to produce popular Polartec items due to a fire. In 2001, unions representing 1200 workers voted to accept a reduction in pay and benefits in an effort to keep Freightliner in Portland, Oregon (Freightliner Union Approves Reduced Pay, 2001).

Heckscher (1989) suggests that the union model is outdated because of trends that have made the public-policy framework of unionization less useful. Porter-O'Grady (2001) takes a much different perspective. "The union isn't the enemy; it's a new reality for nurse leaders" and he suggests that through partnering the formal requirements of the union contract "advances the practice of managing well and maintains the foundation of good management" (p. 32).

Changes in labor law have had a direct impact on the level of union activity in the healthcare sector. The federal role in labor relations is a dynamic, evolving one. The 1935 Wagner Act (National Labor Relations Act) established election procedures for employees to be able to choose their collective bargaining representatives freely. Two years later, the ANA included provisions for improving nurses' work and professional lives. The 1947 Taft-Hartley Act placed curbs on some union activity and excluded employees of not-for-profit hospitals from coverage. The Labor Management Reporting and Disclosure Act of 1959, the Landrum-Griffin Act, provides greater internal democracy within unions. The 1974 amendments to the Taft-Hartley Act removed the exemption of not-for-profit hospitals, and employees of these types of organizations have the same rights as industrial workers to join together and form labor unions. The removal of the exemption for not-for-profit hospitals created a frenzy of activity as traditional industrial unions targeted healthcare facilities. The National Labor Relations Board (NLRB) administers the National Labor Relations Act. State laws further define labor law.

Why is there an increase in organizing nurses and other healthcare professionals? Health care is a "hot" topic at the state and federal levels. The morning newspaper, nightly news, and a continuous parade of "news magazines" have featured countless articles related to health and illness. One may paraphrase Willie Sutton when he was asked why he robbed banks: "That is where the money is." Why organize nurses and other healthcare workers? That is where potential members are.

As technology replaces unskilled workers, a smaller pool of workers is available for trade-union organizing. Declining union membership has been the catalyst for unions to explore other membership bases. In 2003, 12.9% of wage and salary workers were union members, down from 13.3% in 2002. The union membership rate has steadily declined from a high of 20.1% in 1983 (U.S. Department of Labor, 2005). With numerous groups seeking to represent nurses, nurses seeking collective bargaining should carefully consider the representing agent. (See Box 18-4 for suggested screening criteria.)

Traditional industrial unions are increasingly seeking opportunities to represent nurses for the purpose of collective bargaining and to speak for nursing with boards of nursing, regulatory agencies, and legislatures. Organizing nurses and other healthcare workers for the purpose of collective bargaining is very attractive because of the large numbers of people involved and the decrease in organizing in other sectors. Additionally, nurses have a low rate of unionization: 19.1% of the 2,074,741 employed nurses, although the

BOX 18-4

Suggested Criteria for Selecting a Bargaining Agent

- A strong commitment to nursing practice, legislation, regulation, and education
- A well-prepared practice, policy, and labor staff: a minimum of a bachelor's degree in nursing
- Representative of those they represent in both gender and ethnic makeup
- National in scope and local in implementation
- Control by individual members over bargaining unit activities

profession is viewed as a prime target for membership growth. The United American Nurses (UAN) represents 32.9% of nurses covered by a union contract (U.S. Department of Labor, 2001).

Historically, nurses were reluctant to be identified with unions; however, that view has changed. Working together in a cooperative, collaborative manner is important for the safety and quality of care, especially when strain occurs between management and unions. Nurses have a legal right to bargain. The American Hospital Association has spent millions of dollars challenging the appropriateness of all-RN bargaining units or a unit separate from other organized employees. In a 1991 unanimous opinion, the U.S. Supreme Court upheld the NLRB's ruling that provides for RN-only units. This decision was critical for nursing. At stake was the ability of nurses to control nursing practice and the quality of patient care. Employees, including nurses, must be accorded workplace rights and the protection that allows them to practice. Nurses must have the freedom to do what the profession and their licensure status require them to do.

Labeling all RNs as supervisors is a second challenge to the right of nurses to organize. RNs monitor and assess patients as a part of their professional practice, not as a statutory supervisor within the definition of the National Labor Relations Act. A 1996 NLRB ruling held that RNs were not statutory supervisors and were protected by federal labor law; the decision was upheld in 1997 by the U.S. Court of Appeals for the Ninth Circuit (Nguyen, 1997). However, a 2001 Supreme Court decision (National Labor Relations Board v. Kentucky River Community Care, Inc., 2001) upheld a lower court's decision to classify RNs as supervisors, though this decision was later appealed.

Nurses as Knowledge Workers   The change from producing a product to providing a service has many implications for management and labor. In the past, employees in manufacturing were treated like interchangeable cogs: When a cog was broken, it was replaced. A large pool of unskilled workers was available to step forward in the steel mill, the coal mine, and the shop floor. The move from an industrial model in society requires a "knowledge worker." The unskilled worker of yesterday did not have a high school diploma. Today, knowledge workers may have multiple college degrees and certifications. When knowledge workers unionize, they develop organizations that are more similar to associations than traditional industrial unions. They become involved in activities such as lobbying and coalition building. Today's nurses are knowledge workers. The tools of knowledge workers differ from the workers of the past. As the knowledge content of the work increases, the practice of the worker (nurse) is guided more by science than by procedure. Nurses may ask, "Why be represented for collective bargaining?" A collective bargaining contract requires management to bargain, a requirement not present in noncontract organizations. Several factors influence nurses to seek collective bargaining: working conditions, including mandatory overtime, nurse-patient ratios, limited opportunities to participate in decision-making; and the successes that have been achieved by nurses in other healthcare organizations. In addition, many nurses identify the lack of good communication as a major factor in their decision to seek representation for the purposes of collective bargaining.

Nurses have observed a decline in the quality of care, attributable in large measure to decreased professional nurse staffing; they have observed that dividends to stockholders and plan officers have escalated (Appleby, 2004). The increase in the number of healthcare conglomerates has coincided with a diminished concern with humanistic factors (Shindul-Rothschild, Berry, & Long-Middleton, 1996). The focus is shifting from the expectations of the patient to the expectations of the stockholder. The public and the providers become the losers in this shift in focus. Health care is a labor-intensive industry that manifests many of the ills of other labor-intensive industries: impersonal management, discrimination, favoritism, and arbitrary termination. Nursing as a profession, and nurses as individuals, have a distinguished record of "going beyond the call of duty" in emergency situations. However, when extraordinary effort is demanded as ordinary effort, nurses resist the expectation and resent a system that takes advantage of them and their commitment to patient care.

Union or At-Will   The fear of arbitrary discipline and dismissal may be the catalyst for nurses to seek ways to protect themselves from what are perceived to be arbitrary actions. Nurses are seeking assistance from external sources in an effort to balance the assistance available to the organization's administrative personnel. A collective bargaining contract typically alters a balance of power. The discipline structure provided by contract treats all employees in the same manner and may decrease the manager's flexibility in designing or selecting discipline. Although there is **whistleblower** legislation (Box 18-5), the current environment in health care places the **at-will employee** who voices concern about the quality of care in a vulnerable position. Managers of at-will employees have greater latitude in selecting disciplinary measures for specific infractions. State and federal laws do provide a level of protection; however, an at-will employee may be terminated at any time for any reason except discrimination. At-will employees, in essence, work at the will of the employer. An at-will "employee can be terminated . . . for any reason as long as the reason is not unlawful" (Wright, 2004, p. 17). It is critical for nurses to know their rights regarding discipline and termination (Smith, 2002).

Contract language requires management to follow "due process" for represented employees. That is, management must provide a written statement outlining disciplinary charges, the penalty, and the reasons for the penalty. Management is required to maintain a record of attempts to counsel the employee. Employees have the right to defend themselves against charges and the opportunity to settle disagreements in a formal grievance hearing. They have the right to have their representative with them during the process. Management must prove that the employee is wrong or in error. In a nonunion environment, the burden of proof is on the employee. However, Carson and Franklin

---

BOX 18-5

Whistleblower Protection

Whistleblowing "refers to a warning issued by a current or former employee of an organization to the public about a serious wrongdoing or danger created or concealed within the organization" (Hunt, 1995, p. 155). The 1989 Whistle Blower Protection Act protects federal workers. The law does not cover the private sector. Some states have specific laws. It is imperative that the whistleblower understand the consequences of action, and inaction as the shield is an imperfect one (Solomon, 2004). Whistleblowing is often a result and symptom of organizational failure (Fletcher, et al., 1998).

(2001, p. 56) cited changes in the interpretation of the law: "The ability to avail oneself of protection does not depend on whether the employees are represented by a union to the interpretation of the law."

Management maintains the record of counseling. The commitment to nursing requires the manager to be clear about the charge. Although all disciplinary charges are important, those directly related to patient care have a more critical dimension. Clarity in describing the situation is important because it affects patient care, the individual nurse, and nurse colleagues.

Many nurses continue to be intimidated by those individuals who charge that "unions are unprofessional." A labor contract, a collective bargaining agreement/union contract, is unrelated to being professional. Sociologists have characterized the responsibilities of the professional as a respect for the duty to perform, respect for the duty to learn, respect for the public interest, and preservation and enhancement of the image (Moore, 1970). Many physicians and many faculty members have collective bargaining contracts. Why? They want to have greater control of their practice, improve working conditions, and influence their compensation. Contracts are a usual part of our current environment.

It is ironic that a contract between an employer and employee is considered unusual. Replacing the adversarial system should be the goal of efforts to redesign the workplace. A new social order in the workplace must be based on a spirit of genuine cooperation between management and nurses.

Selecting a Bargaining Agent   The ANA represents the interests of the profession, nurses, and health care at the state, federal, and international levels. In 1999 the House of Delegates of the ANA created the UAN to ensure that nurses have a meaningful access to collective bargaining. Subsequently, the UAN affiliated with the AFL/CIO. The collective bargaining program of the UAN is designed to implement strategies that maintain or attain improvement in nursing practice in addition to addressing the economic issues. In addition, nurses may be represented by more traditional unions, including the Service Employees International Union, the American Federation of State, County and Municipal Employees, and the American Federation of Teachers.

Exercise 18-8

If you practice in a setting with a collective bargaining agreement, secure a copy. Identify the articles of this contract. Are they practice issues or economic issues? What is the relationship between the two? If you work in a setting that does not have a collective bargaining agreement, secure dispute resolution policies. Identify the areas that may be disputed. Are they practice issues or economic issues? What is the relationship between the two?

Not all nurses are eligible to participate in collective bargaining. The nurse who is a statutory supervisor is excluded. Statutory supervisors are those nurses who have the authority to act in the interest of the employer, including the power to hire, terminate, reward, and discipline. These functions are stipulated in the statute (the law). These acts differ from those of nonsupervisory nurses,

who act in the interest of the patient. Supervisory nurses share a concern for working conditions, practice standards, and the care delivery environment with nonsupervisory nurses. Many supervisory nurses may think that they are unnecessarily placed in an adversarial relationship with nonsupervisory nurses in the hospital who are represented by the union.

FRAMEWORKS FOR COLLECTIVE ACTION

Nurses practice in multiple settings; some have collective bargaining (union) contracts, and others do not. Collective bargaining and noncollective bargaining environments espouse safe, quality care. Both environments exist within the context of state and federal laws. Professional practice models may exist in both environments. Nurses may feel valued in both environments. There is a critical difference. A contract requires the employer to negotiate within a legally binding framework. Noncollective bargaining environments do not provide that assurance.

The future may hold new relationships, and public policy may continue to include provisions that were formally negotiated through contracts. Nurses practice in highly competitive environments. Decision-making is at the core of nursing practice. Nurse involvement in decision-making contributes to higher levels of job satisfaction for the nurse and higher satisfaction with care for the patient, and it also has a positive influence on health outcomes. Nurses, and those they serve, benefit from collective action that uses a wide range of strategies.

The Solution

In any redesign effort, involving the staff is critical. I began by meeting with the staff and telling them why I wanted to begin a redesign process and what I hoped to accomplish from such efforts. I then set up redesign teams that have a great deal of staff involvement.

Involving the staff is critical for several reasons. First, the individuals who are actually taking care of patients most of the time think of the most creative solutions for redesign. Second, staff members are more likely to embrace redesign activities if they feel that they have been actively involved in the process. Finally, staff can often anticipate issues or problems with these efforts and help develop solutions before the implementation of redesign.

If I worked in a unionized environment, my approach would not differ, except I would meet with the union representatives before initiating the redesign efforts. Again, I would explain what I hoped to accomplish through these efforts, answer any questions or concerns, and ask for their support of the project.

— Peggy Reiley

 Would this be a suitable approach for you? Why?

CHAPTER CHECKLIST

Collectively, nurses possess the knowledge, skills, abilities, and numbers to influence decisions. Collective action may take many forms. Geographic and organizational contexts influence the formal and informal structures in which nurses participate. An organization's structure establishes the parameters for participation in decision-making. Managers establish the context for participation. The decision to organize for the purpose of collective bargaining represents an important decision for nurses and for the organization in which they practice. A level of tension exists when an external group becomes a part of an organization's decision-making processes. External groups may enter as a new management consultant, as a part of a merger, as a new owner, or as a union representing registered nurses. The acceptance and appreciation of the external group are influenced by understanding the rationale for the group's entry and by the respect between the constituencies.

- The purposes of collective participation by nurses are to do the following:
  - Promote the practice of professional nursing
  - Establish and maintain standards of care
  - Allocate resources effectively and efficiently
  - Create satisfaction and support in the practice environment (Minarik & Catramabone, 1998)
- Increased autonomy and diversification decrease the following:
  - Fear of ridicule
  - Fear of punishment
  - Fear of loss of job
  - Fear of favors
- Governance strategies dictate levels of participation. The type and level of participation in decision-making influences job satisfaction.
- Shared governance is characterized by partnerships, equity, accountability, and ownership.
- The framework for advocacy includes mutuality, facilitation, protection, and coordination. The manifestations of advocacy are as follows:
  - Ensuring relevant information
  - Enabling the selection of information
  - Disclosing a personal view
  - Providing support for making and implementing decisions
  - Helping determine personal values
- The goal of workplace advocacy is to equip nurses to practice in a rapidly changing environment.
- Collective bargaining is an effective, legal mechanism used by nurses to obtain the right to participate in decisions regarding their practice.
- Represented nurses are supported by the resources of the union. Unrepresented nurses do not have these resources.
- Representation for the purpose of collective bargaining (belonging to a union) is neither professional nor unprofessional.
- Nurses who are statutory supervisors are excluded from representation.

TIPS FOR COLLECTIVE ACTION

- An understanding of the culture and the organization's approach to any collective action strategy are important for managers and staff.
- Some states have laws that are more supportive of whistleblowing than others.
- Where collective bargaining is the appropriate strategy, develop criteria for the selection of the appropriate collective-bargaining agent.

TERMS TO KNOW

at-will employee
Centers for Disease Control and Prevention (CDC)
collective action
collective bargaining
culture
empowerment
followership
governance
labor law
mentor
OSHA
role model
shared governance
subculture
whistleblower
workplace advocacy

REFERENCES

Agency for Healthcare Research and Quality. (2006, February). *Patient safety indicators overview. AHRQ quality indicators.* Rockville, MD: The Agency.

Aiken, L., Clarke, S., & Sloane, D. (2000, October). Hospital restructuring: Does it adversely affect care and outcomes? *Journal of Nursing Administration, 30*(10), 457–465.

American Nurses Association (ANA). (2001). *The code of ethics for nurses with interpretive statements.* Washington, DC: Author.

Appleby, J. (2004, September 4). Non-profit hospitals' top salaries may be due for a check up: 6 largest systems paid more than $1.2 M, plus perks. Retrieved July 24, 2006, from www.USAToday.com/money/industries/health/2004-09-29-nonprofit-salaries-x.htm.

Bachman, J. (2001). *Alternative dispute resolution.* Washington, DC: ANA.

Carson, W., & Franklin, P. (2001, February). Workplace advocacy: How can it help you? *American Journal of Nursing, 101*(2), 55–57.

Chinn, P., & Kramer, M. (1999). *Theory and nursing: Integrated knowledge development* (5th ed.). St. Louis: Mosby.

Dock, L., & Stewart, A. (1920). *A short history of nursing.* N.Y.: Putnam & Sons.

Duchscher, J., & Cowin, L. (2004, November/December). The experience of marginalization in new nursing graduates. *Nursing Outlook,* 289–296.

Fletcher, J., Sorrell, J., & Silva, M. (1998). Whistleblowing as a failure of organizational ethics. *Online Journal of Issues in Nursing,* December 31, 1998.

Freightliner union approves reduced pay. (2001, October 6). *The Columbian.* p. E1.

Gadow, S. (1990). Existential advocacy: Philosophic foundations of nursing. In T. Pence & J. Cantrell (Eds.), *Ethics in nursing: An anthology.* New York: NLN.

Gerardi, D. (2004). Using mediation techniques to manage conflict and create healthy work environments. *AACN Clinical Issues: Advanced Practice in Acute Critical Care, 15*(2), 182–195.

Gladwell, M. (2005). *Blink: The power of thinking without thinking.* New York: Little Brown and Co.

Hascup, V. (2003). Organizational silence: The threat to nurse empowerment. *Journal of Nursing Administration, 33*(11), 562–563.

Heckscher, D. (1989). *The new unionism: Employee involvement in the changing corporation.* New York: Basic Books.

Hunt, G. (1995). *Whistleblowing in the health service: Accountability, law and professional practice.* London: Edward Arnold.

Institute of Medicine. (2003). *Health professions education: A bridge to quality.* Washington, DC: The National Academies.

Kalisch, B., & Kalisch, P. (1975). Slaves, servants, or saints: An analysis of the system of nurses training in the United States, 1873–1948. *Nurse Forum, 14*(3), 114.

Kennerly, S. (2000). Perceived worker autonomy: The foundation for shared governance. *Journal of Nursing Administration, 30*(12), 611–617.

Kramer, M., & Schmalenberg, C. (2004). Development and evaluation of essentials of Magnetism tool. *Journal of Nursing Administration, 34*(7–8), 365–378.

Kupperschmidt, B. R. (2004). Making a case for shared accountability. *Journal of Nursing Administration, 34*(3), 114–116.

Levitan, S., & Johnson, C. (1983, September/October). Labor and management: The illusion of cooperation. *Harvard Business Review, 61,* 8–16.

Lewis, F., & Batey, M. (1982, October). Clarifying autonomy and accountability in nursing service: Part 2. *Journal of Nursing Administration, 12*(10), 10–15.

Manion, J. (2000, Fall). Emergence of the Free Agent Nurse Workforce. *Nursing Administration Quarterly, 26*(5), 68–78.

Mills, D. (1983, May/June). When employees make concessions. *Harvard Business Review, 61,* 103–113.

Minarik, P., & Catramabone, C. (1998). Collective participation in workforce decision-making. In D. Mason, D. Talbot, & J. Leavitt (Eds.), *Policy and politics for nurses: Action and change in the workplace, government, organizations and community* (3rd ed.). Philadelphia: Saunders.

Moore, W. (1970). *The professions: Roles and rules.* New York: Russell Sage Foundation.

Moss, R., & Rowles, C. (1997, January). Staff nurse job satisfaction and management style. *Nursing Management, 29,* 32–34.

Mrayyan, M. T. (2004), Nurses' autonomy: Influence of nurse managers' actions. *Journal of Advanced Nursing, 45*(3), 326–336.

National Labor Relations Act (NLRA) Sec. 8(5), 29 U.S.C.A. §158 (5).

National Labor Relations Board v. Kentucky River Community Care, Inc., 121 S. Ct. 1861; No. 99-1815 (Argued February 21, 2001; decided May 29, 2001).

Nguyen, B. (1997, September/October). Long-awaited Providence ruling upholds right of charge nurses to bargain. *The American Nurse, 29,* 1, 14.

Parker, M., & Gadbois, S. (2000). Building community in the health care workplace: Part 3. *Journal of Nursing Administration, 30*(10), 466–473.

Porter-O'Grady, T. (2001, June). Collective bargaining: The union as partner. *Nursing Management, 32,* 30–32.

Porter-O'Grady, T. (2001). Is shared governance still relevant? *Journal of Nursing Administration, 31,* 468–473.

Porter-O'Grady, T., Hawkins, M., & Parker, M. (1997). Whole systems shared governance: Architecture for integration. Gaithersburg, MD: Aspen.

Porter-O'Grady, T., & Malloch, K. (2002). *Quantum leadership: A textbook of new leadership.* Gaithersburg, MD: Aspen.

Restifo, R., & Yoder, L. (2004, April 26). Partnership: Making the most of mentoring. *Nurseweek,* 30–33.

Roberts, S. J. (2000). Development of a positive professional identity: Liberating oneself from the oppressor within. *Advances in Nursing Science, 22*(4), 71–82.

Rogers, B. (1996). *Nursing injury, stress, and nursing care. In Nursing staff in hospitals and nursing homes: Is it adequate?* Washington, DC: IOM.

Shindul-Rothschild, J., Berry, D., & Long-Middleton, E. (1996, November). Where have all the nurses gone? Final results of our patient care survey. *American Journal of Nursing, 96,* 25–39.

Smith, M. (2002). Protect your facility and staff with effective discipline and termination. *Nursing Management, 33*(7), 15–16.

Solomon, D. (2004, October 4). Risk Management: For financial whistle-blowers, new shield is an imperfect one. *The Wall Street Journal.*

U.S. Department of Health and Human Services. (1988). *Secretary's commission on nursing: Final report.* Washington, DC: U.S. Government Printing Office.

U.S. Department of Labor. (2001, January 18). *Union members in 2000. Current population survey.* Washington, DC: U.S. Government Printing Office.

U.S. Department of Labor. Bureau of Labor Statistics. Retrieved January 10, 2005, from at www.bls.gov.

Wright, L. (2004, November–December). Employer-employee dynamics for nurses. *The American Nurse,* 17.

SUGGESTED READINGS

Collins, J. (2001). *Good to Great: Why some companies make the leap . . . and others don't.* New York: Harper Business.

Fisher, R., Ury, W., & Patton, B. (1991). *Getting to yes: Negotiating agreement without giving in.* New York: Penguin Books.

Forman, H., & Merrick, F. (2004). Arbitration: A final step in the dispute resolution process. *Journal of Nursing Administration, 34,* 261–263.

Museler, M. C. (2004). Negotiation skills in the practice of dietetics. *Topics in Clinical Nutrition, 19*(4), 303–307.

Perlow, L., & Williams, D. (2003). Is silence killing your organization? *Harvard Business Review, 81,* 52–58.

Slaikeu, K. A., & Hasson, R. H. (1998). *Controlling the costs of conflict: How to design a system for your organization.* San Francisco: Jossey-Bass.

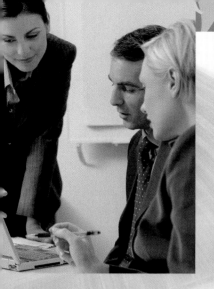

Managing Quality and Risk

Victoria N. Folse

*T*his chapter explains key concepts and strategies related to quality and risk management. All health-care professionals, including nurses, must be actively involved in the continuous improvement of patient care.

Objectives

- Apply quality management principles to clinical situations.
- Use the six steps of the quality improvement process.
- Practice using select quality improvement strategies to do the following:
  - Identify customer expectations.
  - Diagram clinical procedures.
  - Develop standards and outcomes.
  - Evaluate outcomes.

- Incorporate roles of leaders, managers, and followers to create a quality management culture of continuous readiness.

- Apply risk-management strategies to an agency's quality-management program.

Questions to Consider

- *How can a staff nurse make effective suggestions to improve nursing practice?*
- *How can a culture of assigning blame for errors be transformed into an environment invested in improving patient care?*
- *How can patients' expectations be used to improve nursing care and promote optimal outcomes?*

The Challenge

Theresa Finerty, MS, RN, CNA, BC
Director, Emergency/Trauma Services, OSF Saint Francis Medical Center, Peoria, Illinois

Joint Commission on Accreditation of Healthcare Organizations (JCAHO) site surveys are now unannounced. Historically, "ramp up" started about a year in advance of the survey, and the medical center went into intense preparation immediately preceding the visit. With unannounced JCAHO site surveys, the entire medical center needs to be in a continual state of readiness. It was difficult enough to keep the staff focused for a scheduled visit. The current challenge involves changing the culture to be "ever ready" and for the staff to be engaged in thinking how their daily activities meet the quality standards of patient care set forth by JCAHO.

 What do you think you would do if you were this nurse?

INTRODUCTION

Healthcare agencies and health professionals strive to provide the highest quality, safest, most efficient, and cost-effective care possible. The philosophy of quality management and the process of quality improvement need to shape the entire healthcare culture and provide specific skills for assessment, measurement, and evaluation of patient care. The goal of an organization committed to quality care is a comprehensive, systematic approach that prevents errors before they occur or identifies and corrects errors so that adverse events are decreased and safety and quality outcomes are maximized (Gantz, Sorenson, & Howard, 2003). Therefore, quality management and risk management are focused on optimizing patient outcomes and emphasize the prevention of patient-care problems and the mitigation of adverse events.

QUALITY MANAGEMENT IN HEALTH CARE

Healthcare systems that demand quality recognize that survival and competitiveness are built on improved patient outcomes. Success depends on a philosophy that permeates the organization and values a continuous process of improvement. It is essential to integrate patient safety and risk management into broader quality initiatives. Quality

necessitates maintaining safety in patient care, with a continual focus on clinical excellence from the entire multidisciplinary team. Patient safety is a key component of quality improvement and clinical governance (Woodward, 2004a). Moreover, the prevention of adverse events is paramount to improved patient outcomes (Considine & Botti, 2004). The quality management philosophy differs from other evaluation techniques because it focuses on the patient instead of the provider, prevention instead of inspection, and the process instead of the person.

The terms **quality management (QM), quality improvement (QI), performance improvement (PI), total quality management (TQM),** and **continuous quality improvement (CQI)** are often used interchangeably in health care. Quality-related terminology continues to evolve. Table 19-1 lists past, present, and evolving quality terms.

In this chapter, quality management refers to a philosophy that defines a healthcare culture emphasizing customer satisfaction, innovation, and employee involvement. Similarly, quality improvement refers to an ongoing process of innovation, prevention of error, and staff development that is used by institutions that adopt the quality management philosophy. Nurses maintain a unique role in quality management and quality improvement because of the amount of direct patient care provided at the bedside and because they have an understanding of the day-to-day issues involved in delivery of care (Gantz et al., 2003).

Table 19-1 PAST, PRESENT, AND EVOLVING QUALITY TERMS

Past Quality Terms	Present Quality Terms	Evolving Quality Terms
Quality control	Total quality management	Quality management
Quality assurance	Continuous quality improvement	Quality improvement
		Performance improvement

BENEFITS OF QUALITY MANAGEMENT

Healthcare systems employing a comprehensive QM program benefit in a number of ways. First, greater efficiency and proactive planning may overcome some of the resource constraints, including limited reimbursement imposed by prospective payment plans and key staff shortages. Second, successful malpractice suits could be reduced with quality care because QM is based on the philosophy that things should be done right the first time and that improvement is always possible. Third, job satisfaction could be enhanced because QM involves everyone on the improvement team and encourages everyone to make contributions. This style of participative management makes employees feel valued as team members who can really make a difference.

PLANNING FOR QUALITY MANAGEMENT

Multidisciplinary planning is integral to the quest for quality. Issues are examined from various perspectives using a systematic process. Planning takes time and money; however, the price of poor planning can be very expensive. Costs of inadequate planning might involve correcting a patient care error, resulting in extended length of stay and added procedures. In turn, this increases the risk of liability for what was originally done, it risks a negative public image, and magnifies employee frustration and turnover. The costs of errors and ineffective nursing actions are avoidable costs.

EVOLUTION OF QUALITY MANAGEMENT

Non–healthcare industries have excelled in focusing on process improvement as part of their core operating strategies. Numerous business management philosophies have been expanded and modified for use in healthcare organizations. For example, Six Sigma, a data-driven approach targeting a nearly error-free (3.4 defects per 1 million opportunities) environment, empowers employees to improve processes and outcomes. To achieve this, Six Sigma uses a methodology known as DMAIC which stands for define opportunities, measure performance, analyze opportunity, improve performance, and control performance (Vonderheide-Liem & Pate, 2004).

Define opportunities
Measure performance
Analyze opportunity
Improve performance
Control performance

In health care, emphasis is placed in the areas of patient safety and patient satisfaction. Leadership development is fostered; the role of the leader or manager in this TQM method is to enable the team, remove barriers, and instill accountability.

Within healthcare systems, QI combines the assessment of structure (e.g., adequacy of staffing, effectiveness of computerized charting, availability of unit-based medication delivery systems), process (e.g., timeliness and thoroughness of documentation; adherence to critical pathways or care maps), and outcome (e.g., patient falls; hospital-acquired infection rates; patient satisfaction) standards. These three factors are usually considered interrelated, and research has been conducted to determine the characteristics of effective structures and processes that would result in better outcomes.

Recognizing the relationship between quality patient care and nursing excellence, the American Nurses Credentialing Center (ANCC) created a process called the *Magnet™ Recognition Program*. The term *Magnet hospital* was chosen to describe a hospital that attracts and retains nurses even in times of nursing shortages. Magnet hospital research has examined the characteristics of hospital systems that impede or facilitate professional practice in nursing and also promote quality patient outcomes (Upenieks, 2003). Common organizational characteristics of Magnet hospitals include structure factors (e.g., decentralized organizational structure; participative management style; and influential nurse executives) and process factors (e.g., professional autonomy and decision-making; ongoing professional development/education).

QUALITY MANAGEMENT

The combination of QI ideas from theory and research is sometimes referred to as total quality management (TQM) or, more simply, quality management (QM). The basic principles of QM are summarized in Box 19-1 and are developed further in the next section of this chapter.

Involvement

Leaders, managers, and followers must be committed to QI. Top-level leaders and managers retain the ultimate responsibility for QM but must involve the entire organization in the QI process. Although some healthcare organizations have achieved significant QI results without system-wide support, total organizational involvement is necessary for a culture transformation. If all members of the healthcare team are to be actively involved in QI,

---

BOX 19-1

Principles of Quality Management and Quality Improvement

1. Quality management operates most effectively within a flat, democratic, organizational structure.
2. Managers and workers must be committed to quality improvement.
3. The goal of quality management is to improve systems and processes, not to assign blame.
4. Customers define quality.
5. Quality improvement focuses on outcomes.
6. Decisions must be based on data.

---

clear delineation of roles within a non-threatening environment must be established (Table 19-2).

To work effectively in a democratic, quality-focused corporate environment, nurses and other healthcare workers must accept QI as an integral part of their role. Nursing must be recognized and empowered to mobilize performance improvement knowledge and practice measures throughout the organization (Gantz et al., 2003). When a separate department controls quality activities, healthcare managers and workers often relinquish responsibility and commitment for quality control to these quality specialists. Employees working in an organizational culture that values quality freely make suggestions for improvement and innovation in patient care. Exercise 19-1 may help nurses make QI suggestions.

▌ *Exercise 19-1*

Think of a problem or potential problem that exists in the agency where you practice. Define the problem, using as many specific facts as possible. List the advantages to the staff, patients, and agency of correcting this problem. Describe several possible solutions to the problem. Decide whom you would contact about these suggestions.

Goal

The goal of QM is to improve the system, not to assign blame. Managers strive to provide a system in which workers can function effectively. To encourage commitment to QI, nurse managers must clearly articulate the organization's mission and goals. All levels of employees, from nursing assistants to hospital administrators, must be educated about QI strategies.

Communication should flow freely within the organization. To enhance communication, the nurse manager uses a participative or transformational management style. The nurse leader, charged with the responsibility for guiding not only nursing staff but also a multidisciplinary team, must ensure deliberate, intelligent, shared, and data-driven methodology (Gantz et al., 2003). Because QM stresses improving the system, detection of employees' errors is not stressed, and if errors occur, reeducation of staff is emphasized rather than imposition of punitive measures.

Customers

Customers define quality. Successful organizations measure the factors that are most important to

Table 19-2 ROLES/RESPONSIBILITIES IN QUALITY IMPROVEMENT PLAN

Role of Senior Leader	Role of Nurse Manager	Role of Follower
Leads culture transformation	Is accountable for quality and safety indicator performance within areas of responsibility	Follows policies, procedures, and protocols to ensure quality and safe patient care
Sets priorities for house-wide activities, staffing effectiveness, and patient health outcomes	Communicates performance priorities and targets to staff	Remains current in the literature on quality and safety specific to nursing; promotes evidence-based practice standards
Builds infrastructure, provides resources, and removes barriers for improvement	Meets regularly with staff to monitor progress and help with improvement work	Communicates with and educates peers immediately if they are observed not following quality and safety standards
Defines procedures for immediate response to errors involving care, treatment, or services and contains risk	Uses data to measure effectiveness of improvement	Reports quality and safety issues to supervisor/manager
Assesses management and staff knowledge of quality management process regularly, and provides education as needed	Works with staff to develop and implement action plans for improvement of measures that do not meet target	Invests in the process by continually asking self, "Why is this indicator important to measure?" "What has been done to improve it?" "What can I do to improve it?"
Implements and monitors systems for internal and external reporting of information	Provides time for unit staff to participate in quality-improvement measures	Participates actively in the quality-improvement activities
Defines and provides support system for staff who have been involved in a sentinel event	Performs direct observation of staff and coaches as needed	
	Consults Quality Management Team (e.g., Six Sigma) or Risk Management Team as appropriate	
	Writes and submits to senior leaders periodic action plan including performance measures and plans for improvement	
	Shares information and benchmarks with other units and departments to improve organization's performance	

their customers and focus their energies on enhancing quality in these areas. As patients become more sophisticated and view themselves as "consumers" who can take their business elsewhere, they want input into treatment decisions. Although typical patients may not be knowledgeable about a specific treatment, they know if they were satisfied with their experience with the health care provider.

Every nurse and healthcare agency has internal and external customers. Internal customers are people or units within an organization who receive products or services. A nurse working on a hospital unit could describe patients, nurses on the other shifts, and other hospital departments. External customers are people or groups outside the organization who receive products or services. For nurses, these external customers may include patients' families, physicians, managed care organizations, and the community at large. Managers and staff nurses can use Exercise 19-2 to identify their internal and external customers.

Exercise 19-2

For 1 week, list every person with whom you interact as a nurse. The internal customers are those people who work for, or receive care in, your organization. External customers come from outside the organization. What is the best method to obtain feedback from each of these customers?

Consumer satisfaction with health care can be assessed through the use of questionnaires, interviews, focus group discussions, or observation. Patients' perspectives should be a key component of any quality improvement initiative (Woodward, 2004b). However, patients cannot always adequately assess the competence of clinical performance and, therefore, patient feedback and patient satisfaction surveys must serve as only one data source for QI initiatives.

Focus

QI focuses on outcomes. Patient outcomes are statements that describe the results of health care. They are specific and measurable and describe patients' behavior. Outcome statements may be based on patients' needs, ethical and legal standards of practice, or other standardized data systems. Sources for outcome statements are described further in the next section of this chapter.

Decisions

Decisions must be based on data. The use of statistical tools enables nurse managers to make objective decisions about QI. It is imperative that data are not merely collected to support a preconceived idea. Quality information must be gathered and analyzed without bias before improvement suggestions and recommendations are made.

THE QUALITY IMPROVEMENT PROCESS

QI involves continual analysis and evaluation of products and services to prevent errors and to achieve customer satisfaction. The work of continuous QI never stops because products and services can always be improved.

The QI process is a structured series of steps designed to plan, implement, and evaluate changes in healthcare activities. Many models of the QI process exist, but most parallel the nursing process, and all contain steps similar to those listed in Box 19-2. The six steps can easily be applied to clinical situations. In the following example, staff at a community clinic use the QI process to handle patient complaints about excessive wait times.

BOX 19-2

Steps in the Quality Improvement Process

1. Identify needs most important to the consumer of healthcare services.
2. Assemble a multidisciplinary team to review the identified consumer needs and services.
3. Collect data to measure the current status of these services.
4. Establish measurable outcomes and quality indicators.
5. Select and implement a plan to meet the outcomes.
6. Collect data to evaluate the implementation of the plan and the achievement of outcomes.

A community clinic receives a number of complaints from patients about waiting up to 2 hours for scheduled appointments to see a licensed practitioner. The clinic secretary and staff nurses suggest to the clinic manager that scheduling clinic appointments be investigated by the QI committee, which is composed of the clinic secretary, two clinic nurses, one physician, and one nurse practitioner. The clinic manager agrees to the staff's suggestion and assigns the problem to the QI committee. At their next meeting, the QI committee uses a flow chart to describe the scheduling process from the time a patient calls to make an appointment until the patient sees a physician or nurse practitioner in the examining room. Next, the committee members decide to gather and analyze data about the important parts of the process: the number of calls for appointments, the number of patients seen in a day, the number of canceled or missed appointments, and the average time each patient spends in the waiting room. The committee discovers that too many appointments are scheduled because many patients miss appointments. This overbooking often results in long waiting times for the patients who do arrive on time. The QI committee also gathers information on clinic waiting times from the literature and through interviews with patients and colleagues. A measurable outcome is written: "Patients will wait no longer than 30 minutes to be seen by a licensed practitioner." After a discussion of options, the team recommends that appointments be scheduled at more reasonable intervals, that patients receive notification of appointments by mail and by phone, and that all clinic patients be educated about the importance of keeping scheduled appointments. The committee communicates its suggestions for improvement to the manager and staff and monitors the results of the implementation of their improvement suggestions. Within 3 months, the average waiting room time per patient decreases to 90 minutes, and the number of missed patient appointments decreases by 20%.

Identify Consumers' Needs

The QI process begins with the selection of a clinical activity for review. Theoretically, any and all aspects of clinical care could be improved through the QI process. However, QI efforts should be concentrated on changes to patient care that will have the greatest effect. To determine which clinical activities are most important, nurse managers or staff nurses may interview or survey patients about their healthcare experiences or may review unmet quality standards. The results of the research study (Defloor & Grypdonck, 2005) highlighted in this chapter's Research Perspective box identify prevention of pressure ulcers as an area on which to focus.

Assemble a Team

Once an activity is selected for possible improvement, a multidisciplinary team implements the QI process. QI team members should represent a cross-section of workers who are involved with the problem. Team members may need to be educated about their roles before starting the QI process.

To develop effective unit-based quality councils, the workplace environment must promote teamwork. Some departments within healthcare facilities are more open to teamwork than others. Nurse leaders and managers can use Exercise 19-3 to decide whether their clinical unit is ready for a unit-based QI team.

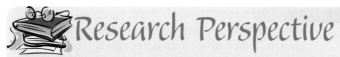

Research Perspective

Defloor, T., & Grypdonck, M. (2005). Pressure ulcers: Validation of two risk assessment scales. *Journal of Clinical Nursing, 14,* 373-382.

This study compared the predictive value of two widely used pressure ulcer risk-assessment scales (Braden and Norton) to the clinical judgment of nurses. In the 1772 participating older patients, neither the Norton nor the Braden scales adequately predicted risk for pressure ulcers. Alarmingly, nurses predicted pressure-ulcer development even less well than the two instruments. Only activity, sensory perception, skin condition, and the existence of old sores were significant predictors of pressure-ulcer lesions (grade 2 and higher).

IMPLICATIONS FOR PRACTICE

Although the performance of the risk-assessment scales is poor, using a risk-assessment tool appears to be a better quality indicator than relying solely on the clinical judgment of nurses. The development of new instruments with higher predictive value of actual risk is needed. If the nurses relied only on the results of the Braden or Norton, 80% of the patients would have unnecessarily received preventive measures. Much needless work is done, and expensive material (i.e., pressure-reducing mattresses) is wrongly allocated. In a climate of limited resources, it is imperative to direct clinical efforts to quality-management and risk-management initiatives that have emerged through research and to incorporate evidence-based practice into daily routines.

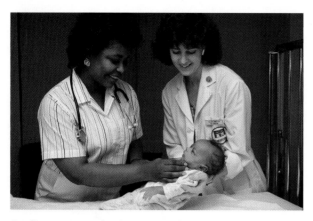

Quality nursing is both caring and compassionate.

Exercise 19-3

Ask yourself the following questions about your department:

1. Is communication between nurses and other professionals promoted? If so, how?
2. Could the communication process be improved in any way?
3. Does your system encourage nurses to act as a team?
4. Are other disciplines/departments included in team activities?
5. Can the team focus be improved in any way?

Collect Data

After the multidisciplinary team forms, the group collects data to measure the current status of the activity, service, or procedure under review. Various data tools may be used to analyze and present this information. These data tools include flow charts, line graphs, histograms, Pareto charts, and fishbone diagrams. The use of empirical tools to organize QI data is an essential part of the QI process.

A detailed flow chart is used to describe complex tasks. The flow chart is a data tool that uses boxes and directional arrows to diagram a process or procedure. Sometimes, just diagramming a patient-care process in detail reveals opportunities for improvement. The flow chart in Figure 19-1 depicts the process of a home health agency receiving a new patient referral.

Line graphs present data by showing the connection among variables. The dependent variable is usually plotted on the vertical scale, and the independent variable is usually plotted on the horizon-

tal scale. In QI this technique is often used to show the trend of a particular activity over time, and the result may be called a trend chart. The line graph in Figure 19-2 illustrates the number of referrals a home health agency receives during a year.

The histogram in Figure 19-3 illustrates the number of home health referrals that come from five different referral sources during a select year. A histogram is a bar chart that shows the frequency of events.

A bar chart that identifies the major causes or components of a particular quality control problem is called a Pareto chart. Used often in QI, the Pareto chart helps the QI team determine priorities. The Pareto chart in Figure 19-4 demonstrates that on a medical-surgical unit over a 1-month period, omission of vital signs was the most common type of documentation error.

The fishbone diagram is an effective method of summarizing a brainstorming session. A specific problem or outcome is written on the horizontal line. All possible causes of the problem or strategies to meet the outcome are written in a fishbone pattern. Figure 19-5 uses a fishbone diagram to present possible causes of patients' complaints about extended waits for clinic appointments.

Although QI teams should be able to use these basic statistical tools, more complex analysis is sometimes necessary. In this situation, a statistical expert could be included on the QI team, or the team may use a statistician as a consultant.

Establish Outcomes

After analyzing the data, the team next sets a goal for improvement. This goal can be established in a number of ways but always involves a standard of practice and a measurable **patient-care outcome.** The multidisciplinary team should use accepted standards of care and practice whenever possible. Clinical practice guidelines and standards should reflect evidence-based practice and should be updated as new research merges. Sources that establish these standards include the following:

1. American Nurses Association (ANA) Standards of Nursing Practice/state nurse practice acts
2. Accrediting bodies such as the Joint Commission on Accreditation of Healthcare Organizations (JCAHO) or recognition bodies such as the American Nurses Credentialing Center (ANCC)

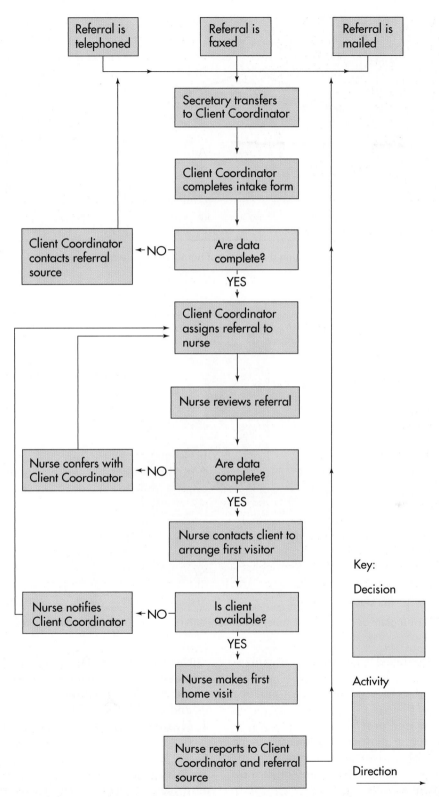

Figure 19-1 Steps in a flowchart diagramming process, starting with the time a home health referral is made and ending with the first home visit.

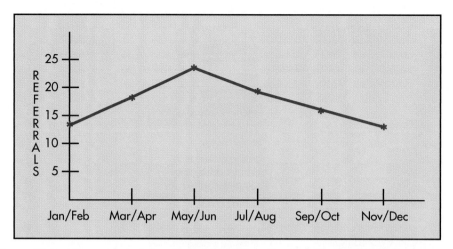

Figure 19-2   Line graph depicting the number of home health referrals received during 1 year.

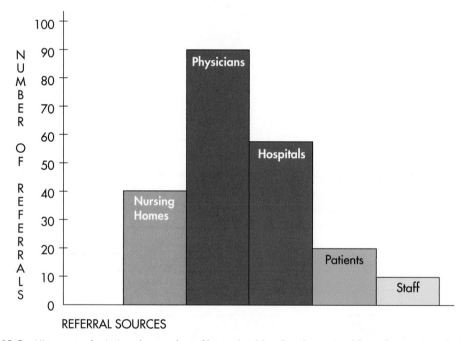

Figure 19-3   Histogram depicting the number of home health referrals received from five sources during 1 year.

3. Nationally recognized professional organizations
4. Nursing research/evidenced-based, best-practice standards
5. Internal policies and procedures
6. Internal or external performance measurement data such as patient-satisfaction surveys, employee-opinion surveys, safety-assessment surveys, and patient rounds
7. Governmental bodies such as the Agency for Healthcare Research and Quality (AHRQ) and the Centers for Disease Control's Division of Healthcare Quality and Promotion (DHQP) and the National Institute for Occupational Safety and Health (NIOSH)
8. Healthcare advisory groups such as the Institute of Medicine (IOM)

Although individual healthcare organizations may have unique patient needs related to their specific population or environment, many targeted outcomes are similar. One way to evaluate the

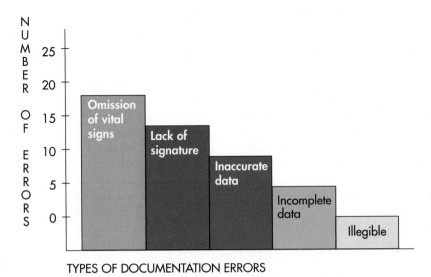

Figure 19-4   Pareto chart presenting major types of documentation error that occurred on a medical/surgical unit over a 1-month period.

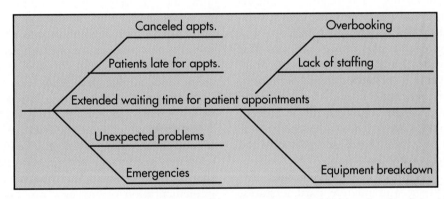

Figure 19-5   Fishbone diagram showing possible causes of extended waiting time for clinic patients.

quality of outcomes is to compare one agency's performance against that of similar organizations. In a process called **benchmarking,** a widespread search is conducted to identify the best performance against which to measure others. Through this process of comparing the best practices against your practice and process, your organization learns to identify desired standards of quality performance. Available data include all reported hospital-acquired infection rates in other institutions as well as specific data, such as postoperative infection rates in adult surgical intensive-care units of similar-size institutions. However, recent mandates in select states to publicly disclose nosocomial infection rates highlight potential issues with disclosure

of data. Specifically, simply reporting hospital infection rates is not enough to promote hand-hygiene practices and may do little to improve outcomes and reduce hospital-acquired infections. Unfortunately, the usefulness of the information from other institutions continues to be hampered by differences in terminology. Information technology plays a vital role in QI by increasing the efficiency of data entry and analysis. A consistent information system that trends high-risk procedures and systematic errors would provide a useful database regarding outcomes of care and resource allocation. The purpose of the National Quality Forum is designed to standardize measures so that true comparisons can be made.

Nursing has been a leader in the information system field by developing standardized nursing-classification systems. The availability of standardized nursing data enables the study of health problems across populations, settings, and caregivers. Consistent use of standardized language enhances the process of QI and also demonstrates the contributions of nursing to lawmakers, healthcare policy makers, and the public. Three leading nursing-classification systems have been identified: the North American Nursing Diagnosis Association's (NANDA) nomenclature (NANDA, 2003), the Nursing Intervention Classification (NIC) System (Dochtermann & Bulechek, 2004), and the Nursing Outcomes Classification (NOC) System (Moorhead, Johnson, & Maas, 2004).

Each classification system focuses on one component of the nursing process. Nursing diagnoses can be labeled using NANDA. These diagnosis labels represent clinical judgments about actual or potential health problems. Each diagnosis contains a definition, major and minor defining characteristics, and related factors (NANDA, 2003).

The NIC System consists of interventions that represent both general and specialty nursing practice. Each intervention includes a label, definition, and a set of activities that nurses perform to carry it out. For example, pain management is defined, and specific activities are listed to alleviate pain or reduce the pain to a level that is acceptable to the patient (Dochtermann & Bulechek, 2004).

The NOC system consists of outcomes that focus on the patient and include patient states, behavior, and perceptions that are sensitive to nursing interventions. Each outcome includes a definition, a five-point scale for rating outcome status over time, and a set of specific indicators to be used in rating the outcomes (Moorhead et al., 2004). Clinical testing for validation and refinement has occurred in various settings, and the standardization of terms continues to develop to reflect current knowledge and changes in nurses' roles and the structure of healthcare systems. The consistency of terms is essential in providing a large database across healthcare settings to predict resource requirements and establish outcomes of care.

Discuss Plans

The team discusses various strategies and plans to meet the new outcome. One plan is selected for implementation, and the process of change begins. Because QM stresses improving the system rather than assigning blame to employees, change strategies emphasize open communication and education of workers affected by the new standard and outcome. Blaming or reprimanding staff for actual or potential mistakes does not encourage an open and safe culture in which to work (Woodward, 2004a). QI is impossible without continual education of all managers and followers.

Policies and procedures may need to be written or rewritten during the QI process. Policies should be reviewed frequently and updated so that they reflect best practice standards and do not become barriers to innovation. Communication about the change or improvement is essential.

Evaluate

As the plan is implemented, the team continues to gather and evaluate data to document that the new outcomes are being met. If an outcome is not met, revisions in the implementation plan are needed. Sometimes improvement in one part of a system presents new problems. For example, nurses wanted to implement screening for suicide risk in adolescents and adults presenting to the emergency department. A result of this improvement in care was a greatly increased number of referrals for counseling, which overwhelmed the existing hospital and community resources. The interdisciplinary team may need to reassemble periodically to handle the inevitable obstacles that develop with the implementation of any new process or procedure. Furthermore, individuals outside the medical center (external customers) may need to be included in the process. The example that follows also illustrates this idea.

A hospital is implementing a pneumatic tube system to dispense medications. A multidisciplinary team is assembled to discuss the process from various viewpoints: pharmacy, nursing, pneumatic tube operation managers, aides who take the medications from the pneumatic tube to the patient medication drawers, administrators, and physicians. The tube system is implemented. A nurse on one unit realizes that several patients do not have their morning medications in their medication drawers. The nurse borrows medications from another patient's drawer and orders the rest of the medications stat from pharmacy. Other nurses on that unit and other units have the same problem and are doing the same or similar things. Several problems are occurring—some of the medications are being given late, nurses waste precious time by searching other medication drawers, the pharmacy charges extra for the stat medications and is overwhelmed with stat requests, and the situation increases the nurses' frustration level. In some cases, patients suffer due to late administration of medications. QM principles would encourage the nurses to report the problems to the nurse manager or appropriate team member. The pneumatic tube team could compile data such as frequency of missing medications, timing of medication orders, and nursing units involved. The problems are analyzed with a system perspective to solve the late medication problem effectively.

In some organizations, when the change is implemented successfully, the QI team disbands. One of the crucial tasks of the nurse manager is to publicize and reward the success of each QI team. The nurse manager must also evaluate the work of the team and the ability of individual team members to work together effectively.

Some organizations that have used the QM philosophy for several years establish permanent QI teams or committees. These QI teams do not disband after implementing one project or idea but rather may meet regularly to focus on improvements in specific areas of patient care. The use of permanent QI teams or the adoption of a culture driven by QM can provide continuity and prevent duplication of efforts within the quality teams.

QM organizations stress system-level change and the evaluation of outcomes; however, in recent years, the need for process/performance improvement, including individual performance appraisal, has reemerged within healthcare organizations. Peer review and self-evaluation are performance-assessment methods that fit within the QM philosophy.

Any nurse can use the six steps of the QI process to self-evaluate and improve individual performance. For example, a nurse on a medical unit who wants to improve documentation skills might study past entries on patient records; review current institution policies, professional standards, and literature related to documentation; set specific performance-improvement goals after consultation with the nurse manager and expert colleagues; devise strategies and a timeline for achieving per-formance goals; and after implementing the strategies, review documentation entries to see whether self-improvement goals have been met.

QUALITY ASSURANCE

Although QI is a comprehensive process to prevent problems, it is naive to suggest the total abandonment of periodic inspection. One method used to monitor health care is **quality assurance (QA)** programs. QA focuses on clinical aspects of the provider's care, often in response to an identified problem. Many QA activities focus on process standards (e.g., documentation; adherence to practice standards). The focus may be asking questions such as, "Did the nurse document the response to the pain medication within the required time period?" instead of, "Did the patient receive adequate pain relief postoperatively?" In contrast, quality improvement (QI) may examine process, structure, and outcome standards. The similarities and differences between QI and QA are summarized in Table 19-3.

One of the methods most often used in QA is chart review or chart auditing. Chart audits may be conducted using the records of active or discharged patients. Charts are selected randomly and reviewed by qualified healthcare professionals. In an internal audit, staff members from the same hospital or agency that generated the records examine the data. External auditors are qualified professionals from outside the organization who conduct the review. An audit tool containing specific criteria based on standards of care is applied to each chart under review. For example, auditors might compare documentation related to use of restraints for medical-surgical purposes with the criterion, "Licensed independent practitioner evaluates patient in person within 4 hours of application." Auditors note compliance or lack of compliance with each audit criterion and report a summary of these findings to the appropriate manager or committee for corrective action.

Because the focus of the chart audit is on detecting errors and determining the person responsible for them, many staff members tend to view QA negatively. The nurse manager must reinforce that QA is not intended to be punitive, but instead is an opportunity to improve patient care at the unit level. For example, to reinforce the importance

Table 19-3 COMPARISON OF TRADITIONAL QUALITY ASSURANCE AND QUALITY IMPROVEMENT PROCESSES

	Quality Assurance (QA) Process	Quality Improvement (QI) Process
Goal	To improve quality	To improve quality
Focus	Discovery and correction of errors	Prevention of errors
Major tasks	Inspection of nursing activities Chart audits	Review of nursing activities Innovation Staff development
Quality team	QA personnel or department personnel	Multidisciplinary team
Outcomes	Set by QA team with input from staff	Set by QI team with input from staff and patients

of documentation, providing the standard of care for documentation and assisting the RN in reviewing several charts is an appropriate educational tool to reinforce policies and procedures or standards regarding documentation. It is the responsibility of the manager to communicate the importance of daily QA activities and how unit-based monitoring ties into the overall quality improvement program. Moreover, many institutions incorporate both the participation in and the results of QA into annual performance appraisals or clinical ladders.

RISK MANAGEMENT

QM and **risk management** are related concepts and emphasize the achievement of quality-outcome standards and the prevention of patient-care problems. Risk management also attempts to analyze problems and minimize losses after an adverse event occurs. These losses include incurring financial loss as a result of malpractice or absorbing the cost of an extended length of stay for the patient, negative public relations, and employee dissatisfaction. Moreover, the inclusion of safety standards in the JCAHO guidelines further emphasizes the importance of risk management. See Box 19-3 for National Patient Safety Goals.

The risk management department has several functions. These include:

- Defining situations that place the system at some financial risk, such as medication errors or patient falls

Box 19-3

National Patient Safety Goals for Hospitals

- Improve the accuracy of patient identification.
- Improve the effectiveness of communication among caregivers.
- Improve the safety of using medications.
- Reduce the risk of health care-associated infections.
- Accurately and completely reconcile medications across the continuum of care.
- Reduce the risk of patient harm resulting from falls.
- Encourage patients' active involvement in their own care as a patient safety strategy.
- The organization identifies safety risks inherent in its patient population.

From Joint Commission on Accreditation of Healthcare Organizations. Retrieved August 7, 2005, from www.jointcommission.org/patientsafety/nationalpatientsafetygoals.

- Determining the frequency of occurrence of those situations
- Intervening and investigating identified events
- Identifying potential risks or opportunities to improve care

Each individual nurse is a risk manager. Each nurse has the responsibility to identify and report unusual occurrences and potential risks. Active involvement in quality and risk management by direct caregivers, however, is a challenge complicated by staffing issues. Data show that a high patient-to-nurse ratios (Aiken, Clarke, Sloane, Sochalski, & Silber, 2002) and a smaller proportion of RNs among a hospital's staff (Clarke, 2003) are associated with higher rates of serious complications or adverse events. Another barrier to improving patient safety is fear of punishment, which inhibits people from acknowledging, reporting, or discussing errors. One way to minimize errors is to monitor threats to patient safety continually and to recognize that individual errors often reflect organizational and system failures. For example, targeting nurse-to-patient load and work schedules including 12-hour shifts and overtime will reduce potential errors from human factors such as fatigue, stress, and distractions (Hughes, 2004).

Both risk management and quality management deal with changing behavior, prevention, focus on the customer, and attention to outcomes (Henry & Ginn, 2002). The following clinical examples illustrate how quality management and risk management complement each other. First, the implementation of lift teams reduces employee injuries associated with lifting heavy or fully dependent patients and simultaneously, for the patient, decreases adverse events associated with difficult transfers. The implementation of lift teams reflects managing both quality and risk. Second, violence prevention in healthcare organizations can also be approached within a TCM framework. Establishing a culture that is committed to protecting employees and patients from violence is important for all, but particularly so for healthcare professionals working in areas of greatest risk for violence, such as critical care and emergency departments (Henry & Ginn, 2002). Although nursing managers would prefer that all staff intrinsically embrace risk management practices aimed at patient and staff safety, accountability for safety can be one aspect of performance evaluations. Active involvement of staff in risk management activities is key to prevention of adverse events. Nurse managers should conduct safety rounds and praise employees for employing safe practice as part of best practice standards. This philosophy reinforces that risk management not only benefits the patient, but also works to keep individual employees safe in the workplace.

Adverse-event reduction is a key strategy for reducing healthcare mortality and morbidity because patients who suffer adverse events are more likely to die or suffer permanent disability. Nurses have always played a pivotal role in the prevention of adverse events and can reduce negative outcomes with a focus on accurate physical assessment and early identification and correction of physiologic abnormality (Considine & Botti, 2004). Also, adherence to best-practice standards and assurance of quality standards for high-risk/high-volume practices (e.g., restraint use, medication management) can reduce adverse events. A comprehensive program would proactively identify and reduce risks to patient safety through completion of a failure mode and effects analysis (FMEA) on select high-risk situations as advanced by JCAHO. If an adverse event occurs, nurses should also be able to recognize **near-misses** and **sentinel events** and participate with a multidisciplinary team in the **root-cause analysis.** A sentinel event is a serious, unexpected occurrence involving death or physical or psychologic harm, such as suicide, infant abduction, or wrong-site surgery. Similarly, a near-miss may have resulted in no harm, but highlights an imminent problem that must be corrected and can provide useful lessons in terms of risk analysis and reduction (Woodward, 2004b). JCAHO calls for voluntary self-reporting of sentinel events by both inpatient institutions and home health agencies. See Box 19-4 for the most common sentinel events reported in the healthcare arena. After a sentinel event is identified, a root-cause analysis is performed by a team that includes those directly involved in the event and those in leadership positions. A root-cause analysis is very similar to the QI process described in this chapter except that the root-cause analysis is a retrospective review of an incident to identify the sequence of events with the goal of identifying the root causes (Woodward, 2004c). The root-cause analysis leads to the development of specific risk-reduction strategies, and in certain situations, the plan must be reported to JCAHO.

While reporting to JCAHO illustrates external reporting to regulatory or accrediting agencies, an internal method of communicating risks or adverse events is through incident reporting. Incident reports are kept separate from the patient's medical record and should serve as a means of communicating an incident that did cause or could have caused harm to patients, family members, visitors, or employees. Aggregated incident reports should be

BOX 19-4

Most Common Healthcare Sentinel Events

Patient suicide
Operative/postoperative complications
Wrong-site surgery
Medication error
Delay in treatment
Patient fall
Patient death/injury in restraints
Assault/rape/homicide
Perinatal death/loss of function
Patient elopement
Infection-related event
Fire
Anesthesia-related event
Maternal death
Ventilator death
Medical equipment related
Infant abduction/wrong family
Utility systems related event

From Joint Commission on Accreditation of Healthcare Organizations. Retrieved July 11, 2005, from www.jcaho.org.

used to improve quality of care and decrease future risk. Trending data can illuminate systems issues that need to be modified to reduce risk and achieve quality patient care. Although an incident report is not warranted for a unit-specific problem or an interdepartmental issue in which no adverse event occurred (e.g., delay in diagnosis or treatment), communication at the appropriate chain of command is essential to improve quality.

Evaluating Risks

In gathering data about unusual occurrences, the risk-management team may involve perspectives from numerous disciplines to discover underlying problems that a single discipline might miss. Risk managers also use multiple data sources, data collection techniques, and perspectives to collect and interpret the data. Quantitative methods such as questionnaire or records of medication administration are combined with qualitative methods such as open-ended question interviews. To illustrate, Cook, Hoas, Guttmannova, & Joyner (2004) administered open-ended questions to nurses to identify the types of errors that were recognized and reported and conducted audits to determine those errors that were actually reported or charted. Both data-collection methods identified the three most common errors: medication errors (wrong patient, time, dose, drug, or mode of delivery), patient falls, and errors caused by illegible handwriting on orders.

However, recognizing errors does not always translate into reporting errors. The lack of agreement as to what constitutes error influences the willingness of healthcare professionals to report errors and subsequently affects whether or not they develop strategies that could reduce future risk (Cook et al., 2004). Moreover, a lack of consensus exists regarding whether or not patients and families should be informed about healthcare errors.

Exercise 19–4

Describe an error that occurred in the agency where you practice that resulted in harm to the patient and one that did not. What would you suggest to avoid a reoccurrence? Decide under what circumstances you would inform the patient and family and under what circumstances you would withhold the information.

Approaches to patient safety and risk management require healthcare providers to challenge their attitudes that errors are an unfortunate but inevitable part of patient care. Diminished resources have the potential to compromise communication among providers and to contribute to an environment in which unsafe practices are overlooked or excused (Cook et al., 2004). A team approach to quality management and risk management is needed to promote optimal outcomes. Nurses have a responsibility to provide quality care, and thus, must serve in leadership roles to ensure a culture of integrated quality management and risk management.

The Solution

Although it is still evolving, part of the solution will be to maintain monthly unit site surveys using the JCAHO tracer methodology. The administrative team, as well as key unit staff, will be included in these rounds as patients are tracked through the entire healthcare process from admission to discharge. Findings will be reported to staff and the unit council for quality review. The unit council will report both problems and solutions as part of the quality report to the medical center's governing nursing body, the Professional Nursing Congress.

— Theresa Finerty

 Would this be a suitable approach for you? Why?

CHAPTER CHECKLIST

Many healthcare organizations are in the process of transforming their system to QM. Greater efficiency with improved quality is the goal of this approach. Effective QI includes identifying consumer expectations, planning, using a multidisciplinary approach, evaluating outcomes, and changing the system to provide an environment in which employees can perform their best.

- The main principles of QM and QI are as follows:
  - QM operates most effectively within a flat, democratic, organizational structure.
  - Leaders and followers must be committed to QI.
  - The goal of QM is to improve systems and processes without assigning blame.
  - Customers define quality.
  - QI focuses on outcomes.
  - Decisions must be based on facts.
- QM strives to prevent errors. Initial planning requires both time and money, but QM contributes to the bottom line in the long run.

- The major steps in the continuous QI process to evaluate and improve patient care are as follows:
  - Identify needs most important to the consumer of healthcare services.
  - Assemble a multidisciplinary team to review the identified consumer needs and services.
  - Collect data to measure the current status of these services.
  - Establish measurable outcomes and quality indicators.
  - Select and implement a plan to meet the outcomes.
  - Collect data to evaluate the implementation of the plan and the achievement of outcomes.
- Any process can be improved.
- Risk management focuses on ensuring safety and on minimizing loss after a patient-care error occurs.
- QA is the responsibility of all nurses and provides an opportunity to improve patient care at the unit level.

TIPS ON QUALITY MANAGEMENT

- QM is based on data; anything measured and recorded can be improved.
- Concentrate QI energies on factors that are most important to your patients.
- Working together to prevent problems is more effective than fixing problems after they occur.

TERMS TO KNOW

benchmarking
continuous quality improvement (CQI)
near-miss
patient-care outcome
performance improvement (PI)
quality assurance (QA)
quality improvement (QI)
quality management (QM)
risk management
root-cause analysis
sentinel event
total quality management (TQM)

REFERENCES

Aiken, L., Clarke, S. P., Sloane, D., Sochalski, J., & Silber, J. H. (2002). Hospital nurse staffing and patient mortality, nurse burnout and job dissatisfaction. *Journal of American Medical Association, 288*(16), 1987–1993.

Clarke, S. P. (2003). Balancing staffing and safety. *Nursing Management, 34*(6), 44–48.

Considine, J., & Botti, M. (2004). Who, when and where? Identification of patients at risk of an in-hospital adverse event: Implications for nursing practice. *International Journal of Nursing Practice, 10*, 21–31.

Cook, A. F., Hoas, H., Guttmannova, K., & Joyner, J. C. (2004). An error by any other name. *American Journal of Nursing, 104*(6), 32–43.

Defloor, T., & Grypdonck, M. (2005). Pressure ulcers: Validation of two risk assessment scales. *Journal of Clinical Nursing, 14*, 373–382.

Dochtermann, J. M., & Bulechek, G. M. (2004). *Nursing interventions classification (NIC)* (4th ed.). St. Louis: Mosby.

Gantz, N. R., Sorenson, L., & Howard, R. L. (2003). A collaborative perspective on nursing leadership in quality improvement: The foundation for outcomes management and patient/staff safety in health care environments. *Nursing Administration Quarterly, 27*(4), 324–329.

Henry, J., & Ginn, G. O. (2002). Violence prevention in health care organizations within a total quality management framework. *Journal of Nursing Administration, 32*(9), 479–486.

Hughes, R. G. (2004). First, do no harm: Avoiding the near misses taking into account one ever-present factor: Human fallibility. *American Journal of Nursing, 104*(5), 81–84.

Joint Commission International Center for Patient Safety. Retrieved July 11, 2005, from www.jcipatientsafety.org.

Joint Commission on Accreditation of Healthcare Organizations. Retrieved July 11, 2005, from www.jcaho.org.

Moorhead, S., Johnson, M., & Maas, M. (2004). *Nursing outcomes classification (NOC)* (3rd ed.). St. Louis: Mosby.

North American Nursing Diagnosis Association. (2003). *NANDA nursing diagnoses: Definitions and classifications, 2003–2004.* Philadelphia: Author.

Upenieks, V. V. (2003). What constitutes effective leadership? Perceptions of Magnet and nonmagnet nurse leaders. *Journal of Nursing Administration, 30*(9), 456–467.

Vonderheide-Liem, D., & Pate, B. (2004). *Applying quality methodologies to improvement health care: Six sigma, lean thinking, balanced scorecard, and more.* Marblehead, MA: Hcpro, Inc.

Woodward, S. (2004a). Achieving a safer health service. Part 1: Making safety a way of life. *Professional Nurse, 19*(5), 265–268.

Woodward, S. (2004b). Achieving a safer health service. Part 2: Reporting Requirements. *Professional Nurse, 19*(6), 328–332.

Woodward, S. (2004c). Achieving a safer health service. Part 3: Investigating root causes and formulating solutions. *Professional Nurse, 19*(7), 390–394.

SUGGESTED READINGS

Institute of Medicine. (2000). *To err is human: Building a safer health system.* Washington, DC: National Academies Press.

Institute of Medicine. (2001). *Crossing the quality chasm: A new health system for the 21st century.* Washington, DC: National Academies Press.

Joint Commission on Accreditation of Healthcare Organizations. (2001). *Front line of defense: The role of nurses in preventing sentinel events.* Oak Brook, IL: Joint Commission Resources, Inc.

Joint Commission on Accreditation of Healthcare Organizations. (2002). *Health care at the crossroads: Strategies for addressing the evolving nursing crisis.* Oak Brook, IL: Joint Commission Resources, Inc.

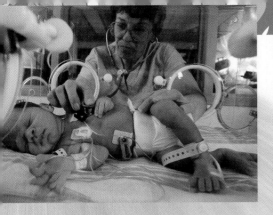

20

Translating Research into Practice

Margarete Lieb Zalon

*T*he importance of research in the development of the scientific basis for nursing practice is described in this chapter. The role of the nurse as a follower, manager, and leader of a healthcare organization in applying research to practice is delineated in the context of twenty-first century demands for providing health care based on the best available scientific evidence. The practical aspects of evaluation and utilization of research and the development of evidence-based practice in nursing are described. Strategies for translating research into practice that can be used by the individual nurse as a follower, leader, and manager in the context of the organization are outlined.

Objectives

- Value the individual nurse's obligation to use research in practice.
- Analyze the difference between research utilization and evidence-based practice.
- Formulate a clinical question that can be searched in the literature.
- Evaluate resources for the best available evidence.
- Identify resources for critically appraising evidence.
- Assess organizational barriers to and facilitators of the implementation of research findings.
- Identify strategies for implementing evidence-based practices within the context of an organization.

Questions to Consider

- What is the scientific basis for the nursing care provided in your clinical setting?
- What are the consequences of providing care that is not based on the best available evidence?
- What would you do if you knew that a particular practice in your organization was not based on the best available scientific evidence?
- How can research-based protocols be implemented in an environment in which nurses are uncomfortable or unsure about their ability to read and understand research reports?
- How would you go about developing a scientifically based approach to address a particular practice problem?

The Challenge

Holly Olsen, BSN, RN, CCRN
Staff Nurse, LifeFlight®, Miami Children's Hospital, Miami, FL

I had been a staff nurse in neonatal intensive care units for 10 years, first in Miami and then Dallas, prior to returning to my hometown of Miami. I have been a member of the neonatal/pediatric transport team for LifeFlight®, which transports critically ill infants from the outlying community hospitals in Florida as well as some international hospitals, back to our medical center. I was concerned about the care that we were able to provide to these fragile neonates. During the emergency of getting an airway at the referral hospitals, using the correct endotracheal tube size and tube placement were not always done according to the Neonatal Resuscitation Program (NRP) guidelines. Sometimes, we would need to reinsert a tube, wasting precious time. We knew that not selecting an appropriate-size endotracheal tube for extremely low birth-weight infants could possibly lead to complications. We were not confident that everyone was familiar with best practices regarding neonatal resuscitation. I felt very strongly that there had to be a way that we could improve on what we were doing.

 What do you think you would do if you were this nurse?

INTRODUCTION

If you or a loved one required nursing care, you would want that care to be based on the best research evidence available. For example, if a family member needed to be on a ventilator, you would want to be sure that the nurses providing the care were using best practices to prevent ventilator-associated pneumonia. You would want to know that there is good communication between nurses and physicians on the clinical unit where your family member has been placed, because you know that research demonstrates that teamwork and collaboration lead to lower mortality and fewer errors. If that family member also had a central venous catheter, you would want to be sure that the nurse who removes that catheter is using an established procedure that minimizes the risk for introducing an air embolism into the circulation. And, when that family member is discharged, you would want to know that the nurses are using well-tested strategies to help that person transition to home and recover from his or her illness. As a follower, a leader, and a manager, you should be concerned about incorporating research not only into clinical practices but also into the management of systems of care. The challenge is how to (1) find the best research evidence, (2) incorporate the best evidence into practice in a meaningful manner, and (3) motivate nurses, nursing leadership, and organizational leadership to care about using evidence in practice in the midst of all the other challenges faced in delivering high-quality nursing care.

Research is an integral part of professional practice. Research is the "diligent, systematic inquiry or investigation to validate and refine existing knowledge and generate new knowledge" (Burns & Grove, 2005, p. 2). Nurses, as professionals, have an obligation to society that involves rights and responsibilities as well as a mechanism for accountability. These obligations are outlined in *Nursing's Social Policy Statement* developed by the American Nurses Association (ANA). "To refine and expand the knowledge base and science of the discipline, nurses generate and use theories and research findings that are selected on the basis of their fit with professional nursing's values of health and health care, as well as their relevance to professional nursing practice" (2003, p. 5).

The *Code of Ethics for Nurses* (ANA, 2001, p. 22) directs that the "nurse participates in advancement of the profession through contributions to practice, education, administration and knowledge development." Furthermore, the global importance of nursing research is illustrated by an

International Council of Nurses (ICN) position statement indicating that it supports "national nurses' associations in their efforts to enhance nursing research, particularly through improving access to education which prepares nurses to conduct research, critically evaluate research outcomes and promote appropriate application of research findings to nursing practice" (1999, ¶ 3). Nursing research is designed to refine and expand the scientific foundation for nursing, which is defined as the "protection, promotion, and optimization of health and abilities, prevention of illness and injury, alleviation of suffering through the diagnosis and treatment of human response, and advocacy in the care of individuals, families, communities, and population" (ANA, 2003, p. 6). Because the practice of nursing draws on nursing science and the physical, economic, biomedical, behavioral, and social sciences (ANA, 2003), nurses need to apply findings of nursing research and research conducted by members of other disciplines that have relevance for their own practice.

The translation of research into practice is not only a concern for nursing, but also for all health disciplines. The National Institutes of Health (NIH) created a *Roadmap* to harness scientific discovery to improve the health of all people. The roadmap has three major themes: (1) new pathways to discovery, (2) research teams of the future, and (3) re-engineering the clinical research enterprise (NIH, n.d.). The focus of new pathways to discovery is on new strategies for diagnosing, treating, and preventing disease, and includes building blocks, biologic pathways and networks, molecular libraries and imaging, structural biology, bioinformatics and computational biology, and nanomedicine. The research teams of the future focus on high-risk research, interdisciplinary teams, and public-private partnerships. Re-engineering the clinical research enterprise focuses on clinical research networks, policy analysis and coordination, dynamic assessment of patient-reported chronic disease outcomes, and translational research. Overall, the emphasis is getting the research into the hands of practitioners who use it to better patient care.

The oft-quoted statistic of taking 17 years to apply research discoveries to clinical practice (Balas & Boren, 2000) suggests that healthcare professionals need to accelerate the integration of research with practice. We might believe that once the results of a research study are published in a journal, it is then read by clinicians and subsequently used by nurses and/or policymakers to improve practice. Often, that is not the case. For example, Norma Metheny has been researching techniques for testing nasogastric tube placement for many years. She and her colleagues have demonstrated that listening for a "swoosh" sound with a stethoscope could be dangerous. Her recommendation is to test gastric contents for pH, with a pH of 0 to 4 indicating gastric placement. When the pH is greater than 4, additional testing of the aspirate for bilirubin or pepsin at the bedside is recommended. Yet, many nurses may not be familiar with the technique, nor do they have access to bedside testing methods (Metheny & Titler, 2001). Thus, the problem is twofold, using ineffective strategies that might harm patients and not using effective strategies that would help patients.

Research has provided the foundation for many improvements in nursing practice. Examples include preoperative teaching, pain management, assessment of child development, falls prevention, pressure-ulcer risk detection, incontinence care, and family-centered care in intensive care units (ICUs) and neonatal intensive care units (NICUs), among others. Nurses need to evaluate nursing studies systematically to decide what interventions should be implemented to improve the **outcomes** of care. Practices that were once thought to be the standard of care may quickly become out-of-date. There may be practices that have been carried out for many years without ever having been examined for scientific basis or effectiveness. Furthermore, the latest research findings need to be incorporated into procedures using an evidence-based model when they are being evaluated or updated by an organization. The Research Perspective provides one example of incorporating research into organizational practices.

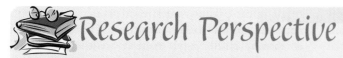

Research Perspective

Reising, D. L., & Neal, R. S. (2005). Enteral tube flushing: What you think are best practices may not be. *American Journal of Nursing, 105*(3), 58-64.

This article describes the research evidence for various practices related to flushing enteral tubes. The authors conducted a literature search for research and nonresearch articles over a 10-year period, which yielded 19 articles. They also reviewed 19 textbooks used in nursing courses and contacted 19 Indiana hospitals regarding policies and procedures related to enteral-tube flushing. The review included (1) flushing during enteral-tube feedings, (2) flushing between enteral-tube feedings, (3) checking feeding residual, (4) flushing fluids, (5) unclogging occluded enteral tubes, and (6) evaluating syringe size for flushing. Within each topic, the authors describe different practices and whether the information is derived from research or textbooks. The authors did not evaluate the strength of the evidence in the research studies they reviewed. Based on their review, the authors created a table of recommendations from their review that includes "*Dos*" and "*Don't*s."

IMPLICATIONS FOR PRACTICE

This article illustrates the lack of standardization of practices related to enteral-tube flushing and the importance of using research for the development of procedures. However, there is also considerable variation in recommended techniques, which the authors attribute to conflicting evidence in the literature. This review illustrates the importance of investigating assumptions about common nursing practices and the need for more specific research.

> ### Exercise 20-1
> Identify a common activity that is part of your nursing practice, and determine whether there is any research to support that particular intervention or nursing care activity.

Nursing research designs can be categorized in several ways, such as basic versus applied, qualitative versus quantitative, cross-sectional versus longitudinal, experimental versus descriptive, and retrospective versus prospective. Regardless of the design, some research is ready for implementation, and some research may not yet be ready to warrant a change in practice. Some decisions should not be based on the results of quantitative data alone, but should be integrated with data from qualitative research to apply it to a particular practice situation. The quality of care and the quality of the outcomes of care can be dramatically improved with the implementation of evidence-based practice. Patients, those entrusted to our care, are deserving of practices that are based on the best available evidence. Examining the evidence for a particular practice will generally need to go beyond examining the results of a single study. There are times when a single, well-designed study is adequate for recommending and implementing a practice change. However, developing an evidence-based practice requires the development of a clearly written clinical question and a more thorough search of the literature, the review of single studies, **meta-analyses,** critically appraised topics, systematic reviews, and **clinical guidelines.**

Appraising the evidence and placing it in the context of patient, family, and community values must also be done. Nurse managers/leaders may not necessarily be the ones actually conducting research, evaluating research evidence, or developing evidence-based guidelines, but they will be facilitating the application of research findings in practice. Key concepts for facilitating evidence-based nursing care include **research utilization, evidence-based practice (EBP), diffusion of innovations, translation of research into practice (TRIP),** evaluation of evidence, organizational strategies (for translating research into practice), and issues for nurse leaders and managers faced with implementing these processes.

RESEARCH UTILIZATION

Research utilization is the process of synthesizing, disseminating, and using research-generated knowledge to make an impact or change in existing practices (Burns & Grove, 2005). Research utilization is different from, but complementary to, research. Although individual nurses may apply research findings to their own practice, nurses' broader responsibilities to society presuppose the activation of the change process in translating research into practice. The use of research can be in a variety of forms from enlightenment, to the implementation of a research-based protocol, to the widespread adoption of standards based on research findings. Ultimately, several factors influence the adoption of a particular research finding and how it is translated into and sustained in practice.

Nurse researchers have a distinguished record of identifying the importance of utilizing research as a basis for practice. Nurses have gone beyond the traditional mode of disseminating research through publication in research journals. In the 1970s, three major federally funded demonstration projects facilitated the utilization of key research findings: the Western Interstate Commission on Higher Education in Nursing Project (WICHEN), 1975; the Conduct and Utilization of Research in Nursing Project (CURN) at the University of Michigan in 1976; and the Nursing Child Assessment Satellite Training (NCAST), 1976 to 1985 (Table 20-1). These early initiatives spawned the growth of many demonstration projects in an effort to implement research findings in practice as well as research studies conducted to identify factors that facilitate or create barriers to research utilization. The NCAST program illustrates the far-reaching and enduring effects of research utilization. This program, developed by Kathryn Barnard in 1976, is widely used today by home health nurses and public health departments across the country and even internationally (Kennedy, 2002). More than 21,000 healthcare professionals have been trained in the use of the NCAST assessment materials, with 200 of them actively providing education at any given time.

Many research utilization models in nursing were developed in the 1970s and 1980s. One of the first of these research utilization models was the

Table 20-1 EARLY NURSING RESEARCH UTILIZATION PROJECTS

Title	Activities	Selected Reference
Western Interstate Commission on Higher Education in Nursing (WICHEN), 1975	Used workshops to pair a nurse clinician with an educator to work together in developing research utilization protocols. Developed a preoperative teaching program, a care plan for grieving spouses, diabetes education, and a program to prevent constipation in nursing home residents.	Krueger, J. C., Nelson, A. H., & Wolanin, M. O. (1978). *Nursing research: Development, collaboration and utilization* (pp. 350-351). Germantown, MD: Aspen.
Conduct and Utilization of Research in Nursing (CURN), 1976	Developed protocols for preoperative teaching, reducing diarrhea in tube-fed patients, urinary catheterization and catheter care, pressure ulcer prevention, pain management, sensory preparation for procedures, intravenous catheter changes, and mutual goal setting.	Horsley, J. A., Crane, J., Crabtree, M. K., & Wood, D. J. (1983). *Using research to improve nursing practice: A guide.* New York: Grune & Stratton.
Nursing Child Assessment Satellite Training (NCAST), 1976-1985	Created evidence-based assessment of child development through a series of feeding and teaching scales to measure caregiver and child interaction between birth and 36 months of age. Information gathered then used to provide parent education and support.	King, D., Barnard, K. E., & Hoehn, R. (1981). Disseminating the results of nursing research. *Nursing Outlook, 29,* 164-169. NCAST-AVENUW www.ncast.org

Stetler-Marram model (2001) developed in 1976, which now includes the facilitation of evidence-based practice. Other research utilization models developed by nurses are listed in Table 20-2.

The 1990s were witness to dramatic change. Although research utilization had consisted of evaluating research and determining its applicability to practice, it was largely a process that focused on a single research study or several related studies. In the 1990s, the focus changed to finding a research-based solution to a problem. Large healthcare institutions began to use research and began to evaluate the changes instituted. The forerunner of the federal Agency for Healthcare Research and Quality (AHRQ) issued consensus-based clinical guidelines for common healthcare problems, such as acute pain, incontinence, pressure ulcers, depression, and HIV prevention. Professional associations and other groups also began to issue clinical guidelines. The *National Guideline Clearinghouse* for clinical guidelines was created on the Web by the AHRQ in partnership with the American Medical As-

sociation and the American Association of Health Plans. The AHRQ guidelines as well as guidelines developed by other groups are included (www.guidelines.gov). The twenty-first century ushers in an era of collaboration between researchers and clinicians to solve particular problems and advance health care. For example, health maintenance organizations are looking to develop strategies to facilitate their patients' adherence to screening guidelines, such as diabetic patients having a hemoglobin A1C drawn every 3 months. Voluntary organizations that provide support services for individuals not covered by health insurance are attempting to strengthen the research foundation—that is, the evidence for the types of services they fund, to more effectively meet community needs.

Stetler's research utilization model (2001) provides direction for an individual and for group members and, therefore, has implications for the leadership roles of nurses responsible for managing patient care. According to Stetler, it is the prepara-

Table 20-2 RESEARCH UTILIZATION MODELS

Model	Selected Source
Dracup-Breu (WICHEN Project)	Dracup, K. A., & Breu, C. S. (1978). Using nursing research findings to meet the needs of grieving spouses. *Nursing Research, 27,* 212-216.
Goode Research Utilization Model	Goode, C. J., Lovett, M. K., Hayes, J. E. & Butcher, L A. (1987). Use of research-based knowledge in clinical practice. *Journal of Nursing Administration, 17*(12), 11-18.
Quality Assurance Model Using Research	Watson, C., Bulecheck, G., & McCloskey, J. (1987). QAMUR: A quality assurance model using research. *Journal of Nursing Quality Assurance, 2*(1), 21-27.
University of North Carolina Model	Funk, S. G., Tornquist, E. M., & Champagne, M. T. (1989). A model for improving the dissemination of nursing research. *Western Journal of Nursing Research, 11,* 361-372.
Multidimensional Framework of Research Utilization	Kitson, A., Harvey, G., & McCormack, B. (1998). Enabling the implementation of evidence based practice: A conceptual framework. *Quality in Health Care, 7,* 149-158.
Change to Evidence-Based Practice Model	Rosswurm, M. A., & Larrabee, J. H. (1999). A model for change to evidence-based practice. *Image: Journal of Nursing Scholarship, 31,* 317-322.
Iowa Model of Evidence-Based Practice to Promote Quality of Care	Titler, M. G., Kleiber, C., Steelman, V. J., Rakel, B. A., Budeau, G., Everett, L. Q., et al. (2001). The Iowa Model of Evidence-Based Practice to promote quality care. *Critical Care Nursing Clinics of North America, 13,* 497-509.
Collaborative Research Utilization Model	Dufault, M. (2004). Testing a collaborative research utilization model to translate best practices in pain management. *Worldviews on Evidence-Based Nursing, 1*(3), S26-S32.
Ottawa Model of Research Use	Graham, K., & Logan, J. (2004). Using the Ottawa Model of Research Use to implement a skin care program. *Journal of Nursing Care Quality, 19,* 18-24.

tory steps of research utilization that sustain evidence-based practice. Stetler's model consists of five phases: preparation, validation, evaluation/decision-making, translation/application, and evaluation (Figure 20-1). The preparatory phase involves searching, sorting, and selecting sources of evidence as well as defining external factors that can influence the application of a research finding and internal factors that can diminish objectivity. The second phase, validation, is based on a utilization focus with an appraisal of study findings rather than the critique of a study's design. An integral component of this phase is the completion of review tables to facilitate understanding each study and to facilitate decision-making. The third phase, comparative evaluation, involves making a decision about the applicability of the studies reviewed by synthesizing cumulative findings; evaluating the degree and nature of other criteria, such as risk, feasibility, and readiness of the finding; and actually making a recommendation about using the research. The fourth phase, translation and application, involves practical aspects of implementing the plan for translating the research into practice at the individual, group, department, or organizational level. The recommendation here includes multiple strategies for the implementation of change and being sure that the translation of the research finding into practice does not exceed what is warranted by the evidence. The last phase includes an evaluation, which can be informal or formal, and may include a cost-benefit analysis. The evaluation can be conducted on an individual or institutional level. Evaluation can include whether the research innovation was implemented as intended and whether the particular goals were achieved. Stetler's

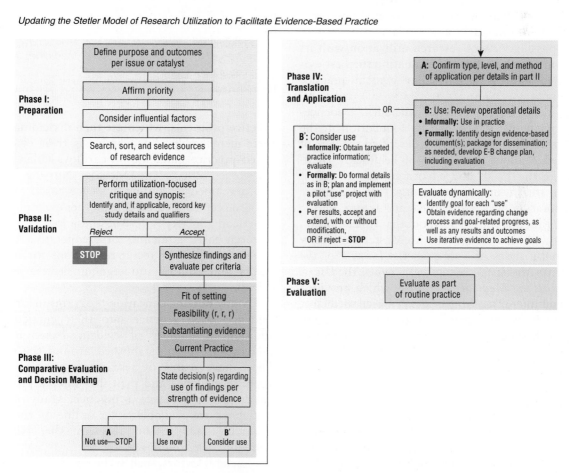

Figure 20-1   Stetler's Model. (From Stetler, C. B. (2001). Updating the Stetler Model of Research Utilization to facilitate evidence-based practice. *Nursing Outlook, 49,* 272-279, Figure 3A, p. 276.)

model focuses heavily on the change process to facilitate the successful translation of research findings into practice.

EVIDENCE-BASED PRACTICE

Evidence-based practice is the integration of the best research evidence with clinical expertise and the patient's unique values and circumstances in making decisions about the care of individual patients (Straus, Richardson, Glasziou, & Haynes, 2005, p. 1). Evidence-based nursing practice is "the conscientious, explicit, and judicious use of theory-derived, research-based information on making decisions about care delivery to individuals or groups of patients and in consideration of individual needs and preferences" (Ingersoll, 2000, p. 151). In evidence-based practice, clinical problems drive the search for solutions based on the best available evidence that is then translated into practice. Evidence-based practice is a broader, more encompassing view of research utilization with its focus on searching for and evaluating the best evidence to address a particular clinical practice problem.

Evidence-based practice includes evidence-based medicine, which had its foundation in the work of Archie Cochrane. He described the lack of knowledge about the effects of healthcare treatments in the 1970s and advocated for the use of proven treatments. Subsequently, the Cochrane Collaboration was established at Oxford in the United Kingdom in 1993. About that time, Gordon Guyatt and his colleagues at McMaster University authored a series of articles in the *Journal of the American Medical Association* known as the *Users' Guides to the Medical Literature,* which provided a foundation for teaching evidence-based medicine. Since then, the evidence-based practice movement has grown exponentially with the establishment of centers, resources on the web, and grants given specifically to advance the translation of research into practice. Resources for evidence-based health care are listed in Box 20-1.

Various organizations have developed evidence-based standards of practice and clinical guidelines. Specialty associations have begun testing research-based interventions for use by their members. The Association of Women's Health Obstetrical and Neonatal Nurses (AWHONN) tests research-based

BOX 20-1

Resources for Evidence-Based Health Care

Agency for Healthcare Research and Quality (AHRQ): www.ahrq.gov/clinic/epcix.htm
Bandolier: www.ebandolier.com
The Cochrane Collaboration: www.cochrane.org
   Cochrane Database of Systematic Reviews (CDSR)
Center for Evidence-Based Medicine at University of Toronto: www.cebm.utoronto.ca
Centre for Reviews and Dissemination (CRD) www.york.ac.uk/inst/crd
   Database of Abstracts of Reviews of Effects (DARE)
   Health Technology Assessment Database (HTA)
   NHS Economic Evaluation Database (EED)
National Guideline Clearinghouse: www.guidelines.gov
National Institute for Health and Clinical Excellence in the United Kingdom: www.nice.org.uk
National Institute of Clinical Studies in Australia: www.nicsl.com.au
Oxford-Centre for Evidence-Based Medicine: www.cebm.net

practice protocols, which are then disseminated to their membership. An example is their evidence-based practice guideline on cardiovascular health for women (2003). The Oncology Nursing Society has developed an online evidence-based practice resource center (Box 20-2). Another example is the American Society of Anesthesiologists' (ASA) research-based guideline for preoperative fasting, which standardizes recommendations for healthy adults and children undergoing elective surgery (1999).

Many nursing education programs incorporate evidence-based practice into their curricula. In addition, a number of evidence-based nursing centers have been established around the world. These have teams of researchers who critically appraise evidence and then disseminate protocols for the use of evidence in practice. Many of these guidelines are available either online on the organization's website or through the *National Guideline Clearinghouse.*

Societal factors, such as the rising cost of health care, quality improvement initiatives, and the pressures to avoid errors, have resulted in an increased emphasis on research as a basis for practice decisions. Nurses and other healthcare professionals are increasingly called upon to use evidence in practice in the midst of an exponentially expanding scientific knowledge base. The Institute of Medicine calls for all healthcare professionals to be educated in evidence-based practice. Specifically, professionals should be able to (1) know where and how to find the best possible sources of evidence, (2) formulate clear clinical questions, (3) search for relevant answers to those questions from the best possible sources, including those that evaluate or appraise evidence for its usefulness with respect to a particular patient or population, and (4) determine when and how to integrate those findings into practice (Greiner & Knebel, 2003).

Nursing research exists on a continuum, and not all research is ready for, or of a quality that is appropriate for, implementation, or it may not be ready for implementation in a particular setting. However, the quality of care and the quality of the outcomes of care can be dramatically improved with the implementation of evidence-based nursing practices. Nurses are heeding the call to develop evidenced-based practices. Nurse leaders and managers have a critical responsibility in promoting the use of the best evidence for practice. Resources for evidence-based nursing are listed in Box 20-2.

Exercise 20-2

Select a clinical guideline that is appropriate for implementation in your clinical setting (See *National Guideline Clearinghouse [www.guideline.gov]* or the University of Iowa Gerontological Nursing Interventions Research Center, Research Dissemination Core *[www.nursing.uiowa.edu/centers/gnirc/protocols.htm]*). Identify as many strategies as possible for disseminating the key points in the guideline to staff nurses at your facility or a facility where you have your clinical experiences. Compare your list of strategies with that of a colleague.

BOX 20-2

Resources for Evidence-Based Nursing

Arizona State University College of Nursing Center for the Advancement of Evidence-Based Practice (CAEP): http://nursing.asu.edu/caep

Sarah Cole Hirsch Institute, Frances Payne Bolton School of Nursing, Case Western Reserve University: http://fpb.cwru.edu/HirshInstitute

Centre for Evidence Based Nursing at the University of York (UK): www.york.ac.uk/healthsciences/centres/evidence/cebn.htm

Gerontological Nursing Interventions Research Center: Research Dissemination Core, University of Iowa: www.nursing.uiowa.edu/centers/gnirc/

The Joanna Briggs Institute for Evidence-Based Nursing and Midwifery: www.joannabriggs.edu.au/about/home.php

Oncology Nursing Society: http://onsopcontent.ons.org/toolkits/ebp/index.htm

The Registered Nurses Association of Ontario Nursing Best Practices Guidelines: www.rnao.org/bestpractices/

University of Texas Health Science Center at San Antonio's Academic Center for Evidence-Based Nursing (ACE): www.acestar.uthscsa.edu/

DIFFUSION OF INNOVATIONS

The theory of diffusion of innovations (Rogers, 2003), describes how innovations spread through society. This theory, highlighted in the Theory Box, provides a useful model in planning for the integration of evidence into practice over time. According to Rogers, the diffusion of innovations occurs in stages: knowledge, persuasion, decision, implementation, and confirmation.

Theory Box

ROGERS' DIFFUSION OF INNOVATIONS THEORY (2003)

STAGE	KEY IDEA	ACTIVITIES
Knowledge	Exposure to an innovation and how it functions	The process includes seeking and analyzing information. Literature reviews are focused on addressing practice problems. Information can be disseminated through journals, conferences, educational programs, audiovisual or electronic media, journal clubs, and/or other outlets.
Persuasion	Development of attitudes about an innovation through psychological involvement and selective perception	Informal communication networks are used to facilitate change. Positive or negative attitudes can develop. An event or activity can be used to spark interest in moving from a favorable attitude to behavior change.
Decision	Commitment to adoption	The innovation can be adopted, adopted and then discontinued, rejected outright, or not even considered by the organization at this stage.
Implementation	Putting the innovation into practice	Change agents provide support for the implementation process. Behavior changes as the innovation is adopted. Key features of an innovation are identified in order to evaluate its effectiveness. Problems with implementing the innovation are addressed. Change and modification (reinvention) occur in order to use the innovation in a particular practice environment. Reinvention facilitates the sustainability of the innovation.
Confirmation	Evaluate the innovation	A decision is made about continuing or discontinuing the innovation. The innovation, if adopted, is integrated into the organization's practices.

Adapted from Rogers, E. (2003). *Diffusion of innovations* (5th ed., pp. 171-195). New York: Free Press.

An innovation might be continued because of the positive reinforcement received when there are favorable outcomes. An innovation also might be discontinued—for example, when a better idea is adopted or when disenchantment occurs due to dissatisfaction with the process or outcome.

An intervention's characteristics can influence its adoption. These include the relative advantage (whether it is better than what it replaces), compatibility (consistency with values, experiences, needs), complexity (difficulty in understanding its use), trialability (the degree to which it can be easily tested), and observability (the ease of seeing the results) (Rogers, 2003).

Rogers' (2003) diffusion of innovations theory provides a framework for determining how to best facilitate the adoption of an innovation. For example, widespread media attention to a particular finding can be instrumental in publicizing a research study. This is illustrated by the media publicity regarding the results of a study on the impact of family presence during emergency procedures and resuscitation (Meyers et al., 2000). When the study was first published, it was accompanied by press releases and publicized in television news stories.

Nurse researchers write clinical articles in addition to research articles. Many journals that are directed toward clinicians provide nurses with easy to understand summaries of studies from the general healthcare and nursing research literature. Nursing schools develop press releases when researchers publish studies that are then used by the media for their news articles. For example, research conducted by Lipman and her colleagues (2004) on the accuracy of height measurements in primary-care practices was described in the *New York Times*. Parents, as consumers, when reading the article were able to understand the importance of obtaining an accurate height measurement of their child in their healthcare provider's office. Sufficient information about the methodology for obtaining an accurate height was described so that parents would know whether the correct technique was used to measure their child's height.

▪ Exercise 20–3

Locate a research column in a clinical nursing journal. Identify one study that has implications for your practice. Retrieve the original article to learn more about the patient population, details of the study design, and results.

The translation of research into practice requires that nurse leaders and managers understand group dynamics, individual responses to innovation and change, and the culture of their healthcare organization. Rogers (2003) categorizes people according to how quickly they are willing to adopt an innovation. Box 20-3 describes these categories. Understanding the characteristics of innovation adopters is critical when planning to introduce new practices based on research evidence.

Nursing, as a profession, has an obligation to the public to condense the 17-year typical time frame from discovery to the adoption of a research finding. Those committed to the evidence-based practice movement in nursing have attempted to speed the adoption of innovations. Rogers' (2003) theory of diffusion of innovations is useful in helping us understand how research can be disseminated to the larger community and how to take advantage of organizational dynamics to accelerate the process.

The diffusion of an innovation does not necessarily follow a linear path. There are times when external factors may contribute to the adoption of an innovation. These may include the development of standards regarding the practice that are widely disseminated, cost-effectiveness studies, changes in the products or technology, the publication of clear and compelling evidence, and changes in staff members and leadership at an institution. This was illustrated with the Women's Health Initiative study demonstrating a higher rate of heart disease and breast cancer in women who had estrogen plus progestin therapy (Rossouw et al., 2002). Women learning about the study's findings rushed to their healthcare providers' offices and discontinued their use of estrogen replacement therapy.

A well-known example of an innovation in nursing is that of the use of a weak heparin solution to flush capped angiocatheters. Although the use of heparin or saline had been debated for many years, in 1991 a meta-analysis published in *Nursing Research* provided compelling evidence for the use of saline and the elimination of the low-dose heparin flush for capped angiocatheters (Goode et al., 1991). A meta-analysis statistically combines similar studies investigating a particular issue to determine whether the findings are significant across settings and multiple studies. The accompanying editorial declared that it was time to "remove this outmoded, expensive and potentially harmful

BOX 20-3

Characteristics of Innovation Adopters

TYPE	CHARACTERISTICS
Innovators	Active in seeking new information. Organization's visionaries.
Early adopters	Organization's opinion leaders who learn about an innovation and apply it to their practice. Can be effective in communicating the value of an innovation.
Early majority	Will not bring forth an innovation, but will readily adopt it when brought forth by others.
Late majority	Skeptics who do not adopt something unless there is pressure. Feel safe when there is limited uncertainty.
Laggards	Most secure in holding on to the past. Most comfortable when an idea cannot fail.

From Rogers, E. (2003). *Diffusion of innovations* (5th ed.). New York: Free Press.

procedure from clinical practice" (Downs, 1991, p. 323). Although a number of institutions continued to use heparin flushes for a number of years, its use became less common and all but disappeared in the late 1990s. This was considerably later than one would expect, given the compelling nature of the evidence. This example illustrates the particular challenges in implementing an evidence-based practice when more than one discipline is involved. Not only did the innovation need to be communicated to nurses, but also nurses needed to convince physicians and the institutional hierarchy that using heparin was no longer appropriate. For some institutions, it was not until the costs were analyzed and concerns were raised about complications from small doses of heparin that the transition to saline flushes was finally accomplished.

Another example of innovation diffusion is the evidence-based protocol for intramuscular injections developed by Nicoll and Hesby (2002). The extent to which this guideline is used by nurses and nurse educators is not known. The guideline is an excellent basis for the administration of intramuscular injections. The practice of administering intramuscular injections for pain management in adults in acute care settings has virtually disappeared with the use of the intravenous and epidural routes for analgesic administration. However, intramuscular injections are still widely used in many settings throughout the world to deliver certain long-acting antibiotics; biologicals such as immune globulins, vaccines, and toxoids; and hormonal agents. Nicoll and Hesby emphasize that the first decision to be made by the nurse is whether the intramuscular route is appropriate. The protocol is important because it establishes an evidence-based standard of practice. This is particularly significant because of wide variation among nurses in their technique and anecdotal reports of organizations providing only subcutaneous needles for nurses to administer influenza vaccinations when the product literature states the intramuscular route is required.

Fetzer's (2002) metaanalysis of 20 studies demonstrated that the pain of venipuncture and intravenous line insertion could be reduced in 85% of the population (adults and children), with the use of eutectic mixture of local anesthetics (EMLA) cream. But, today this practice has not been widely adopted, particularly with adults. A stumbling block described by practitioners is the length of time required for the EMLA to take effect. This is indicative of the relative value placed on patient comfort and patient satisfaction and the challenge in changing pain management practices because starting an intravenous line or performing a venipuncture is not always done during emergency circumstances.

More recently, Madsen and colleagues (2005) questioned the practice of listening to the bowel sounds of abdominal surgery patients in order to assess the return of gastrointestinal motility. They concluded that the presence or absence of bowel sounds was not associated with any interventions. The authors recommend that problems experienced by abdominal surgery patients indicative of the absence of bowel motility (e.g., nausea, abdominal distention) can be treated with specific interventions such as the administration of an antiemetic or the insertion of a nasogastric tube. A practice guideline was developed and evaluated by the research team outlining the steps in gastrointestinal assessment. Astute practitioners should observe for the subsequent adoption of these guidelines by nurses in other healthcare facilities and whether textbooks continue to mention the assessment of bowel sounds for postoperative abdominal surgery patients.

TRANSLATION OF RESEARCH INTO PRACTICE (TRIP)

The science of how research is adopted is known as translation science, the science of translating research into practice (TRIP). Translation research involves scientifically investigating the methods and variables that affect adoption of evidence-based healthcare practices by individual practitioners and healthcare systems to improve clinical and operational decision-making and includes testing the effects of strategies to promote and sustain evidence-based practices (Titler, 2004).

Research takes a very long time to be translated into practice. This is illustrated by the classic example of scurvy. Lancaster demonstrated that lemon juice supplements eliminated scurvy in sailors in 1601, and Lind replicated that finding in 1747. However, it was not until 1795 that the British navy added a citrus-juice supplement to the diet of its sailors (Brown, 2003, p. 228). In nursing, we have medication tickets or small cards that were first used in 1910 to facilitate the administration of medications. Nearly 100 years later, some institutions are still using these tickets as reminders for some aspects of their medication- and/or treatment-administration systems despite evidence of the potential for error through their loss or duplication. This issue is indicative of a much broader problem related to the limited use of electronic health records. According to Geibert (2006, p. 132), "technology is the bridge to integrating EBP [evidence-based practice] into patient care."

Although the interest in research utilization in nursing paralleled the development of nursing as a research-based discipline, the actual translation of research into practice has not been as rapid. Nurses have chronicled the difficulties in using research. Funk, Champagne, Wiese, & Tornquist (1991) developed an instrument, *Barriers to Research Utilization*. They categorized nurses' responses (N = 1989) regarding barriers to research utilization according to the research itself, the nurse, the setting or organization, and how the research is presented. The most important factor was perceived to be organizational support, particularly the provision of time to use and conduct research. Retsas (2000) found that barriers to using research in Australia included access to research, anticipated outcomes of research use, organizational support, and support from others. Estabrooks (1999) examined the conceptual structure of research utilization indicating that there are direct, indirect, and persuasive aspects of research utilization. An example of direct research utilization consists of actually using recommended interventions to prevent ventilator-associated pneumonia. An indirect research utilization example would be when a nurse has greater understanding of a person's response to diabetic teaching because of reading a research report. An example of persuasive research utilization is when nurses work to implement an institutional change in practice such as using pH paper to test nasogastric tube placement. Estabrooks (1999) suggests that different strategies are needed to achieve different types of research utilization and that researchers need to approach the study of how research is adopted more systematically.

When planning an initiative to translate a research finding into practice, it is important to know what types of strategies have been most successful. Not only that, it is also helpful to know how much time-commitment was involved (the dose), how often the strategy was used (frequency), how long the treatment lasted (length of the prescription), and whether the results lasted (sustainability). Therefore, the next frontier is testing the effectiveness of specific interventions within an organizational context and evaluating adherence to the evidence-based practice. For example, although there may be good results from a particular protocol used in a randomized controlled trial to decrease ventilator-associated pneumonia, those same results might not be as dramatic when the protocol is implemented at institutions with varying resources and degrees of commitment to implementing the protocol on a regular basis. Therefore, it would be important to know what kinds of strategies are the most effective for translating research into practice. The American Pain Society published a quality assurance standard for pain management in 1995. However, there are still many challenges faced by nurse managers and pain-management clinical specialists as they attempt improve the assessment and management of pain (Stenger, Schooley, & Moss, 2001).

Nurses need to not only pay careful attention to the development of a clinical protocol or an evidence-based guideline, but also address the implementation process. For example, in a study implementing pilot interventions related to lipid management for coronary heart disease patients, barriers to successful implementation were found to be related primarily to the intervention process and secondarily to the characteristics of the intervention itself (Sharp, Pineros, Hsu, Starks, & Sales, 2004). In this instance, the intervention involved discussions of the guidelines and involving the clinicians in selecting the strategies to facilitate their implementation. The results indicated that more effort needed to be put into the initial planning and actual implementation of the intervention.

Some research has been done on the effectiveness of various strategies in facilitating the use of research. Dobbins, Ciliska, Estabrooks, and Hayward (2005) evaluated the strength of the research evidence for various strategies that promote behavioral change among health professionals. Consistently effective strategies included academic detailing or educational outreach visits (providing healthcare providers with accurate information in face-to-face visits), reminders, multi-faceted interventions, and interactive education meetings and workshops. Strategies having mixed effects included

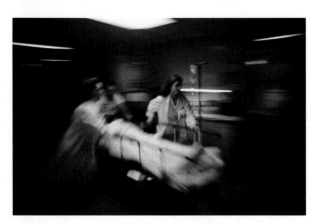

The purpose of gathering and analyzing evidence is to improve care.

audit and feedback, local opinion leaders, local consensus processes, and patient-mediated interventions. Strategies having little or no effect included the distribution of educational materials and didactic educational programs. The key point here is that active involvement leads to greater success.

According to Ferlie and Shortell (2001), the translation of research into practice operates at four levels: the individual healthcare professional, healthcare groups or teams, organizations, and the larger healthcare system or environment in which individual organizations are embedded. They go on to describe strategies for change that are appropriate at each level, such as protocol and guideline development at the individual and team level, knowledge management at the organizational level, and the establishment of evidence-based practice centers at the systems level. This implies a multifaceted approach to disseminating evidence-based practices and the responsibility to the larger healthcare community in fostering evidence-based practice. Various funding agencies are now supporting TRIP projects designed to evaluate the effectiveness of strategies to implement research findings because of the societal need to implement scientific findings in a timely manner. TRIP science has the potential to speed up the adoption of innovations and sustain their use over time.

For research to be translated into practice, it needs to reach the nurse, nurse leaders, nurse man-

agers, and administrators in an institution, as well as policymakers who can provide the infrastructure and support necessary for the implementation of research results. Changing widespread practices can be very challenging. For example, Brooten and her colleagues (2002) have consistently demonstrated that interventions by advanced practice nurses have improved patient outcomes and reduced healthcare costs for very low birth-weight (VLBW) infants; women with unplanned cesarean births, high-risk pregnancies, and hysterectomy surgery; and elders with cardiac medical and surgical diagnoses. But, this research was being conducted and disseminated during the same time period that hospitals were eliminating clinical nurse specialist positions! However, the public and government agencies will increasingly expect that research findings are implemented, particularly when there are significant improvements in patient outcomes and cost-savings.

Evidence-based nursing involves a fundamental shift in philosophy. Rather than relying on nurses, be they clinicians, managers, or administrators, to read the research and apply it to practice, we are now called upon to analyze practice problems and identify the research that will help us to answer questions about how we should go about delivering care. Translation science takes evidence-based practice a step further in accountability for using evidence-based strategies to implement scientifically based practices.

EVALUATING EVIDENCE

Evidence is best evaluated with a systematic process. The steps of evidence-based practice are illustrated in Box 20-4.

The first step in the implementation of evidence-based practice is identifying the problem so that the relevant information can be obtained. Melnyk and Fineout-Overholt (2005) recommend putting the clinical question into the widely used *PICO* format of *patient, intervention, comparison, and outcome* to facilitate searching for the appropriate evidence. This format is illustrated in Box 20-5.

Identifying the question may be the most challenging part of the process. Different strategies can be used to identify practice problems. For example, one might wish to conduct a survey of staff members or use a focus group methodology. However, conducting a staff survey would necessitate that staff members have sufficient knowledge of research and evidence-based practice to understand what is desired. The data from surveys or focus groups, or even informal interviews with staff, can be examined along with patient outcome data for a particular setting in order to address relevant practice problems. Collaborating with nurses and extending that to interdisciplinary collaboration to identify desired outcomes will enhance the ultimate success of an evidence-based project. This is because the staff members who will eventually be involved in implementing the practice are involved in its design

and conception. Once the clinical question has been identified, writing it down will help in moving on to the next step of gathering evidence.

Exercise 20–4

Develop a clinical question using the PICO (patient, intervention [interest], comparison, and outcome) format. Do a search in *PubMed* with the key PICO terms.

The second step of the process is searching for evidence. A number of databases is available for searching for evidence. Some databases contain preprocessed evidence, such as abstracts of studies and systematic reviews of evidence. Other databases contain citations for original single studies. Commonly used databases are listed in Box 20-6. In this instance, it is helpful to obtain the assistance of a librarian to navigate the databases. This is important because databases are constantly being upgraded with the addition of new features that facilitate the search process. Several of the suggested readings include more detailed information on locating research evidence. Preprocessed evidence can also be located in the evidence-based resources listed in Boxes 20-1 and 20-2.

The evidence for a particular practice problem can come from a single research study, an integrative review of the literature, a meta-analysis, a meta-synthesis, a clinically-appraised topic, a clinical guideline, or a systematic review. Sometimes a single research study might be very appropriate for application to a particular problem. For other clinical questions, there might be multiple guidelines from different organizations on essentially the

BOX 20-4

Steps of Evidence-Based Practice

1. Asking the relevant clinical question.
2. Searching for the best evidence.
3. Appraising the evidence critically.
4. Integrating evidence with clinical expertise, patient preferences, and values in making a practice decision or change.
5. Evaluating the practice decision or change.

From Melnyk, B. M., & Fineout-Overholt, E. (2005). Making the case for evidence-based practice. In Melynk, B. M,. & Fineout-Overholt E. (Eds.), *Evidence-based practice in nursing and health care.* (p. 9). Philadelphia: Lippincott, Williams & Wilkins.

BOX 20-5

Asking the Right Question: The PICO Format

Patient population	What is the patient population or the setting? This could be adults, children or neonates with a certain health problem, or home care versus an acute care setting.
Intervention/**I**nterest Area	What is the intervention? This can be an intervention or a specific area of interest (e.g., postoperative complications, the experience of postoperative pain).
Comparison	What is a comparison intervention? This is what the intervention might be compared with, such as a treatment, or the absence of a risk factor.
Outcome	What are the results? There might be multiple strategies to measure the results, such as complication rate, satisfaction, a nursing diagnosis, or a nursing quality indicator.

BOX 20-6

Commonly Used Databases for Nursing

CINAHL: Cumulative Index to Nursing and Allied Health Literature www.cinahl.com www.epnet.com	An abstract database that also includes some full-text material such as state nursing journals, nurse practice acts, research instruments, government publications, and patient education material from 1982 to the present. By institutional or personal subscription.
EMBASE www.embase.com	Biomedical and pharmaceutical studies. By institutional subscription.
OVID www.ovid.com	A search process for a variety of databases including Medline in the OVID platform. By institutional subscription and individual pay per view.
PsychINFO www.apa.org/psycinfo/	Abstract database of the behavioral sciences and mental health literature from the 1800s to the present. By institutional subscription or individual article purchase.
PubMed www.ncbi.nlm.nih.gov/entrez	The abstract database of the National Library of Medicine providing access to over 15 million citations from the 1950s to the present. Links to publishers' websites for many articles. Free.

same clinical problem with slightly different recommendations. DiCenso, Ciliska, and Guyatt (2005) describe a hierarchy for rating the strength of evidence for treatment decisions: (1) unsystematic clinical observations, (2) physiologic studies (e.g., blood pressure, bone density), (3) single observational study addressing important patient outcomes, (4) systematic review of observational studies addressing important patient outcomes, (5) randomized trial, and (6) systematic review of randomized trials. A hierarchy of pre-processed evidence (that is, evidence from a single research study to research analyzed by evidence-based practice groups such as the Cochrane Collaboration or the Joanna Briggs Institute) originally developed by Haynes (2001) and adapted by Collins, Voth, DiCenso, and Guyatt (2005) is illustrated in Figure 20-2. The AHRQ has identified 19 different rating systems for evidence that include key quality domains (2002). It is clear that this is a rapidly growing field and that there is no single-established method of rating evidence that is best for every situation. Ultimately, whoever conducts the analysis, be it an individual or a team, will have to make some decisions about the strength of the evidence and its applicability to the particular patient population. What is important is that once the evidence has been located, an appropriate and systematic

method for rating or appraising the evidence is used. This rating system should include an analysis of whether the evidence can be applied to a particular clinical situation.

Appraisal tools exist for evaluating different types of evidence from a single qualitative study, qualitative meta-syntheses, descriptive studies, and randomized clinical trials to systematic reviews. The suggested readings provide examples. These appraisal tools generally include a series of steps for evaluating the quality of the research that is specific to the study design, type of review or guideline, or strategy for determining the applicability of the evidence to one's practice. The *AGREE Collaboration* provides a tool specifically for evaluating clinical guidelines (www.agreecollaboration.org). Key elements of such appraisal tools include an assessment of the reliability and validity of the evidence.

Much of the evidence-based practice literature has been devoted to evaluating randomized clinical trials. A **randomized controlled trial (RCT)** includes at least two groups and the random assignment of study participants to one group or another either by a coin toss or some other strategy to test a treatment's effectiveness. Generally, it is preferable that such studies are double-blinded, meaning that the participants and those who are evaluating the

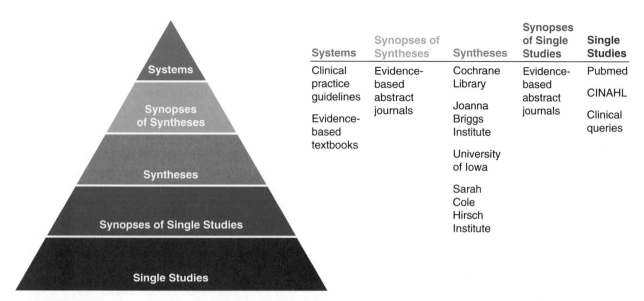

Figure 20-2   Hierarchy of Preprocessed Evidence. (Adapted from Collins, S., Voth, T., DiCenso, A., & Guyatt, G. [2005]. Finding the evidence. In A. DiCenso, G. Guyatt, & D. Ciliska [Eds.], *Evidence-based nursing: A guide to clinical practice* [pp. 20-43]. St. Louis: Elsevier.)

outcomes do not know who has received the treatment. Although this design is generally considered the gold standard in terms of ranking individual studies, the number of RCTs conducted in nursing has been limited. Also, in certain clinical trials, blinding the recipients to a nursing intervention may be difficult to accomplish effectively. Aside from that, an RCT is not always an appropriate design for answering a particular research question. Hence, it is important that the appraisal method examine the rigor or the quality of the research in accordance with standards for that type of study.

Once the evidence has been appraised, this information needs to be integrated with clinical expertise, and the preferences and values of patients, families, and communities in making the change. For example, in evaluating a research-based protocol for teaching oncology patients about preparing for a bone marrow transplant, consideration needs to be given to the amount and type of information that would be desired by the patient. In this instance, a qualitative research study might provide guidance for decision-making. For certain types of interventions, the inclusion of patient preferences might not be appropriate, as in the example of implementing a protocol for the reduction of ventilator-associated pneumonia. Determining patient preferences is dependent on the nature of the intervention or change that is proposed.

The sheer quantity and complexity of information available indicates that nurses in direct practice need to collaborate with researchers. Nurses bring their clinical expertise, their assessment of clinically relevant questions and their understanding of the patient population. Researchers bring their capacity to appraise evidence critically to facilitate its application to the clinical setting. Together, nurses and researchers can forge a partnership in the development of an evidence-based solution to a clinical practice problem.

ORGANIZATIONAL STRATEGIES

The partnership between nurses and researchers needs to be extended to top leaders and stakeholders within an organization. To implement evidence-based practices, an organization needs to be committed to the process. The key points are that staff and management need to partner with researchers to identify the appropriate evidence and to present it to key decision-makers within the organization in a usable format. For example, in deciding whether it is best for nurses to administer pre-procedure sedation, or for parents to administer sedatives to children prior to their arrival in a department for a procedure, one needs to consider the evidence, the safety of the procedure, and the risks of unmonitored or parent-administered sedation. Providing key organizational decision-makers with evidence regarding the safety of such a practice would be critical in reaching a decision.

Nurse leaders and managers need to understand the organizational context for implementing research evidence. Lomas (2004) identifies the specific tasks that need to be accomplished: (1) under-standing the research and the decision-making environment, (2) ability to find and assess relevant research, (3) mediation and negotiation skills, (4) communication skills, and (5) credibility. He recommends that healthcare organizations place themselves on the mailing lists for key alerts from agencies concerned with healthcare quality improvement, such as the AHRQ, distribute easy-to-read summaries to key decision-makers, and have researchers brief senior management and board members directly.

The Registered Nurses Association of Ontario (2002) developed a very comprehensive toolkit to assist nurses in maximizing their guideline-implementation efforts. The toolkit recommends

---

BOX 20-7

Implementation of Clinical Practice Guidelines (CPG): Environmental Readiness Assessment Worksheet

ELEMENT	QUESTION	FACILITATORS	BARRIERS
Structure	To what extent does decision-making occur in a decentralized manner? Is there enough staff to support the change process?		
Workplace culture	To what extent is the CPG consistent with the values, attitudes and beliefs of the practice environment? To what degree does the culture support change and value evidence?		
Communication	Are there adequate (formal and informal) communication systems to support information exchange relative to the CPG and the CPG implementation processes?		
Leadership	To what extent do the leaders within the practice environment support (both visibly and behind the scenes) the implementation of the CPG?		
Knowledge, skills, and attitudes of target group	Does the staff have the necessary knowledge and skills? Which potential target group is open to change and new ideas? To what extent are they motivated to implement the CPG?		
Commitment to quality management	Do quality improvement processes and systems exist to measure results of implementation?		
Availability of resources	Are the necessary human, physical, and financial resources available to support implementation?		
Interdisciplinary relationships	Are there positive relationships and trust between the disciplines that will be involved or affected by the CPG?		

Reprinted with permission from Registered Nurses Association of Ontario. (2002). *Toolkit: Implementation of clinical practice guidelines*. Toronto, Canada: Author. Available online at www.rnao.org/bestpractices.

strategies for working with key stakeholders and particularly stresses their early involvement because of their understanding of the extent of the problem, unmet needs, and motivation required to address the problem (p. 18). An environmental assessment included in the toolkit appears in Box 20-7. Stetler (2003) emphasizes that to sustain evidence-based practice in an organization, the leadership needs to support a research culture, the organization needs the capacity to engage in evidence-based practice, and an infrastructure needs to be created to facilitate evidence-based practice. The latter includes the integration of a research focus into documents, creation of expectations and roles, recognition, and technical support.

Exercise 20-5

Use the environmental readiness assessment in Box 20-7 to assess the capacity of your agency to implement an evidence-based guideline. Identify one strategy to address a specific barrier to implementation.

The Magnet™ Recognition Program developed by the American Nurses Credentialing Center (ANCC) to recognize excellence in nursing services includes an expectation related to the support of research and its integration into the delivery of nursing care and nursing administration (ANCC, 2005). In addition, research-based practices can be used to demonstrate how an institution meets a number of the other Magnet criteria (Messmer, Jones, & Rosillo, 2002). As more hospitals seek Magnet designation, greater emphasis will be placed on the integration of research with the delivery of nursing care. Accordingly, Magnet designation requires persistent development of evidence-based practices in the delivery of nursing services (Steinbinder & Scherer, 2006).

The adoption of evidence-based practices ultimately depends on a complex interaction of individual and organizational factors. Individual determinants of research utilization are related to (1) beliefs and attitudes, (2) involvement in research activities, (3) information seeking, (4) professional characteristics, (5) education, and (6) other socioeconomic factors (Estabrooks, Floyd, Scott-Findlay, O'Leary, & Gushta, 2003). Organizational determinants influencing the adoption of innovation have generally not been studied in nursing. However, outside of nursing, factors associated with the adoption of innovation include larger organizational size, presence of a research champion, less traditionalism, and uncommitted organizational resources. Factors inhibiting research adoption include lack of time, centralization, and access to research and resources (Estabrooks, 2003). Research utilization also depends on professional autonomy and support from peers, nursing administration, and other healthcare professionals (Estabrooks, 2003). Nurse managers and administrators increasingly will be called upon to provide support to individual nurses, to implement strategies to enhance individuals' use of evidence, and to participate in creating an organizational infrastructure that promotes evidence-based practice.

ISSUES FOR NURSE LEADERS AND MANAGERS

Some of the issues faced by nurse leaders and managers include a lack of resources, limited expertise of staff members with respect to evidence-based practice, lack of knowledge about nursing research, and limited time for advance planning. Not all organizations can hire a full-time nurse researcher. Some organizations may not employ clinical nurse specialists. One could argue that this is shortsighted in view of the potential benefits of improved patient outcomes and cost-savings due to a reduction in adverse outcomes. However, this resource limitation is a reality faced in many organizations. Regardless, it is important to remember that using the best available evidence can be most successful in a partnership model. Therefore, working with nurse researchers at a local college or university could be very valuable. An example of a partnership between second-degree nursing students and clinicians facilitated by Patricia Stone at Columbia University is illustrated in Box 20-8. Faculty can partner with staff in a facility to provide consultation for a specific patient-care problem. Agencies can partner together to address a specific practice problem.

Another issue is that many nurses might not have had research and/or statistics courses in their basic nursing education, or they had it many years before and have not used their research knowledge since then. Even if they did have a course, nurses, nurse managers, and administrators might not be familiar with how to appraise evidence critically for use in practice. Nurses on a clinical unit might not be familiar with reading research or with using

BOX 20-8

Collaboration in Developing an Evidence-Based Protocol for Kangaroo Care

CLINICIAN PERSPECTIVE

We discovered there was interest in, but not common practice of, kangaroo care for premature babies. Many of the staff members in our facilities have a wealth of clinical experience. But, they really did not have the chance to learn about evidence-based practice in school. The students came to us to talk about our needs. When they finished their work, they presented their findings about the evidence for kangaroo care and thermoregulation at our regional perinatal center nursing leadership retreat. Initially, they were intimidated about presenting to a group of such experienced nurses. However, it was rewarding to see them become more confident about their work.

Since the student presentation, we have had an upsurge of interest in providing kangaroo care. It has helped us in overcoming resistance to its use. We are now working on how to most effectively implement kangaroo care because it takes concerted work and staff time to teach and prepare the parents. One of our hospitals is using the poster developed by the students as a training tool. I enjoyed working with the students in a way that produced a tangible outcome for everyone involved. Learning how to conduct research for evidence-based practice gave the students a skill that they will have as new nurses and can offer as a complement to their more experienced nursing colleagues as they begin their professional careers.

Sally Girvin, MPH, BS, RN, NP
Coordinator, New York Presbyterian Regional Perinatal Centers New York, NY

STUDENT PERSPECTIVE

The eight of us who worked on this project were in the middle of our accelerated nursing program when it was assigned to us. We had to come up with an answerable clinical question, but due to our lack of clinical experience, we had only a vague idea of what to ask. We were able to develop our question after we talked with Sally and listened to her needs. We had spent some time in the neonatal intensive care unit and realized how hard it would be for the already busy nurses to take on this project. As students, we had the time.

When we went to the retreat to present our project, we thought no one would be interested in what we had done, that it might not be applicable, or that we had discovered something they already knew. The response was incredible. Our presentation created open debate. Some hospitals had kangaroo-care policies, some did not, some had them and did not follow them, and some people were unsure what they had in place. It really prompted people to look at their practices. It was a great experience to work with Sally and her colleagues and to see that what we did had an influence on policy. It was an experience that we can take with us wherever we go.

Elizabeth K. Kelly, BS, RN
Student at Columbia University School of Nursing, New York, NY, when this project was developed.

advanced search strategies to locate the evidence for a particular practice problem. This might be especially true for nurses who have been out of school for a long time and have not had the opportunity to develop computer literacy skills in searching for research evidence. Information on evidence-based nursing as an approach has only recently been incorporated into nursing research textbooks. Therefore, a first step in developing the

capacity to evaluate evidence for practice can be facilitated by starting a journal club that meets once a month. This involves reading a relevant research article and discussing how it might be applied to the practice situation. Although there are a number of general and specialty nursing research journals, *Evidence-Based Nursing* and *Worldviews on Evidence-Based Nursing* are specifically devoted to evidence-based nursing practice. The latter

BOX 20-9

Strategies for Implementing Evidence-Based Practices

1. Talk with colleagues to identify challenges in providing care.
2. Ask questions about agency practices.
3. Ask about the research evidence underlying agency practices.
4. Identify clinical practice problems.
5. Join a professional and a specialty association to have ready access to the latest news, research, and standards.
6. Subscribe to journals that have synopses of clinical research evidence.
7. Sign up for alerts from key agencies for research and patient outcome news.
8. Start a journal club for discussion of research articles.
9. Incorporate research into the revision of procedures and agency guidelines as they come up for review.
10. Search for and use existing guidelines for practice problems if possible.
11. Incorporate the use of evidence into performance and evaluation processes.
12. Identify key stakeholders.
13. Involve as many people as possible in the process of developing an evidence-based practice.
14. Put as much time into the planning for implementation as evaluating and developing the evidence-based protocol.
15. Evaluate the results to see if the practice continues to be used and what needs to be improved.
16. Partner with researchers at local colleges and universities.
17. Partner with faculty and nursing students to gather evidence.
18. Publicize nursing research to nurses, healthcare professionals, and the public.
19. Publicize your successes.

includes the archives of the *Online Journal of Knowledge Synthesis in Nursing.* The resulting discussion at a journal club can be used as a springboard for the identification of clinical practice problems. Even small hospitals have libraries and perhaps a part-time librarian who can assist with gathering information and identifying useful articles for the journal club's agenda.

Nurses, other healthcare professionals, and the public might not be very familiar with nursing research or evidence-based nursing. Therefore, it is important to publicize key nursing research findings. When nursing research is publicized in the media or through news alerts, be sure to communicate these findings to key decision-makers within the organization. Sending e-mails, posting articles, and providing people with the resources helps others learn for themselves. Research has a much better chance of being implemented if key persons have the opportunity to see its relevance. Multiple strategies are needed to implement research findings, and multiple strategies are needed to change a culture to one that is driven by research and evidence-based standards for practice. Suggested strategies are listed in Box 20-9. Finally, if one should have the opportunity to implement an evidence-based practice, as much consideration needs to be given to planning for implementation as protocol development (see Chapter 16). Advance planning should include a thorough and frank discussion of the barriers and facilitators as well as how to minimize the barriers and maximize the facilitators. In addition, consideration needs to be given to strategies to sustain the adoption of the practice over time. Although the implementation of evidence-based practice is a very complex process, the increased emphasis on the use of scientifically based evidence creates an exciting opportunity for nurses to demonstrate the value of nursing in improving patient care and healthcare outcomes.

The Solution

I began by working with a team that included a fellow staff nurse, a nurse researcher, and a nurse practitioner. We reviewed the literature and found that there was a lack of clarity in the guidelines for selecting an appropriate-size endotracheal tube for extremely low birth-weight infants. We also decided to do a retrospective chart audit to determine what, if any, were the effects of size variations of the endotracheal tube and the depth of endotracheal tube placement on oxygen saturation and carbon dioxide levels on intubation. We used guidelines from the Neonatal Resuscitation Program (NRP).

Conducting research is not without its challenges. I have not had a lot of experience with data collection. It was also very hard to get the time to do the study. However, we really wanted to carry out this project.

Sometimes, we would take our laptop on transport with us and do data entry during the "dead leg" (on the way to get the patient), as well as during our down times between transports. We shared the results with the staff at our hospital and with our community partners. Subsequently, we made large charts to be used by everyone who would be involved in neonatal resuscitation. We had a very positive response. I believe that the work we did was really important in improving the quality of care provided by the staff of our transport team and our outlying community hospitals for these tiny, fragile babies.

— Holly Olsen

 Would this be a suitable approach for you? Why?

CHAPTER CHECKLIST

Society increasingly demands that health care be based on the best available evidence. Nurses have a societal obligation to use practices that are based on sound scientific evidence. The length of time from scientific discovery or publication of research to implementation in practice is lengthy and needs to be shortened. Nurses can speed this process by using scientifically based strategies to facilitate the translation of research into practice. The nurse manager needs to understand the organizational context for the implementation of evidence-based protocols. Multiple strategies need to be developed to enhance the use of evidence as the foundation for nursing-care delivery.

- Research is an integral part of professional nursing practice and part of every nurse's obligation under the *Code of Ethics for Nurses* (2001).
- Research utilization is critical to an organization.
  - Synthesis, dissemination, and use of research are three distinct efforts.
  - Nurse researchers have a long history of developing demonstration projects to enhance research utilization.
  - A number of research utilization models have been developed in nursing.

- The Stetler Model (2001) incorporates elements of evidence-based practice and focuses heavily on the change process to facilitate translation of research into practice. The model's steps include preparation, validation, evaluation/decision-making, translation/application, and evaluation.
- Evidence-based nursing practice is the driving force in today's healthcare approaches.
  - Research-based information is used to make decisions.
  - Patient needs and preferences need to be considered.
  - Evidence-based practice is broader in scope in that it involves appraising the evidence to address a specific clinical practice problem whereas research utilization involves applying the findings from a particular study in practice.
- Rogers' *Diffusion of Innovations Theory* (2003) is a useful framework for understanding how innovations are diffused throughout an organization. The phases of the innovation adoption process include knowledge, persuasion, decision, implementation, and evaluation.
- According to Rogers (2003), innovation adopters can be classified in the following categories: innovators early adopters, early majority, late majority, and laggards.

- The science of how research is adopted is the science of translating research into practice (TRIP). Once an evidence-based protocol has been developed, research-based methods need to be used to enhance its implementation and sustain its adoption over time.
- Evaluating research evidence should be done in a systematic manner:
  - Asking the relevant clinical question
  - Searching for the evidence
  - Appraising the evidence
  - Integrating the evidence with clinical expertise, patient, family and community preferences, and values
  - Evaluating the outcomes
- Developing a relevant clinical question is enhanced by using the PICO format:
  - Patient population
  - Intervention/interest
  - Comparison
  - Outcome
- An organizational assessment of the capacity for evidence-based practice will facilitate the translation of research into practice. An organization assessment includes:
  - Access to resources for evidence
  - Capacity to appraise evidence
  - Adaptability in providing key leaders with summarized evidence
  - Capacity to demonstrate applicability of the evidence to key leaders
- Skills required for translating research into practice include:
  - Understanding the research and decision-making environment
  - Ability to find and assess relevant research
  - Mediation and negotiation skills
  - Communication skills
  - Credibility
- Strategies to enhance individuals' abilities in using evidence, support for individual nurses' efforts to use research, as well the establishment of an organizational infrastructure will promote the use of evidence-based practices.

TIPS FOR DEVELOPING SKILL IN USING EVIDENCE

- Make a personal commitment to read research articles.
- Obtain assistance from researchers, advanced practice nurses, and nurse leaders.
- Complete an online tutorial in evidence-based practice.
- Use your clinical experiences to develop relevant clinical questions.
- Encourage your colleagues to join you in learning about evidence-based practice.

TERMS TO KNOW

clinical guidelines
diffusion of innovation
evidence-based practice (EBP)
meta-analysis
outcomes
randomized clinical/controlled trial (RCT)
research
research utilization

REFERENCES

Agency for Healthcare Research and Quality (AHRQ). (2002). *Systems to rate the strength of scientific evidence. Evidence report/technology assessment No. 47* (AHRQ Publication #02-E016). Retrieved April 15, 2006, from www.ahrq.gov/clinic/epcsums/strengthsum.htm.

The AGREE Collaboration. (2001). *Appraisal of Guidelines for Research & Evaluation (AGREE) Instrument.* Retrieved July 24, 2006, from www.agreecollaboration.org

American Nurses Association (ANA). (2003). *Nursing's social policy statement.* Washington, DC: Author.

American Nurses Association (ANA). (2001). *Code of ethics for nurses with interpretive statements.* Washington, DC: Author.

American Nurses Credentialing Center. (2005). *What is magnet?* Silver Spring, MD: Author. Retrieved April 15, 2006, from www.ana.org/ancc/magnet/consumer/whatis4.html.

American Society of Anesthesiologists Task Force on Preoperative Fasting and the Use of Pharmacologic Agents to Reduce the Risk of Pulmonary Aspiration.

(1999). *Practice guidelines for preoperative fasting and the use of pharmacologic agents to reduce the risk of pulmonary aspiration: Application to healthy patients undergoing elective procedures.* Park Ridge, IL: Author. Retrieved April 15, 2006, from www.asahq.org/publicationsAndServices/npoguide.html.

Association of Women's Health, Obstetrical and Neonatal Nurses. (2003). *Evidence-based clinical practice guidelines. Cardiovascular health for women: Primary prevention.* Washington, DC: Author.

Balas, E., & Boren, S. (2000). Managing clinical knowledge for health care improvement. In J. vanBemmel & A. McCray (Eds.). *Yearbook of medical informatics 2000—Patient-centered systems* (pp. 65–70). Stuttgart, Germany: Schattauer.

Brooten, D., Naylor, M. D., York, R., Brown, L. P., Munro, B. H., Hollingsworth, A. O., et al. (2002). Lessons learned from testing the quality cost model of Advanced Practice Nursing (APN) transitional care. *Journal of Nursing Scholarship, 34,* 369–375.

Brown, A. (2003). *Scurvy.* New York: St. Martin's Press.

Burns, N., & Grove, S. K. (2005). *The practice of nursing research: Conduct, critique, and utilization* (5th ed.). St. Louis: Elsevier Saunders.

Collins, S., Voth, T., DiCenso, A. & Guyatt, G. (2005). Finding the evidence. In A. DiCenso, G. Guyatt, & D. Ciliska (Eds.), *Evidence-based nursing: A guide to clinical practice* (pp. 20–43). St. Louis: Elsevier Mosby.

DiCenso, A., Ciliska, D., & Guyatt, G. (2005). Introduction to evidence-based nursing. In A. DiCenso, G. Guyatt, & D. Ciliska. (Eds.), *Evidence-based nursing: A guide to clinical practice* (pp. 3–19). St. Louis: Elsevier Mosby.

Dobbins, M., Ciliska, D., Estabrooks, C., & Hayward, S. (2005). Changing nursing practice in an organization. In DiCenso A., Guyatt G., & Ciliska, D. (Eds.), *Evidence-based nursing: A guide to clinical practice* (pp. 172–200). St. Louis: Elsevier Mosby.

Dobbins, M., DeCorby, K., & Twiddy, T. (2004). A knowledge transfer strategy for public health decision makers. *Worldviews on Evidence-Based Nursing, 1,* 120–128.

Downs, F. S. (1991). How to make a difference. *Nursing Research, 40,* 323.

Dracup, K. A., & Breu, C. S. (1978). Using nursing research findings to meet the needs of grieving spouses. *Nursing Research, 27,* 212–216.

Dufault, M. (2004). Testing a collaborative research utilization model to translate best practices in pain management. *Worldviews on Evidence-Based Nursing, 1(3),* S26–S32.

Estabrooks, C. A. (1999). The conceptual structure of research utilization. *Research in Nursing and Health, 22,* 203–216.

Estabrooks, C. A. (2003). Translating research into practice: Implications for organizations and administrators. *Canadian Journal of Nursing Research, 3,* 53–68.

Estabrooks, C. A., Floyd, J. A., Scott-Findlay, S., O'Leary, K. A., & Gushta, M. (2003). Individual determinants of research utilization: A systematic review. *Journal of Advanced Nursing, 43,* 506–520.

Ferlie, E. B. & Shortell, S. M. (2001). Improving the quality of health care in the United Kingdom and the United States: A framework for change. *Milbank Quarterly, 79,* 281–315.

Fetzer, S. J. (2002). Reducing venipuncture and intravenous insertion pain with eutectic mixture of local anesthetic: A meta-analysis. *Nursing Research, 51,* 119–124.

Funk, S. G., Champagne, M. T., Wiese, R. A. & Tornquist, E. (1991). Barriers: The Barriers to Research Utilization Scale. *Applied Nursing Research, 4,* 39–45.

Funk, S. G., Tornquist, E. M., & Champagne, M. T. (1989). A model for improving the dissemination of nursing research. *Western Journal of Nursing Research, 11(3),* 361–372.

Geibert, R. C. (2006). The journey to evidence: Managing the information infrastructure. *In* Malloch K., & Porter-O'Grady, T. (Eds.), *Introduction to evidence-based practice in nursing and health care.* Boston: Jones & Bartlett, pp. 125–148.

Goode, C. J., Lovett, M. K., Hayes, J. E., & Butcher, L. A. (1987). Use of research based knowledge in clinical practice. *Journal of Nursing Administration, 17(12),* 11–18.

Goode, C. J., Titler, M., Rakel, B., Ones, D. S. Kleiber, C., Small, S., et al. (1991). A meta-analysis of effects of heparin flush and saline flush: Quality and cost-implications. *Nursing Research, 40,* 324–330.

Graham, K., & Logan, J. (2004). Using the Ottawa Model of Research Use to implement a skin care program. *Journal of Nursing Care Quality, 19,* 18–24.

Greiner, A. C., & Knebel, E. (Eds.), Board on Health Care Services, Committee on the Health Professions Summit, Institute of Medicine. (2003). *Health Professions Education: A Bridge to Quality.* Washington, DC: National Academies Press.

Haynes, R. B. (2001, March-April). Of studies, syntheses, synopses, and systems: The "4S" evolution of services for finding current best evidence. *ACP Journal Club, 134,* A11–A13.

Horsley, J. A., Crane, J. Crabtree, M. K., & Wood, D. J. (1983). *Using research improve nursing practice: A guide.* New York: Grune & Stratton.

Ingersoll, G. (2000). Evidence-based nursing: What it is and what it isn't. *Nursing Outlook, 48,* 151–152.

International Council of Nurses. (1999). *Nursing Research* [Position Statement]. Retrieved April 15, 2006, from www.icn.ch/psresearch99.htm.

Kennedy, M. S. (2002). Nurses making a difference: Rock on: Kathryn Barnard, champion of newborns. *American Journal of Nursing, 102(6),* 110–111.

King, D., Barnard, K. E., & Hoehn, R. (1981). Disseminating the results of nursing research. *Nursing Outlook, 29,* 164–169.

Kitson, A., Harvey, G., & McCormack, B. (1998). Enabling the implementation of evidence based practice: A conceptual framework. *Quality in Health Care, 7,* 149–158.

Krueger, J. C., Nelson, A. H., & Wolanin, M. O. (1978). *Nursing research: Development, collaboration and utilization.* Germantown, MD: Aspen.

Lipman, T. H., Hench, K. D., Benyi, T., Delaune, J., Gilluly, K. A., Johnson, L., et al. (2004). A multicentre randomised controlled trial of an intervention to improve the accuracy of linear growth measurement. *Archives of Disease in Childhood, 89,* 342–346.

Lomas, J. (2004). It takes two to tango: The importance of joint knowledge production for research use. *Canadian Health Services Research Foundation.* Presentation at the Ministerial Summit on Health Research and Global Forum, Mexico City, Mexico, November, 2004.

Madsen, D., Sebolt, T., Cullen, L., Folkedahl, B., Mueller, T., Richardson, C., et al. (2005). Listening to bowel sounds: An evidence-based practice project. *American Journal of Nursing, 105*(12), 40–49.

Melnyk, B., & Fineout-Overholt, E. (2005). Making the case for evidence-based practice. *In* Melnyk B., & Fineout-Overholt E. (Eds.). *Evidence-based practice in nursing and healthcare: A guide to best practice.* (pp. 3–24). Philadelphia: Lippincott.

Messmer, P. R., Jones, S. G., & Rosillo, C. (2002). Using nursing research projects to meet Magnet Recognition Program standards. *Journal of Nursing Administration, 32,* 538–543.

Metheny, N. A., & Titler, M. G. (2001). Assessing placement of feeding tubes. *American Journal of Nursing, 101*(5), 36–46.

Meyers, T. A., Eichhorn, D. J., Guzzetta, C. E., Clark, A. P., Klein, J., Taliaferro, E., et al. (2000). Family presence during invasive procedures and resuscitation: The experience of family members, nurses, and physicians. *American Journal of Nursing, 100*(2), 32–43.

National Institutes of Health. (n.d.). *NIH Roadmap; Accelerating medical discovery to improve health.* Retrieved April 15, 2006, from http://nihroadmap.nih.gov.

Nicoll, L. H., & Hesby, A. (2002). Intramuscular injection: An integrative research review and guideline for evidence-based practice. *Applied Nursing Research, 16,* 149–162.

Registered Nurses Association of Ontario. (2002). *Toolkit: Implementation of clinical practice guidelines.* Toronto, Canada: Author. Retrieved April 15, 2006, from www.rnao.org/bestpractices.

Reising, D. L., & Neal, R. S. (2005). Enteral tube flushing: What you think are best practices may not be. *American Journal of Nursing, 105*(3), 58–64.

Retsas, A. (2000). Barriers to using research evidence in nursing practice. *Journal of Advanced Nursing, 31,* 599–606.

Rogers, E. (2003). *Diffusion of innovations* (5th ed.). New York: Free Press.

Rossouw, J. E., Anderson, G. L., Prentice, R. L., LaCroix, A. Z., Kooperburg, C., Stefanick, M. L., et al. (2002). Risks and benefits of estrogen plus progestin in healthy postmenopausal women: Principal results from the Women's Health Initiative randomized control trial. *Journal of the American Medical Association, 288,* 321–333.

Rosswurm, M. A., & Larrabee, J. H. (1999). A model for change to evidence-based practice. *Image: Journal of Nursing Scholarship, 31,* 317–322.

Sharp, N. D., Pineros, S. L., Hsu, C., Starks, H., & Sales, A. E. (2004). A qualitative study to identify barriers and facilitators to implementation of pilot interventions in the Veterans Health Administration (VHA) Northwest Network. *Worldviews on Evidence-Based Nursing, 1,* 129–139.

Steinbinder, A., & Scherer, E. (2006). Creating nursing system excellence through the forces of magnetism. In K. Malloch & T. Porter-O'Grady (Eds.), *Introduction to evidence-based practice in nursing and health care.* Boston: Jones & Bartlett, pp. 235–266.

Stenger, K., Schooley, K., & Moss, L. (2001). Moving to evidence-based practice for pain management in the critical care setting. *Critical Care Nursing Clinics of North America, 13,* 319–327.

Stetler, C. B. (2001). Updating the Stetler Model of Research Utilization to facilitate evidence-based practice. *Nursing Outlook, 49,* 272–279.

Stetler, C. B. (2003). Role of the organization in translating research into evidence-based practice. *Outcomes Management, 7*(3), 97–103.

Straus, S. E., Richardson, W. S., Glasziou, P., & Haynes, R. B. (2005). *Evidence-based medicine: How to practice and teach EBM* (3rd ed.). Edinburgh: Churchill Livingston.

Titler, M. G. (2004). Methods in translation science. *Worldviews on Evidence-Based Nursing, 1,* 38–48.

Titler, M. G., Kleiber, C., Steelman, V. J., Rakel, B. A., Budeau, G., Everett, L. Q., et al. (2001). The Iowa Model of Evidence-Based Practice to promote quality care. *Critical Care Nursing Clinics of North America, 13,* 497–509.

Watson, C. A., Bulecheck, G., & McCloskey, J. (1987). QAMUR: A quality assurance model using research. *Journal of Nursing Quality Assurance, 2*(1), 21–27.

SUGGESTED READINGS

Bakken, S., Cimino, J. J., & Hripcscak, G. (2004). Promoting patient safety and enabling evidence-based practice through informatics. *Medical Care, 42*(Suppl. 2), 49–56.

Brown, S. J. (1999). *Knowledge for health care practice: A guide to using research evidence.* Philadelphia: W. B. Saunders.

Cronenwett, L. (February 19, 2002). Research, practice and policy: Issues in evidence based care. Online Journal of

Issues in Nursing, 7(2). Retrieved April 15, 2006, from http://nursingworld.org/ojin/keynotes/speech_2.htm.

DiCenso, A., Guyatt, G., & Ciliska, D. (Eds.). (2005). *Evidence-based nursing: A guide to clinical practice.* St. Louis: Elsevier Mosby.

Duffy, M. E. (2004). Resources for building a research utilization program. *Clinical Nurse Specialist, 18,* 279–281.

Hutchinson, A. M., & Johnston, L. (2004). Bridging the divide: A survey of nurses' opinions regarding barriers to, and facilitators, of research utilization in the practice setting. *Journal of Clinical Nursing, 13,* 304–315.

Malloch, K., & Porter-O'Grady, T. (Eds.). (2006). *Introduction to evidence-based practice in nursing and health care.* Boston: Jones & Bartlett.

Melnyk, B., & Fineout-Overholt, E. (Eds.). (2005). *Evidence-based practice in nursing and healthcare: A guide to best practice* (pp. 3–24). Philadelphia: Lippincott.

Interpersonal and Personal Skills

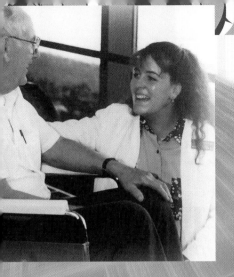

21

Consumer Relationships

Margarete Lieb Zalon

This chapter explores the changes that have altered consumer relationships with healthcare providers and looks specifically at nurses' responsibilities to the consumer. Nurses set the tone for effective staff-patient interaction. Because nurses are the healthcare providers who spend the most time with the consumer, this chapter provides concepts and strategies to assist in developing effective nurse-consumer relationships.

Objectives

- Categorize health consumers' interactions into three relationship structures.
- Interpret the results of selected changes that have influenced consumer relationships in health care.
- Examine the importance of a service-oriented philosophy to the quality of the nurse-consumer relationship.
- Apply the four major responsibilities of nursing—service, advocacy, teaching, and leadership—to the promotion of successful nurse-consumer relationships.

Questions to Consider

- Why is the consumer perspective so important to nursing leaders?
- What changes have taken place that have altered the relationships between consumers and healthcare providers?
- What concepts must be applied to provide service-oriented nursing care to consumers?
- How are cultural diversity and individual differences taken into consideration when practicing nursing?
- What is consumer advocacy, and who is responsible for it?

The Challenge

Suzanne Freeman, RN, MBA
President of Carolinas Medical Center, Charlotte, North Carolina

Customer satisfaction is the number one goal in our healthcare facilities. The hospital board officially acknowledged this goal, and systems were set in place to measure, monitor, and improve customer satisfaction. The staff ultimately defined principles to illustrate their commitment to this goal: teamwork, integrity, caring, commitment, and communication. Each individual would be treated with dignity and as a valued member of a "family."

The husband of a patient seen in the emergency department (ED) some time ago called the nurse manager a few days after her visit. When his wife arrived at the ED, her chief complaint was intermittent chest pain for 2 days. She had indicated that she did not have pain upon arrival to the ED and was ultimately admitted to the hospital with the diagnosis statement "Chest pain, rule out MI [myocardial infarction]."

The husband complained that his wife had been required to "sign herself in," even though he had asked the nurse to have his wife seen immediately. He felt the nurse had not taken his wife's complaints seriously, and the resulting delay had caused her condition to worsen. He attributed this issue to the fact that his wife required coronary artery bypass surgery the following day.

The nurse manager immediately met with the triage nurse involved. They talked through the encounter and examined the documentation. The triage nurse felt her assessment of "nonemergent" was valid. She noted that the patient was registered by the patient registration

personnel, and the physician saw her within 30 minutes of her arrival. The triage nurse's assessment indicated "Vital Signs stable, no history of heart disease, right-sided chest pain × 2 days." The pain scale records indicated "No pain now." The assessment made by the triage nurse appeared valid to the nurse manager. The nurse manager also noted that the nurse's competency in assessing patients for triage was historically reliable. The triage nurse did not recall the husband asking for his wife to be seen immediately.

The nurse manager visited the patient and her spouse in the coronary care unit. She apologized for their expectations not being met during the triage process. She assured the couple that their concerns were taken seriously and offered her sincerest apologies. Her words seemed to be well received by the couple. Each thanked her for her concern and visit.

Apparently, the couple was not satisfied, however, because the Vice President for Patient Services received a call from the husband that same day. He related the story, including the nurse manager's visit. He added that he had recently viewed a news report about how women were undertreated and misdiagnosed with regard to chest pain. The vice president listened carefully and promised to follow up quickly with a response.

 What do you think you would do if you were this nurse?

INTRODUCTION

A *Dilbert* cartoon declared that there are two essential rules of management: (1) Customers are always right, and (2) they must be punished for their arrogance! The days of thinking that a patient or consumer who becomes actively engaged in healthcare decisions is stepping out of bounds, a mind-set often referred to as *paternalism*, are fortunately coming to an end.

Consumer relationships in healthcare delivery refer to the multitude of encounters between the

consumer (client, patient, or customer) and healthcare system representatives. Who are the consumers of health care, and what do they expect from providers? What are their likes and dislikes, and how do they evaluate their health care?

Today, hospitals and other healthcare organizations are concerned with protecting consumer rights and are actively engaged in assessing patient/consumer satisfaction as a strategy to improve quality, enhance market share, and meet regulatory and/or accreditation requirements. The role of nurses as trusted professionals in the development of consumer relationships in healthcare organizations is increasingly recognized for its importance.

Consumers hold nurses in high regard. They view nurses as knowledgeable, worthy of respect, concerned for others, honest, caring, confidential, friendly, hardworking, and especially trustworthy. In the 2003 Harris Poll, 49% of Americans reported that they perceived nurses to have very great prestige (Taylor, 2003). Nurses are at the top of the list in the 2005 Gallup poll of the public's ratings of honesty and ethical standards of various professions. Nurses have been at the top of the list in all but one year since they were added to the annual survey in 1999. The public has a very positive view of nurses, with 82% of the public rating nurses' ethical standards and honesty as high or very high (Ulrich, 2006). Nurses, by virtue of this favorable status with the public, occupy positions of influence and can foster and promote successful consumer relationships across health care settings.

We are all consumers of health care—friends, neighbors, families, people like us, and people very different from us. Consumers are diverse culturally, ethnically, socially, physically, and psychologically. Consumers are indeed becoming better connoisseurs of health care than they were in the past. One sure sign of the healthcare industry's response to that fact is direct marketing of pharmaceuticals and other health-related products. Between 1996 and 2000, the annual spending on direct-to-consumer advertising for prescription drugs in the United States tripled to nearly $2.5 billion (Rosenthal, Berndt, Donohue, Frank, & Epstein, 2002). Chronic health conditions require that consumers take an active role in managing their health. In fact, chronic illnesses account for 60% of global mortality and one-third of the world's disease burden (World Health Organization, nd). Consumerism is increasingly seen by employers as a vehicle for reducing healthcare costs and for improving quality by empowering employees to make more appropriate choices about their use of healthcare services while improving health care. The Leapfrog Group, a consortium of more than 160 employers and organizations that buys health care, is working to prevent mistakes in health care and improve the quality and affordability of health care. Data from the 2000 U.S. census indicate that 42% of households had a computer; approximately 40% of those individuals with Internet access reported using it to search for health or healthcare

advice or information, and one third of those reported that it affected a healthcare decision (Baker, Wagner, Singer, & Bundorf, 2003). Although these data have implications for access to healthcare information, they also reflect changes that impact the nature of the relationship between consumers and nurses, consumers and other **healthcare providers**, and consumers and healthcare organizations.

Consumers have access to limitless amounts of information about health; however, such access may vary to some degree by ethnicity and socioeconomic status. Although some information that is available from the Internet and other resources might not be valid, **healthcare consumers** tend to be better informed now more than they ever have been. Publicity about medical errors and the nursing shortage as well as information campaigns directed toward consumers to promote safety have heightened consumer awareness about the importance of being involved in all aspects of one's health care. Consumers question providers regarding the care they receive or do not receive, and they ask, "Why are you doing that?" "Where can I get the best care?" "Why did my nurse do that differently yesterday?" and "How do I know what is the best decision for me?"

RELATIONSHIPS

The Consumer Focus

Consumer relationships are constantly changing and thus affect the providers of health services: primary care and public health services, managed care organizations, hospitals, home health agencies, and nursing homes, as well as individual providers such as nurses and physicians. As inpatient services have become more complex and outpatient services have grown, competition for patients becomes fiercer. This has resulted in a shift in focus from **healthcare providers** to healthcare consumers. As noted in *The Challenge*, consumers drive what happens in our healthcare settings. Healthcare processes are being redefined with the consumer as the center. How consumers view and value their care becomes important data. Consumers enter into distinct relationships to meet their healthcare needs, including relationships with healthcare agencies, insurers or payers, nurses, physicians, and allied health providers. Changes in access to service, insurance coverage, nurses' roles and responsibilities, and physician services are a few of the significant factors that have influenced these relationships.

Health Literacy   Consumers rely on information from a variety of sources to make decisions about their health. The relationships that consumers develop with their healthcare providers, including nurses, are important in helping them navigate the healthcare system. However, nearly half of America's adults—that is, 90 million people—have difficulty in understanding and using health information (Nielson-Bohlman, Panzer, & Kindig, 2004). The definition of **health literacy** used by *Healthy People 2010* is "the degree to which individuals have the capacity to obtain, process, and understand basic health information and services needed to make appropriate health decisions" (Ratzan & Parker, 2000, p. vi).

Understanding consumers' health-literacy needs goes beyond just examining reading ability. Health literacy arises from merging expectations, preferences, skills of those seeking health information and services with the expectations, and preferences and skills of those providing the information and skills (Nielson-Bohlman et al., 2004). Promoting health literacy involves education, but social and cultural factors and the context of the situation also need to be considered. For example, a nurse who is an expert clinician in a specialty practice area, when diagnosed with a serious chronic illness, may not have the appropriate background to make informed healthcare decisions. Promoting health literacy is an important component of health care because individuals with limited literacy are vulnerable. They are more likely to be sicker when they enter into the healthcare system and are more likely to consume more healthcare services.

HealthCare Provider–Consumer Relationships

Healthcare provider–consumer relationships have changed as physicians' typical mode of practice moved from a single, private enterprise to multi-group practices that also include nurse practitioners, certified nurse-midwives, certified registered nurse anesthetists, clinical nurse specialists, registered nurse first assistants, physicians' assistants, and other healthcare professionals. Some group practices are incorporated into health maintenance organizations (HMOs), managed care programs, or physician-hospital organizations. When consumers visit a group practice, they might not have the option of selecting a specific healthcare provider. Patients no longer know their healthcare providers as they did in the past, and the providers may be less familiar with their patients, resulting in decreased opportunity for the development of mutual respect and trust. However, trust still is an important component of consumer relationships. For example, elderly patients' satisfaction with their care is related to trust in their healthcare providers (Hupcey, Clark, Hucheson, & Thompson, 2004; Scotti & Stinerock, 2003). These results indicate the importance of treating patients with respect and being attentive to their concerns.

Rural consumers of health care have seen local hospitals close and have had to seek care in regional health centers. They may not have a relationship with the healthcare providers to whom they are directed to seek care, which often leads consumers to be more critical and less accepting of the care delivered. They often feel alienated and insecure in unfamiliar circumstances, even if they are receiving the best health care. Patients' perceptions are becoming an increasingly valued outcome of care. Consumers may be caught in the middle without a healthcare provider when physicians leave communities because of malpractice premiums, when insurance companies limit access to certain types of healthcare providers, or when the providers change their healthcare facility affiliations.

Agency–Consumer Relationships

Consumers of healthcare services may have been accustomed to receiving acute care in an inpatient setting. In many situations, this option is no longer available. Patients may be angry and frightened at the thought of being on their own or with receiving very limited services from home health agencies. When inpatient services are deemed appropriate, the type of insurance coverage and the insurance carrier will most likely dictate the specific hospital or healthcare agency chosen. Managed care options require that the consumer use particular and specific healthcare facilities or be responsible for all or a larger portion of the bill.

No longer is a trip to the emergency department an option for a sore throat at midnight. The price tag for that service is prohibitive. Unfortunately, the emergency department may provide the only access to care for various groups. Consumers' options for seeking care are shrinking, and the costs are increasing. The insurance plans available to most people include a co-payment or a deductible clause requiring the consumer to meet a certain dollar amount before the insurance companies will pay their 60% to 90% of the bill, resulting in a significant impact on the consumer. Medicare and Medicaid recipients also find themselves in the midst of changes in terms of how healthcare costs are managed. Understanding the new Medicare prescription drug benefit is a daunting task for many seniors.

Consumer-directed healthcare plans with high-deductibles are being developed to provide consumers with information about various choices in an effort to decrease healthcare costs by empowering them to make informed choices about risks, benefits, and relative costs (Nolin & Killackey, 2004). Predictions indicate a greater emphasis on case management, disease management, and patient education. These plans use report cards, risk assessments, nurse-help telephone lines, websites, and an array of other consumer education materials. Consumers will be comparison-shopping for healthcare services just as they might comparison-shop for prescription drugs. Despite this growth in consumer awareness, the impact of consumer-directed healthcare plans on patient satisfaction and healthcare costs are not known. Critics of consumer-directed health plans are concerned that these plans shift costs to consumers without offering any true reductions in healthcare spending. Consumers have come to expect high technology and the latest treatments. Requiring consumers to make decisions about their health care may place additional strain on consumers' relationships with healthcare professionals and healthcare organizations.

Many healthcare organizations are still operating under an outmoded paradigm with the needs of physicians and third-party payers driving the agency's priorities. In increasingly competitive healthcare markets, executives need to focus on their patients/customers who are becoming more knowledgeable and assertive (Ford & Fottler, 2000).

Nurse-Consumer Relationships

Nurses are the healthcare providers who spend the most time with the consumer. These encounters are generally personal and intensely meaningful. Therefore, the nurse is in a distinct position to influence and promote positive consumer relationships. The nurse manager sets the tone for effective staff-patient interactions with exciting opportunities presented in care that is centered on the patient.

Changes from hospital or nursing home care to outpatient and in-home care have particularly altered the nurse-consumer relationship. Nurses are taking leadership roles as primary care providers (e.g., nurse practitioners, midwives), teachers and educators, and home healthcare managers and advocates, particularly in compensation and insurance areas. Nurses may emerge as the **gatekeepers** of the healthcare system, the liaisons between the consumer and a complex healthcare market. The nurse in the role of gatekeeper can be an influential advocate for consumers who could receive less than desired care in a complicated healthcare system. This group includes those who receive no care and need it most, such as those who are homeless, uninsured or underinsured persons, persons who abuse drugs or alcohol, children of poverty, migrant workers, and people with AIDS. Some institutions and private corporations have capitalized on the case-management skills of nurses by developing the "nurse navigator" or "patient navigator" roles, which are designed to assist patients through a complex healthcare system, or with healthcare decisions.

Nursing has long valued the integral nature of the nurse–patient relationship and the value of caring as an element of that relationship. The *Code of Ethics for Nurses* holds that the "nurse's primary commitment is to the patient" with an expectation that the nurse involves patients in planning for care (American Nurses Association [ANA], 2001, pp. 9-10). This reciprocal nature of the relationships between nurses and patients has been examined. The evolution of the nurse–client relationship has been described as a result of a growth in democratic thinking and a strategy to promote human rights in healthcare relationships and the embodiment of power sharing and negotiation, resulting in client empowerment (Gallant, Beaulieu, & Carnevale, 2002). Wylie and Wagenfeld-Heintz (2004), in reviewing the literature on relationship-centered care, note the evidence for nurses' receptiveness to mutuality and reciprocity in relationships that honor all persons. Mutuality balances power and respect and promotes productive communication.

Nurses have four major responsibilities in promoting successful consumer relationships. They are:

1. Service
2. Advocacy
3. Teaching
4. Leadership

Exercise 21-1

List as many ways as you can think of that the nurse might carry out the four aforementioned responsibilities. Compare your list with those of your peers.

SERVICE

A **service** orientation responds to the needs of the customer. In The Challenge, activities centered on the patient and family, including how nursing care and all other services are delivered so that patient care is a "whole" concept. The Institute of Medicine's (IOM) aims for the improvement of the healthcare system are that health care is safe, effective, patient-centered, timely, efficient, and equitable (Committee on Quality of Health Care in America, 2001). Healthcare professionals, including nurses, want to deliver patient-centered care. However, assessing how well that is being accomplished in an organization is challenging. The Picker Institute, a nonprofit organization, has done extensive research on the evaluation of care from the patient's perspective. Its model of patient-centered care, no matter where the services are delivered, focuses on the consumer's perspective, as illustrated in Box 21-1. Each of these dimensions is an important part of the consumer's interaction with the healthcare system and provides guidance in promoting consumer relationships.

A service orientation is different from the concept of **service lines,** in which all related types of services are grouped into single functional management units. These are commonly related to clinical specialties, such as women's health, cardiovascular care, or orthopedics. More recently, we have seen the growth of specialty hospitals, for example, in cardiovascular care or orthopedics. Although the concept of providing all services related to a particular specialty is appealing, it has created controversy when the other hospitals in the community are financially burdened and must

---

BOX 21-1

Seven Primary Dimensions of Patient-Centered Care

- **Respect for patient's values, preferences, and expressed needs:** includes attention to quality of life, involvement in decision-making, preservation of a patient's dignity, and recognition of patient's needs and autonomy
- **Coordination and integration of care:** involves clinical care, ancillary and support services, and "frontline" patient care
- **Information, communication, and education:** includes information on clinical status, progress, and prognosis; information on processes of care; and information and education to facilitate autonomy, self-care, and health promotion
- **Physical comfort:** considers pain management, help with activities of daily living, and hospital environment

- **Emotional support and alleviation of fear and anxiety:** demands attention to anxiety over clinical status, treatment, and prognosis; anxiety over the effect of the illness on self and family; and anxiety over the financial impact of the illness
- **Involvement of family and friends:** recognizes the need to accommodate family and friends and involve family in decision-making; to support the family as caregiver; and to recognize family needs
- **Transition and continuity:** addresses patient anxieties and concerns about information on medication, treatment regimens, follow-up, danger signals after leaving the hospital, recovery, health promotion, and prevention of recurrence; coordination and planning for continuing care and treatment; and access to continuity of care and assistance

From Gerteis, M., Edgman-Levitan, S., Daley, J., & Delbanco, T. L. (2002). *Through the patient's eyes: Understanding and promoting patient-centered care.* San Francisco: Jossey-Bass.

eliminate services that are not cost-effective. Thus, access to health care might be further compromised. Using a service line model requires that the manager monitor data from a variety of sources to meet consumer needs including (1) demographic data, (2) clinical **quality indicators**, (3) customer satisfaction (patient, healthcare provider and staff), (4) technology trends, (5) financial performance, (6) market share, and (7) competitor analysis (Clancy, 2002).

Even with an increasing emphasis on customer **service,** most healthcare facilities are not as "customer-friendly" as they could be; that is, they are built and organized in a manner that best serves the organization, not the consumer. They are compartmentalized with each department having specialized functions. Patients are transported from department to department to receive services. They risk loss of privacy, excessive exposure, and increased discomfort and fatigue during the transfer and waiting episodes. On an average day, a seriously ill hospitalized patient may have encounters with up to 50 or more different personnel in the course of receiving treatment and care. This approach is not "service-oriented." A service orientation means delivering services in a manner that is least disruptive to the consumer. When possible, services should come to the patient and should be as easy, comfortable, pleasant, and effective as possible. The consumer is interested in high-quality care that is technologically advanced and compassionate (Doucette, 2003). It is important to distinguish between the quality of care and service. The quality of care refers to the outcomes of care in relation to a standard, whereas the service is a measure of perception of what matters to the patient (Doucette, 2003).

▌ Exercise 21-2

List the things that you think are not consumer-friendly in your nursing situation. (Example: Patients admitted to healthcare facilities being asked to repeat information several times to different staff members such as admissions clerks, nurses, and radiograph technicians.)

Providing satisfying and meaningful service is not easy. Every consumer is different, and every situation is different. How things are done and how needs are met vary in each situation. Service is not a prescribed set of rules and regulations and is not a unidimensional concept. Service means placing a premium on the design, development, and delivery of care. For example, a home-care patient needs intravenous (IV) antibiotic therapy. Inserting the IV catheter is the task-oriented, production part of the care. The service aspect involves taking into consideration the special needs of the patient, such as placing the needle in the left arm so that he can continue to use his cane with his right arm, or using a local anesthetic before inserting the needle to reduce discomfort.

Delivering nursing care includes both service and product characteristics. In the context of health care, a service involves interaction between a consumer and the healthcare system related to the provision of needs, whereas a product is a tangible item with physical characteristics. Some nursing actions require clearly prescribed rituals—the actual physical act of production, such as insertion of a Foley catheter. In performing this act, certain physical characteristics are apparent, and the outcome is predictable. At the same time, no two patients are alike; human interaction alters the situation, and unforeseen variables demand spontaneity. Caring, concern, and respect for the individual are intangible characteristics that affect the ultimate success or failure of the physical nursing action. Quality nursing care must be both clinically correct and satisfying to the customer. "Clinically correct" is the product aspect and "satisfying to the consumer" is the service orientation.

Healthcare agencies, as service organizations, must be sensitive to whether the agency milieu is indeed a healing environment that supports and reinforces the actual quality of clinical care. The challenge in the busy, unpredictable, cost-constrained world of health care is to provide settings of care that meet or exceed customer expectations. People are looking for an environment that meets their needs for safety and security, support, and psychological and physical comfort. Such needs are best addressed in healthcare organizations that deliver clinically competent care within a service orientation (Fottler, Ford, Roberts, & Ford, 2000). Hospital leaders value the role of Magnet™ recognition in terms of promoting competent care and a service orientation. Magnet status as a quality indicator demonstrates the importance of excellence in nursing care and service for the patient as customer (Tropello, 2003).

A service orientation is consumer-driven and consumer-focused, and it places the emphasis on the quality of the nurse–patient relationship. The importance of relationships is reflected in current nursing theory in the caring philosophy. Caring has been described as the essence of nursing. It denotes a special concern, interest, or feeling capable of fostering a therapeutic nurse–patient relationship. Caring is important, but it is not enough to simply care. The ability to think critically and take appropriate, timely action must be a part of the therapeutic process. The nurse must do the right thing right at the right time.

The concept of nursing as a caring service is seen in the reality of "high tech–high touch." **High tech** denotes a mechanistic perspective, whereas **high touch** denotes a caring, humanistic perspective. Caring for patients is challenging in an environment driven by technology. At the same time, patients depend on nurses to deliver high-tech care in a caring, humanistic manner. The more high technology is used in health care, the more the patient wants and needs high touch—someone who is trusted and respected and who will add human touch to the experience. The quality of these human contacts becomes the measure by which the consumer forms perceptions and judgments about nursing and the health agency. In health care, consumers are frequently unable to judge or evaluate the quality of interventions, but they always have the ability to evaluate the quality of the relationship with the person delivering the service.

Patient satisfaction ratings, along with measurable healthcare outcomes, are important data used by healthcare organizations to provide quality care and to maintain a competitive edge. Nurses, because of their 24-hour accountability for patient care, are integral to high patient-satisfaction ratings. According to Urden (2002), **patient satisfaction** was for a long time considered to be "soft" data. However, this is no longer true; healthcare organizations are collecting patient satisfaction data and are very much interested in having high patient-satisfaction ratings, so much so that they are advertising their ratings to the community. Standard-setting organizations, such as the Joint Commission on the Accreditation of Healthcare Organizations (JCAHO), and the National Quality Forum include patient satisfaction as a quality indicator. Urden further notes that satisfaction with nursing care is an integral component of patient satisfaction.

Hospitals and other healthcare organizations contract with vendors to measure patient satisfaction or use their own instruments. Nurses need to realize that, very often, patient-satisfaction ratings are clustered together at the high end of the scale, making it difficult to interpret the results and make improvements. One needs also to consider the range and the depth of the information that is collected. For example, some hospitals may only collect data on the hotel amenities, such as the cleanliness of the room. Other hospitals may collect more specific data on satisfaction with nursing care, including such elements as how promptly the call light was answered and if patients were satisfied with a specific aspect of nursing care, such as pain management. The National Database of Nursing Quality Indicators (NDNQI) is a national repository for unit-based quality data that can be used by organizations to benchmark their outcomes against those of other institutions (ANA, 2004). Unit-based quality indicators, including satisfaction with nursing care, is a key feature of the NDNQI database, enabling nurse managers and nurses to make improvements.

It is important for nurses to keep in mind that they have a responsibility to exercise critical-thinking and decision-making with respect to patient satisfaction with nursing care. For example, a postoperative patient may not want to cough and deep breathe, yet we know that failure to do so can result in harm to the patient if he or she develops pneumonia. Similarly, one of the challenges in providing effective pain management is that patients can be quite satisfied with poor pain management. In fact, research has demonstrated that patients can experience severe postoperative pain, yet be quite satisfied with their pain management (Sauaia et al., 2005). This paradox illustrates the responsibility that nurses have for (1) advocating on behalf of their patients, (2) ensuring that their patients' pain is relieved, (3) correcting patient misconceptions, and (4) implementing pain-management strategies that are consistent with established standards. Reviewing and analyzing patient satisfaction survey results are an invaluable tool in improving consumer relationships.

An essential component of a strong customer service program is a **service recovery** element (Bendall-Lyon & Powers, 2001). Service recovery is a strategy for identifying complaints and rectifying service failures to retain or "recover" dissatisfied customers. Six steps in using complaint management as an effective service recovery tool include (1) encouraging complaints as part of the quality-improvement process, (2) establishing a team to address the complaints, (3) resolving consumer issues quickly and effectively, (4) developing a database of complaints to analyze trends and generate information for management and staff, (5) committing to the identification of failure points in the system, and (6) using information to improve service processes (Bendall-Lyon & Powers, 2001). This concept has extended to encouraging healthcare providers, rather than just hospital administrators, to talk with patients when a serious error has occurred. In the past, healthcare organizations have been concerned with the potential risk for liability when the person making an error talks with the patient or family about it. However, recent research suggests that the content of the message has a significant effect on how the person feels about an error. Specifically, messages that contain both an apology and an effort to address the problem in the future are the most productive (Kiger, 2004). Furthermore, when offering an apology, consideration must be given to deciding which person in the organization is the most appropriate to offer it. For example, a nurse making a medication error that has not harmed a patient is probably the best person to talk with the patient. On the other hand, if a patient's discharge is delayed by a day because of an omission or error in preparation for a diagnostic test, then the nurse manager or nurse administrator might be the more appropriate person to initiate discussion with the patient.

Exercise 21–3

Make a "what-if" list of things that would enhance services to the consumers of health care. (Example: What if patients were referred to nurses at the same time that they were referred to physicians?)

Each individual nurse is responsible for providing quality patient care. The nurse manager is accountable for quality management. The term *patient-focused care* was created in the 1990s by Booz-Allen, a consulting firm of organizational strategists (Lathrop, 1993). However, there is no clearly explicated model or one widely accepted definition for this concept. Subsequently, hospitals across the nation introduced the concept of *patient-focused* care, with the goal of decentralizing services, reducing inefficiencies and decreasing the number of staff members interacting with patients. Some strategies in this delivery model include bringing care to the patient—that is, providing point of care (POC) services performed directly at the bedside whenever possible, decreasing the number of transfers, and using wireless technology to track patients and their data. Intuitively, this model of care-delivery is very appealing from the consumer perspective. Unfortunately, the concept of patient-focused care in the 1990s developed a negative connotation as it was coupled with downsizing, substitution of less qualified personnel for registered nurses, and disruption of care processes. More recently, Ingersoll and colleagues (2002) demonstrated that management and staff had different expectations about patient-focused care, thus highlighting the importance of managers assessing the perceptions of their employees regarding initiatives to improve customer service.

ADVOCACY

Nurses today practice in a healthcare environment that is dominated by unrest and insecurity. Some of these forces are shown in Box 21-2. Such forces

---

BOX 21-2

Forces of Unrest and Insecurity in the Healthcare Environment

1. Increased costs
2. Shift to outpatient services
3. Complex social problems (AIDS, violence, poverty)
4. Decreased access to health care
5. Aging population (increasing life span)
6. Technologic and genetic advances
7. Shortage of nurses and other healthcare professionals
8. Culturally and ethnically diverse work/consumer groups
9. Underrepresentation of women and ethnic groups in health-related research

bring about ethical and moral questions: Who gets care? Where do they get care? How much care? Who has the right to die? Who has the right to live? Who makes the decisions? Differing values and beliefs, along with economic constraints and limited resources, affect decisions that are made.

Consumers have some basic rights that need to be protected—the right to individualized care; the right to their own values, beliefs, and cultural ways; and the right to be informed and participate in care decisions. The unresolved issue of two levels of care that are based on economics but may tend to result in racial-cultural discrimination remains within the healthcare system. Not only has care been on a two-tiered basis but also minorities and women have been significantly underrepresented in health-related research, which results in additional healthcare disparities.

Who in the healthcare system is in a position to be the guardian of these rights for the consumer? The nurse is! The nurse acts as the primary person to be alert to circumstances that may prevent a successful outcome for the patient and to intervene on the patient's behalf. The nurse is in the position to address the issues of cultural, ethnic, and racial sensitivity.

The definition of nursing includes advocacy in the care of individuals, families, communities, and populations (ANA, 2003b). Nurses, in accordance with the ANA *Code of Ethics for Nurses,* have the responsibility to promote, advocate, and strive to protect the health, safety, and rights of the patient (2001). Advocacy is a multidimensional concept and has many different meanings and applications. An **advocate** is one who (1) defends or promotes the rights of others, (2) changes systems to meet the needs of others, (3) empowers and promotes self-determination in others, (4) promotes autonomy of diverse cultures and social groups, (5) ensures respect, equality, and dignity for others, and (6) cares for the humaneness of all.

Nursing practice involves interacting with consumers who are culturally, economically, and socially diverse. Diversity encompasses more than differences in nationality or ethnicity and may include a variety of ways that a patient is different from the dominant group of healthcare providers. Nurses are responsible to consumers to assist them in successfully accessing and participating in the system. Some patients enter the healthcare system much like immigrants entering a foreign country.

The result may be culture shock for such patients as they enter a system with a set of values, beliefs, behaviors, and language unlike their own. Patients who speak little or no English and those who may have low health literacy are particularly vulnerable for poor health outcomes in their encounters with the healthcare system. Nurses need to recognize the culture of their work setting, realizing that it may differ markedly from the culture of the consumer who enters the system, and move beyond ethnocentrism to provide culturally competent care. **Cultural competence** brings together attitudes, behaviors, and policies within an organization in such a way that allows people to work effectively in cross-cultural situations (National Alliance for Hispanic Health, 2000). Camphina-Bacote (2002) emphasizes the importance of the fluid nature of cultural competence, with nurses perceiving themselves as becoming culturally competent rather than seeing themselves as having cultural competence, a static attribute. Cultural competence is critical to reducing the potential impact of healthcare disparities and is an integral component of providing consumer service.

The advocate role requires the nurse to perceive and be comfortable with conflict and then mediate, negotiate, clarify, explain, and intervene. The nurse can advocate by being a liaison between the consumer and the system. The nurse's role is to interpret the rules and customs of the agency to the consumer. The role is also to negotiate changes when the consumer and agency differ in values and beliefs. An example is shown in Box 21-3.

To provide culturally appropriate care, the nurse must possess knowledge about various culturally diverse groups (see Chapter 8). It takes time to develop cultural sensitivity and awareness. Some guidelines that are useful in learning to appreciate and value diversity are:

1. Avoid stereotyping.
2. Avoid making assumptions.
3. Learn by observing interactions of minority group members.
4. Adjust expectations to be culturally sensitive.
5. Create a more level playing field—modify your behavior to accommodate diversity.

Powerlessness or an imbalance in power between the consumer and the system can result in value systems being forced on the recipient of care.

BOX 21-3

Racial and Cultural Differences

A young adult African-American male, shot while running from the police, had been hospitalized for more than 3 weeks. A psychiatric clinical nurse specialist made the following assessment:

PERSPECTIVE OF NURSING STAFF

1. No one wants to take care of this patient. Avoiding him is common. His call light goes unanswered.

2. The patient is loud, rude, and uses vulgar language.

3. Nursing staff suspects that sexual activity is occurring between the man and his girlfriend in the hospital.

4. Nurses feel physically and sexually threatened when trying to provide care.

PERSPECTIVE OF PATIENT OF COLOR

1. Patient feels isolated and forgotten. His room is at the end of the hall. He infrequently sees nurses and physicians, has little information about his gunshot wounds, and fears he is never going to walk again. He fears he will die in his room and no one will know.

2. Patient speaks loudly and uses vulgar talk to emphasize his concerns.

3. Patient makes comments with sexual overtones and spends hours with his girlfriend when she visits; he seeks comfort and affirmation through sexuality.

4. Patient's family only comes on weekends and then in large numbers.

Summary: Stereotypes about black males were operational on the unit. The staff members avoided the patient because of the sexual overtones, and they withheld information regarding his condition. Overt and covert battles of will with the patient resulted in further patient isolation.

Modified from Malone, B. L. (1993). Caring for culturally diverse racial groups: An administrative matter. *Nursing Administration Quarterly, 17*(2), 21-29.

Consumers who lack economic means by being uninsured, underinsured, or undocumented often become powerless in the healthcare delivery system. They are at the mercy or will of those who control the power and the money. These consumers (described earlier) may be denied access to care, or if they achieve access, they may not receive equal care.

Consumers interacting with our healthcare systems, regardless of their status, have a right to know about their eligibility for services and care. The nurse must be willing to ensure that economic constraints do not prevent consumers from receiving what they need. Some advocacy for the recipients of inequality in our healthcare system is done on the here-and-now level—initiating a referral to a social agency, appealing on behalf of the consumer to the ethics committee. On a broader scale, advocacy means becoming involved professionally and politically to change the systems and policies to provide equality and access to health care.

Exercise 21-4

Using the scenario in Box 21-3, determine how the culturally competent nurse can mediate the cultural differences between the staff and the patient.

Race and ethnicity as factors in health and health care have been the subject of concern, yet very often people may erroneously assume that members of a particular minority group have the same beliefs, attitudes, and values about health when, in fact, there is extraordinary diversity. Further research is needed on the effectiveness of healthcare organizations and encouraging cultural competency in clinical interactions.

The nursing profession continues to strive for greater diversity among its ranks, with only very modest progress. The U.S. Census of 2000 revealed remarkable increases in the diversity of our population. However, in the *2004 National Sample Survey of Registered Nurses* (Department of Health and Human Services, 2006), only 11.6% of registered nurses identified themselves as minorities in comparison to 32.1% of the population in the United States. Cultural knowledge and educational preparation of healthcare workers influence cultural skills (Jones, Cason, & Bond, 2004). Diversity in the healthcare workforce strengthens cultural competence and cultural competence influences how healthcare professionals deliver health care (Sullivan Commission, 2004). The Census Bureau predicts that by 2040, more than half the U.S. population will comprise ethnic minorities. Currently, residents of the United States speak at least 329 languages (Agency for Healthcare Research and Quality, 2001)! It is most useful to define diversity broadly, to include not only race and ethnicity but also age, gender, socioeconomic status, religion, sexual orientation, physical characteristics, or disability. Thus, cultural competence will play an increasingly important role in nurse-consumer relationships.

Some of the keys to becoming a successful nurse advocate are (1) developing networking systems within work agencies, (2) being involved in professional associations to enhance awareness of issues impacting practice and, thus, consumers, (3) acquiring the knowledge needed to access systems, (4) learning about community resources and support networks, and (5) developing skill in referring and engaging patients.

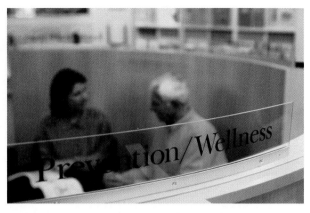

A nurse acts as a consumer advocate by empowering patients.

A patient advocate's ultimate aim is to empower patients (i.e., the consumers of health care) to help them use their own abilities to promote health. Patient empowerment is a critical component of health care today and is seen as integral to the reduction of errors. Although the conceptual definition of empowerment in the literature is unclear, it generally includes elements of providing patients with information and involving them in decision-making (Williams, 2002). Nurses must be sensitive to patient preferences for information and decision-making, as illustrated in the Research Perspective.

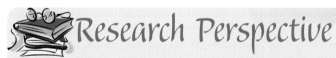

Research Perspective

Sobo, E. J. (2004). Pediatric nurses may misjudge parent communication preferences. *Journal of Nursing Care Quality, 19,* 253-262.

This study was designed to develop an instrument to assess patients'/parents' communication preferences that could be easily used by nurses. The author used a rapid cycle improvement (RCI) process that follows the Shewhart-Deming model of plan, do, study, and act for instrument development. The final version of the instrument involves plotting the degree of information against the degree of involvement in decision-making desired. Two thirds of the nurses misjudged patients'/parents' communication preferences ($n = 51$). Nurses were equally likely to overestimate or underestimate the involvement desired. They also underestimated preferences for information 51% of the time. Although Spanish-speaking patients/parents preferred less information, no differences were found between nurse attributions and patients'/parents' language or gender.

IMPLICATIONS FOR PRACTICE

This study illustrates the importance of communicating with patients and their families about their preferences regarding information and decision-making. Nurses need to be attentive to potential cultural differences in information and decision-making preferences.

The nurse manager should keep in mind the most basic element of empowerment—helping people assert control. In the healthcare industry, control applies to factors that affect health. For example, when a county hospital closed, a network of community-based providers was developed, emphasizing preventive care and appropriate utilization of health care services (Wolff et al., 2003). A nurse telephone service was added to the network to provide patient education and triage to appropriate services, resulting in improved patient confidence in illness management. Melnyk and her colleagues (2004), in a well-designed clinical trial, evaluated the effects of a preventive intervention program, the Creating Opportunities for Parent Empowerment (COPE) program. This program, initiated early during intensive care unit hospitalization, was designed to produce positive mental health/psychosocial outcomes in critically ill young children and their mothers. The mothers who received the COPE program experienced improved maternal functional and emotional coping outcomes resulting in fewer child-adjustment problems in the year following discharge. This work is now being extended to hospitalized elders and their families. The information that patients receive influences their preferences for involvement in healthcare decisions, which in turn affects decision-making opportunities and ultimately, perceptions of health status (Valimaki et al., 2004).

In healthcare facilities, nurses can evaluate the consumer's quality of care by comparing it with quality indicators or critical pathways in the quality-review process. For example, if patient care standards indicate that patients with a particular bronchial condition need a chest radiograph examination on day 2 and another on day 5, all patients should receive this same level of care. In agencies using critical pathways to prescribe the plan of care, patients who cannot pay for services should not be denied treatment, therapy, or tests if the pathway requires specific action. Organizations are increasingly examining nurse-sensitive quality indicators as important outcomes. For example, pressure ulcers and nosocomial infections, such as hospital-acquired pneumonia, are indicators of the quality of nursing care. Nurse managers are in a distinct position to ensure that all patients receive appropriate care. The tone set by the manager signals staff to report and document discrepancies and omissions.

Nurse managers must acknowledge and respect the legal, ethical, and moral responsibilities of the staff to advocate for patients. For example, if a patient receives the wrong medication just before being discharged, the patient needs to be informed, and this information needs to be included in the patient's record. Therefore, should the patient have an adverse reaction and need to return to the emergency department, there is a record that would aid in diagnosis and facilitate the institution of an appropriate treatment promptly. Pennsylvania passed legislation to require written notification to consumers regarding a serious error. Although efforts have been made to increase error-reporting to facilitate the institution of system changes to decrease errors, managers predominantly use blame and reprimand in addressing errors (Wolf & Serembus, 2004). This situation represents a major challenge for nurse managers who are attempting to identify problematic practices to reduce error and promote patient safety.

The savvy manager knows that the way in which consumers define quality may not always match the way "experts" define it. However, patient perception of nurse staffing is a strong predictor of the nursing care received and that it in turn is a significant predictor of overall patient satisfaction (Schmidt, 2004).

Quality health care and quality nursing care are not dependent on the ability to pay or social acceptance. Good care occurs irrespective of the economic circumstance of the consumer. Nurses are the guardians of that right for consumers. Nurses have historically been the champions for the poor and the underserved. It is no different today.

TEACHING

Consumers of health care have a right to know and a need to know how to care for their own health needs. Nurses have an obligation to teach the consumer. Patient teaching is included in the standards of nursing practice (ANA, 2003a) and is often included in the definitions of professional nursing found in state nurse practice acts. Accrediting organizations, such as JCAHO, also mandate patient teaching in their family and patient education standards. *Nurses as Teachers* is one of the fourteen Forces of Magnetism in ANCC's Magnet Recognition Program (Steinbinder & Scherer,

2006). Consumers are demanding information about their health status and plan of care. Consumers are entitled to information regarding health concerns, to participate in caring for their health needs, and to contribute to finding solutions to their health problems. Education empowers consumers to exercise self-determination. It allows them to have greater control over what happens, to make informed decisions, and to choose wisely from options. An ancient proverb says that if you give a man a fish, you feed him for a day, but if you teach a man to fish, you feed him for a lifetime. Knowledge is power. Sharing knowledge means sharing power. Research supports the value of providing health-related education to consumers (Broom, 2001). Health-related education needs also to consider patient preferences for information and decision-making in different situations.

The changes in health care actively affect the way nurses teach consumers. Probably the most significant changes are shorter hospital stays with more care being provided in outpatient settings and transitional care facilities. This requires that patients be able to manage their own health care earlier and more independently. Hands-on, technical training is needed in many instances. Nurses' perceptions of their patients' understanding of post-discharge treatment plans differ from the perceptions of patients themselves. Nurses often perceive patients to be much more knowledgeable than the patients themselves report. Teaching prevention and health promotion will increase the consumer's quality of life. Three *P*'s for a successful consumer education focus are shown in Box 21-4.

Nurses need to be sensitive to the teaching needs of those at risk for disparities in health care: persons of a different race or ethnic group, women, children, the elderly, rural residents, and those with limited or no health insurance and/or low socioeconomic status. Nurses may unintentionally communicate lower expectations for persons who are disadvantaged, have a low literacy level, or have limited English proficiency.

Patients may be hesitant to ask for help with language skills. Some healthcare agencies include an assessment of a patient's ability to learn. However, the lack of assessment criteria may hinder nurses' efforts to institute appropriate teaching. Pope (2005) recommends that nurses use the U.S. Census language screening questions. The person is asked if a language other than English is spoken

---

BOX 21-4

Three P's for a Successful Consumer Education Focus

1. **Philosophy**—Patient education is an investment with a significant positive return. Money invested in teaching is money well spent. Time and energy invested are time and energy well spent.
2. **Priority**—Education is important. Quality nursing care always has an educational component. Informed consumers want to participate and look to nurses to teach them.
3. **Performance**—Clinical teaching excellence is a required nurse competency. Nurses must be skilled in using a variety of techniques and methods to meet the needs of the diverse consumers served.

---

at home and if the answer is *yes*, the person is asked to rate how well he or she speaks English: very well, well, not well, or not at all (Shin & Bruno, 2003). The Office of Minority Health (2001) recommends the adoption of the National Standards for Culturally and Linguistically Appropriate Standards (CLAS), which include standards for cultural competence, language access and organizational support.

Teaching can be simple or complex. In teaching elemental, task-oriented behaviors, the nurse uses basic materials, simple relationships, guides, sequencing of steps, and cause-and-effect relationships. Chronic disease self-management education programs, for example, have an impact on health behaviors, health care, and health care utilization (Lorig, Ritter, & Gonzalez, 2003). Patients with chronic illnesses are often hospitalized for complications related to those illnesses. Therefore, nurses need to be prepared to provide patient education. The nurse manager role is to ensure that staff members have the resources to provide patient teaching, that it is done effectively, and that it is appropriately documented on the plan of care. Teaching behaviors should be addressed in performance evaluations.

In addition to being easy to read, written teaching materials need to reflect relevance, accuracy, and thoroughness and need to be updated regularly. The tone needs be warm and personal and in an inviting format (Winslow, 2001).

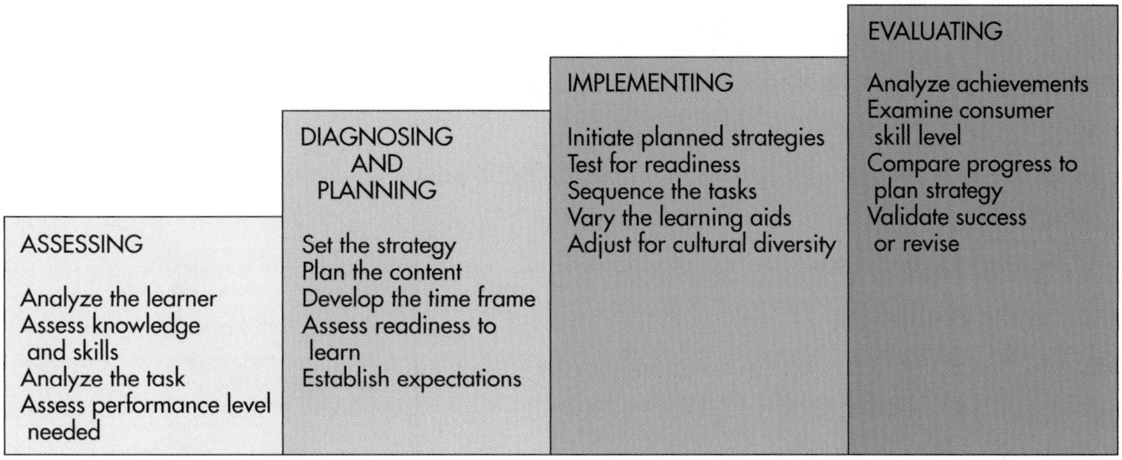

Figure 21-1 Teaching model adapted to the nursing process.

As a step-by-step process, teaching can be adapted to the problem-solving process model shown in Figure 21-1.

The following example uses the nursing process model in teaching a patient about diabetes.

Assess
: Patient is a 16-year-old, Hispanic boy with no previous knowledge of diabetes or skill in drug administration. English is a second language. He needs to administer insulin by the time he is discharged from the hospital.

Plan
: Begin with a demonstration and return demonstration of basic subcutaneous injection. Progress step-by-step to basic understanding of diabetes, blood sugar, hypoglycemia, and insulin dosage by the time of discharge. He is to return to a nurse-managed health center for follow-up care.

Implement
: Set times to spend in instruction with patient. Begin with a demonstration, a return demonstration, and repeat instructions. Adjust learning materials to accommodate language barrier and age.

Evaluate
: Patient has met minimal skill level of subcutaneous technique. He can administer insulin safely but has limited disease and cause-and-effect understanding. To be followed per nurse-managed health center with continued teaching.

Conceptually, teaching also fits into the general systems theory model as shown in Figure 21-2. The following example uses the general systems theory model in teaching a patient with diabetes:

Input
: Present information about the disease, the procedures to be learned, the skills necessary for successful achievement, and the cause-and-effect relationships. Have patient-education materials written in Spanish. Demonstrate injection preparation and administration.

Throughput
: Language barrier eased with materials printed in Spanish. Fear threat to macho image typical of 16-year-old boy. Allow time for practice of technique.

Output
: Return demonstration successful. Give posttest to assess knowledge (in Spanish).

Feedback
: Praise for successful return demonstration. Provide examples of sports heroes or movie stars with diabetes. (Search the Internet with the term *diabetes* and type of hero.)

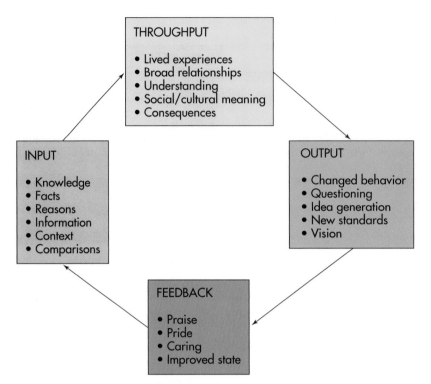

Figure 21-2 Teaching model adapted to general systems theory.

Teaching is one of the most positive experiences nurses can have. Teaching can be fun and rewarding, but it is hard work.

Nurses need to be prepared and skilled to teach. They must be able to adapt to the learning styles of the consumer by using a variety of styles and flexible approaches in meeting the educational goals. For example, cancer detection and screening toolboxes were developed for migrant and seasonal farm workers with community input (Meade, Calvo, Rivera, & Baer, 2003). Selected learning preferences are shown in Box 21-5. Being knowledgeable in the subject, understanding consumer preferences, and being able to individualize the information to meet the consumer's ability to learn are critical to quality teaching.

BOX 21-5

Selected Learning Preferences

Auditory (words)	Visual (sight)
Active (participate)	Passive (contemplate)
Linear (step-by-step)	Circular (model, picture)
Rational (reasoning)	Abstract (global)

with discharge planning was continuity of care and the extent to which they felt prepared to manage care (Bull, Hansen, & Gross, 2000). Numerous patient- and family-satisfaction instruments are available to institutions, which can aid in understanding patient and family concerns. See the *Research Perspective* for an illustration of the importance of considering patient and family preferences.

■ Exercise 21–5

Using either the nursing process model or the general systems theory model as presented to prepare a teaching plan based on your actual nursing experience.

The family should also be included when providing patients with information. The best predictors of elders' and family caregivers' satisfaction

LEADERSHIP

Nurses are critically positioned to provide leadership for the 21st century changes in health care.

Factors that will have an impact on the healthcare organization of the future include:

1. Changing societal demographics in relation to age and diversity.
2. Globalization with changes in the workforce and international migration.
3. Interdisciplinary collaboration.
4. Consumerism and patient expectations.
5. Evidence-based practice.
6. Linkages between cost and outcomes.
7. Full integration of nursing into quality and information systems.
8. Technology in the delivery of interventions and transfer of information.

Understanding paradigm shifts in health care and the need to be responsive to change will prepare nurse managers to participate fully in shaping healthcare organizations of the future. Porter-O'Grady (2003) points out that our future nursing leaders need to be able to adapt continuously, to celebrate accomplishments, to refuel, and to move on to the next wave of transformation while being sensitive to the issues within a particular practice environment.

Nurses, according to the Institute of Medicine, play a pivotal role in patient safety (Page, 2004). Nurse managers are well-positioned to influence the quality of care delivered by the staff. They set the tone for the vision and mission of the unit and the focus for the staff. They must believe in and model the consumer-based service philosophy. One who truly believes in the need to provide service that is satisfying to the consumer knows that each and every consumer is different. What will satisfy one person will not satisfy another. Nurse managers, because they receive referrals when patients are dissatisfied with some aspect of their care, are in a unique position to not only find a solution, but also understand the types of problems being experienced by the patients on a unit and suggest strategies for solving them. Being successful as leaders in nursing requires being open and flexible; leaders are expected not only to do things right but also to do the right things. According to Fitzpatrick (2000), leadership requires (1) giving individualized attention to followers; (2) offering intellectual stimulation; (3) providing inspirational motivation; and (4) serving as a role model (idealized influence). Leadership also involves the ability to relinquish

control and a tolerance for ambiguity, as well as sudden and sometimes dramatic change.

Change is the modus operandi of the nursing environment in any healthcare setting. What works today may not work 6 months from now. Given the rapidly changing environment, the pressure to control costs, and advances in technology, science, and information, nurse managers need a whole new set of beliefs, behaviors, and skills. Selected examples of these are as follows:

1. Keep the consumer as the center of focus.
2. Recognize that each staff member has a specific contribution to make to the success of the unit. Allow staff to be creative and flexible in their work, ask for suggestions and new approaches to old problems, and seek participation in decision-making. Managers set the tone and create the environment, enabling staff to deliver the service.
3. Promote dignity, worth, caring, individual contributions, and cultural sensitivity in the staff. Successful managers recognize individual accomplishments and support failures. They accept that human beings are not perfect at all times and that it is okay to take a risk, look foolish, and fail. They implement hiring practices that foster selection of qualified and culturally diverse applicants.
4. Understand the economic value of service. Managers must believe that service will pay real dollar dividends to justify the cost in terms of adequate quality and quantity of staff.
5. Evaluate patient outcomes and perceptions of care. It is imperative to ask patients about the services provided and how it felt to them, not only after the fact but also while they are receiving the service.

Patient outcomes, standards of care, and evidence-based practice are attracting greater attention and receiving much more public scrutiny. The focus of healthcare reform in the marketplace, the managed care movement, and consumer-directed health plans focus on the provision of quality care along with controlling costs. With this comes the realization that the evidence for certain nursing practices is limited and that nursing, as a profession, needs to be much stronger in making the case for value of the services provided by nurses.

In the area of consumer relations, patient satisfaction with care is a particularly relevant measure. Patient satisfaction has been evaluated in the past with varying degrees of success. Current research efforts are aimed at developing valid and reliable patient outcome measures, including patient satisfaction. The National Quality Forum (2005), an organization focused on a national strategy for healthcare quality measurement, has recently endorsed a standardized survey of patients' perceptions of the quality of hospital care known as Hospital CAHPS. This was developed by the Centers for Medicaid and Medicare Services and the Agency on Healthcare Research and Quality (AHRQ) and is ultimately intended for public reporting. Nursing-services researchers are particularly interested in responses to and satisfaction with nursing care. However, valid measurement of patient satisfaction is an evolving science; nurses do not always accurately gauge what factors are most important to patients, and satisfaction measures are often skewed in a positive direction, with scores clustered at the top of the scale. These issues are addressed by Lynn and McMillen (2004), who used a qualitative methodology to develop a patient satisfaction instrument based on factors considered important by patients. Subsequently, they used a sophisticated methodology that resulted in a survey instrument yielding greater variation in the scores. These improvements will make it much easier to interpret the results and more importantly, take appropriate action for improvement. Selected items appear in Box 21-6. Another strategy to address patient concerns is the development of a patient satisfaction instrument for persons with low literacy (Weiner et al., 2004).

A number of patient satisfaction initiatives have also been instituted in the international community. In a Taiwanese study, Chou, Chen, Woodard, and Yen (2005) found that responsiveness was related to overall patient satisfaction and that reliability was related to satisfaction with nursing care. A European cancer care organization developed a patient satisfaction measure for use across cultures to appraise doctors, nurses, organizations and services (Bredart et al., 2005). The International Hospital Federation (2006) is in the process of developing an international patient satisfaction index with the goal of providing benchmarking within hospitals and across industries. Managers need to share the results of such surveys

> ### BOX 21-6
>
> ## Sample Items from Patient's Perception of Quality Scale-Acute Care Version (PPQS-ACV)
>
> - The nurse uses touch to reassure or support me.
> - The nurse knows who I am as a person.
> - The nurse makes sure that I have plenty of time to talk to her/him.
> - The nurse shows me that I am her/his first concern.
> - The nurse helps me take care of my daily physical needs.
> - The nurse frequently checks on me.
> - The nurse is patient.
> - The nurse is able to talk to me.
> - The nurses see me as an individual, a real person.
> - The nurse is attentive and responsive to my needs.
> - The nurse is clear when teaching me about my care.
> - The nurse gives me my medications on time.
> - The nurse knows what she/he is doing.
>
> From Lynn, M R., & McMillen, B. J. (2004). The scale product technique as a means for enhancing the measurement of patient satisfaction. *Canadian Journal of Nursing Research, 36,* 66-81.

with their staff, examine what they are doing right to keep on doing it, and determine how improvements could be made to address areas of concern.

Managers must be willing to give up direct control of every process. Staff must be given power and permission to be in control and to make decisions at the consumer-staff level of interaction. Some of our greatest successes derive from spontaneous actions. Giving up control involves being willing to take a risk and having a belief in the other person's ability to perform.

Leadership behaviors contributing to individual and personal excellence include (1) allowing professionals more influence over their practice, (2) giving staff opportunities to learn new and varied skills, (3) giving recognition and reward for success and support and consolation for lack of success, and (4) fostering motivation and belief in the importance of each individual and the value of his or her contribution. The leader's role is to create within the worker a passion to do and contribute to the work effort successfully. This is supported by the

Staff Member	Skill Level	Commitment Level	Suggested Action
(1) S. Baker, RN	High technical competence Able to teach others Learns quickly Needs improved people skills	Appears bored Does only what is assigned No enthusiasm Critical of any change	Assign challenges to utilize technical strengths Provide situations in which teaching others occurs Plan: Team assign with D. Carroll
(2) D. Carroll, RN	6-mo post basic program Learns quickly Slow with technical skills Needs technical supervision Excellent people skills	Excited about work Asks for new experiences Accepting of new ideas Volunteers to help others	Improve technical skills Provide safe and successful learning experiences Plan: Team assign with S. Baker
(3) J. Ratke, RN	Moderate technical competence Works best alone Not interested in teaching co-worker Good people skills	Restless, distracted Looking for a change Accepts new ideas Self-commitment—not group-oriented	Set up an independent project of her choosing (e.g., unit research idea) Provide some special technical training to increase skills
(4) C. Thomas, RN	High level technical skills Enjoys helping others Excellent people skills Looks for challenges	Team player Interested in welfare of group Critical of poor performers Acts as cheerleader for change	Utilize willingness and group skills to plan and present a unit activity (e.g., inservice education production, unit open house)

Figure 21-3   Staff-assessment tool.

work of Aiken, Clarke, and Sloane (2002), who indicate that nurse staffing and organizational/managerial support for nursing are key to improving the quality of patient care.

Focusing on Consumers

We do best those things that we know how to do skillfully and those things about which we feel passionately. Fitting the right person to the right job is important. Maximum contribution is required from each staff member in today's healthcare agencies. Because the leader is the one who sets the standard for the success or failure of the staff's contributions, it is important to assess each staff member carefully—what is his or her skill level and commitment level, and what can be done to assist in making a maximum contribution? Figure 21-3

is an example of a completed staff assessment tool. Nurse managers can compile similar information for their staff members. Subsequently, the information can be used to form staff development plans.

Exercise 21–6

Form small groups and assess each member of the group using the headings shown in the staff assessment tool (see Figure 21-3).

When staff members know the leader is sincerely concerned about their welfare, they are better able to use their time, energy, and talents to serve the needs of the consumer. Staff members who are nurtured and cared for will be better able to nurture and care for the consumer.

The Solution

The vice president immediately met with the triage nurse and nurse manager. The nurse manager was surprised that her visit had not resolved the complaint. The vice president asked the triage nurse if she would have assessed a man with the same profile differently. Her immediate answer was "no." She stated that the staff was aware of the literary documents related to gender bias but that the protocol for assessing chest pain was well-designed and very objective, without bias to gender. With the approval of the nurse manager and triage nurse, the vice president invited the husband into the meeting. The husband and the nurse talked through the scenario of events and conversation that occurred during triage, especially the husband's perception that the triage nurse dismissed his request for immediate attention. They agreed that the husband might have said, "Does she really have to register herself?" The triage nurse had not interpreted his statement as a request for immediate action. Each realized that a miscommunication had occurred. Furthermore, the nurse responded to the husband's concern about gender bias. She explained that there had been information in the medical literature, but that cardiologists, ethicists, and other healthcare experts had reviewed and approved the chest pain assessment protocol, ensuring no bias of gender. This situation was brought to resolution by an open line of communication. The result can often be "service recovery."

Several important points may be learned from this incident:

Effective communication is a critical success factor. Clarification is always appropriate in situations of intensity and high emotion. Active listening is an essential component of effective communication.

Imagine yourself in the patient's situation and environment when analyzing a communication exchange.

Engage the involved persons in the evaluation and solution related to a miscommunication.

Healthcare practices, policy, and procedure should be updated regularly to reflect new knowledge.

Consumers are increasingly knowledgeable about health care; therefore, expectations are more sophisticated, and maintaining public trust is of great concern.

Leadership must exude missionary zeal in educating personnel to the expectations for behavior in terms of consumer satisfaction.

— Suzanne Freeman

 Would this be a suitable approach for you? Why?

CHAPTER CHECKLIST

Times have changed, as has the role of the nurse manager. The trend of health care moving into the community, home, clinic, and outpatient setting has placed a whole new perspective on how to provide quality, cost-effective nursing care. Patients must participate in their care and need service-oriented nurses to be teachers, advocates, and leaders on their behalf. Managing care delivery in these diverse settings requires the use of flexible and creative skills. The key is to keep the patient as the center of focus and provide cultural and racially sensitive nursing care.

- Consumer relationships in health care typically involve interactions between the consumer and the following:

The healthcare provider
- Healthcare provider-patient relationships are changing because of changes in the way health care is delivered.

The nurse
- Nurses, as the healthcare providers who spend the most time with the consumer, set the tone for effective staff-patient interactions.

The healthcare agency
- The agency's approach to care is determined by its mission and philosophy.

The healthcare payers
- Insurance coverage and carriers usually dictate the services patients receive and where they receive them.

- Because of their favorable status with consumers, nurses are in a unique position to promote positive consumer relationships.

- Four major responsibilities of nurses in promoting successful consumer relationships are as follows:
  - Service
  - Advocacy
  - Teaching
  - Leadership
- A service orientation is consumer-driven and consumer-focused, emphasizing the quality of the nurse–patient relationship and the delivery of services in a caring atmosphere.
  Services differ from products:
  - Services are intangible, unpredictable, created and consumed simultaneously, and personal.
  - Products are tangible, predictable, produced and stored, and impersonal.
- The nurse can advocate by serving as a liaison between the consumer and the healthcare system.

  Nurses can interpret the agency's rules and customs for the consumer and negotiate if conflicts arise.

  Nurses also help secure culturally appropriate care and mediate cultural differences.

- Teaching is the sharing of information and education to help consumers become independent, self-responsible, and self-determining.

  Nurses have an obligation to teach the consumer.

The three P's for successful consumer education are as follows:

- Philosophy: Patient education is an investment with a significant positive return.
- Priority: Education is important.
- Performance: Clinical teaching excellence is a required skill for nurses.

Teaching can follow the five-step nursing process or a general systems model.

- Leadership fosters decision-making at the consumer–staff level of interaction. Effective leadership strategies for the nurse manager include the following:
  - Keeping the central focus on the consumer and remembering that the consumer may be a whole population
  - Recognizing staff members' unique contributions and helping them maximize their personal excellence
  - Promoting staff members' sense of dignity, worth, caring, cultural diversity, and sensitivity
  - Understanding the economic value of service
  - Valuing interdisciplinary approaches to care
  - Evaluating patient outcomes, patients' perceptions of care, and patient satisfaction

TIPS FOR PROMOTING A CONSUMER FOCUS

- Greet the patient by introducing yourself by full name and role.*
- Recap previous treatments or encounters.*
- Explain what to expect next.*
- Ask for questions.*
- Tell patients when they can expect you back.*
- Ask yourself if this service or approach is one you would wish to receive.
- Remember that in the pyramid of health services, it is the consumer who is the apex—the rest is there to support that person.
- Enter care relationships with the mindset of how to make care better from the recipient's perspective.
- Treat fellow employees, other healthcare professionals, families, and visitors with courtesy and respect.

- Ask staff members what they need to help them incorporate a customer service approach to care.
- Use the service, advocacy, teaching, leadership approach.

*From Baird, K. (2000). Customer service in health care: A grassroots approach to creating a culture of service excellence. San Francisco: Jossey-Bass.

TERMS TO KNOW

advocate	high tech
consumer focus	high touch
cultural competence	patient satisfaction
gatekeeper	quality indicator
health care consumer	service
health care provider	service line
health literacy	service recovery

REFERENCES

Agency for Healthcare Research and Quality. (2001, January). Health plans need culturally and linguistically appropriate materials for non-English speaking patients. *AHRQ Research Activities, 245,* 11. Retrieved May 29, 2006, from www.ahrq.gov/research/resact.htm.

Aiken, L. H., Clarke, S. P., & Sloane, D. M. (2002). Hospital staffing, organization, and quality of care: Cross-national findings. *Nursing Outlook, 50,* 187–194.

American Nurses Association (ANA). (2001). *Code of ethics for nurses with interpretive statements.* Washington, DC: Author.

American Nurses Association (ANA). (2003a). *Nursing: Scope and standards of practice.* Washington, DC: Author.

American Nurses Association (ANA). (2003b). *Nursing's social policy statement* (2nd ed.). Washington, DC: Author.

American Nurses Association (ANA). (2004). *NDNQI: National Database of Nursing Quality Indicators.* Washington, DC: Author. Retrieved May 29, 2006, from www.ana.org/quality/ndnqi.pdf.

Baird, K. (2000). *Customer service in health care: A grassroots approach to creating a culture of service excellence.* San Francisco: Jossey-Bass.

Baker, L., Wagner, T. H., Singer, S., & Bundorf, M. K. (2003). Use of the Internet and e-mail for health care information: Results from a national survey. *Journal of the American Medical Association, 289,* 2400–2406.

Bendall-Lyon, D., & Powers, T. L. (2001). The role of complaint management in the service recovery process. *Joint Commission Journal on Quality Improvement, 27(5),* 278–286.

Bredart, A., Bottomley, A., Blazeby, J. M., Conroy, T., Coens, C., D'Haese, S., et al. (2005). An international prospective study of the EORTC cancer in-patient satisfaction with care measure (EORTC IN-PATSAT32). *European Journal of Cancer, 41,* 2120–2131.

Broom, B. L. (2001). Assessing the value of the follow-through family project for students and families. *Journal of Nursing Education, 40,* 79–85.

Bull, M. J., Hansen, H. E., & Gross, C. R. (2000). Differences in family caregiver outcomes by their level of involvement in discharge planning. *Applied Nursing Research, 13,* 76–82.

Camphina-Bacote, J. (2002). The process of cultural competence in the delivery of health care services: A model of care. *Journal of Transcultural Nursing, 13,* 181–184.

Chou, S. M., Chen, T. F., Woodard, B., & Yen, M. F. (2005). Using SERVQUAL to evaluate quality disconfirmation of nursing service in Taiwan. *Journal of Nursing Research, 13,* 75–84.

Clancy, T. R. (2002). Defining lines. Service-line management helps community hospitals draw up a plan for a healthy database. *Nursing Management, 33(4),* 25–26.

Committee on Quality of Health Care in America. (2001). *Crossing the quality chasm: A new health system for the 21st century.* Washington, DC: National Academies Press.

Department of Health and Human Services, Health Resources and Services Administration, Bureau of Health Professions. (2006, March). *Preliminary findings: 2004 National Sample Survey of Registered Nurses.* Retrieved May 29, 2006, from http://bhpr.hrsa.gov/healthworkforce.

Doucette, J. N. (2003). Serving up uncommon service. *Nursing Management, 34(11),* 26, 28–30.

Fitzpatrick, J. J. (2000). Reflections on achieving professional leadership. *Nursing Leadership Forum, 5(1),* 25–27.

Ford, R. C., & Fottler, M. D. (2000). Creating customer focused health care organizations. *Health Care Management Review, 25(4),* 18–33.

Fottler, M. D., Ford, R. C., Roberts, V., & Ford, E. W. (2000). Creating a healing environment: The importance of the service setting in the new consumer-oriented health care system. *Journal of Healthcare Management, 45,* 91–107.

Gallant, M. H., Beaulieu, M. C., & Carnevale, F. A. (2002). Partnership: An analysis of the concept within the nurse-client relationship. *Journal of Advanced Nursing, 40,* 149–157.

Geron, S. M. (2002). Cultural competency: How is it measured? Does it make a difference? *Generations, 26(3),* 39–45.

Gerteis, M., Edgman-Levitan, S., Daley, J., & Delbanco, T. L. (2002). *Through the patient's eyes: Understanding and promoting patient-centered care* (2nd ed.). San Francisco: Jossey-Bass.

Hupcey, J. E., Clark, M. B., Hucheson, C. R., & Thompson, V. L. (2004). Expectations for care: Older adults' satisfaction with and trust in health care providers. *Journal of Gerontological Nursing, 30(11),* 37–45.

Ingersoll, G. L., Wagner, L., Merck, S. E., Kirsch, J. C., Hepworth, J. T., & Williams, M. (2002). Patient-focused redesign and employee perception of work environment. *Nursing Economics, 20,* 163–170, 187.

International Hospital Federation. (2006). *IHF Projects. Patient satisfaction (IPSI).* Retrieved May 30, 2006, from www.hospitalmanagement.net/ihf/projects.html.

Jones, M. E., Cason, C. L., & Bond, M. L. (2004). Cultural attitudes, knowledge, and skills of a health workforce. *Journal of Transcultural Nursing, 15,* 282–290.

Kiger, P. J. (2004). The art of the apology. *Workforce Management, 81(10),* 57–58, 60–62.

Lathrop, J. P. (1993). *Restructuring health care: The patient-focused paradigm.* New York: John Wiley.

Lorig, K M., Ritter, P. L., & Gonzalez, V. M. (2003). Hispanic chronic disease self-management: A randomized community-based outcome trial. *Nursing Research, 52,* 361–369.

Lynn, M. R., & McMillen, B. J. (2004). The scale product technique as a means of enhancing the measurement of patient satisfaction. *Canadian Journal of Nursing Research, 36,* 66–81.

Malone, B. L. (1993). Caring for culturally diverse racial groups: An administrative matter. *Nursing Administration Quarterly, 17*(2), 21–29.

Meade, C. D., Calvo, A., Rivera, M. A., & Baer, R. D. (2003). Focus groups in the design of prostate cancer screening information for Hispanic farmworkers and African-American men. *Oncology Nursing Forum, 30,* 967–975.

Melnyk, B. M., Alpert-Gillis, L., Feinstein, N. F., Crean, H. F., Johnson, J., Fairbanks, E., et al. (2004). Creating opportunities for parent empowerment: Program effects on the mental health/coping outcomes of critically ill young children and their mothers. *Pediatrics, 113,* 597–607.

National Alliance for Hispanic Health. (2000). *Quality health services for Hispanics: The cultural competency component.* Washington, DC: Department of Health and Human Services.

National Quality Forum. (2005, May). National Quality Forum endorses survey of patient perception of care. Washington, DC: Author. Retrieved May 29, 2006, from www.qualityforum.org/news.

Nielson-Bohlman, L., Panzer, A. M., & Kindig, D. A. (Eds.). Committee on Health Literacy, Board on Neuroscience and Behavioral Health, Institute of Medicine. (2004). *Health literacy: A prescription to end confusion.* Washington, DC: National Academies Press.

Nolin, J., & Killackey, J. (2004). Redirecting health care spending: Consumer-directed health care. *Nursing Economics, 22,* 251–253, 257.

Office of Minority Health. (2001). *National standards for culturally and linguistically appropriate services in health care (CLAS).* Washington, DC: U.S. Department of Health and Human Services. Retrieved July 22, 2006, from www.omhrc.gov/assets/pdf/checked/finalreport.pdf.

Page, A. (Ed.), Committee on the Work Environment for Nurses and Patient Safety. Board on Health Care Services. (2004). *Keeping patients safe: Transforming the work environment of nurses.* Washington, DC: National Academies Press.

Pope, C. (2005). Addressing limited English proficiency and disparities for Hispanic postpartum women. *Journal of Obsteric, Gynecologic, and Neonatal Nursing, 34,* 512–520.

Porter-O'Grady, T. (2003). Of hubris and hope: Transforming nursing for a new age. *Nursing Economics, 21,* 59–64.

Ratzan, S. C., & Parker, R. M. (2000). Introduction. In Selden C. R., Zorn M., Ratzan S. C., Parker R. M., (Eds.), *National Library of Medicine Current Bibliographies in Medicine: Health Literacy.* NLM Pub. No. CBM 2000-1. Bethesda, MD: National Institutes of Health. U.S. Department of Health and Human Services. Retrieved May 29, 2006, from www.nlm.nih.gov/pubs/cbm/hliteracy.pdf.

Rosenthal, M. B., Berndt, E. R., Donohue, J. M., Frank, R. G., & Epstein, A. M. (2002). Promotion of prescription drugs to consumers. *New England Journal of Medicine, 346,* 498–505.

Sauaia, A., Min, S. J., Leber, C., Erbacher, K., Abrams, F., & Fink, R. (2005). Postoperative pain management in elderly patients: Correlation between adherence to treatment guidelines and patient satisfaction. *Journal of the American Geriatrics Society, 53,* 274–282.

Schmidt, L A. (2004). Patients' perceptions of nurse staffing, nursing care, adverse events, and overall satisfaction with the hospital experience. *Nursing Economics, 22,* 295–306.

Scotti, D. J. & Stinerock, R. N. (2003). Cognitive predictors of satisfaction with hospital inpatient service encounters among the elderly: A matter of trust. *Journal of Hospital Marketing and Public Relations, 14*(2), 3–22.

Shin, H. B., & Bruno, R. (2003, October). *Language use and English speaking ability: 2000* (Census 2000 brief). U.S. Census Bureau, U.S. Department of Commerce, Economics and Statistics Administration. Retrieved July 22, 2006, from www.census.gov/prod/2003pubs/c2kbr-29.pdf.

Sobo, E. J. (2004). Pediatric nurses may misjudge parent communication preferences. *Journal of Nursing Care Quality, 19,* 253–262.

Steinbinder, A., & Scherer, E. (2006). Creating nursing system excellence through the forces for Magnetism. In K. Malloch & T. Porter-O'Grady (Eds.), *Introduction to evidence-based practice in nursing and health care.* Boston: Jones & Bartlett.

Sullivan Commission. (2004). *Missing persons: Minorities in the health professions.* A report of the Sullivan Commission on diversity in the workforce. Retrieved May 29, 2006, from www.amsa.org/advocacy/Sullivan_Commission.pdf.

Taylor, H. (2003). Scientists, firemen, doctors, teachers and nurses top list as "Most Prestigious Occupations." The Harris Poll # 57, October 1, 2003. Retrieved May 29, 2006 from http://www.harrisinteractive.com/harris_poll/index.asp?PID = 406.

Tropello, P. G. D. (2003). Magnet status as a competitive strategy of hospital organization: Marketing a culture of excellence in nursing services. *Journal of Hospital Marketing and Public Relations, 14,* 53–57.

Ulrich, B. (2005, December 19). Looking back, looking forward. *Nursing Spectrum.* Retrieved May 29, 2006, from http://community.nursingspectrum.com.

Urden, L. (2002). Patient satisfaction measurement: Current issues and implications. *Lippincott's Case Management, 7,* 194–200.

Valimaki, M., Leino-Kilpi, H., Gronroos, M., Dassen, T., Gasull, M., Lemonidou, C., Scott, P. A., et al. (2004). Self-determination in surgical patients in five European countries. *Journal of Nursing Scholarship, 36,* 205–311.

Weiner, J., Aguirre, A., Ravenell, K., Kovath, K., McDevit, L., Murphy, J., et al. (2004). Designing an illustrated patient satisfaction instrument for low-literacy populations. *American Journal of Managed Care, 10,* 853–860.

Williams, T. (2002). Patient empowerment and ethical decision making: The patient/partner and the right to act. *Dimensions of Critical Care Nursing, 21,* 100–104.

Winslow, E. H. (2001). Patient education materials. *American Journal of Nursing, 101*(10), 33–38.

Wolf, Z. R., & Serembus, J. F. (2004). Medication errors: Ending the blame-game. *Nursing Management, 35*(8), 41–48.

Wolff, M., Spens, R., Young, S. Lucey, P., Cooper, J., Ahmed, S. et al. (2003). Patient empowerment strategies for a safety net. *Nursing Economics, 21,* 219–225.

World Health Organization. (nd). Cross-cutting: Noncommunicable dieases. Retrieved May 30, 2006, from www.who.int/mdg/cross_cutting/noncommunicable_diseases/en.

Wylie, J. L., & Wagenfeld-Heintz, E. (2004). Development of relationship-centered care. *Journal of Healthcare Quality, 26*(1), 14–21, 45, 60.

SUGGESTED READINGS

Aday, L. (2001). *At risk in America: The health and health care needs of vulnerable populations in the United States* (2nd ed.). San Francisco: Jossey-Bass.

Geron, S. M., Smith, K., Tennstedt, S., Jette, A., Chassler, D., & Kasten, L. (2000). The home care satisfaction measure: A client-centered approach to assessing the satisfaction of frail older adults with home care services. *Journals of Gerontology Series B, 55,* S259–S270.

Lipson, L. G., & Dibble, S. L. (Eds.) (2005). *Culture and clinical care.* San Francisco: UCSF Nursing Press.

Osborne, L. (2003). *Resolving patient complaints: A step by step guide to service recovery* (2nd ed.). Boston: Jones-Bartlett.

Press, I. (2002). *Patient satisfaction: Defining, measuring and improving the experience of care.* Chicago: Health Administration Press.

Radwin, L., Alster, K., & Rubin, K. M. (2003). Development and testing of the Oncology Patients' Perceptions of the Quality of Nursing Care Scale. *Oncology Nursing Forum, 30,* 283–290.

Woodring, S., Polomano, R. C., Haagen, B. F., Haack, M. M., Nunn, R. R., Miller, G. L., et al. (2004). Development and testing of patient satisfaction measure for inpatient psychiatry care. *Journal of Nursing Care Quality, 19,* 137–148.

WEBSITES

Agency on Healthcare Research and Quality Information for Consumers and Patients: www.ahrq.gov/consumer/

Cultural Diversity in Health Care: www.ggalanti.com/index.html

Cultural Diversity in Nursing: www.culturediversity.org/

EurasiaHealth Knowledge Network: www.eurasiahealth.org

FirstGov for Consumer Health: www.consumer.gov/health.htm

Health Canada: www.hc-sc.gc.ca/index_e.html

Health on the Net Foundation: www.hon.ch

Healthsites: Your Portal to Medical Information on the Net: www.healthsites.co.uk/index.php

Institute of Medicine: www.iom.edu

Medline Plus: Trusted Health Information for You: www.nlm.nih.gov/medlineplus/

National Health Information Center, U. S. Department of Health and Human Services: http://healthfinder.gov/

National Institutes of Health, Health Information: http://health.nih.gov/

Office of Minority Health: www.omhrc.gov

World Health Organization: www.who.int

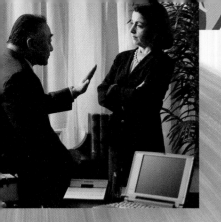

Chapter

22

Conflict: The Cutting Edge of Change

Mary Ann T. Donohue

To resolve conflicts, nurse leaders must be able to determine the nature of a particular issue, choose the most appropriate approach for each situation, and implement a course of action. Therefore, an understanding of organizational culture, personality theory, and stress will help the nurse leader and manager accept the nature of individual differences and capitalize on the group members' collective strengths. This chapter focuses on maximizing the nurse leader's and manager's ability to deal with conflict by providing effective strategies for conflict resolution. Because some conflicts are, by nature, unresolvable, an understanding of polarities and polarity management will also help the nurse leader and manager capitalize on the positives in any difficult situation.

Objectives

- Use a model of the conflict process to determine the nature and sources of hypothetical and actual conflict.
- Assess your preferred approaches to conflict and commit to be more effective in resolving future conflict.
- Determine which of the five optional approaches to conflict is the most appropriate in hypothetical and real situations.

- Diagram the structure and dynamics of important polarities (unresolvable conflicts) and identify ways to manage them.

Questions to Consider

- *What situations, issues, and people trigger conflict for you? Why? How do you trigger conflict for others?*
- *How do you usually determine why people are having conflict? How do you usually react to and resolve conflict?*
- *What typical consequences occur from conflicts in which you are involved?*
- *How have you tended to handle unresolvable or recurring conflicts in the past? How could you handle them in the future?*

The Challenge

Midge Grady, RN, BC, Nurse Manager; Sandra Gauker, MSN, RN, APN, C., Advanced Practice Nurse; Diego Coira, MD, Chairman, Department of Psychiatry and Behavioral Medicine, Hackensack University Medical Center, Hackensack, New Jersey

During the past several years, the census on our 24-bed, acute in-patient psychiatric unit has been extremely labile. At our multidisciplinary Behavioral Health Performance Improvement Service Line meetings, we began to discuss the possibility of providing care to the psychiatric patient who is also medically compromised. In terms of the medical center at-large, we were very much aware that the volume and average daily census often exceeded bed capacity for the medical-surgical (med-surg) patient. We thought that our unit could be of assistance in offering the capability to transfer patients with a primary psychiatric diagnosis who also had medical or surgical issues. Prior to this, we had not been able to provide the appropriate level of care for this type of patient.

We knew that our nursing staff, all of whom had always incorporated the medical diagnosis of our psychiatric population into their existing treatment plans, had never before taken care of patients with intravenous lines, Foley catheters, and more complicated physical assessment needs, to name a few. There were at least several nurses who had never worked on a med-surg unit, but had come directly into the specialty of psychiatric mental health nursing after graduation.

When we held our round-the-clock meetings with the staff, their responses to the change varied. At least one staff member opted for early retirement, and many expressed the thought that perhaps the unit would gradually take on so many patients with medical illnesses that, at some point, it would give up its identity and licensure as a psychiatric unit. Most staff responses, however, fell somewhere in between: expressing the lack of confidence in obtaining or regaining their med-surg skills, and recognizing that this change would not have been anyone's preference in the first place.

The conflict was this: How would the staff balance the needs of the medically ill psychiatric patient, continue to serve the needs of the acutely ill psychiatric patient, and assimilate both into the existing treatment activities and groups—how to manage for example, the patient who is experiencing active suicidal or psychotic thinking into a group alongside patients with IVs and other medical devices?

 What do you think you would do if you were a nurse in this team?

INTRODUCTION

Conflict. We all say we would like to *know* how conflict can be resolved rationally, logically, and effectively; however, most of us would rather not "deal" with it at all—we would much rather busy ourselves with just about anything else. When confronting the problem becomes unavoidable, however, it is indeed tempting to turn to simple solutions to be done with it. It would follow, then, that defining conflict and then exhorting managers to follow fail-proof strategies to address comprises much of the literature on the topic: A quick look at this week's business bestsellers, or a search engine review, for instance, on the subject of conflict reso-

lution yields numerous illustrations of this point. The error in formulaic approaches, however, is the assumption that conflict is inherently negative. Second, following a series of steps rarely leads to permanent solutions and, finally, resolution is not always desirable or tenable in every situation.

Before we can try to resolve conflict, we must understand its nature. **Conflict** primarily stems from a clash in individuals' or groups' values, differences in beliefs, attitudes, and expectations (Conerly & Tripathi, 2004). Conflicts are about much more than simple disagreements. Conflict arises from a strong sense, a feeling of incompatibility. It represents an escalation of everyday competition and discussion into an arena of emotional or even hostile encounters that put a strain on personal or interpersonal tranquility, or both (Scott, 1990, p. 1). Perhaps the most difficult to accept is the idea that conflict can be a strategic tool when addressed appropriately, and that it can actually serve to deepen and develop human relationships (Porter-O'Grady, 2003). Some of the first authors on **organizational conflict** (Blake & Mouton, 1964), for example, claimed that a complete resolution of conflict might in fact be undesirable because conflict also stimulates growth, creativity, and even a refreshing change for the better.

As human beings leading increasingly complicated and stressful lives, we naturally bring with us to the workplace a certain preoccupation with events of the home and heart. Depending on the enormity of the issue in the worker's own personal life, complicated matters on the job may produce compounding stress that is significant (Berstene, 2004). In the corporate world, there is no shortage of issues from which conflict may arise. For example, many employees are faced with an ever-present threat to lifetime job security that used to be the mainstay of many American workers. One current threat is the practice of outsourcing, e.g., obtaining needed technical talent and goods from foreign countries and shifting career opportunities away from the United States itself. The healthcare environment is also not without its stressful effects. Here, workers are exposed to very high stress levels from increased demands on an ever-limited and aging workforce, a decrease in available resources, and a more acutely ill and underinsured patient population. A groundbreaking body of literature has tied the stress of poorer nursing staffing patterns to correspondingly higher levels of job dissatisfaction and burnout, significantly higher levels of risk-adjusted mortality, and failure to rescue (Aiken, Clarke, Sloane, Sochalski & Silber, 2002). Indeed, Dr. Linda Aiken's research team has examined the relationship between stress on the nurse (burnout) as well as the patient (Vahey, Aiken, Sloane, Clarke, & Vargas, 2004), and found that, among other critical variables, patients cared for on units with good relations (as in diminished episodes of conflict) between their own doctors and nurses were more than twice as likely to be satisfied with their care and, as an added "bonus," their nurses also reported lower burnout and dissatisfaction with their jobs.

An important ingredient to the successful management of stress and conflict is a better understanding of its context within the specific workplace. Today, as in the past, members of the healthcare team have not been forthright about their feelings of stress and fatigue. Furthermore, nursing administrators have not been accustomed to making changes that show respect for staff members' concerns about how such factors contribute to conflict in the workplace. Instead, we have unfortunately created a culture of "shame and blame" whereby the overwhelmed nurse is left feeling alone, angry, and somehow single-handedly responsible for the structural weakness of an entire organization. Other stressful occupations, such as the aviation field, have conscientiously created a culture whereby fatigue, stress, and errors are readily identified as areas for continuous improvement (Sexton, Thomas, & Helmreich, 2000). Such strategies, borrowed from business and industry, are just beginning to permeate the healthcare arena, perhaps because the performance improvement and quality literature is now able to establish the connection between caregiver stress and patient safety (Rogers, Hwang, Scott, Aiken, & Dinges, 2004). The landmark Institute of Medicine publication, *Keeping Patients Safe: Transforming the Work Environment of Nurses* (Page, 2004), declared that even voluntary overtime is potentially dangerous to the well-being of hospitalized patients.

At the practitioner level, the partnerships we have with one another vis-a-vis the larger organization may often threaten the quality of full participation and unity as well as the ability to fully connect with each other in a meaningful way (Cloke & Goldsmith, 2000). The organizations that tolerate and perhaps even promote or endorse destructive behaviors have not yet fully integrated such everyday variables such as gender (Valentine, 2001), culture (von Glinow, Shapiro, & Brett, 2004), ethics (Dubler & Liebman, 2004), and even to the degree one uses politeness strategies (Jameson, 2004). Women, for example, are more known for their use of compromise and avoidance, as opposed to a more open acknowledgment of the factors contributing to the issues causing the conflict and may thus be unwitting saboteurs of the resolution process. Kramer and Schmalenberg (2005), commenting on their analysis of the quality of the relationship between nurses and physicians, pointed out that physicians work best with nurses who demonstrate that they "know their patients" (p. 197). Given the wide variation in staffing patterns and the looming nursing shortage that exists in hospitals today, the root cause of some nurse–physician relationship conflicts may very well lie at the heart of the nurse–patient relationship instead. Unfortunately, one report (Farrell, 1999) indicated that nurses were actually more fearful and concerned about staff-staff, that is colleague-colleague, aggression as a distress factor when compared with other workplace issues.

TYPES OF CONFLICT

Conflict occurs in all areas of our lives and in three broad categories. Conflict can be intrapersonal, interpersonal, or organizational in nature.

Intrapersonal conflict occurs within a person. Questions often arise that create a conflict over priorities, ethical standards, and different ways to act. When a nurse manager decides what to do about the future (e.g., "Do I really want to study for a higher degree or should we start our family now?"), there are conflicts between personal and professional priorities. Some issues present a conflict over comfortably maintaining the status quo (e.g., "My relationship with the experienced nurses on the unit is pretty smooth right now, so why would I want to rock the boat?") or taking risks to make suggestions and confront people when needed (e.g., "Would telling them their way of doing things could use a little fine-tuning and recommending some improvements that I learned about in school jeopardize my rapport with them?").

Interpersonal conflict occurs when we realize that everybody does not see the world in exactly the same way. There are conflicts between and among patients, nurses, care teams, family members, physicians, one's own staff members, and members of other departments. A manager may be called upon to assist two nurses in resolving a scheduling conflict or to determine whether sharing particularly sensitive information would be a violation of confidentiality. Patients—and indeed most of us—resist suggestions for making changes to diet, exercise, and health habits. Members of healthcare teams often have disputes over the best way to treat particular cases or how much information is necessary for patients and families to have about their illness or other factors regarding their hospitalization. Yet, interpersonal conflict is part of life, is quite common, can serve as the impetus for needed change, and can accelerate innovation (Hagel & Brown, 2005).

Organizational conflict occurs when there is discord, as when there is dissonance between policies and procedures, or formal personnel codes of conduct, and informally accepted norms of behavior and patterns of communication. Some organizational conflict is related to hierarchical structure and role differentiation among employees, such as in labor and management negotiations or financial administrators' and department heads' arguments over budgetary matters. Nurse managers, as well as their staffs, often become embattled in institution-wide conflict concerning staffing patterns and how they affect the quality of care for which they are also held ultimately responsible. Increasingly, they may become troubled by the consequences of a greater emphasis on technology, research, and the financial bottom line when it appears to come at the price of limiting access to care for the poor and underprivileged. Complex ethical and moral dilemmas often arise when profitable services are increased and unprofitable ones are downsized or even eliminated.

A major source of organizational conflict now stems from new systems that promote more participation and autonomy of staff nurses. Increasingly, nurses are charged with determining as well as carrying out direct patient care and acting to meet institutional goals to bring about quality patient care improvement. The Magnet™ Recognition Program of the American Nurses Credentialing Center (2005) identifies autonomy as one of the fourteen "Forces of Magnetism", based on the belief that staff nurses who share in the governance process of an institution experience job satisfaction, an important measure of personal fulfillment and organization success. Yet, an empowered nursing staff simultaneously revise their roles and relationships with nurse managers (Keenan, Hurst, & Olnhausen, 1993). As staff nurses assume more autonomy and accountability for identifying areas for quality improvement in patient care, they may desire a greater voice in organization-wide politics and openly campaign for diversity and inclusiveness. At the same time, managers' span of control steadily increases, so previously clear (and perhaps, more manageable?) roles become even more blurred and subsequently cry out for redefinition, particularly in multidisciplinary workgroups with its demand for one to develop the ability to hold expanding perspectives, without judgment (Swanson, 2004). Internal change such as this involves not only organizational conflict, but also intrapersonal and interpersonal conflict, requiring deft management of once unimagined variables.

Another source of conflict has to do with the **allocation of scarce resources.** In the past, it was assumed that moral and ethical standards would nearly always override financial concerns in health care. In the United States, however, increased expenditures have failed to demonstrate the best results. The "One Hundred K Lives" campaign of the Institute for Healthcare Improvement (IHI) is established to reduce harm and save lives caused by faulty patient-care systems (IHI, 2005; McCue, 2005a; McCue, 2005b). Nurse leaders must provide the best example of advocacy to their staff by coaching newer nurses to think differently than ever before—daily drawing the link between nursing practice and quality outcomes:

- How can we quantify it?
- What can we do about it?
- What evidence will show that we have achieved the desired outcome? (Porter-O'Grady, 1999).
- Are we committed to implementing change that is proven to save lives? (IHI, 2005).

THE CONFLICT PROCESS

Conflict proceeds through four stages: frustration, conceptualization, action, and outcomes (Hurst & Kinney, 1989; Kinney & Hurst, 1989). The ability to resolve conflicts productively depends on understanding this process (Figure 22-1) and on developing creative ways to deal with conflict. Notice how the arrows in Figure 22-1 flow both ways between stages. This illustrates that moving into a subsequent stage may lead to a return to and change in a previous stage. For instance, two nurses view the conflict (conceptualize it) as a fight, a battle to control. A third nurse thinks it is all about professional standards. They have expressed much frustration and mistrust. A nurse leader/manager gets them all to talk. All agree that the real conflict comes from a difference in goals or priorities, which leads to less negative emotion and ends with a much clearer understanding of all the issues.

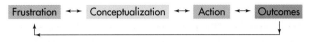

Figure 22-1   Stages of the conflict process.

Frustration

When people or groups perceive that their goals may be blocked, they feel frustrated. This frustration may escalate into stronger emotions, such as anger and deep resignation. This frustration comes from what people believe to be true, even though there may not be a real conflict at all! For example, a nurse may perceive that a patient is uncooperative when in reality the patient is afraid or has had a different set of priorities at the start from those of the nurse. At the same time, the patient may view the nurse as controlling and insensitive. When such frustrations occur, it is a cue to stop and clarify the nature of major differences.

Conceptualization

Everyone involved develops an idea or picture of what the conflict is about. This may be an instant "snapshot," or it may develop over time. This concept of the conflict may be very clear in people's minds, or it may be very fuzzy. Everyone involved has an individual interpretation of what the conflict is and why it is occurring. Most often, these interpretations are different and involve the person's own perspective, which is based on personal values, beliefs, and culture.

Regardless of its clarity or accuracy, however, conceptualization forms the basis for everyone's reactions to the frustration. The way the individuals perceive and define the conflict has a great deal of influence on the creative resolution and productive outcomes to follow. For example, within the same conflict situation, some individuals may see the conflict as insubordination, become angry at the threat to his/her role, and fall back upon rigid reliance on policy and procedure. Others may view it as trivial bickering and voice criticism, as in "We've been over this subject already, why can't you just drop it" and complain or withdraw. Such differences in conceptualizing the issue block its resolution. Thus, it is important for each person to clarify "the conflict as I see it" and "how it makes me feel" before all the people involved can define the conflict (i.e., develop an accurate conceptualization together) and proceed to resolve their differences.

People are not likely to reach outcomes that truly resolve the conflict and satisfy them unless their own leaders promote clear and ethical values themselves and permit understanding of the differences among their own workgroups. During the conceptualization process, we can ask several very powerful questions:

1. What is the nature of our differences?
2. What are the reasons for those differences?
3. Does our leader endorse behaviors that add to the conflict?
4. If so, do I need to be mentored by someone else, even if they are outside of my own department or work area?

People may differ on four aspects of a conflict: facts; goals; methods to achieve goals; and the values or standards used to select goals, priorities, and methods. Providing accurate information is usually easier than working out differences in values, priorities, methodology, and standards. Disagreements over facts may uncover conflicts over goals, means, and values, which may lead to the conflict expanding or even escalating out of control. Values, opinions, and beliefs are much more personal, thus generating disagreements that can be threatening and adversarial. The more accurately any conflict is defined, the more likely it will be resolved, but this is often where attempts at resolution fail.

Action

Intentions, strategies, plans, and behavior "flow" out of the conceptualization. A pattern of interaction among the individuals involved is set in motion (e.g., "Let's work together" or "We're not getting any place this way"). As actions are taken to resolve the conflict, the way that some or all parties conceptualize the conflict may change. The important point is that people are always taking some action regarding the conflict, even if that action is **avoiding** it or deciding to do nothing.

There are five distinct action-oriented approaches to resolving conflict. The longer ineffective actions continue, the more likely people will experience frustration, resistance, or even hostility. Bacal (2004) uses the term "ugly" to refer to attempts to downplay and pretend conflict does not exist:

When it is part of the organizational culture to pressure staff to "smile and nod" when asked "everything's ok, right?" when everyone knows it isn't (Ugly Strategy One: Nonaction)

A common, although no less troubling, way for managers to avoid conflict in the workplace is to not respond to colleagues' attempts at professional communication in voice mails or e-mail messages or making a habit of canceling meetings. If this behavior is known by his or her leader and continues, the avoiding behavior is said to be endorsed or approved. Worse, a leader may make mention of another team member's failure in a particular area, while remaining silent about another's well-known transgressions, giving rise to a distressing double standard (Ugly Strategy Two: Administrative Orbiting).

Another means of getting around conflict is having secrets. Not letting people know where you are during the day; having back-stage discussions about, rather than with, the involved parties; and playing favorites all amount to scenarios with a high potential for fueling, rather than dealing with, the actual conflict in the first place (Ugly Strategy Three: Secrecy).

A most unfortunate choice, yet one painfully recalled by anyone who has ever worked as a staff nurse, is the leader who relies on regulations, power, policy, and procedure. Destructive because it thwarts healthy discussion and challenge to the status quo, the manager who uses it most frequently thinks that by quoting line and verse, conflict can actually go away (Ugly Strategy Four: Law and Order).

The more the actions appropriately match the nature of the conflict, the more likely it will be resolved with desirable results. There is room for improvement, when there is plenty of discord, complaining, gossiping, and time spent on self-preservation instead of resolving differences (p. 22).

Outcomes

Tangible and intangible consequences, or "outcomes," result from the actions taken. The conflict may be resolved with a new plan that incorporates the goals of two or more people to ensure that no one loses. Productivity and efficiency may increase, decrease, or stay the same. Emotions may be high, and anger and resistance may remain, resulting in further conflicts. Relationships may be strengthened, weakened, or ended. Such outcomes have very important consequences in the work setting. Assessing the degree of conflict resolution (Box 22-1) is useful for improving individual and group skills in resolutions.

Exercise 22-1

Recall a situation in which conflict was apparent. Note arguments each person/side made and how each responded to the other's comments. What was the outcome? Was the conflict resolved? Was anything left unresolved?

Two general outcomes are considered when assessing the degree to which a conflict has been resolved: the degree to which important goals were achieved and the nature of the subsequent relationships among those involved (Boxes 22-2 and 22-3). Four questions can be asked about the nature of the subsequent relationships (Johnson & Johnson, 1997): (1) Are the relationships stronger, and are people better able to interact? (2) Do the members like and trust each other more? (3) Are all the members satisfied with the results of the conflict? (4) Have group members become more able to resolve future conflicts with one another?

Exercise 22-2

It is time to assess your tendencies to approach conflict. As you read and answer the 30-item conflict survey in Box 22-3, think of how you face and respond to conflict in professional situations. After completing the survey, tally, total, and reflect on your scores for each of the five approaches. Consider the following questions:

- Which approaches do you prefer? Which do you use least?
- Why do you think you tend to act that way?
- Considering the types of conflicts you tend to have, what are the strengths and weaknesses of your pattern?
- Have others mentioned information that could be valuable to you?
- As you read the rest of this section, use this pattern of scores and your reflections to examine the appropriate uses of each approach, assess your use of each approach more extensively, and commit to new behaviors to increase your future effectiveness.

BOX 22-1

Assessing the Degree of Conflict Resolution

I. Quality of decisions
   A. How creative are resulting plans?
   B. How practical and realistic are they?
   C. How well were intended goals achieved?
   D. What surprising results were achieved?
II. Quality of relationships
   A How much understanding has been created?
   B. How willing are people to work together?
   C. How much mutual respect, empathy, concern, and cooperation has been generated?

Modified from Hurst, J., & Kinney, M. (1989). *Empowering self and others.* Toledo, OH: University of Toledo.

MODES OF CONFLICT RESOLUTION

Five general, distinct approaches can be used in conflict resolution: avoiding, accommodating, **competing, compromising,** and collaborating (Johnson & Johnson, 1997; Thomas & Kilmann, 1973). These approaches can be viewed along two different continua: from uncooperative to highly cooperative and from unassertive to highly assertive (Thomas, 1975). (See the Conflict Self-Assessment in Box 22-3.)

On the cooperative continuum, actions can range from complete competition to total cooperation. Two nurses might compete for a manager position on the one extreme while teaming cooperatively to institute the practice of multidisciplinary rounding on their unit. On the assertiveness continuum, actions range from ignoring one's own goals (highly unassertive) to doing what it takes to get what one wants (highly assertive). A nurse might forgo asking for time to attend an outside conference, class, or professional meeting (unassertive) because the clinical manager predicts the unit might be understaffed and overly busy (assertive).

It is unlikely that anyone would select any one approach to the exclusion of the rights of others. In fact, as we will examine later in the discussion of polarity management, people tend to move

BOX 22-2

Snapshot of Two Conflicts

UNPRODUCTIVE

Suppose I perceive a conflict between you and me because you disagree with my ideas about how to motivate others to achieve 100% patient satisfaction. Looking at the four stages in the process of conflict, we might find the following in an unproductive conflict:

1. I am **frustrated** working together on the patient satisfaction committee because you usually put down my ideas for change. **You** are frustrated because you perceive that I do not support your goals for improved patient care.

2. I see **(conceptualize)** the conflict as your ignorance of new concepts and research findings. Besides, you want things pretty much your way. **You** see it as my eagerness to "shake up" people, promote myself as a leader, and increase my power.

3. **My** view leads to my being forceful (action) with you and sharing new research studies and articles that I have found to prove my point, which confirms your judgment of me. **You** resist me with your considerations about why the new techniques will not work and by refusing to read the articles and not answering my e-mail or telephone calls.

4. The **outcome** is that **we** have created a **defensive climate** and a lack of desire to work together. We have clouded the real issue and generated hostility among all members of the group. The committee submits a compromise plan to which no one is committed and it then disbands. **The project essentially has failed.**

PRODUCTIVE

The same conflict could present itself and evolve through the same process with different outcomes:

1. I feel **frustrated** that we have to work on the same committee together because I believe that you tend to resist and disagree with my ideas for change. **You** seem to think that what the organization is doing now works just fine because you have not come up with any innovations in response to our scores.

2. As **we talk,** we realize **(conceptualize)** that we want the same thing: incentives to support patient satisfaction.

3. Our commitment to getting these incentives spurs us to identify critical areas for study. At the same time, **we decide (action)** that we need to look at new plans and research to suggest improvements and additions for our patient satisfaction initiatives. I say, "If you look at current and new plans, I will work on securing supporting research." We agree and others on the committee agree to do other necessary tasks.

4. The committee then prioritizes areas for study and develops a time frame **(outcomes).** It creates an incentive program **combining the strengths** of our plan with some new ideas to promote internal motivation and productivity and recommends it to the personnel committee. The committee continues, and the **project is successful**.

horizontally or vertically between these continua in some combined set of actions that are appropriately assertive and cooperative, depending on the nature of the conflict situation.

Avoiding

Avoiding, or withdrawing, is very unassertive and uncooperative because avoiders neither pursue their own needs, goals, and concerns immediately nor assist others to pursue theirs. The positive side of withdrawing may take the form of diplomatically side-stepping or postponing an issue until a better time or simply walking away from a "no-win" situation (Box 22-4). The self-assessment in Box 22-5 will help you recognize your own avoidance behaviors and use them more effectively.

Accommodating/Smoothing

When accommodating, people neglect their own needs, goals, and concerns (unassertive) while trying to satisfy those of others (cooperative). This approach has an element about it of being self-sacrificing and simply obeying orders or serving other people. For example, sometimes we do not care where we eat, but others in our group do. So we say, "Fine, let's eat there! I like all kinds of food. I'm really hungry, so let's go." Box 22-6 lists some appropriate uses of **accommodation.**

Accommodators often feel disappointment and resentment because they "get nothing in return." This is a built-in by-product of the overuse of this approach. The self-assessment in Box 22-7 asks you to examine your current use of accommodation and challenges you to think of new ways to use it more effectively.

Competing/Coercing

During competition, people pursue their own needs and goals at the expense of others. Sometimes

---

BOX 22-3

Conflict Self-Assessment

Directions: Read each of the following statements. Assess yourself in terms of how often you tend to act similarly during conflict at work. Place the number of the most appropriate response in the blank in front of each statement. Put 1 if the behavior is never typical of how you act during a conflict, 2 if it is seldom typical, 3 if it is occasionally typical, 4 if it is frequently typical, or 5 if it is very typical of how you act during conflict.

_____ 1. Create new possibilities to address all important concerns.

_____ 2. Persuade others to see it and/or do it my way.

_____ 3. Work out some sort of give-and-take agreement.

_____ 4. Let other people have their way.

_____ 5. Wait and let the conflict take care of itself.

_____ 6. Find ways that everyone can win.

_____ 7. Use whatever power I have to get what I want.

_____ 8. Find an agreeable compromise among people involved.

_____ 9. Give in so others get what they think is important.

_____ 10. Withdraw from the situation.

_____ 11. Cooperate assertively until everyone's needs are met.

_____ 12. Compete until I either win or lose.

_____ 13. Engage in "give a little and get a little" bargaining.

_____ 14. Let others' needs be met more than my own needs.

_____ 15. Avoid taking any action for as long as I can.

_____ 16. Partner with others to find the most inclusive solution.

_____ 17. Put my foot down assertively for a quick solution.

_____ 18. Negotiate for what all sides value and can live without.

_____ 19. Agree to what others want to create harmony.

_____ 20. Keep as far away from others involved as possible.

_____ 21. Stick with it to get everyone's highest priorities.

_____ 22. Argue and debate over the best way.

_____ 23. Create some middle position everyone agrees to.

_____ 24. Put my priorities below those of other people.

_____ 25. Hope the issue does not come up.

_____ 26. Collaborate with others to achieve our goals together.

_____ 27. Compete with others for scarce resources.

_____ 28. Emphasize compromise and trade-offs.

_____ 29. Cool things down by letting others do it their way.

_____ 30. Change the subject to avoid the fighting.

Continued

BOX 22-3

Conflict Self-Assessment—cont'd

Conflict Self-Assessment Scoring

Look at the numbers you placed in the blanks on the conflict assessment. Write the number you placed in each blank on the appropriate line below. Add up your total for each column, and enter that total on the appropriate line. The greater your total is for each approach, the more often you tend to use that approach when conflict occurs at work. The lower the score, the less often you tend to use that approach when conflict occurs at work.

COLLABORATING	COMPETING	COMPROMISING	ACCOMMODATING	AVOIDING
1. _____	2. _____	3. _____	4. _____	5. _____
6. _____	7. _____	8. _____	9. _____	10. _____
11. _____	12. _____	13. _____	14. _____	15. _____
16. _____	17. _____	18. _____	19. _____	20. _____
21. _____	22. _____	23. _____	24. _____	25. _____
26. _____	27. _____	28. _____	29. _____	30. _____
Total _____	Total _____	Total _____	Total _____	TOTAL _____

Throughout the rest of this section, there are descriptions of each approach and related self-assessment and commitment-to-action activities. Use these totals to stimulate your thinking about how you do and could handle conflict at work. Most important, consider if your pattern of frequency tends to be consistent, or inconsistent, with the types of conflicts you face. That is, does your way of dealing with conflict tend to match the situations in which that approach is most useful?

From Hurst, J. B. (1993). Human Resource Development Center, University of Toledo, OH.

BOX 22-4

Appropriate Uses for the Avoiding Approach

1. When facing trivial and/or temporary issues, or when other far more important issues are pressing (e.g., tangential issues are only symptoms of deeper conflicts)
2. When there is no chance to obtain what one wants or needs, or when others could resolve the conflict more efficiently and effectively
3. When the potential negative results of initiating and acting on a conflict are much greater than the benefits of its resolution
4. When people need to "cool down," distance themselves, or gather more information, perhaps gaining a hindsight or meaningful view

people use whatever power, creativeness, or strategies are available to "win." Competing may also take the form of standing up for your rights or defending important principles, as when we contend for limited funds (Box 22-8).

People who compete so well so often may not even be able to hear the truth, or have much tolerance when others disagree and challenge them, even when they are wrong. They often react by feeling threatened or acting defensively or aggressively, or even resort to cruelty in the form of razor-sharp remarks ("We may as well call the Joint Commission on ourselves, you've all done such a bad job, and you'd better start writing your resignation letters") or well-aimed gossip or hurtful innuendo ("Did you see that outfit that consultant was wearing? How can we possibly take her observations about us very seriously?"). Competition within work groups can generate ill will, favor a win-lose stance, and commit people to a stalemate. Such behaviors force people into a corner from which there is no easy or graceful exit, a "damned if I do and damned if I don't" form of a double-bind that gives rise to the unfortunate culture of a so-called "shame and blame" mentality. Use Box 22-9 to help you learn to use competing more effectively.

Negotiating/Compromising

Negotiating involves both assertiveness and co-operation on the part of everyone and requires

BOX 22-5

Avoidance: Self-Assessment and Commitment to Action

If You Tend to Use Avoidance Often, Ask Yourself the Following Questions:
1. Do people have difficulty getting my input into and understanding my view of conflicts?
2. Do I block cooperative efforts to resolve issues?
3. Am I distancing myself from significant others?
4. Are important issues being left unidentified and unresolved?

If You Seldom Use Avoidance, Ask Yourself the Following Questions:
1. Do I find myself overwhelmed by a large number of conflicts and a need to say "no"?
2. Do I assert myself even when things do not matter that much? Do others view me as an aggressor?
3. Do I lack a clear view of what my priorities are?
4. Do I stir up conflicts and fights for some reason?

Commitment to Action
What two new behaviors would increase your effective use of avoidance?
1.
2.

BOX 22-6

Appropriate Uses of Accommodation

1. When other people's ideas and solutions appear to be better or when you have made a mistake
2. When the issue is far more important to the other(s) than it is to you (This is a natural, logical step to cooperation and collaboration.)
3. When you see that accommodating now "builds up some important credits" for later issues
4. When you are outmatched and/or losing anyway; when continued competition would only damage the relationships and productivity of the group and jeopardize accomplishing major purpose(s) and maintaining credibility
5. When preserving harmonious relationships and avoiding defensiveness and hostility are very important
6. When letting others learn from their mistakes and/or increased responsibility is possible without severe damage, no "shame and blame" (and you are able to avoid saying, "I told you so!" or "Everybody knows *that*.")

BOX 22-7

Accommodation: Self-Assessment and Commitment to Action

If You Use Accommodation Often, Ask Yourself the Following Questions:
1. Do I feel that my needs, goals, concerns, and ideas are not being attended to by others?
2. Am I depriving myself of influence, recognition, and respect?
3. When I am in charge, is "discipline" lax?
4. Do I think people are using me?
   Infrequent use of accommodation may result in your being viewed as unreasonable or insensitive.

If You Seldom Use Accommodation, Ask Yourself the Following Questions:
1. Am I building goodwill with others during conflict?
2. Do I admit when I've made a mistake?

3. Do I recognize legitimate exceptions?
4. Do I know when to give in, or do I assert myself at all costs?
5. Am I hiding behind a leader who may be endorsing my "bad" behavior?
6. What would a "360-degree" evaluation (soliciting others' candid and anonymous) opinion of me reveal?

Commitment to Action
What two new behaviors would increase your effective use of accommodation?
1.
2.

BOX 22-8

Appropriate Uses of Competing

1. When quick, decisive action is necessary
2. When important, unpopular action needs to be taken, or when trade-offs may result in long-range, continued conflict
3. When an individual or group is right about issues that are vital to group welfare
4. When an individual or group has had others take advantage of the individual's or group's noncompetitive behavior and now feel obliged to compete

BOX 22-9

Competing: Self-Assessment and Commitment to Action

If You Use Competing Often, Ask Yourself the Following Questions:
1. Am I surrounded by people who agree with me all the time and who avoid confronting me?
2. Are others afraid to share themselves and their needs for growth with me?
3. Am I out to win at all costs? If so, what are the costs and benefits of competing?
4. What is the honest assessment of me (or the department to which I report) by others, the "word on the street?"

If You Seldom Compete, Ask Yourself the Following Questions:
1. How often do I avoid taking a strong stand and then feel a sense of powerlessness?
2. Do I avoid taking a stand so that I can escape risk?
3. Am I fearful and unassertive to the point that important decisions are delayed and people suffer?

Commitment to Action
What two new behaviors would increase your effective use of competition?
1.
2.

maturity and confidence. It is a learned skill, developed over time. The *Theory Box* illustrates the key ideas behind negotiation. A give-and-take relationship results in conflict resolution, with the result that each person is able to meet his or her most important priorities as much of the time as possible. Compromise is very often the exchange of concessions as it creates a middle ground, inviting everyone to join in. This is the preferred means of conflict resolution during union negotiations, in which each side is appeased to some degree. In this mode, nobody gets everything they think they need, but there is a sense of energy that is necessary to build important relationships and teams.

Theory Box

NEGOTIATING THEORIES

THEORY/CONTRIBUTOR	KEY IDEA	APPLICATION TO PRACTICE
Getting to Yes: Negotiating agreement, principled negotiation, or negotiation on merits theories were developed by Fisher and Vry (1991).	Principled negotiation can produce mutually acceptable agreements in every type of conflict. The method involves four steps: (1) Separate the people from the problem; (2) focus on interests, not positions; (3) invent options for mutual gain; and (4) insist on using objective criteria.	Negotiation requires extra efforts to communicate: Speak and listen for mutual understanding. Getting to yes comes from building a working relationship and creatively developing options from which those involved will benefit.

From Fisher, R. S., Ury, W., & Patton, B. Copyright 1981, 1991 by Fisher, R., and Ury, W. *Getting to yes: Negotiating agreement without giving in.* Houghton Mifflin Company. Reprinted with permission. All rights reserved.

Negotiation and compromise are valued approaches. They are chosen when less accommodating or avoiding is appropriate (Box 22-10). Compromising is a blend of both assertive and cooperative behaviors, although it calls for less finely honed skills for each behavior than does **collaboration**. Negotiation is more like trading (e.g., "You can have this if I can have that" as in "I

BOX 22-10

Appropriate Uses of Compromise

1. When two powerful sides are committed strongly to perceived mutually exclusive goals
2. When temporary solutions to complex issues need to be implemented
3. When conflicting goals are "moderately important" and not worth a major confrontation (coercion/competing)
4. When time pressures people to expedite a workable solution
5. When collaborating and competing fail

BOX 22-11

Negotiation/Compromise Self-Assessment and Commitment to Action

If You Tend to Use Negotiation Often, Ask Yourself the Following Questions:

1. Do I ignore large, important issues while trying to work out creative, practical compromises?
2. Is there a "gamesmanship" in my/our negotiations?
3. Am I sincerely committed to compromise or negotiated solutions?

If You Seldom Use Negotiation, Ask Yourself the Following Questions:

1. Do I find it difficult to make concessions?
2. Am I often engaged in strong disagreements or do I withdraw when I see no way to get out?
3. Do I feel embarrassed, sensitive, self-conscious, or pressured to negotiate, compromise, and bargain?

Commitment to Action

What two new behaviors would increase your compromising effectiveness?

1.
2.

promise to come to your monthly meetings with the float pool staff if you call me immediately with any problems you are hearing about how my managers treat them"). Compromise is one of the most frequently selected behaviors used by nurse leaders because it supports a balance of power between themselves and others in the work setting. The self-assessment in Box 22-11 will help you become more aware of your own use of negotiation and compromise and improve it.

Collaborating

Collaborating, the opposite of both avoiding and competing, is the most creative stance. It is both assertive and cooperative because people work creatively and openly to find the solution that most fully satisfies all important concerns and goals to be achieved. Collaboration involves analyzing situations and defining the conflict at a higher level where shared "superordinate" goals are identified and commitment to working together is generated (Box 22-12). For example, when nurses and physicians work together, they can collaborate by replacing the statement "I'm in charge" with "What is the best thing we can do for the patient and family right now?" and "How does each of us fit into the plan to meet their needs?" This requires discussion about the plan (superordinate goals), how it will be accomplished, and who will make what contributions toward its achievement and proposed outcomes.

BOX 22-12

Appropriate Uses for Collaboration

1. When seeking creative, integrative solutions where both sides' goals and needs are important, thus developing group commitment and a consensual decision
2. When learning and growing through cooperative problem solving, resulting in greater understanding and empathy
3. When identifying, sharing, and merging vastly different viewpoints
4. When being honest about and working through difficult emotional issues that interfere with morale, productivity, and growth; compromise supports a balance of power between self and others in the workplace

The same scenario fits for patients and families as well. What is their superordinate goal? Who will do what so that they can reach this goal? The stakes are high (quality patient care) when all stakeholders (e.g., patient, nurse, family, physician) work together.

Trivial issues do not require collaboration and consensus seeking. Some people favor collaboration to reduce their risk-taking and to spread responsibility, particularly in "shame and blame" environments, when self-protection is the order of the day. Use the self-assessment in Box 22-13 that follows to determine your own use of collaboration.

At the onset of conflict, involved individuals can carefully analyze situations to identify the nature and reasons for conflict and choose an appropriate approach for promoting collaboration. In other words, we can collaborate on the decision to withdraw, compete, or negotiate. For example, suppose you and I are disagreeing about the timing of procedures for patients under your care. At the point that we both agree that it is your responsibility and decision to make, we collaborate and agree. I say, "I see your point, so let's do it that way." Or we might talk and subsequently agree that you are too emotionally involved with a patient's problem and that it may be time for you to withdraw from providing the care and enlist the support of another nurse, even temporarily. Discussion can result in collaboration aimed at allowing you to withdraw appropriately. Another, less desirable choice could be to compete and let the winner's position stand (e.g., "Do as I say, I know I'm right" or "I'm in charge of this patient, I took care of him or her last time"). The decision to compete or collaborate depends on both parties involved.

The nature of the differences, underlying reasons, importance of the issue, strength of feelings, commitment, and goals involved all have to be considered when selecting an approach to resolving conflict. Preferred and previously effective approaches can be considered, but they need to match the situation. Sometimes, a third party may be introduced into a conflict so that **mediation** can occur. Mediation is a learned skill for which advanced training and/or certification is available. The mediator is usually an impartial helper who assists each party in the conflict to better hear and understand the other. This is thought to work in many situations because successful resolution is more apt to happen when people get a "feel" for this style and when individuals can be adapt to

---

BOX 22-13

Collaboration Self-Assessment and Commitment to Action

If You Tend to Collaborate Often, Ask Yourself the Following Questions:

1. Do I spend valuable group time and energy on issues that do not warrant or deserve it?
2. Do I postpone needed action to get consensus and avoid making key decisions?
3. When I initiate collaboration, do others really respond that way? (Are there hidden agendas, unspoken hostility, and/or manipulation in the group?)

If You Seldom Collaborate, Ask Yourself the Following Questions:

1. Do I ignore opportunities to cooperate, take risks, and creatively confront conflict?
2. Do I tend to be pessimistic, distrusting, withdrawing, and/or competitive?
3. Am I involving others in important decisions, eliciting commitment, and empowering them?

Commitment to Action

What two new behaviors would increase your collaboration effectiveness?

1.
2.

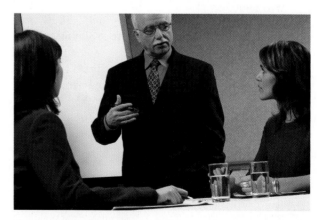

Compromise supports a balance of power between self and others in the workplace. (Copyright 2005 by JupiterImages Corporation.)

conflict as well as to the parties who are involved (Ross, 2003). According to Kritek (2002), an internationally known nurse scholar and consultant on the art of conflict resolution through her company, *"Courage,"* mediation is not so easy. In our society, for example, there is much focus on who can control whom and on who is the "winner." The successful individual involved in conflict resolution and negotiation often moves beyond avoidance, accommodation, and compromise, which are more about trying not to disturb the status quo. In the nursing practice arena, there is often the added difficulty in negotiating conflicts when at least one of the parties, which has historically been the physician over quality of care issues, is on an unequal or uneven playing field. This disadvantage is made even worse when the other party to the conflict does not even acknowledge the disparities involved (Kritek, 2002; Marcus, Dorn, Kritek, Miller, & Wyatt, 2004). However, as the Research Perspective points out, we must address conflicts or suffer negative outcomes.

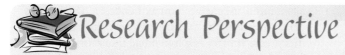

Research Perspective

Meyer, S. (2004). Organizational response to conflict: Future conflict and work outcomes. *Social Work Research,* *28*(3), 183-190.

The purpose of this study was to examine an organization's response to conflict and evaluate how its response affected future conflict and work outcomes. Conflict handling styles were studied in 3374 government employees in one organization. The organizational conflict survey was divided into three subsections: the employee's perceptions of their supervisor's conflict handling styles; the employees' rating of the frequency, resolution, and intensity of conflict in their work area during the past year; and demographic data. The sample consisted of men and women with 12.7 average years of service, with representation of the overall organization in terms of gender, race, and job title.

The key dependent variables identified by the primary investigator were rate of accidents, absenteeism, and use of overtime as identified by organizational reports. Five conflict-handling styles were identified for use in the study: integrating, compromising, obliging, avoiding, and forcing (p. 183), with the assumption that the integrating style is generally the best, and the forcing style, the worst.

RESULTS

The findings suggested that there is a relationship between conflict-handling styles and conflict rating. Supervisors with a style that tried to force one way of doing things over another generally experienced more conflict with greater intensity. Supervisors who abused their subordinates and/or avoided conflict altogether also found themselves in greater conflict. As expected, participants with high levels of collaboration had fewer conflicts than those who reported lower levels of collaboration.

A significant finding was the correlation with individual and summed work indicators, meaning that when the amount and intensity of a conflict on the job escalates, the result is inefficiencies and poor performance. Furthermore, the relationship of supervisor conflict-handling strategies and work indicators was mediated by the actual degree (how bad) of conflict reported.

IMPLICATIONS FOR PRACTICE

Tensions and stress in modern healthcare settings will undoubtedly continue, and even escalate. Organizations must recognize the relationship between conflict in the workplace and poor outcomes. Endorsement of an adaptive stance allows both parties in a disagreement to respect the other's point of view and limit the recurrence of problems in the future. Initiatives to reduce unacceptable behaviors, such as shouting, cursing, and threats, must be developed so that a zero-tolerance policy prevails at all levels of the organization. Because training in crisis intervention, anger management, and employee assistance programs are so readily available, managers should resolve conflict, decrease stress, and thus, help to avoid loss in productivity. In this way, negative outcomes such as the rate of errors, call-ins (absenteeism), overtime, and even incidents of violence in the workplace may be reduced.

MANAGING UNRESOLVABLE CONFLICTS

Not all of the conflicts confronting people are resolvable. In fact, most of our own current problems and conflicts, especially the continuing or reappearing ones, are most probably unresolvable. Such conflicts cannot be resolved by the right amounts of money, time, resources, staff, support networks, state-of-the-art technology, diet, exercise, vacation time, teamwork, courage, training, rational thinking, and/or leadership (Box 22-14). They are inherently unresolvable (Johnson, 1992).

Many conflicts (and problems) are unresolvable because they consist of two interdependent, dynamic polar opposites that require a shifting emphasis from pole to pole over time, rather than the selection of the one "best" option. Resolvable conflicts (and solvable problems) tend to be "either/or" choices that lead to some end. Unresolvable conflicts, or **polarities,** involve a "both/and" decision of when to emphasize one pole and when to emphasize its opposite. For instance, a manager's need to give clear direction to a team automatically places less emphasis on the team deciding on the direction themselves. However, for the team to be successful, sooner or later that manager will experience the need for the team to work on its own, setting its own direction. Johnson (1992) has identified several common polarities with which people deal continually. These include self and others, individual and team, individual and organizational responsibility, control and participatory management, specific and general communication, tasks and relationships, centralization and decentralization, and stability and change. Others you are probably confronting include "me and my department," personal life and professional life, stimula-tion (stress) and tranquility, conditional acceptance (love) and unconditional acceptance (love), cost and quality, efficiency and effectiveness, management and leadership, and planning and acting. Lencioni (2006) refers to this tug between parties as silos and turf wars.

Polarity Structure

Polarities have six important elements (Figure 22-2), including two neutral, interdependent poles; two sets of resulting positive consequences ("upsides"), one for each pole; and two sets of associated negative consequences ("downsides"). To determine the nature of the unresolvable conflicts, one has to ask five basic questions, as shown in Box 22-15.

By answering the basic questions in Box 22-15, an individual or team can diagram the specifics of any polarity situation. Typically, people see only half of the situation—the upside of their preferred pole and the downside of its opposite—and are

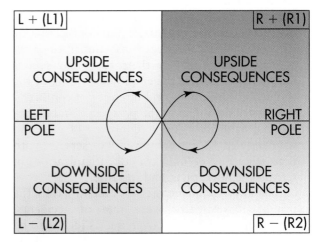

Figure 22-2 Generic structure and predictable flow of polarities.

How to Tell if a Conflict May Be Unresolvable

PROBABLY IS UNRESOLVABLE	ASK THESE QUESTIONS ABOUT THE SITUATION	PROBABLY IS RESOLVABLE
Answer is yes	Is this difficulty ongoing?	Answer is no
Answer is yes	Are there two interdependent poles?	Answer is no
Answer is yes	Does one choice need to incorporate the other to succeed?	Answer is no
Answer is yes	Is this really a both/and decision?	Answer is no

BOX 22-15

Basic Polarity Questions

1. What neutral terms describe the two polar opposites involved?
2. What are the positive consequences of actions emphasizing the first pole?
3. What are the negative consequences of action overemphasizing that pole to the exclusion of its opposite?
4. What are the positive consequences of actions taken toward the second pole?
5. What are the negative consequences of action overemphasizing the second pole while excluding the first?

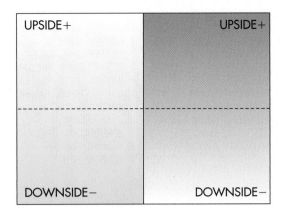

Figure 22-3 Polarity diagram.

therefore blind to the other two quadrants—their preferred pole's downside and its opposite's upside (Johnson, 1992). This blindness, coupled with the need to be right, leads to much conflict with those who favor the opposite pole and see only the other two quadrants. The awareness that there are such things as polarities and diagramming important ones tend to increase collaboration and "win-win" thinking because people learn that fighting over one pole leads to experiencing its downside consequences (Johnson, 1992).

Polarity Dynamics

Visually, a polarity diagram consists of the two polar opposites on a horizontal axis divided into four quadrants of results by a vertical line. Although simple in form, polarity diagrams clearly picture the consequences to be experienced and the nature of its historical and predictable flow.

Notice in Figure 22-2 that polarities naturally and predictably "flow" (arrows represent a plot of changes in results) from the downside of pole L toward the upside of pole R, then into the downside of pole R, then toward the upside of pole L, and finally back to the downside of L where it all began. For example, a nurse manager was confronted by an angry team because they felt they were being treated like children and told what to do all the time (control management's downside, L2). Working together, they initiated team meetings and decision-making procedures (actions emphasizing participatory management, as in self-scheduling

practices) that resulted in more ideas, a sense of ownership, and a noticeable self-direction from the team and its individual members (participatory upside, R1). However, after a few months of continually emphasizing participation, the team began to lose its focus and cohesiveness (participatory downside, R2) and once again came to the manager for more direction. The manager listened and provided clarification (action emphasizing control management), and the team regained its focus and efficiency (upside of control management, L1). Polarities have this infinite-type swing to them, as represented by the shape of the flow of the arrows in Figure 22-2.

Wide, rapid, or very prolonged swings usually lead to disruptions in the smooth conduct of activity. When any polar opposites, such as change and stability, are approached as separate, independent problems or conflicts—as they generally are—the outcomes tend to reflect the greater amount of time and intensity of consequences in the downside "quadrants" (Figure 22-3). Sometimes people hang onto one pole so long—usually for fear of the other pole's downside—that they either are forced to change their emphasis or do so very rapidly and extremely. This leads to a "flip" from the downside of the original pole to the downside of the new pole, almost without experiencing the upside on the way (Johnson, 1992). This hanging onto one pole to reap the benefits of its upside and avoid its opposite's downside is what Johnson (1992) calls "the one pole myth," or being "stuck" (p. 156).

The polarity diagram in Figure 22-4 was generated by a team of college students working on assertiveness ("crusading" away from the passive downside toward the assertive upside). They drew

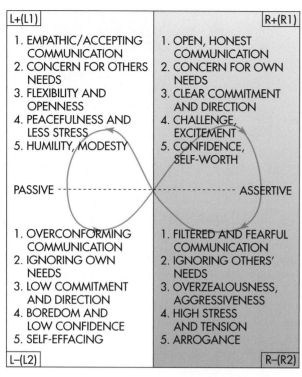

Figure 22-4   The passive acceptance and assertive polarity.

this on a chart pad by asking these questions: (L2) With what negative results of passiveness are we dissatisfied? (R1) To what positive outcomes of assertiveness are we committed? (R2) What negative consequences would occur from overemphasizing assertiveness (excluding any passive acceptance)? (L1) What are the positive consequences of being passively accepting?

▪ *Exercise 22-3*

After rereading the section on polarity dynamics, answer the questions listed in Box 22-15 and fill out the blank polarity diagram shown in Figure 22-3 in relation to a conflict you would describe as "ongoing" in a clinical setting. Be specific about the upside and downside consequences of each pole. Then draw a time line through the quadrants, starting in the lower left quadrant and moving through the upper right, down into the lower right, up toward the upper left, and finally back into the lower left. Shape the line to conform with how the organization has moved through this polarity over time. Talk to some people who have been around for a while to get their historical perspective on this issue. Then consider the following questions:

• Who tends to crusade for what pole? What are their positions and years of experience?
• How are resources, time, and personnel wasted on mismanaging this polarity?

• What blocks the effective management of this polarity?
• What already aids in its management?
• What new things and actions would add to its management in the future?

By seeing the total picture, the involved parties can take steps to make changes flexibly, without overemphasizing any one pole for too long. Most important, they can draw the results line (arrows) that best represented how this polarity usually flowed. They can see how stuck they had been, especially with almost every assertive act "feeling" negative and being resisted by others and almost every positive passive act lumped in with the negatives of "giving in." Input from as many people as possible is important when drawing such diagrams.

Polarity Management

Once people determine that their conflict is a polarity, they can act to maximize both poles' upsides and minimize both poles' downsides. This is called *polarity management*, which requires a shifting focus from pole to pole when cues of approaching downside consequences are noted. The key to effective polarity management is to sense oncoming downside consequences, or to be sensitive to feedback that there are negative consequences occurring, and take action toward the opposite pole. One nurse manager noticed that two teams had been functioning so long that individual members were complaining about being overlooked and that their creativity was stifled by the group. The manager scheduled a luncheon party, presented individual awards to each member, and initiated a creative suggestion box for staff to contribute individual and team ideas for improving quality and efficiency.

Polarity management involves two opposing groups that usually are in conflict. "Crusaders" are dissatisfied with the downsides of the present pole and advocate action toward its opposite. "Tradition bearers" prefer the present pole, citing its upsides, and point to the downsides of the crusaders' preferred pole as reasons to keep the emphasis where it is. Typically, the communication between crusaders and tradition bearers is argumentative, competitive, and defensive. Both sides know they are right and the other side is wrong. Polarity management alters this communication to a mood of cooperation, collaboration, and support because

BOX 22-16

Actions for Managing a Polarity

The Following List of Actions Exemplifies Steps in the Management of Any Polarity:

- Note that the situation involves at least one, continuous both/and polarity.
- Diagram, in writing, the polarity's poles, upsides, and downsides.
- Draw a timeline (arrows representing its past, present, and predictable future flow) with dates to identify the history of this particular polarity.
- Listen carefully to people with preferences for the opposite pole. Solicit their input regularly.
- Identify key individuals and groups who are "crusading" for the new pole and "traditionally supporting" staying at the present pole. Involve them in analyzing and managing this polarity.
- State major goals and objectives in terms of maximizing the upside consequences.

- Determine what present policies, procedures, committee structures, and typical actions (1) block the effective management of this polarity (shifting from pole to pole) and (2) exemplify and/or support managing this polarity effectively. Then create new ones that would facilitate managing this polarity in the future.
- Note which people are most accurately sensitive to any changes in results toward either downside and encourage and listen to their ongoing feedback.
- Identify and create flexible ways to shift resources to either pole and to monitor results.
- Diagram polarities and monitor their flow continually.
- Value crusaders' and tradition bearers' viewpoints, their ongoing collaboration, and healthy competition between them.

both sides realize that any decision to emphasize one pole results in everyone experiencing the downside of that pole and, if stuck at that pole long enough, experiencing the downsides of both poles at once (Johnson, 1992).

A manager and an organization can do several things to begin managing polarities more collaboratively and effectively. Many of them are listed in Box 22-16.

As a rule, the more skilled people are at problem-solving and conflict-resolution, the more likely they will mismanage polarities. This happens when people treat both/and decisions like either/or ones, thus looking for the right choice. Yet no one right choice exists, at least in the long run. Partnering with others and shifting action to what is needed next in a timely manner are important to manage polarities effectively.

The Solution

The nurse manager, medical director (psychiatrist-leader) and advanced practice nurse collaborated to address the conflict. We met with the nurse educator and together designed a medical-surgical orientation program, complete with skills lab and physical assessment training, and reassured the staff that we would not allow the admission of patients who required care beyond their capability. We created a policy by which all admissions would first have to be approved by both the nurse manager and psychiatric medical director on a 24-hour basis. The staff psychiatrists, in conjunction with the staff nurses, committed themselves to holding each medical specialist accountable for the care of each patient. Currently, there is a medical chain of command in place, which starts with

the psychiatric medical director of the unit to ensure that this happens in a timely fashion. We also provided a forum within the multidisciplinary treatment team to identify and prioritize the medical and psychiatric problems of each patient. All staff maintain their clinical competency in the care of the psychiatric patient with concomitant medical-surgical problems and have adapted successfully to the change in their nursing practice.

— Midge Grady, Sandra Gauker, and Diego Coira

Would this be a suitable approach for you? Why?

CHAPTER CHECKLIST

Conflicts may be resolvable or unresolvable, and they are common in health care and when dealing with people. To resolve conflict, parties need to identify their differences, priorities, and common goals; determine which approach to conflict is most appropriate; and act in that way to resolve it. When conflicts involve polarities, parties need to analyze their structure and dynamics, identify ways to shift emphasis among opposite poles, and partner with others concerned.

- The three types of conflict are as follows:
  - Intrapersonal
  - Interpersonal
  - Organizational
- The conflict process flows among four stages:
  - Frustration
    - Blocked goals lead to frustration.
    - Frustration is a cue to stop and clarify differences.
  - Conceptualization
    - The way a person perceives a conflict determines how he or she reacts to the frustration.
    - Differences in conceptualizing an issue can block resolution.
  - Action
    - Intentions, strategies, plans, and behavior flow out of conceptualization.
  - Outcome (may be both tangible and intangible)
- When assessing how well a conflict has been resolved, one must consider the following:

- The degree to which important goals were achieved by assessing the outcomes
- The nature of subsequent relationships among those involved in the conflict
- The five modes of conflict resolution are as follows:
  - Avoiding
  - Accommodating
  - Competing
  - Compromising
  - Collaborating
- Each mode of conflict resolution can be viewed along two different continua:
  - From uncooperative to highly cooperative
  - From unassertive to highly assertive
- A conflict probably is unresolvable in the following circumstances:
  - The difficulty is ongoing.
  - There are two interdependent, polar-opposite positions.
  - One pole needs to incorporate the other to succeed.
  - It is a both/and rather than either/or decision.
- Polarities are unresolvable conflicts.
  - Polarities have six important elements:
    - Two neutral, interdependent poles
    - Two sets of resulting positive consequences (upsides)
    - Two sets of associated negative consequences (downsides)

Polarity management requires a shifting focus from one pole to the other when cues of the approaching downside consequences become evident.

TIPS FOR ADDRESSING CONFLICT

- Communicate to yourself and others that conflict is a necessary and beneficial process typically marked by frustration, different conceptualizations, a variety of approaches to resolving it, and ongoing outcomes.
- Assess the work environment to see what behaviors are endorsed and fostered by the leaders at the executive, administrative, and less senior levels. Are these behaviors worthy of imitation? Do you need to go outside the usual group for appropriate mentorship and support?

- In sorting out the different conceptualizations of a conflict situation, determine any similarities and differences in facts, goals, methods, and values.
- To assess the degree of conflict resolution, ask questions about the quality of decisions (e.g., creativity, practicality, achievement of goals, breakthrough results) and quality of the relationships (e.g., understanding, willingness to work together, mutual respect, and cooperation).
- Remind yourself of your preferences for perceiving and resolving conflict (e.g., which of the five approaches do you avoid and which do you overuse?) and assess each situation to match the best approach

for that type of conflict regardless of which is your favorite approach.

- Assist others around you in assessing conflict situations and determining how they can best approach them. Utilize non-work relationships, such as in professional organizations such as state nurses' associations, to learn and practice.

- Persistent and recurring problems and conflicts often are polarities that inherently are unresolvable. Approach them by mapping their upsides and downsides and creating ways to balance actions toward each pole when appropriate.

TERMS TO KNOW

accommodation
allocation of scarce resources
avoiding
collaboration
competing
compromising
conflict
interpersonal conflict
intrapersonal conflict
mediation
negotiating
organizational conflict
polarities

REFERENCES

Aiken, L. H., Clarke, S. P., Sloane, D. M., Sochalski, J., & Silber, J. H. (2002). Effects of nurse staffing on nurse burnout and job dissatisfaction, and patient deaths. *Journal of the American Medical Association, 288,* 1987–1993.

Aiken, L. H., Sloane, D. M., Lake, E. T., Sochalski, J., & Weber, A. L. (1999). Organization and outcomes of inpatient AIDS care. *Medical Care, 37*(8), 760–772.

American Nurses Credentialing Center. (2005). *The Magnet Nursing Recognition Program.* Washington, DC: ANCC.

Bacal, R. (2004). Organizational conflict: The good, the bad and the ugly. *The Journal for Quality & Participation, 27*(2), 21-22.

Berstene, T. (2004). Conflict and change: Conflict can be managed to create a positive force for change. *The Journal for Quality & Participation, 27*(2), 5-9.

Blake, R. R., & Mouton, J. S. (1964). *The managerial grid.* Houston: Gulf.

Cloke, K., & Goldsmith, J. (2000). Conflict resolution that reaps great rewards. *The Journal for Quality & Participation, 23*(3), 27-30.

Conerly, K., & Tripathi, A. (2004). What is your conflict style? *The Journal for Quality & Participation, 27*(2), 16–20.

Dubler, N. N., & Liebman, C. B. (2004). Bioethics: Mediating conflict in the hospital environment. *Dispute Resolution Journal,* 32–39.

Farrell, G. A. (1999). Aggression in clinical settings: Nurses' views—A follow-up study. *Journal of Advanced Nursing, 29*(3), 532–541.

Hagel, J., & Brown, J. S. (2005). Productive friction: How difficult business partnerships can accelerate innovation. *Harvard Business Review, 83*(2), 82-91

Hurst, J., & Kinney, M. (1989). *Empowering self and others.* Toledo, OH: University of Toledo.

Institute for Healthcare Improvement. (2005). The 100K lives campaign: Some is not a number. Soon is not a time. Retrieved May 24, 2006, from http://www.ihi.org/IHI/Programs/Campaign.

Jameson, J. K. (2004). Negotiating autonomy and connection through politeness: A dialectical approach to organizational conflict management. *Western Journal of Communication, 68*(3), 257–277.

Johnson, B. (1992). *Polarity management: Identifying and managing unsolvable problems.* Amherst, MA: HRD Press.

Johnson, D. W., & Johnson, F. P. (1997). *Joining together: Group theory and group skills* (6th ed.). Englewood Cliffs, NJ: Prentice Hall.

Keenan, M. J., Hurst, J. B., & Olnhausen, K. (1993). Polarity management for quality care: Self-direction and manager direction. *Nursing Administrator Quarterly, 18*(1), 23–29.

Kinney, M., & Hurst, J. (1989). *Group process in education.* Lexington, MA: Ginn Custom Publishers.

Kramer, M., & Schmalenberg, C. (2005). Revising the essentials of magnetism tool. *Journal of Nursing Administration, 35*(4), 188–198.

Kritek, P. B. (2002). *Negotiating at an uneven table: Developing moral courage in resolving our conflicts* (2nd ed.). San Francisco, CA: Jossey-Bass.

Lencioni, P. (2006). *Silos, politics and turf wars: A leadership fable.* San Francisco: Jossey Bass.

Marcus, L. J., Dorn, B. C., Kritek, P. B., Miller, V. G., & Wyatt, J. B. (2004). Renegotiating health care: Resolving conflict to build collaboration. San Francisco, CA: Jossey-Bass.

McCue, M. T. (2005a). For your benefit: Converting political fervor for the benefit of everyone. *Managed Healthcare Executive.* Retrieved from www.ihi.org/NR/rdonlyres/73125243-4DD8-4CF7-97CC-75027F762031/0/MHE25705e.pdf.

McCue, M. T. (2005b). I'm losing my patience. *Managed health care executive.* Retrieved from www.ihi.org/NR/rdonlyres/73125243–4DD8–4CF7–97CC–75027F762031/0/MHE25705e.pdf.

Meyer, S. (2004). Organizational response to conflict: Future conflict and work outcomes. *Social Work Research, 28*(3), 183–190.

Page, A., (Ed.). (2004). *Keeping patients safe: Transforming the Work Environment for Nurses.* Washington, DC: National Academies Press.

Porter-O'Grady, T. (2003). Managing conflict in the workplace. *Imprint, 50*(4), 66–68. TPOG Associates, Inc., Emory University, Atlanta. PMID: 14596190. (PubMed, indexed for MEDLINE).

Porter-O'Grady, T. (1999). The leader as mediator. *Aspen's Advisor for Nurse Executives, 14*(7), 1–5.

Rogers, A. E., Hwang, W., Scott, L. D., Aiklen, L. H., & Dinges, D. F. (2004). The working hours of hospital staff nurses and patient safety. *Health Affairs, 23*(4), 202–212.

Ross, O. (2003). *Situational mediation: conflict resolution.* Riverdale, WA: Issues Press.

Scott, G. G. (1990). *Resolving conflict with others and within yourself.* Oakland, CA: New Harbinger.

Sexton, J. B., Thomas, E. J., & Helmreich, R. L. (2000). Error, stress and teamwork in medicine and aviation: Cross sectional surveys. *British Medical Journal, 320,* 745–749.

Thomas, K. (1975). Conflict and conflict management. In M. Dunnette (Ed.), *The handbook of industrial psychology.* Chicago: Rand McNally.

Thomas, K. W., & Kilmann, R. H. (1973). Thomas-Kilmann conflict mode instrument. In J. W. Pfieffer, R. Heslin, & J. E. Jones (Eds.), *Instrumentation in human relations training* (pp. 266–268). San Diego: University Associates.

Vahey, D. C., Aiken, L. H., Sloane, D. M., Clarke, S. P., & Vargas, D. (2004). Nurse burnout and patient satisfaction. *Medical Care, 42*(2, suppl), 57–66.

Valentine, P. E. B. (2001). A gender perspective on conflict management strategies of nurses. *Journal of Nursing Scholarship,* 69–74.

von Glinow, M. A., Shapiro, D. L., & Brett, J. M. (2004). Can we talk, and should we? Managing emotional conflict in multicultural teams. *Academy of Management Review, 29*(4), 578–592.

SUGGESTED READINGS

Burkhalter, D. K., Farmer-Dougan, V. A., & Nordstrom, C. R. (1997). Targeted goal setting: Helping nurses manage a turbulent work environment. *Journal of Nursing Management, 5,* 89–96.

Bush, R. A. B., & Folger, J. P. (2003). *The promise of mediation: The transformative approach to conflict* (revised edition). San Francisco, CA: Jossey-Bass.

Couch, M. Z. (1999). Is there an elephant in the copy room? Bold remedies for resolving hidden issues at work. Lubbock, TX: Perelandra.

Covey, S. R. (2004). *The 7 habits of highly effective people.* New York: The Free Press.

Curtin, L. (1993). Empowerment: On eagle's wings. *Nursing Management, 24*(6), 7–9.

Daley, K. (2004). How to disagree: Go up against your boss or a senior executive and live to tell the tale. *Journal of the American Society of Training and Development, 4,* 82–84.

Davidson, J., & Wood, C. (2004). A conflict resolution model. *Theory Into Practice, 43*(1), 6–13.

Gerardi, D. (2004). Using mediation techniques to manage conflict and create healthy work environments. *AACN Clinical Issues, 15*(2), 182–195.

Gordon, J., (Ed.). (2003). *Pfeiffer's classic activities: Managing conflict at work.* San Francisco, CA: Jossey-Bass/Pfeiffer.

Heim, P., & Murphy, S. (2001). *In the company of women: Turning workplace conflict into powerful alliances.* New York: Putnam.

Maruping, L. M., & Agarwal, R. (2004). Managing team interpersonal processes through technology: A task-technology fit perspective. *Journal of Applied Psychology, 89*(6), 975–990.

Menkel-Meadow, C., & Wheeler, M. (Eds). (2004). *What's fair: Ethics for negotiators.* San Francisco, CA: Jossey-Bass.

Sioukas, T. (2003). *The solution path: A step-by-step guide to turning your workplace problems into opportunities.* San Francisco, CA: Jossey-Bass.

Tschannen, D. T. (2004). The effect of individual characteristics on perceptions of collaboration in the work environment. *MedSurg Nursing, 13*(5), 312–318.

Ursiny, T. E. (2003). *The coward's guide to conflict: An expert's guide to facing conflict head-on and building confidence along the way.* Naperville, IL: Sourcebooks.

WEBSITES

Conflict Resolution Institute: www.crinfo.org

CPR Institute for Dispute Resolution: www.cpradr.org

Program on Negotiation at Harvard Law School: www.pon.harvard.edu/main/home/

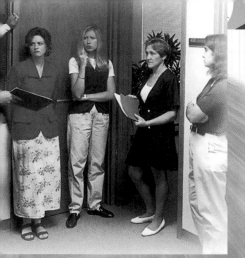

23

Delegation: An Art of Professional Practice

Patricia S. Yoder-Wise

*D*elegation is a complex process that can be quite effective in accomplishing work. This chapter defines various aspects of delegation, including legal perspectives and how to make delegation decisions. The emphasis is on the role of the nurse as delegator, irrespective of the formal position an individual may hold.

Objectives

- Define *delegation* and its component parts.
- Evaluate how tasks and relationships influence delegation to a specific individual.
- Comprehend the legal authority for a registered nurse to delegate.

- Value the complexity of decision-making related to delegation.

Questions to Consider

- *How does a registered nurse make delegation decisions?*
- *How complex is delegation?*
- *When is it appropriate to delegate?*
- *To whom can tasks be delegated?*
- *What can be delegated?*

The Challenge

Molly Patteson, RN, BSN
Weekend Supervisor, Rollins Brook Community Hospital, Lampasas, Texas

Weekend staffing is a challenge. As a supervisor, I had a dilemma. The census (16) was rising and the 7-3 staff on Sunday did not have sufficient personnel. I had depleted my call list and reassured my 1-year-out-of-school RN that I would find a solution. We had a seasoned LVN and an aide. We also had one RN assigned to the emergency department. Normally, this sounds good, but our hospital has eight new beds on one unit and the rest of the beds in the older part of the hospital. There is no way of communicating between the two except by phone. A 3-11 RN volunteered to come in at 11 AM. I chose to go home at 9 PM Saturday night and pray for returned calls from the staff I could not reach previously.

 What do you think you would do if you were this nurse?

INTRODUCTION

Delegation is a complex, loophole-ridden, work-enhancing strategy. It can make the difference between caring for a group of patients and experiencing great anxiety and caring for that same group with a controlled expectation of what can be achieved. Used properly, delegation can enlarge the effect you have on patient care; used improperly, it can be frustrating and scary. Delegation is an art and a skill that can be developed and honed into one of the most effective professional management strategies any registered nurse can use. Each of the following sections is designed to foster the best of delegation.

HISTORICAL PERSPECTIVE

Until the early 1970s, registered nurses (RNs) were quite familiar with the art of delegation. Most care occurred in acute care hospitals, which were staffed by RNs (mostly diploma graduates, frequently prepared in the hospital in which they worked), licensed practical/vocational nurses (LPNs/LVNs), and nurse aides (commonly called *unlicensed assistive* or *unlicensed nursing personnel*, or *UAPs* or *UNPs*, today). Team nursing was used, and staffing ratios were such that it was not uncommon for relatively few RNs to be present on a nursing unit. Direct care was provided primarily by LPNs/LVNs and aides. Of course, because there were few complex procedures, the direct care provided was related primarily to physical comfort and to what today would be called *simple treatments*.

As care became far more intricate and monitoring demands and expectations placed on nursing increased, moving to a higher ratio of RNs was logical. Thus, during the 1970s and 1980s, many nurses entered the profession with relatively limited experience or knowledge about the details of delegation—there was no one in the clinical area to whom one could delegate anything related to patient care except the basic physical care. Sometimes, the professional staff even dealt with that. In a study by Standing, Anthony, and Hertz (2001), most nurses identified that they were prepared for delegation mainly by experience rather than by education.

In the mid-1990s, a dramatic shift from primary nursing (an all-professional staff concept) to a multilevel nursing staff occurred. As a result, addressing the topic of delegation in some detail became critical to safe care. This return, however, was not to delegation as it was known earlier. In part, the difference today is based on the sophisticated demand for cost containment and reduction and the new complexities that are present in health care. As the healthcare industry emphasizes community-based care, the challenge of delegation and the resultant supervision become even more difficult. The increase, especially in unlicensed nursing personnel (UNPs), related in the past to a shortage of nurses. Although a shortage exists now, an even more dramatic one is predicted over the next several years (Division of Nursing, 2005). Therefore, in addition to the supply of nurses and healthcare cost control measures, the role of the RN will change to meet the increasing demands for care. Nursing's flexibility to alter how we function based on the changes we find has allowed nursing to survive and sometimes thrive. The consistent element, irrespective of how we function, is care.

During the early part of the 21st century, both the National Council of State Boards of Nursing (NCSBN) and the American Nurses Association (ANA) became increasingly concerned about the quality of delegation decisions. The NCSBN believes that "state boards of nursing should regulate nursing assistive personnel" (NCSBN, 2005, p. 160). This means that they believe the current approach in many states of having certified nursing assistants regulated through the health or hospital division of the state no longer meets the needs of nursing. Additionally, they have added an expectation that basic training for nursing assistive personnel include an emphasis on the concepts related to how to receive delegation. The ANA (2005) has focused on the principles of delegation that an RN must use.

DEFINITION

Delegate, or *delegation,* is defined in multiple ways. However, consistent elements can be found in each definition. Each definition calls for **at least two people** (a **delegator** and a **delegatee**), work, and some kind of transfer of authority and **responsibility** to perform the work. No definition suggests it is an abdication of **accountability** for the overall outcomes or performance or the abdication of the need to be involved. This is an important point because remaining in touch with others who are completing work on behalf of a manager is sometimes difficult. Figure 23-1 shows that accountability remains fixed and that some portion of work is transferred along with the authority and responsibility for that delegated work. The over-arching element of communication suggests that it must be constant to ensure basic, safe care.

A definition of *delegation,* therefore, might be as follows: achieving performance of care outcomes for which you are accountable and responsible by sharing activities with other individuals who have the appropriate authority to accomplish the work. Acceptance of the delegated work must occur,

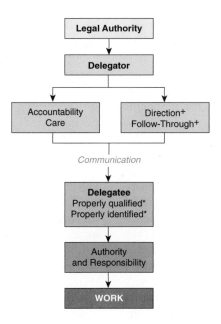

[+]Two common failures identified by Standing, Anthony, and Hertz (2001).
[*]Two key recommendations by Fagin (2001).

Figure 23-1 A delegation framework: delegation to achieve care outcomes.

either passively (i.e., no protest occurs) or actively (i.e., communication indicates acceptance). Therefore, delegation can occur only when two people are involved in a mutual work situation and one of the persons has accountability and the other has some authority for performing specific tasks. When two RNs work together sharing activities, delegation does not occur. However, if one RN has specific accountability for an outcome and that nurse asks another RN to perform a specific component of the overall function, that is delegation (see Assignment versus Delegation for further information).

Delegation occurs when an RN assigns an LPN/LVN or UNP to perform a specific function or aspect of care. The term UNP incorporates a variety of workers, such as nursing assistants, orderlies, nurse associates, and patient care assistants. This role, as the word "assistive" conveys, is an aid to the registered nurse who is accountable for care. Most UNPs today are prepared in some formal program but that program may range from less than a week to several weeks. Consistency in preparation and job descriptions for UNPs is lacking! The NCSBN (www.ncsbn.org) has expressed concern about preparation inconsistency and suggests that programs and UNPs both need greater public accountability.

The RN needs to be aware of individual qualifications needed to perform safely. Authority is a critical component. It may be designated by law, such as the nursing practice act, or it may be designated by educational preparation/certification. Typically, a position description further defines what the nature of the authority is for a specific position. Knowing someone's abilities is critical to successful delegation.

Two of the numerous recommendations Fagin (2001) made that relate to delegating are (1) being certain that delegation is made only to those properly qualified to perform whatever the assignment is and (2) requiring that all staff be properly identified. The first recommendation is evident from the previous discussion in this chapter; the second is designed to help patients, families, and others know the type of personnel providing care to an individual or group. Some states and organizations require name and title identification. Many accrediting agencies expect this minimal element for safety reasons. Unfortunately, in some situations in the 1990s, vague or no identification was fostered to create the impression of greater numbers of nurses. Fortunately, few places continue this practice today.

Finally, in a study about delegation, Standing, Anthony, and Hertz (2001) found the two most common errors associated with poor patient outcomes related to (1) giving improper directions and (2) providing improper follow-through of agency protocol. These findings suggest that communication and agency protocols are crucial to achieving positive performance outcomes. Examples of improper directions could include not indicating when to report important findings or alerting the delegatee to what the important findings might be. Examples of improper follow-through of agency protocol might be found when the delegator fails to validate findings that are not anticipated or when the delegator encourages the individual to perform functions beyond the stated position description for the delegatee. Additionally, failure of the delegatee to report findings is an example of failure to follow through. Figure 23-1 shows the one way of direction and the two ways of follow-through.

Achieving Performance Outcomes

Achieving performance outcomes is the driving force of all health care. If what someone does has little or no benefit in improving the delivery of care, it is, of course, ineffective. Therefore, all care is based on attaining expected outcomes, whether that care is provided directly by an individual or group of professionals or whether that care was shared between professionals and assistants. Performance of care outcomes relates to the profession's keeping its trust with the public, that is, to perform safely and competently. Standing, Anthony, and Hertz (2001) suggest that negative outcomes seem more related to delegation situations in which the nurse is less experienced in practice and the UNP is less experienced in a specific setting. In ever-changing healthcare settings, it is critical to know that you must delegate to achieve all that is expected of you. In essence, this means that if you cannot trust others or if you are frustrated because you cannot do it all yourself, you will be very frustrated with the way in which health care is delivered and your career opportunities will be fairly limited. Learning about another and developing trust are critical to success. Lencioni (2002) cites lack of trust as the number one dysfunction of a team. Comfortable, confident delegation requires considerable trust to function as a smooth pairing.

Accountability and Responsibility

The terms *accountability* and *responsibility* refer to the legal expectation the state has vested in persons with the designation of RN. *Accountability* means that someone must be able to explain actions and results. Legally, the RN is accountable for nursing care. *Responsibility* refers to reliability, dependability, and obligation to accomplish work. It also refers to each person's obligation to perform at an acceptable level. Thus, assistants, whether UNPs or LPNs/LVNs, are obligated to perform that which they can at acceptable quality levels. Those individuals are also responsible for informing the delegator what limitations, if any, would prevent the accomplishment of expected outcomes. The *Code of Ethics for Nurses* (ANA, 2001), Provision 4, states: "The nurse is responsible and accountable for individual nursing practice and determines the appropriate delegation of tasks consistent with the nurse's obligation to provide optimum patient care" (p. 4).

Organizational accountability is another aspect. Making solid decisions depends on how well the organization provides adequate resources, including appropriate staffing and mix. Organizations that function in positive ways, such as Magnet™ organizations, typically have supportive environments that help teams function effectively. The NSCBN concurs with the ANA that the driving principle in decision-making is patient (public) safety.

Sharing Activities

Sharing activities may sound simplistic; however, when someone with the legal accountability for a role shares elements, that individual is not giving away role elements. That individual is sharing activities or functions to ensure total outcomes. Therefore, the delegation definition here emphasizes that care itself is not delegated—only elements (activities) are. Thus, accountability rests with the delegator. Sharing may consist of many strategies ranging from asking an assistant to perform a specific task to expecting the same performance as the day before. For delegation to be effective, the RN must accept that sharing activities is important and provides benefits to patient care. Professional aspects may never be delegated; only basic skills

(frequently thought of as daily living/personal hygiene activities) and some monitoring/technical skills may be delegated. Some organizations provide a two- or three-stage approach to UNP positions with each allowing for more skills to be performed. In the future, we might anticipate that more, rather than fewer, skills might be delegated to others as the stability and predictability of those skills increases and the need to assist nurses in more ways increases.

Other Individuals

Other individuals may include persons with no formal preparation or recognition (e.g., UNPs), those with dependent status (e.g., LPNs/LVNs who function under the direction of a physician or RN), or others who are designated as being accountable to the delegator (e.g., other RNs or healthcare providers who report to a designated delegator, such as a nurse manager).

Span of control is an important concept to keep in mind when interacting with others to achieve care. This term refers to how many people for whom you have responsibility. For example, if a nurse has responsibility for five staff members, each of whom cares for 10 patients, the nurse, in effect, has responsibility for five staff *and* 50 patients. This may not be as overwhelming as it may seem at first if the patients are in stable condition and their needs are predictable; if the staff are well-prepared, experienced providers of routine care; and if the geographic area is restricted. On the other hand, if any of these factors is lacking, this responsibility may be overwhelming, even if each staff member provides care for only five patients. Thus, if others render elements of care, multiple factors must be assessed to determine how manageable the situation is.

Appropriate Authority

Appropriate authority to perform certain functions stems from various sources. For example, the practice of LPNs/LVNs is defined by state titling or practice acts, as well as by institutional policies. UNPs, such as certified nursing assistants, are prepared to meet a specific set of functions. As mentioned, considerable variation exists in the preparation of UNPs. That preparation, coupled with institutional policies, defines what UNPs may do. Position descriptions may provide more specific insight about the authority designated in certain positions. In essence, the term *appropriate author-ity,* as used in the previous definition, refers to a baseline indicator that an individual is expected to be able to perform certain aspects of care and, therefore, may receive an assignment to execute those aspects. In 2005, the NCSBN conducted work to share with individual state boards of nursing. This work included the concept of delegation and its importance in healthcare delivery.

All organizations have descriptors of what tasks may be performed by someone in a particular position. When a position description contains functions that are normally performed or are believed to be an essential part of the practice of a licensed person (e.g., physician, nurse, pharmacist), the person performing in that role is doing so through a passive delegation act. There is, in essence, no active decision being made by the RN in determining what to delegate or to whom. When active delegation occurs, the RN assesses the situation, determines what is best for patient care, directs a UNP to perform certain tasks, and holds the person accountable. Even when organizational protocols indicate that someone else may perform a task on behalf of the RN, the employee must be competent to perform the tasks. This expectation suggests that the delegator will make initial and ongoing assessments related to the delegatees' performance in addition to assessment of patients and their needs. Furthermore, state laws governing the practice of professional nursing typically define what the RN must do when someone else assumes certain tasks.

A FRAMEWORK FOR DELEGATION

In addition to the framework laid out in Figure 23-1, another way to consider the concept of delegation can be found in Hersey and Blanchard's (1988) original work about leadership style. (See the Theory Box.) Although the terms have changed in subsequent revisions, the key concepts have not. These researchers explained followership behavior in the context of two factors: ability and willingness. Both factors relate to specific situations. *Ability* relates to knowledge and skills; *willingness* relates to attitude. Thus, if a delegatee indicates reluctance to perform some work, the delegator assumes more control of the situation to determine whether knowledge is lacking; whether there is some psychomotor interference with performing the work; or whether the delegatee is bored, anxious, or upset and thus unwilling to meet the expectations of the situation. The less able or willing the delegatee is in a situation, the more involvement is needed from the delegator. This theory was not designed for application to delegation, but many nurses find it helpful as they make delegation decisions.

Theory Box

SITUATIONAL THEORY

THEORY/CONTRIBUTOR	KEY IDEAS	APPLICATION TO PRACTICE
Hersey and Blanchard (1988) created this theory to explain how leaders/managers need to behave differently.	A wise leader analyzes how an individual interacts in a specific situation. The analysis consists of the sophistication of the employee and the task itself and the need for interaction. A leader then responds differently based on this analysis.	Treating people equally is unfair. Before delegating, an RN must know what a specific employee needs in a specific situation.

Exercise 23-1

Ask three staff nurses what their top three assessment factors for delegatees are. Compare these cited factors to determine any commonalities among the lists.

So, what strategy does the delegator use to interact with a delegatee? In essence, the greater the ability and willingness of the delegatee is, the more likely it is that the delegator could use delegation as the strategy for interacting with that person in a specific situation. In other words, both the amount of guidance (task behavior) and the amount of support (relationship behavior) would be relatively low. This seems logical for established work relationships. However, not all situations are established. For example, a delegatee may have limited knowledge and ability to perform a task. Such a situation would require more guidance. If the relationship is limited (i.e., these two people are unlikely to work together again), the delegator would likely simply tell the individual what to do and how to perform. Hersey and Blanchard call this "*tell*." In another instance, however, there may be only a new task (i.e., the relationship is an ongoing one or the relationship will become such). In this case, researchers found that the best strategy is to explain what to do and how to do it. This option is called "*sell*." Logically, if producing outcomes in a given situation is the driving force, delegators are much less likely to expend additional time and effort investing in a casual, limited relationship than they are in one that will be repeated. A third behavior described by these researchers is called "*participate*." This behavior is appropriate for situations in which the delegatee has abilities and willingness but the relationship is relatively new. In other words, in such situations both the delegator and the delegatee must determine mutual expectations and conditions of performance. The final behavior is called "*delegate*" and is best used with established relationships and expertise.

When the delegatee has a high degree of ability and willingness and the expected task is familiar, little guidance is needed. If the relationship is new or developing, more support is needed, and, therefore, the delegator and delegatee need to interact in a participating mode. This approach helps each learn more about the other and contributes to advancing to the most developed relationship, a point at which true delegation is possible: The delegatee is willing and able, needs little guidance, and needs relatively little support to accomplish work. Such behavior is evident when people work together in the same situations for some time. The delegatee knows what needs to be done, what needs to be reported, how to prioritize, and when to ask for help.

Delegation can be viewed as a spectrum of behaviors based on the context and needs in a specific situation. Knowing how to interact with a given delegatee is one of the key challenges of a delegator if effective outcomes are desired.

Figure 23-2 integrates the various considerations for delegation. Each registered nurse has assistants available during a designated shift. Mutual trust and shared responsibility must exist between the registered nurse and the assistants and their focus is on the patients at the center of the model. The registered nurse retains accountability for the patient and considers each assistant's abilities, authority, experiences and willingness in relation to various patient care tasks to meet the needs of the patient. This decision process occurs in light of organizational settings and policies and the broader legal and standard perspective.

Exercise 23-2

Ask three nursing assistants/UNPs who are experienced on specific nursing units what they most want to have in an interaction with the RN delegator. Consider the model in Figure 23-2 to determine what type of relationship the delegator should have with these delegatees in relation to specific tasks.

Another way to think about delegation is described in Hansten and Washburn's (1998) work. These authors suggest a "big picture" view that has seven key elements. Knowing your world (the environment in which you practice) provides a context. Knowing yourself and what needs to be done leads to the complex process of knowing the delegatee, communicating, resolving conflict, and providing feedback and evaluating. This should be considered a cyclic process: As you gain various experiences you might have a different understanding of your world and yourself, which leads to new abilities in the other elements of the process.

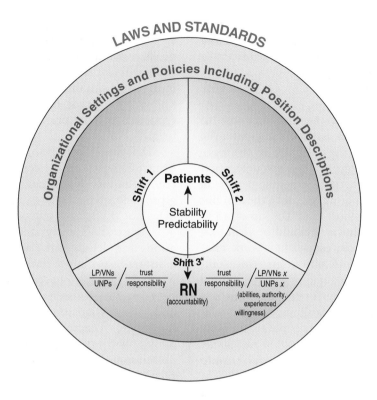

x = Number of LPN/LVNs and UNPs working with a specific RN.

*Repeated for other shifts.

Figure 23-2   Delegation framework.

ASSIGNMENT VERSUS DELEGATION

Two meanings are attributed to the term "assignment." The most common meaning refers to the work each person is to accomplish in a designated work period. This assignment consists of patient care expectations and unit-related activities, which may include such aspects as learning activities, regulation activities, and unit-management activities. The second meaning relates to assignment as the transference of both responsibility and accountability. This strategy is most common when one RN assigns a patient to another. Although nurses typically refer to the way work is distributed as an assignment, in reality, some portions of the work distribution are delegated care, not assigned. Thus, UNPs receive delegated activities, whereas RNs receive assigned care/assignments. When an RN assigns care to another RN, both accountability and responsibility are transferred. When an RN

delegates care to someone, such as a UNP, responsibility is transferred; accountability is not. Table 23-1 depicts the differences. (Note that the state of New York has a different interpretation of the terms, delegation and assignment.)

Table 23-1 DELEGATION VERSUS ASSIGNMENT		
Aspect	**Responsibility**	**Accountability**
Delegation	Yes	No
Assignment	Yes	Yes

IMPORTANCE OF DELEGATING

Delegation is a critical skill for accomplishing care in a timely manner. It usually saves time in the long run and, when effective, is cost effective. At its worst, however, it is exceedingly costly. Therefore, making the best decisions about care is imperative. One of the misconceptions about the profession of nursing that has been a plague is the thinking that defines nursing care in terms of psychomotor tasks. Therefore, professional nurses must convey the consistent message that doing a task is one component of care. Although the performance of a psychomotor task is critical, the critical analyses "behind the scenes" are clearly the precipitators of the actions. Research indicates that it is truly the careful decision-making of nurses and their ability to synthesize information from various sources that matter in terms of effective nursing care (Aiken, Clarke, Cheung, Sloane, & Silber, 2003; Cho, Ketefian, Barkauskas, & Smith, 2003; Clark and Aiken, 2003; and Rogers, Hwang, Scott, Aiken, & Dinges, 2004). Although delegation to others was not cited in these articles, it is logical to consider the importance of the professional role in safe patient care whether that care is performed by an individual RN or by others through delegation.

Delegation has direct patient and professional benefits. One of these is the availability of the professional staff to patients to teach the basics of safe

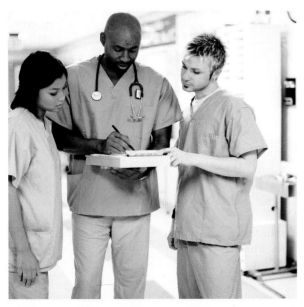

Nursing managers face complex decisions with delegation involving patients and staff. (Copyright 2005 by JupiterImages Corporation.)

activities of daily living (ADL). Seldom should a decision to delegate be based on timesaving considerations alone, but the truth is that in an effective team, delegation can be an effective time-conservation technique.

Exercise 23-3

Ask a staff nurse and a nurse manager about their individual perspectives of the pros and cons of delegation. Now ask a UNP employee the same questions.

LEGAL AUTHORITY TO DELEGATE

Most state practice acts address the concept of delegation; some explicate rules and regulations governing what may be delegated and when. State boards of nursing are vested with protecting the public; therefore, they regulate practice and the educational preparation required to practice nursing. The expectation that specific knowledge about nursing and delegation is needed to perform safely makes the nurse legally accountable and thus liable. Because nursing roles evolve over time, thinking about the scope of liability for the RN is valuable. Many acute care hospitals have decreased their use of LP/VNs, leaving only UNP-type personnel available to assist with care.

Legally, the concept of delegation is complex. First, the individual doing the delegation is personally responsible for prudent action. If delegation is not performed within acceptable standards, malpractice may be the outcome. In addition, according to Guido (1999), failure to delegate and supervise within acceptable standards may extend to direct corporate liability for the institution. Furthermore, whenever care is provided by other than a registered nurse, the accountability for care remains with the manager (of care)/delegator even though others provide various aspects of care. This view of professional liability is consistent with the idea that licensure conveys both privilege and expectations.

Exercise 23-4

Review your state nursing practice act, rules, and regulations. Discuss with two or more classmates what your state provides as direction about delegation. What conclusions can you reach?

SELECTING THE DELEGATEE

In many settings, you are one of a group of professional staff members who have the authority to delegate; therefore you probably will not be able to select the person with whom you will work. On the other hand, opportunities may occur in your career when you have a chance to select your own assistant. Several aspects of selecting an assistant are important. For example, knowing that you can communicate readily is important. If an LPN/LVN who has functioned in a physician's office for some time and is not familiar with working under the directions of an RN or having nursing care supervised is concerned about your supervision, talking about it can eliminate or diminish feelings of concern.

Appreciating and valuing each other's cultural perspectives can help with communication and with care itself. For example, an assistant who does not concur with you about the goals of hospice might actually work at counter purposes to the organizational philosophy. In addition, if the assistant is like you in terms of strengths, you will both want to do the same things, possibly leaving gaps in care. So, selecting someone with strengths that are different from yours enhances the work the two of you can accomplish together. This approach is consistent with strengths theory (Buckingham & Clifton, 2001), which suggests that we all should focus on building our strengths rather than "fixing" our weaknesses to be more effective at what we do. Realistically, however, it is often impossible to balance your strengths through the deliberate selection of a delegatee. In such cases, it is even more important to consider the whole aspect of patient care to be sure that the full spectrum of needs is addressed. An experienced UNP is likely to be able to adapt to changing situations, including changing delegators.

SUPERVISING THE DELEGATEE

Because the RN is always accountable for assessment, diagnosis, planning, and evaluation, it is important that UNPs understand what elements of implementation they may carry out and why the RN is responsible for analyzing data gathered. Thus, RNs are accountable for an initial assessment and then intermittent evaluations. Both elements must be present to ensure effectiveness in entrusting an element of care to someone else.

Delegators may have lessened the amount of direct care work to be done. However, this condition has simultaneously increased their supervisory work. Creating a plan to evaluate how both patients and delegatees are doing throughout the work period is critical and is influenced by factors such as knowledge of and experience with the delegatee, the number of delegatees and patients for whom the delegator is accountable, the geographic design of the unit, the stability of the patients, and other resources available to staff.

DELEGATION DECISION-MAKING

Figure 23-3 illustrates the delegation process, which begins with assessing the patient and the UNP. Four key factors must be considered before an assessment of the UNP's abilities is done. They are safety, critical thinking, stability, and time. If the patient is unsafe for any reason, delegation may be inappropriate. Exceptions tend to focus around monitoring behaviors, for example when patients are assigned suicide precautions. Critical thinking refers to the intensity and complexity of decisions that are needed. For example, simple teaching, such as washing hands can be performed by a UNP; complex teaching, such as diabetic care, can not. Stability suggests that the more stable a patient is, the more likely a UNP could provide care. Finally, time refers to the length and intensity of interaction. Thus, relatively few UNPs are found in emergency departments; many are found in extended-care facilities.

Assuming the patient-assessment outcomes suggest someone could assist with care, the RN next assesses the abilities of the UNP. When a "fit" (elements of work and performance abilities) occurs, tasks can be assigned. If a fit does not occur, tasks can still be assigned, but the delegator will need to educate, monitor, or evaluate more closely to ensure adequate care. Although the UNP is performing tasks (their responsibility), the RN is monitoring (accountability) care and outcomes. The RN should seek information, and the UNP should report information. This two-way follow-through allows alterations in care to be made in a timely manner. At times, especially as new skills are acquired or new relationships are forged, the RN will want to provide feedback during the care process. In all

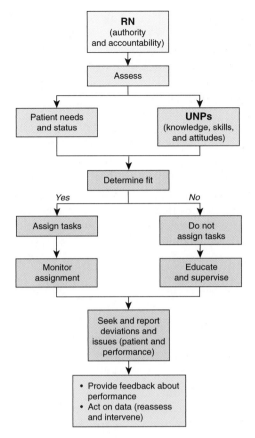

Figure 23-3   The delegation process.

situations, the RN needs to provide feedback about performance at the end of such activity. In addition to making it known that the UNP was monitored and supported, the UNP knows how to perform better next time because feedback should be directed toward quality.

Sometimes we fail to delegate to others. We may think it is too time- or energy-consuming. Sometimes, we frankly believe we can do a better job ourselves or we seek the recognition for specific care. But, when we delegate, we leverage our contributions to care.

Exercise 23–5

Select three patient records from a clinical setting in which delegation occurs. On the basis of the documentation only, evaluate if there are indications/assumptions about safety, critical-thinking, stability, and time. If you are familiar with any UNPs in the setting, use Figure 23-2 to identify how you would work with prospective delegatees to accomplish the care. Finally, in one or two sentences, state the rationale for your conclusions about delegation.

Integrating Factors

Combining these factors into an integrated whole for making decisions is valuable. One factor may be the overriding element. For example, when critical-thinking needs are great, the other factors may be relatively less influential. Thus, reaching decisions about to whom to delegate, what to delegate, and when to delegate is a complex process.

Providing specific feedback about performance is the best strategy for shaping future behavior. Therefore, statements such as "You performed that procedure with ease" are more effective than saying "Nice job." Equally important is the feedback from the person performing the tasks. Was the work completed? How did the patient respond? What changes were noted? These are examples of what the RN must know from the person who performed the delegated portion of care. The wise RN also listens for clues about the UNP's perception of the delegation interaction and uses that information to continue building trust.

Table 23-2 GETTING TO THE RIGHT ANSWERS

Check these Questions	Questions You Might Ask Yourself
The right task	_____ Is it appropriate to delegate (based on legal and institutional factors)? _____ Is the person able and willing to do this specific task?
The right circumstances	_____ Would the delegation process suggest that the circumstances are right? _____ Is staffing such that the circumstances demand delegation strategies?
The right person	_____ Is the prospective delegatee a willing and able employee? _____ Are the patient needs a "fit" with the delegatee?
The right direction/communication	_____ Do you and the delegatee have "common language"? (Do words, such as time frames, needs, and critical, mean the same to both of you?) _____ Does the delegatee know what and when to report? Is your communication based on a "fit" with the situation and culture?
The right supervision	_____ Do you know how and when you will interact about patient care with the delegatee? _____ How often will you need to provide direct observation?

Based on work by the National Council of State Boards of Nursing.

When possible, provide positive feedback; however, it undermines your credibility to convey satisfaction when the performance is less than desirable. Therefore, being honest about feedback is the best strategy. Being honest about the circumstances and performance and what we can do to change them helps the delegatee develop for the future. Attacking the person or personal characteristics not only has little, if any, positive effect on care, but also has the potential to undermine a long-term relationship. The Literature Perspective identifies that communication is critical to positive teamwork. Table 23-2 poses some appropriate questions for reaching decisions about delegation.

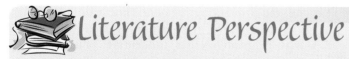

Literature Perspective

Anthony, M. K., Casey, D., Chau, T., & Brennan, P. F. (2000). Congruence between registered nurses and unlicensed assistive personnel perception of nursing practice. *Nursing Economics, 18,* 285-293.

Questionnaires were given to 647 RNs and 241 non-RN staff in three acute-care hospitals. Both RNs and UAPs were asked for their perception about various aspects of nursing practice. There were considerable differences of agreement on various aspects. Communication is especially important to RNs and UAPs working together. Although there was 100% agreement that nurses and UAPs speak throughout the shift, there was only 25% agreement on the nature of that communication. RNs believed that they commonly were asking for help, whereas UAPs perceived the conversation to be about observations of patients (as opposed to a request for help, work management or personal issues).

IMPLICATIONS FOR PRACTICE
Being clear about communication is especially important when working with others.

Finally, keep in mind that some individuals occupy positions for which they are not qualified. One strategy for dealing with this is to lower your expectations so that the individual can be successful. *Before doing that, however, think about the effect on others.* For example, why is one employee held to a standard and another is not? Who becomes responsible for accomplishing the work the one person cannot achieve? Is it fair to compensate for someone who cannot meet performance expectations? What are the potential liabilities of altering the standards of performance? Reaching decisions about delegating elements of care is a complex process. When the professional nurse knows the individual is incapable of appropriate performance and does not intervene, the potential for liability increases. Even eliminating the legal questions, ethical considerations should influence the nurse (ANA, 2001).

DELEGATION-PROCESS CHALLENGES

Delegation clearly is complex, but there are some ways to simplify the process. For example, when possible, selecting the delegatee whose talents match the task is better than merely selecting a competent individual. In large organizations, having a choice about who the delegatee is is more likely to occur than in smaller facilities. In rural settings, the delegatees tend to be more predictable, long-term employees; thus delegation is made easier because more is known about them and their abilities. Delegation also can be underused or overused as the Research Perspective illustrates.

Delegation may be difficult early in careers and in specific circumstances. In those situations, it may be helpful to initiate working together with an oral acknowledgment that the delegatee's abilities are unknown but that together this team is committed to providing the best care for its patients. Stating up front that offense or insult are not intended and then seeking feedback later makes the delegatee more receptive to hearing messages. The key is to seek specific feedback so that messages that are offensive can be changed. The goal, however, remains the same: to focus on the outcomes of patient care.

Letting the delegatee implement the task in his or her own way can be a challenge. Someone else will be unlikely to do a task just as the delegator would. However, assuming no safety or ethical discrepancies are likely, delegation really is a matter of trust. If the delegator intervenes, the delegatee loses confidence or becomes frustrated, and the delegator has lost the benefits of delegating. Curtis and Nicholl (2004) cite staffing levels and pleasantness of the task as two other challenges. "When staff levels are sufficient and pleasant work has to be allocated, delegation is usually easy.

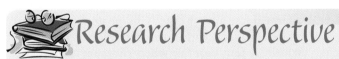

Research Perspective

Spilsbury, K., & Meyer, J. (2004). Use, misuse and non-use of health care assistants: Understanding the work of health care assistants in a hospital setting. *Journal of Nursing Management, 12,* 411-418.

Health care assistants (HCAs) performed care in three primary areas: direct care, housekeeping, and clerical duties, with the greatest emphasis in direct care. HCAs believed that their amount of work at the bedside provided visibility and new relationships for patient interaction. This study revealed that RNs occasionally ask HCAs to exceed their role authority, although HCAs were not rewarded for this additional responsibility.

RNs often used credentials to differentiate roles. They also did not always use the HCAs' full range of capabilities.

IMPLICATIONS FOR PRACTICE

The authors advocate for monitoring and supervising changes in nursing work. Additionally, assessing the competencies of HCAs is important.

Delegation can become more difficult, however, when staff levels are too low, unpleasant work has to be delegated or when delegatees are inexperienced" (p. 28).

Having deadlines helps keep the delegatee on target without oversupervising. Being clear about the need to check quality and effectiveness ensures that monitoring will be ongoing.

In settings other than those of confined geography, such as hospitals, long-term care facilities, and clinics, one of the greatest challenges of delegation relates to supervision. In such situations, it is especially important to be very clear about what is expected of the delegatee. Box 23-1 presents a communication template to use when delegating. The more that is understood between the delegator and the delegatee about a particular delegation situation, the greater the chances are of being effective in patient care.

BOX 23-1

Delegation Communication Template

- State exactly what is being delegated and what the expected outcome is.
- Convey recognition of the authority to perform what is expected.
- Identify priorities.
- Acknowledge monitoring activities you may perform.
- Specify any performance limitations, such as time limits on performing a procedure.
- Specify deadlines, including exact timing if that is important.
- Specify report time lines and data expected.
- Specify parameter deviations, including when immediate action must be taken.
- Identify appropriate resources, including people who may be consulted.
- Be clear about what may not be delegated.

Exercise 23-6

Think about what you could delegate, then use the delegation communication template found in Box 23-1 to practice with a classmate the transfer of specific responsibilities for care.

Finally, situations may occur in which you see issues associated with delegation but you have no authority. Fisher and Sharp (1998) suggest that influencing positive outcomes is still possible. Assuming no negative patient outcomes or safety issues are involved, you can help other delegators achieve positive outcomes by doing three things: asking, offering, and doing. Begin by asking questions related to the problem/issue/mission. This in itself may help the delegator see a situation differently. Making an offer such as an idea to move the process ahead toward a favorable outcome may be necessary or desirable. Finally, whatever you advocate is best valued if you can demonstrate the behavior you propose (doing).

Exercise 23-7

Using the assignments made by a nurse manager or charge nurse where you have a clinical experience, answer the following questions: Was it clear what was delegated? Why or why not? Were delegation decisions logical? Why or why not? From what you know about your nursing practice act and professional standards, did the assignments make sense legally and ethically? What is your rationale?

CHARGE NURSES

If no other RN delegates (usually because of the limited numbers of LVNs/LPNs or UNPs), the charge nurse always does. Charge nurses frequently emerge as such within the first year of practice or within a few months when they are experienced and working in a new situation. Connelly, Yoder, and Miner-Williams (2003) studied this group of people and found that there were four areas of competencies that this group needs to have. The second Research Perspective summarizes this article.

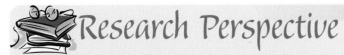

Research Perspective

Connelly, L. M., Yoder, L. H., & Miner-Williams, D. (2003). A qualitative study of charge nurse competencies. *MedSurg Nursing, 12*, 298-305.

Using a stratified, purposeful sampling technique resulted in interviews of 42 nurses at all management levels: staff nurses, charge nurses, head nurses, and supervisors. A constant comparative analysis produced 54 competencies that were classified as clinical/technical (15), critical-thinking (13), organizational (9), and human-relations skills (17). According to the author, the charge nurse role meets the definition of an administrator. The charge nurses were seen as the front-line manager and the representative of the nurse manager for the shift. They were problem solvers and managers of quality. They created the unit culture for the shift they serve as charge nurse. Critical-thinking and troubleshooting were expected abilities. In addition to the competencies, 15 characteristics were defined. They include accountability, positive attitude, confidence, fairness, humor, initiative, maturity, and responsibility.

IMPLICATIONS FOR PRACTICE

Almost every nursing care situation operates with a charge nurse. Choosing the right person to perform this important role affects care, quality, perception, and satisfaction.

INTEGRATED CARE

In the late 1990s, care moved from multidisciplinary, coordinated care to an integrated approach. Again, this move provides an impetus for a multiskilled worker. Having someone who performs "what is needed now" for the patient or the professional staff is the focus rather than the "me and my assistants" approach. This is consistent with the IOM report, *Health Professions Education: A Bridge to Quality* (2003). Patient-centered care is a key factor in redirecting health care to what patients need as opposed to what we offer. However, as McCloskey, Bulechek, Moorhead, and Daly (1996) suggest, the nurse will continue to provide the important "glue role" so that care achieves positive outcomes. In other words, in many settings, nursing's presence on a regular basis predisposes nurses to the "glue" role (holding patient care together) for logical reasons. Integrating care enhances the potential of both for *safe* patient care *and* for *quality* patient care.

The Solution

Sunday morning came. I arrived at 6:30 AM, took report, and sent the unseasoned RN and the seasoned LVN to the eight patients on the older side, where they were assigned the day before. The aide and I went to the eight patients on the new side. We teamed up room to room doing vital signs, passing trays, and conducting quick assessments. At 8:00 AM, the emergency department RN came to that unit to pass the morning medications. Although I do not support such fragmented care, I knew to whom I could delegate what, I knew the abilities of the various people I work with, I knew I could prioritize care and seek additional resources for short periods, I knew that I may not be timely in everything I got done, and I knew my own abilities. Because we truly work as a whole, I had others volunteering to answer phones and call lights. Is this ideal? Absolutely not! Is it sometimes the reality? Absolutely.

— Molly Patteson

Would this be a suitable approach for you? Why?

CHAPTER CHECKLIST

Delegation obviously is a complex issue. It has many facets, each of which by itself is complex. One of the critical roles of RNs is that of the "glue factor," by which the RN coordinates care across the spectrum of providers and affects the quality of care. Current research suggests that many indirect care interventions are not delegated by RNs because of the complexities and quality implications.

- Delegation involves achieving outcomes and sharing activities with other individuals who have the authority to accomplish work for which the delegator is accountable and responsible.

- The ways in which delegation can actually be enacted can be based on a situational leadership model.
- Nursing practice acts, rules, and regulations provide the legal structure for delegation; the *Code of Ethics for Nurses* provides the ethical structure.
- Knowing the skills and abilities of the delegatees is critical to feeling comfortable and confident in delegation.
- The delegation process provides a comprehensive approach to a productive interaction.

Building a trusting relationship takes time and has tremendous value in working effectively.

TIPS FOR DELEGATING

- Be familiar with your nursing practice act and the corresponding rules and regulations.
- Ascertain the skills of unlicensed nursing personnel to whom you may delegate tasks.
- Assess your patients with the perspective that some of their care will be provided by others.
- Use the communication template to enhance successful delegating.
- Use a decision-making framework to screen what can be delegated to unlicensed nursing personnel.

- Evaluate on a regular basis your effectiveness in delegating to others.

TERMS TO KNOW

accountability   delegator
delegatee   responsibility
delegation

REFERENCES

Aiken, L. H., Clarke, S. P., Cheung, R. B., Sloane, D. M., & Silber, J. H. (2003). Educational levels of hospital nurses and surgical patient mortality. *Journal of the American Medical Association, 290,* 1617–1623.

American Nurses Association (ANA). (2005). *Principles for Delegation.* Silver Spring, MD: The Association.

American Nurses Association (ANA). (2001). *Code of ethics for nurses with interpretive statements.* Washington, DC: The Association.

Anthony, M. K., Casey, D., Chau, T., & Brennan, P. F. (2000). Congruence between registered nurses and unlicensed assistive personnel perception of nursing practice. *Nursing Economics, 18,* 285–293.

Buckingham, M., & Clifton, D. O. (2001). *Now, discover your strengths.* New York: The Free Press.

Cho, S.-H., Ketefian, S., Barkauskas, V. H., & Smith, D. G. (2003). The effects of nurse staffing on adverse events, morbidity, mortality, and medical costs. *Nursing Research, 52,* 71–79.

Clark, S. P., & Aiken, L. H. (2003). Failure to rescue. *American Journal of Nursing, 103,* 1–6.

Connelly, L. M., Yoder, L. H., & Miner-Williams, D. (2003). A Qualitative Study of Charge Nurse Competencies. *MedSurg Nursing, 12,* 298–305.

Curtis, E., & Nicholl, H. (2004). Delegation: A key function of nursing. *Nursing Management, 11*(4), 26–31.

Division of Nursing. (2005). *The registered nurse population: National sample survey of registered nurses—March 2004. Preliminary Findings. October 2005.* Washington, DC: U.S. Department of Health and Human Services: Health Resources and Services Administration, Bureau of Health Professions.

Fagin, C. M. (2001). *When care becomes a burden: Diminishing access to adequate nursing.* New York: Milbank Memorial Fund.

Fisher, R., & Sharp, A. (1998). *Getting it done: How to lead when you're not in charge.* New York: Harper Perrenial.

Guido, G. W. (1999). Legal and ethical issues. In P. S. Yoder-Wise (Ed.), *Leading and managing in nursing* (2nd ed.). St. Louis: Mosby.

Hansten, R., & Washburn, M. (1998). *Clinical delegation skills: A handbook for professional practice*, Gaithersburg, MD: Aspen.

Hersey, P., & Blanchard, K. H. (1988). *Management organizational behavior* (5th ed.). Englewood Cliffs, NJ: Prentice Hall.

Institute of Medicine. (2003). *Health Professions Education: A Bridge to Quality.* Washington, DC: National Academies Press.

Lencioni, P. (2002). *The Five Dysfunctions of a Team.* San Francisco: Jossey-Bass.

McCloskey, J. C., Bulechek, G. M., Moorhead, S., & Daly, J. (1996). Nurses' use and delegation of indirect care interventions. *Nursing Economics, 14*, 22–33.

National Council of State Boards of Nursing. (2005). *Business Book, Annual Meeting.* Chicago IL: The NCSBN.

Rogers, A. E., Hwang, W.-T., Scott, L. D., Aiken, L. H., & Dinges, D. F. (2004). The working hours of hospital staff nurses and patient safety. *Health Affairs, 23,* 202–212.

Spilsbury, K., & Meyer, J. (2004). Use, misuse and non-use of health care assistants: Understanding the work of health care assistants in a hospital setting. *Journal of Nursing Management, 12*, 411–418.

Standing, T., Anthony, M. K., & Hertz, J. E. (2001). Nurses' narratives of outcomes after delegation to unlicensed assistive personnel. *Outcomes Management for Nursing Practice, 5*(1), 18–23.

SUGGESTED READINGS

Anthony, M. K., Standing, T., & Hertz, J. E. (2000). Factors influencing outcomes after delegation to unlicensed assistive personnel. *Journal of Nursing Administration, 30,* 474–481.

Habgood, C. M. (2000). Ensuring proper delegation to unlicensed assistive personnel. *AORN, 71,* 1058–1060.

Kenney, P. A. (2001). Maintaining quality care during a nursing shortage using licensed practical nurses in acute care. *Journal of Nursing Care Quality, 15,* 60–68.

McLaughlin, R. E., Barter, M., Thomas, S. A., Rix, G., Coulter, M., & Chadderton, H. (2000). Perceptions of registered nurses working with assistive personnel in the United Kingdom and the United States. *International Journal of Nursing Practice, 6,* 1, 46–57.

Moll, J. A., & Tripp, E. (2002). Nursing delegation: Implications for home care. *Caring, 21,* 9, 24–28, 30, 32.

Munroe, D. J. (2003). Assisted living issues for nursing practice. *Geriatric Nursing, 24,* 2, 99–105.

Sikma, S. K., & Young, H. M. (2001). Balancing freedom with risks: The experience of nursing task delegation in community-based residential care settings. *Nursing Outlook, 49,* 193–201.

Walczak, M. B., & Absolon, P. L. (2001). Essentials for effective communication in oncology nursing: Assertiveness, conflict management, delegation, and motivation. *Journal of Nurses in Staff Development, 17*(2), 159–162.

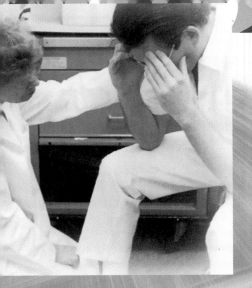

24

Managing Personal/ Personnel Problems

Karren Kowalski with Cynthia Whittig Roach

T he purpose of this chapter is to discuss various personal and personnel problems that a leader must face in all nursing settings. Some specific tips and tools are provided as ways to intervene, coach, correct, and document problem behaviors. Emphasis is placed on effective communication, both written and verbal.

Objectives

- Differentiate common personal/ personnel problems.
- Relate role concepts to clarification of personnel problems.
- Examine strategies useful for approaching specific personnel problems.
- Prepare specific guidelines for documenting performance problems.
- Value the leadership aspects of the role of the novice nurse.

Questions to Consider

- How do you react when you see that an employee is absent often and you or others seem to have a heavier workload as a result?
- Have you ever been in a position in which you were not really sure what was expected of you? How did you feel?
- What would you do if you observed clinical incompetence in a co-worker or peer?
- What is the best approach to deal with someone you believe is chemically dependent or impaired at work?

The Challenge

Cherie Gorby, RN, MSN
Senior Administrator Patient Services, Memorial Hospital, Colorado Springs, Colorado

New monitoring equipment was installed on the pediatric unit in an acute care hospital. This necessitated the instigation of several new standards of care. Everyone who worked in this area had to demonstrate competency in these standards.

The clinical manager and I determined that one competency could be demonstrated through a basic electrocardiogram (ECG) take-home test. Of the 42 nurses who took this test, seven failed with a score of less than 70%. These seven who failed were required to take an 8-hour class focusing on a review of pediatric arrhythmias. This class consisted of a pretest and posttest, along with hands-on didactic exercises. Six of the seven failed the posttest and/or the didactic. These six people were then required to do a 6-week basic ECG class. We also provided a tutor who was a clinical nurse specialist to help them with their homework when necessary. Three of these six failed the basic ECG class.

We thought perhaps these failures might result from test anxiety, and we wanted to be as fair as we possibly could with these individuals. We then permitted them to view the videotapes of all of the classes and review their tests along with the tutor. They were then retested; one person passed, but two failed. Everyone was told at the beginning that it was a job requirement to pass this test, which indicated mastery of the standard of care for this pediatric unit.

How can a manager deal fairly with employees who fail to meet established standards of care despite numerous efforts on the manager's part to assist the employee in meeting these standards?

 What do you think you would do if you were this nurse?

INTRODUCTION

As a novice nurse, the question may be one of perception. "As a new staff nurse, I don't think of myself as a leader, so how is this information applicable?" In reality, even nurses with limited experiences (referred to here as novice) are responsible for and thus lead assistive and support personnel. They often lead a team consisting of licensed practical/vocational nurses and nurse aides who are responsible for a group of patients. The novice nurse must know how to interact with difficult situations, including the decision to involve the unit leadership. It can be quite satisfying to work effectively with people. On the other hand, working with people presents some of the greatest challenges in the work place. Problems such as **absenteeism,** uncooperative or unproductive employees, clinical incompetence, employees with emotional problems, and **chemically dependent** employees are only a few of the issues. If a leader wants to be successful, these problems must be dealt with in ways to minimize their effects on patient care and on staff morale. Just as documentation of patient care is

critical, documentation of performance problems are critical. Overall goals are to assist the employee in the improvement of performance, to maintain the highest standards for the delivery of patient care, and to provide a supportive environment in which all staff members deliver the best care and attain work satisfaction. From this perspective, in this chapter we examine several specific employee problems and address the leader's role and options as well as the responsibilities of the novice nurse.

PERSONAL/PERSONNEL PROBLEMS

Absenteeism

One of the most vexing personnel problems is that of absenteeism. Inadequate staffing adversely affects patient care both directly and indirectly. When an absent caregiver is replaced by another who is unfamiliar with the routines, employee morale suffers, and care may not meet established standards.

Working short-staffed or working overtime to cover for absent workers creates physical and mental stress. Replacement personnel usually need more supervision, which not only is costly but also may decrease productivity and the quality of patient care. Indirectly, co-workers may become resentful about being forced to assume heavier workloads and/or may be pressured to work extra hours. Chronic absenteeism may lead to increased staff conflicts, decreased morale, and eventually to an increase in absenteeism among the entire staff. Given that nurses prefer to avoid conflict and negative behavior and to accommodate or make excuses for these situations (Sportsman, 2005), one way in which to confront persistent absenteeism is to discuss the situation directly with the employee (also see Chapter 17) by verbalizing:

> "I feel concerned when I see that you have been absent three different days this month."
>
> "Can you see how excessive absences affect the smooth functioning of the unit and the work load of other team members?"
>
> "This rate of absences cannot continue. What is your plan for addressing this situation?"

Absenteeism also has a deleterious effect on the financial management of a nursing unit. Replacement of absent personnel by temporary personnel or overtime paid to other employees is very costly, and the cost of fringe benefits used by absent workers is very high. When employee costs are excessive, they compromise the ability to support other creative efforts of the unit such as staff education and new equipment and may impact staff–patient ratios. Also, as care delivery systems become more complex and technically oriented, successful nurse leaders realize that technology is not a replacement for human caregivers. Absent caregivers cannot be replaced with machines.

Absenteeism cannot be totally eliminated. There are always unplanned illnesses, accidents, bad weather, sick family members, a death in the family, and even jury duty, which are legitimate reasons for missing work and beyond the control of management. However, some portion of absenteeism is voluntary and preventable; thus, the cause must be identified so that it may be addressed. Absenteeism may also indicate poor work satisfaction. If the leader believes that the issue is attributable to work dissatisfaction, unit-based focus groups may lead to insight about the sources. Such groups provide an excellent opportunity for the novice nurse to listen, to learn, and to speak to issues. If the underlying cause can be identified, there may be a way to prevent the loss of the employee, should retention of the employee be the goal. Some employees who convey they are never happy with their jobs may continually disrupt the overall unit with their absenteeism and should be terminated. The Research Perspective illustrates some of those factors to consider and that the problem is prevalent in other countries too.

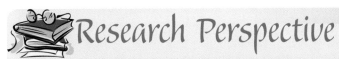

Research Perspective

Sui, O. (2002). Experience before and throughout the nursing career: Predictors of job satisfaction and absenteeism in two samples of Hong Kong nurses. *Journal of Advanced Nursing, 40*, 218-229.

A self-administered questionnaire was used for two samples of nurses. Both groups contained general nurses and psychiatric nurses. Using multiple regression analysis, the investigator found that there were key predictors of job satisfaction. Other factors, specifically age, involvement, psychological distress, and job satisfaction were significant predictors of absenteeism in one group. The other group showed occupational type, organizational relationships, and level of involvement were significant predictors of absenteeism.

IMPLICATIONS FOR PRACTICE

This international study suggests that absenteeism is not a U.S. phenomenon and that many factors need to be considered when absenteeism increases.

With role theory as a framework, absenteeism has been linked to **role stress** and **role strain** (see Theory Box). Absence from work is a way of withdrawing from an undesirable situation short of actually leaving, and many employees increase their absenteeism just before submitting their resignation. If the healthcare worker is experiencing some form of role stress, it might be manifested through absenteeism. Role strain may be reflected by (1) withdrawal from interaction; (2) reduced involvement with colleagues and the organization; (3) decreased commitment to the mission and the team; and (4) job dissatisfaction. All of these could be manifested through absenteeism. With this framework, management of absenteeism is based on the belief that competent role performance requires interpersonal competence. "Role competence is the ability of a person in an interdependent position, which is ongoing in time, to carry out lines of action that are task and interpersonally effective" (Hardy & Conway, 1988, p. 195). Role behavior occurs in a social context rather than in isolation. Therefore, the nurse leader needs to understand the existing situation, when the situation changed to its current status, when it needs to change further, and how to accomplish such change. Because people who are more satisfied in their work usually commit to "be there" for their team, enhancing job satisfaction may be an effective strategy toward reducing absenteeism.

One model for **nonpunitive discipline** can be found in Figure 24-1. This model demonstrates how undesirable behaviors, such as absenteeism, can be successfully altered. Box 24-1 identifies specific steps that are involved in nonpunitive discipline.

This model of nonpunitive discipline allows employees to free themselves from some role stress by clarification of role expectations and assumptons. Employees can receive satisfaction from the realization that a problem may not be inadequate performance due to personal faults, but rather a lack of clarification of role expectations within the organization. The specific steps involved in Box 24-1 are a process in which the novice nurse may be involved with the nurse manager or a support staff member or in extenuating circumstances for herself or himself. Remember, the focus is on the clear understanding of the situation, the growth of the individual, and the smooth and effective functioning of the team.

Exercise 24-1

Review the policy manual at a local healthcare organization. Determine what constitutes excessive absenteeism. What are the identified consequences?

Uncooperative or Unproductive Employees

The problem of uncooperative or unproductive employees is another area of frustration for the nurse leader. Hersey, Blanchard, and Johnson

Theory Box

ROLE THEORY

THEORY/CONTRIBUTOR	KEY IDEA	APPLICATION TO PRACTICE
Role theory is not considered a true scientific theory but more of a perspective or framework to understand individual behavior as it applies to specific roles (Hardy & Conway, 1988).	Professional socialization is a learned behavior and clarifies specific role prescriptions or sets of rules that are inherent within a given profession.	Within each area of practice or within each organization, there are specific rules, behaviors, and expectations that are prescribed and that will direct practice. Each professional nurse has the responsibility to completely understand his or her role. When this does not occur, role ambiguity or role strain may result. Absence of role clarity can also lead to decreased work satisfaction.

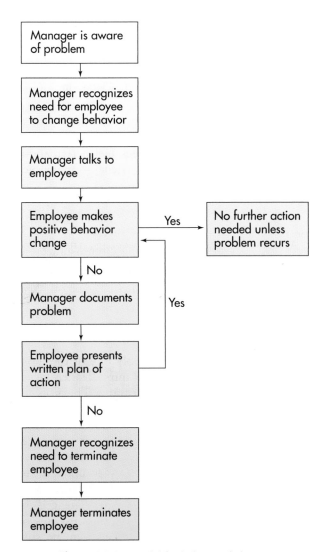

Figure 24-1 Model for behavioral change.

(1996) identified two major dimensions of job performance that relate to this problem: motivation and ability. The type and intensity of motivation vary among employees because of differing needs and goals that employees express. The leader can best handle employees with motivation problems by attempting to determine the cause of the problem and by working to provide an environment that is conducive to increased motivation for the employee. If the employee is uncooperative or unproductive because of a lack of ability, education and training are appropriate interventions.

The manager can determine lack of ability on the part of an employee in various ways. Frequent errors in judgment or techniques are often an indication of lack of knowledge, skill, or critical think-

ing. This illustrates the need for the nurse leader to document all variances or untoward events carefully after discussing these with the employee. When the nurse manager has thorough documentation, trends may be discovered that in turn suggest that a specific employee is having problems. The nurse manager can cite problem behaviors and perhaps even trends to the employee. Corrective action is easier to pursue and resolution is more effective with this strategy. When the problem is determined to result from a need for more education or training, the manager can work with the education department or the clinical specialist for the involved unit to help the employee improve his or her skills. Most employees are extremely cooperative in situations such as this because they want to do a good job but sometimes do not know how. Employees may deny they need help or may be too embarrassed to ask for help. When the manager can show an employee concrete evidence of a problem area, cooperation is enhanced.

Immature Employees

Sometimes, an unproductive employee simply lacks maturity. This lack of maturity may be described as *emotional intelligence underdevelopment* that results in such problems as being socially inept or unable to control one's impulses (Strickland, 2000). The management tips column in *Health Care Manager* describes this situation in "Case in Health Care Management: Managing the Drama Queen" (2004). These employees are frequently defensive and emotional or tearful. They lack self-insight into their behavior. Sometimes, immaturity in an employee may not be readily apparent to the leader but may be manifested in any of the following actions: defiance, testing of workplace guidelines, passivity or hostility, or little appreciation for any management decisions. The challenge for the nurse leader is not to react in kind, but rather to relate to this employee in a positive and mature manner. A sense of humor and the ability to tease the employee into a more receptive, jovial mood is sometimes helpful. However, the leader needs to determine whether the undesirable behaviors are reflecting a state of being uncomfortable or incompetent (LaDuke, 2000). For example, if an employee states, "Administration is always making decisions to make our jobs harder," rather than making a hostile or defensive comment in reply, the manager could take the employee aside and say, "I notice that you seem to be angry about this new policy. Let's talk about it some more." Immature employees either act immaturely all of the time or regress to an immature level when stressed. The nurse leader must recognize immaturity in an employee and react calmly and without anger. The leader must keep in mind that this employee may be displaying dynamics rooted in unresolved personal areas and that the behavior is not a personal attack on the leader. The best way to deal with this behavior is to confront the employee with the specific problem and define realistic limits of acceptable

behavior with consequences for nonadherence. Generally, employees comply with specific limits but will test management in other areas. As this testing occurs, the leader must continue the same limit-setting technique. Remember that the immature employee usually has problems because of a lack of self-worth, power, and self-control. Praise and affirmation are valuable tools that the leader can use to help these employees feel better about themselves. Chapter 2 addresses generational issues if they are factors to consider.

> ## Exercise 24–2
>
> A nurse comes to you, the nurse leader, and states that one of the other nurses is tying a knot in the air vent (pigtail) of nasogastric tubes. This nurse does not know how to approach the employee to discuss the problem. What would you do?

Clinical Incompetence

Clinical incompetence is possibly one of the most frustrating problems that the nurse leader faces, although it may be entirely correctable. The problem may surface immediately in a new employee. At other times, clinical incompetence comes as a surprise if co-workers "cover" for another employee. Some nurses are unwilling to report instances of clinical incompetence because they do not want to feel responsible for getting one of their peers in trouble. When other employees are engaged in enabling behavior by covering for the mistakes of one of their peers, the nurse leader may be surprised to discover that the employee does not know or cannot do what is expected of him or her at work. Sadly, the employee in question has been able to cover incompetence by hiding behind the performance of another employee. The nurse leader must remind employees that part of professional responsibility is to maintain quality care and thus they are obligated to report instances of clinical incompetence, even when it means reporting a co-worker. Ignoring violations of a safety rule or poor practice is unprofessional and cannot be tolerated.

Most healthcare agencies use skills checklists or a competency evaluation program to ascertain that their employees have and maintain essential skills for the job they are expected to do. A skills checklist is one way to determine basic clinical competency (Table 24-1). This checklist typically contains a number of basic skills along with ones that are essential for safe functioning in the specific

Table 24-1 EXAMPLE OF A SKILLS CHECKLIST

Purpose

1. The clinical skills inventory is a three-phase tool to enable the newly hired RN and the nurse manager to determine individual learning needs, verify competency, and plan performance goals.
2. The RN will complete the self-assessment of clinical skills during the first week of employment. The RN will use the appropriate scale to document current knowledge of clinical skills.
3. The nurse manager will document observed competency of the orientee or delegate this to a peer. All columns must be completed on the inventory level.
4. At the end of orientation, the new RN and the manager will use the inventory to identify performance goals on the plan sheet. The skills

inventory will be in a specified place on the nursing unit so that it is available to the manager and other RNs. It should be updated at appropriate intervals as specified by the manager.

Scale for Self-Assessment

1 = Unfamiliar/never done
2 = Able to perform with assistance
3 = Can perform with minimal supervision
4 = Independent performance/proficient

Score for Validation of Competency

1 = Unable to perform at present
2 = Able to perform with assistance
3 = Progressing/repeat performance necessary
4 = Able to perform independently

CLINICAL SKILLS (EXAMPLES)	SELF-ASSESSMENT Scale	Date	COMMENT	VALIDATION Score	Date	Initials	COMMENT
Epidural catheter care							
NG/Dobbhoff							
Insertion							
Management							
Preoperative care/teaching							
Postoperative care/teaching							

Plan Sheet for Skills Inventory

Name _____

Date _____

Goals	Date to Be Completed

Orientee's signature _____

Manager's signature _____

Date _____

area of employment. Any type of skills review should be directly linked to quality-improvement indicators. The employee may be asked to do a self-assessment of the listed skills or competencies and then have performance of the skills validated by a peer or co-worker. This is a very effective method for the leader to assess the skill level of employees and to determine where additional education and training may be necessary. In addition, if the leader discovers that an employee is unable to perform a skill adequately, the skills list can easily be checked and directly observed behaviors can be assessed to determine at what level the employee is functioning. At the completion of the assessment, a specific plan for remediation can be developed. Sometimes, an employee may be able to perform all of the tasks on a skills checklist but is still unable to manage overall patient care effectively. If, in questioning the employee, or in evaluating the employee's performance, the manager/leader determines that there is a lack of knowledge or that there are problems with time management, formal education may be the proper course of action. In either event, the leader must establish a written contract containing a plan of action that sets time limits within which certain expectations must be achieved. This ensures compliance on the part of the employee. A more comprehensive program for competency evaluation might include not only the skills checklist but also unit-specific objectives, an overall framework for evaluation, and critical-thinking exercises that are interactive in nature (Johnson, Opfer, VanCura, & Williams, 2000). The role of the novice nurse leader, particularly with ancillary personnel, is to support the nurse manager as well as be helpful and supportive of the team members who are striving to improve.

Emotional Problems

Emotional problems among nursing personnel may affect not only the involved individual but also co-workers and ultimately the delivery of patient care. The nurse leader must be aware that certain behaviors, such as poor judgment, increased errors, increased absenteeism, decreased productivity, and a negative attitude, may be manifestations of emotional problems in employees.

A nurse manager began hearing complaints from patients about a nurse named Nancy. Patients were saying that Nancy was abrupt and uncaring with them. The manager had not received any complaints about Nancy before this time, so she questioned Nancy about why this was occurring. Nancy reported that her mother was very ill and she was so worried about her and so upset that she could not sleep and was tired all of the time. She went on to say that she was having trouble being sympathetic with complaining patients when they did not seem to be as sick as her mother.

When there is a significant change in an employee's behavior, personal problems with which the person cannot cope may be the cause. The nurse leader is not and should not be a therapist but must intercede, not only to help the individual with the problems but also to maintain proper functioning of the unit. In dealing with the employee who exhibits behaviors that indicate emotional problems, the manager assists the individual to obtain professional help to cope with the problem. Adjustments may need to be made in the individual's work setting and schedule. This may require support from other staff members so there is no negative effect on patient care. The manager acknowledges that an employee is experiencing emotional difficulties and yet the standards of patient care cannot be compromised. It is reassuring for staff to witness the care and concern shown a fellow staff member who is in great difficulty. They can interpret that similar support would be given to them should they be in a difficult situation.

The most important approach that the manager can take with an emotionally troubled employee is to provide support and encouragement and to assist the individual to obtain appropriate help. Many agencies have some kind of employee assistance program (EAP) to which the manager should refer any troubled employee. (The Literature Perspective describes a counseling service and how it helps retain nurses.) During this process, the manager must remember to check with the human resources department about any implications that may occur because of the Americans with Disabilities Act (ADA). If an employee has a documented mental illness, the employing agency may be under certain legal constraints as specified in the ADA. The nurse manager should always remember that many resources are available to assist with personnel problems. The manager should never feel required to know all of the legal implications regarding employment policies. Rather, the manager must know that help is available and how to access it.

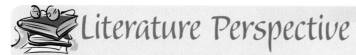

Literature Perspective

Luquette, J. S. (2005). The role of on-site counseling in nurse retention. *Oncology Nursing Forum, 32,* 234-236.

This article describes various aspects of an on-site counseling service and how it demonstrates value to nurses. The key cornerstone beliefs of the service are confidentiality, minimal financial cost, professionalism of the provider, and convenient appointment times and office locations. Services can be both group and individually based. To be effective, the services must be available when nurses work and also be available by phone. The offices need to be in less trafficked areas to help maintain confidentiality. Numerous professional and personal issues are cited. Additionally, the service should include crisis intervention and services devoted to team-building.

IMPLICATIONS FOR PRACTICE
The availability of on-site counseling during any work schedule helps charge nurses and nurse managers refer individuals for help and allows individual nurses to seek the support they may need during challenging times.

Exercise 24-3

As a nurse manager in a community health agency, you have just had a meeting that was called by several of your staff nurses. They expressed concern regarding another nurse colleague who has come to work tearful several times during the past week. They state she often goes into the break room when she is in the agency and appears as if she has been crying when she comes out. She has refused to discuss her distress with her colleagues. These nurses express concern and want you to help her. What is your response? What would you do?

Chemical Dependency

Chemical dependency among nursing personnel places patients and the organization at risk. Such an employee adversely affects staff morale by increasing stress on other staff members when they have to assume heavier workloads to cover for the chemically dependent employee who is not performing at full capacity or who is often absent. As a result, patient care may be jeopardized because staff is focusing more on the problems of a co-worker than on those of the patients. For the novice nurse, it is critical to be aware of the professional responsibilities of reporting incidents in which peers or team members exhibit signs of chemical dependency.

The manager is responsible for early recognition of chemical dependency and referral for treatment when appropriate (McAndrew & McAndrew, 2000). State laws vary as to the reportability of chemical dependency. As is true of all nurses, a nurse manager is responsible for upholding the nurse practice act and should be familiar with the legal aspects of chemical dependency in the state in which he or she is employed. As with the employee with emotional problems, the nurse manager should be aware of ADA issues and check with the human resource department for help with how to handle the employment of a chemically dependent employee. Most states and agencies have reporting requirements regarding substance abuse. The state board of nursing is a key place to determine specific details required by a given state. All nurse

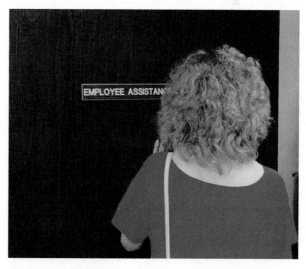

Many agencies have an employee assistance program to which the manager can refer the troubled employee.

managers should familiarize themselves with the nurse practice act in the state in which they reside and with the personnel policies relating to substance abuse in their employing agency. Furthermore, nurse managers should make certain that staff is familiar with legal requirements.

In the present social climate, there is more interest in helping affected individuals than in punishing them, and there is also more empathy and understanding toward them. Identification of an employee with a chemical dependency is usually difficult, especially because one of the primary symptoms is denial. The primary clue to which a manager should be alert when there is a suspicion of chemical dependency is any behavioral change in an employee. This change could be any deviation from the behaviors the employee normally exhibits. Some specific behaviors to note might be mood swings, a change from a tidy appearance to an untidy one, an unusual interest in patients' pain control, frequent changes in jobs and shifts, or an increase in absenteeism and tardiness.

When a manager suspects that an employee may be chemically dependent, the manager must intervene because patient care may be jeopardized. A manager facing a problem with an impaired nurse must be compassionate yet therapeutic. Knowing that denial may be one of the primary signs of substance abuse, the manager must focus on performance problems that the nurse is exhibiting and urge the nurse to seek counseling or treatment voluntarily. EAPs always protect the employee's privacy and are usually available free or at a minimal charge to the employee. The manager should strive to refer any troubled employee to the EAP. This removes the manager from the counseling role and helps employees get the professional help they need without fear of a breach in confidentiality. If a nurse refuses to seek help voluntarily for a substance abuse problem, the manager is responsible for following the established policy for such employees. The manager must remember that if the substance-abusing employee is terminated and not reported, the manager not only may be violating a law but also may be enabling this employee to obtain employment in another agency and potentially be in a position to harm patients and co-workers.

Many states have rehabilitation programs for chemically impaired nurses so that they may return to nursing if rehabilitated. Nurse managers are sometimes asked to assist with monitoring the progress of a chemically impaired nurse. Specific guidelines are established through the rehabilitation program with the cooperation of the employee, the agency, and the manager. The manager is typically asked to provide feedback about the employee's progress to the employee and to the state or rehabilitation program involved. These programs vary, but, for example, a nurse who has been an admitted abuser of meperidine may be allowed to work in a setting in which this drug is never used, or the nurse may not be permitted to administer any controlled substances to patients. This, of course, puts an added burden on other staff members, but it can be a positive experience for all because nurses face some of their professional responsibility by helping another nurse while upholding patient care. Often, as a part of their therapy, these nurses are required to share openly with other staff members what their problem is and what they are doing to control it. When handled in a positive, professional way, the nurse manager can turn a potentially destructive situation into a positive, constructive one.

Regardless of the type of personnel issue, the manager needs to have a plan in place for ongoing monitoring and follow-up of issues/problems.

Exercise 24-4

Review your state's nurse practice act and rules and regulations. What are you required to do if you believe a nurse has a problem with chemical dependency?

DOCUMENTATION

Documentation of personnel problems is unquestionably one of the most important, but also one of the most onerous, aspects of the nurse manager's job. As much as some managers may wish they would, personnel problems probably will not "disappear," and, therefore, will eventually have to be resolved. Through careful, ongoing documentation of problems, the manager makes the task of identifying and correcting problems much less burdensome.

Documentation cannot be left to memory! When an employee is involved in a problem situation or if an employee receives a compliment or does something extremely well, a brief notation to this effect must be placed in the personnel file. This entry includes the date, time, and a brief description of the incident. Adding a small notation as to what was done about a problem when it occurred is also helpful. Along with this, the nurse manager should keep a log or summary sheet of all reported errors, unusual incidents, and accidents. These extremely important data should include the date, time, and names of involved individuals and should be tallied at monthly intervals for analysis by the manager. The few extra minutes each day that the manager spends tracking these data provide invaluable information to the manager about organizational and individual functioning. This tracking can then be used to pinpoint an individual's problem areas, areas of excellence in individual performance, and overall organizational problem areas. The manager who keeps careful records about organizational functioning has greater control in the management of personal and personnel problems. Box 24-2 describes content and format for

such documentation and provides an example as an illustration.

 ## PROGRESSIVE DISCIPLINE

When an employee's performance falls below the acceptable standard, despite corrective measures that have been taken, some form of discipline must be enacted. Most organizations use some form of **progressive discipline** to correct problem behaviors. When the nurse leader suspects that specific behaviors may lead to progressive discipline, it is critical that all interactions be documented and that the human resources department be involved in the process to be certain that all policies are accurately adhered to. Progressive discipline consists of evaluating performance and providing feedback within a specified structure of increasing sanctions. These sanctions, progressing from least severe to most severe, are described in Box 24-3. Examples of the kind of workplace behavior that usually involves

---

BOX 24-2

Documentation of Problems

- Description of incident—an objective statement of the facts related to the incident
- Actions—statements describing the plan to correct and/or prevent future problems
- Follow-up—dates and times that the plan is to be carried out, including required meeting with the employee

Example
Several patients reported to the nurse manager that Becky, one of the night-shift registered nurses, was "curt" and "gruff" and seemed uncaring with them. The manager called Becky into her office and reiterated the complaints that she had received. The nurse manager was specific as to times and incidents. The manager then reminded Becky about what her expectations were relating to patient care, emphasizing the importance of a caring attitude with all patients. She discussed with Becky what the possible cause of Becky's behavior might be, such as problems at home or lack of sleep. Becky

denied being curt or gruff, but agreed that some of her mannerisms might be misinterpreted. The manager suggested to Becky that perhaps she needed to be particularly aware of her body language and to soften her tone of voice. After discussing this incident and reminding Becky of the importance of caring in nursing, the manager told Becky that this behavior would not be tolerated. The manager told Becky she wanted to meet with her every Friday morning at the end of Becky's shift to discuss how the week had gone and to determine how she was interacting with the patients assigned to her. The manager also told Becky that she would be checking with patients to see what they had thought of Becky. The manager routinely asked patients about their nursing care as she made rounds, so this was not an unusual thing for her to do. These weekly meetings were to be conducted for 6 weeks, followed by monthly meetings for a 3-month period. If there were no recurrence of problems, the meetings would be discontinued after this time.

BOX 24-3

Steps in Progressive Discipline

1. Counsel the employee regarding the problem.
2. Reprimand the employee. A verbal reprimand usually precedes a written one, but some organizations issue both a verbal and a written reprimand simultaneously. When the documentation is written, the employee must sign to verify that the problem was discussed. This does not mean that the employee agrees with the reprimand. It means only that the employee is aware of a written reprimand that is to be placed in the employee's personnel file. The employee always receives a copy of a written reprimand.
3. Suspend the employee if the problem persists. The employee will be suspended without pay for a specified period, usually several days or longer according to the agency policy. During this time, the employee may realize the seriousness of the problem based on the resulting discipline.
4. Allow the employee to return to work with written stipulations regarding problem behavior.
5. Terminate the employee if the problem recurs.

progressive discipline and could even result in immediate termination are harassment and chemical abuse (Brennan, 1999).

TERMINATION

At times, even though the manager has done everything possible to gain the cooperation of a problem employee, the problems may persist. In such cases, there is no choice but to terminate the employee. Because termination is one of the most difficult things a manager does, the following guidelines should be adhered to: First, the manager must be confident that everything possible has been done to help the employee correct the problem behaviors. Second, the manager must recognize that if employment continues, this employee will have a deleterious effect on overall organizational functioning and, more importantly, on nursing care. Third, the employee must have been made fully aware of the problem performance and of the fact that all of the correct disciplinary steps have been followed. Finally, a nurse manager should check with the

human resources and legal departments before proceeding to ensure that termination is justifiable legally and that proper steps have been followed. The nurse manager needs to be confident in the knowledge that all policies regarding termination have been followed before having an actual termination meeting with the employee. It is always preferable to err on the side of caution when proceeding with termination of an employee. Remember that termination is something that the employee has caused as a result of persistent problem behaviors or certain behaviors for which the organization has zero tolerance. Termination is not done at the whim of management; it results from failure on the part of the employee to change a problem behavior.

Situations that may warrant immediate dismissal include theft, violence in the workplace, and willful abuse of the patient, to name a few. Again, the manager should use the assistance of the human resource department to ensure that all of the organization's policies are being upheld correctly. The following example illustrates that a manager needs to anticipate a termination to ensure ongoing standards:

Linda has gone through all of the steps in the progressive discipline process as a result of her abusive behavior toward her co-workers. She returned to work and seemed to be doing well until about 6 weeks later, when she slammed down her clipboard during report and angrily accused the charge nurse of always giving her the worst assignments. The nurse manager was present and asked Linda to come into her office. At this point, she told Linda she was relieving her of her assignment that day and asked her to go home to cool off. The manager told her that she would call her the following day about what would be done. Linda went home, and the manager reviewed the incident with her nurse administrator. They both agreed that Linda's behavior not only was intolerable but also violated the terms of her probation and therefore she should be terminated. The manager called Linda the following day as she had agreed to do and asked Linda to come and meet with her. The manager and administrator met with Linda and reviewed the incidents and the disciplinary measures leading up to this incident. The nurse manager asked the administrator to be present at the scheduled meeting because it is a good practice to have a witness in a confrontative situation such as termination. The manager stated to Linda that she regretted it had come to this, but pointed out to her that her behavior had violated all of the agreed-upon stipulations, and as a result she would be terminated immediately. Linda was tearful and had numerous excuses, but the manager remained firm and merely repeated that Linda, in not fulfilling the agreement, had chosen to end her employment.

Exercise 24–5

Review a healthcare organization's policies regarding termination. What are the conditions, such as stealing or violence, that are described as cause for immediate dismissal? Is abusing substances at work one of those conditions?

CONCLUSION

All employees share a role with managers to prevent and control personal/personnel problems in their work setting. Everyone must be willing to refuse to allow unethical behavior from co-workers and to speak out and act appropriately when problems occur.

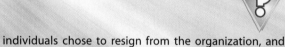

The Solution

As a final step, we met with the two individuals who had not passed, despite all of our efforts, and gave them the opportunity to transfer to another clinical area of their choosing, where they would feel comfortable, if an opening was available. We made it clear to them that they could not work on the pediatric unit because they had not met the established standards of care. One of the individuals chose to resign from the organization, and the other one transferred to another area.

— Cherie Gorby

Would this be a suitable approach for you? Why?

CHAPTER CHECKLIST

To obtain satisfaction from working with people, a nurse manager must be knowledgeable about personal and personnel issues that are likely to occur in the work setting. The nurse manager must be able to detect, prevent, and correct problems that affect nursing care and staff morale in a nursing agency. Proper documentation and follow-up are key elements in the successful management of all personnel issues.

- Absenteeism's detrimental effects are as follows:
  - Patient care may be below standard.
  - Replacement personnel require additional supervision.
  - Absenteeism may increase among the entire staff.
  - Financial management of the unit suffers adverse effects.
- Effective strategies to reduce absenteeism include the following:

- Enhancing nurses' job satisfaction
- Using Haddock's model of nonpunitive discipline:
  - Remind the employee of the problem orally.
  - Follow up with a written reminder if the oral one fails.
  - Grant the employee a day of decision if the written reminder fails.
  - Terminate if the employee decides not to adhere to standards.
- Uncooperative or unproductive employees may lack motivation, ability, or maturity.
  - The nurse manager can try to provide an environment that is more conducive to motivation.
  - Education and training are appropriate interventions for lack of ability.
  - Praise and affirmation are often the most effective strategies for an employee who lacks maturity.
- Clinical incompetence is a highly correctable problem for nurse managers.
  - Clinical incompetence may be masked by co-workers' enabling behavior.

- A skills checklist helps determine basic clinical competency and pinpoint the need for additional training and education.
- A comprehensive competency program may include not only a skills checklist but also a means for evaluating critical-thinking ability of the employee.
- When emotional problems are evident, the nurse manager must assist the employee in getting professional help. The nurse manager is responsible for early recognition of chemical dependency and referral for treatment when appropriate.
  - The manager must do the following:
    - Uphold the state's nurse practice act.
    - Be familiar with state laws on chemical dependency.
    - Know the healthcare organization's personnel policy on chemical dependency.
  - Some warning signs of possible chemical dependency are as follows:
    - Behavioral changes such as mood swings

    - Sudden and unusual neglect for personal appearance
    - Unusual interest in patients' pain control
    - Increased absenteeism and tardiness
- Documentation of problems must include the following:
  - A description of the incident
  - A description of the manager's actions
  - A plan to correct/prevent future occurrences
  - Dates and times of follow-up measures
- Progressive discipline may be used when other corrective measures have failed. Steps in progressive discipline are as follows:
  - Counsel the employee regarding the problem.
  - Reprimand the employee (first verbally, then in writing).
  - Suspend the employee if the problem persists.
  - Allow the employee to return to work, with written stipulations regarding problem behavior.
  - Terminate the employee if the problem recurs.

TIPS IN THE DOCUMENTATION OF PROBLEMS

- Identify the incident and related facts.
- Describe actions taken by the manager when the problem was identified.
- Develop an action plan for everyone involved.
- Schedule a follow-up meeting to evaluate progress of the action plan.

- Remember to document everything objectively and completely!

TERMS TO KNOW

absenteeism	progressive discipline
chemically dependent	role strain
nonpunitive discipline	role stress

REFERENCES

Barnes, B., Leis, S., Brammer, I. M., Gustin, T. J., & Lupo, T. C. (1999). A developmental evaluation process for nurses. Enhancing professional excellence. *Journal of Nursing Administration, 29*(4), 25–32.

Brennan, W. (1999). Bully off! *Nursing Standard, 13*(18), 27–28.

Case in health care management: Managing the drama queen. (2004). *The Health Care Manager, 23*(4), 318–320.

Haddock, C. (1989). Transformation leadership and the employee discipline process. *Hospital Health Service Administration, 34*(2), 185–194.

Hardy, M. E., & Conway, M. E. (1988). *Role theory: Perspectives for health professionals* (2nd ed.). Norwalk, CT: Appleton & Lange.

Hersey, P., Blanchard, K., & Johnson, D. E. (1996). *Management of organizational behavior: Utilizing human resources* (7th ed.). Englewood Cliffs, NJ: Prentice Hall.

Johnson, T., Opfer, K., VanCura, B., & Williams, L. (2000). A comprehensive interactive competency program. Part I: Development and framework. *MedSurg Nursing, 9*(5), 265–268.

LaDuke, S. (2000). Nurses' perceptions: Is your nurse uncomfortable or incompetent? *Journal of Nursing Administration, 30*(4), 163–165.

McAndrew, K. G., & McAndrew, S. J. (2000). Workplace substance abuse impairment: The occupational health care provider's role. *AAOHN Journal, 48*(1), 32–47.

Osborne, J., Blais, K., & Hayes, J. S. (1999). Nurses' perceptions: When is it a medication error? *Journal of Nursing Administration, 29*(4), 33–38.

Sportsman, S. (2005). Build a framework for conflict assessment. *Nursing Management, 36*(4), 32–40.

Strickland, D. (2000). Emotional intelligence: The most potent factor in the success equation. *Journal of Nursing Administration, 30*(3), 112–117.

SUGGESTED READINGS

Quinn, C., & Barton, A. (1999). The implications of drug treatment and testing orders. *Nursing Standard, 14*(27), 38–41.

Wright, D. (1998). *The ultimate guide to competency assessment in health care.* Eau Claire, WI: PESI HealthCare.

Yoder, L. H. (1995). Staff nurses' career development relationships and self-reports of professionalism, job satisfaction, and intent to stay. *Nursing Research, 44*(5), 290–297.

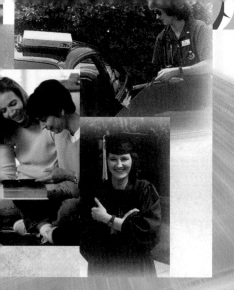

Chapter

25

Role Transition

Diane M. Twedell with Jennifer Jackson Gray

T his chapter provides information about role transition—the process of moving from a clinically focused position to a supervisory position with increased responsibility. The basic overview of management roles illustrates the complexity of managing work done by others and provides a foundation for understanding role transition. The exercises offer opportunities to recognize one's own expectations, resources, and management potential.

Objectives

- Construct the full scope of a manager role by outlining responsibilities, opportunities, lines of communication, expectations, and support (ROLES).
- Analyze specific examples of role transitions as a staff nurse and a nurse manager.
- Describe the phases of role transition by using a past life experience.
- Construct a response to an unexpected role transition.
- Compare strategies to facilitate a successful role transition.

Questions to Consider

- *What do I need to know about a management position before applying and interviewing for it?*
- *What questions do I need to ask prior to accepting a nursing management position?*
- *How can I successfully make the transition from clinical nurse to nurse manager?*
- *Am I currently in a role transition?*

The Challenge

Robin E. Keene, RNC
ICU Nurse Manager, Central Texas Veterans Health Care Services, Temple, Texas

I was a staff nurse for 6 years before becoming nurse manager, the last 4 of which were in the intensive care unit (ICU), where I am now manager. I was motivated to join the management team because I believed I could help to improve working conditions for staff nurses at this facility. I always thought that the nurse managers forgot where they came from and what it is like to be a staff nurse. The management team at my facility comprises mainly older female registered nurses (RNs). I envisioned that by being the youngest and most energetic member of the team, I would be able to motivate them and facilitate a more progressive and positive management team.

My role changed dramatically and quickly once I was put in the management role. I went from caring for patients to writing reports, proficiencies, and time schedules and dealing with personnel conflicts and problems overnight. I had no previous training for this and felt totally lost. My workday quickly became one of policy/procedure and the Joint Commission on Accreditation of Healthcare Organizations rather than providing patient care.

The most difficult part of the transition for me was making the change from patient care provider to management. The second most difficult part of this transition was making the move from staff nurse to administration in the same unit. My former friends could no longer be my friends, and my co-workers became my employees. I already knew their good and bad habits, who I wanted to work for me and who I did not. Everyone looked at me differently immediately (even though I was still the same person). Some of my staff members brought up the word *favoritism* anytime I gave one of my former friends time off. The last part of the transition that has been so difficult is the realization that I cannot make changes at this facility without a struggle. Because I manage in a government facility, making change is extremely difficult, and I was not prepared for that. How could I be comfortable in this new role?

 What do you think you would do if you were this nurse?

INTRODUCTION

Role transition involves transforming one's professional identity. A new graduate makes a transition from the student role to the nurse role. Expectations of students are clearly specified in course and clinical objectives. Expectations for a new nurse as an employee may not be so clear. The new graduate nurse faces the first of several profes-sional transitions. The two Research Perspectives provide further information on role transitions for new graduate nurses, which is helpful for new graduates, their co-workers, and their managers.

Consider the staff nurse who becomes a nurse manager. The staff nurse performs tasks related to the care of patients. As a follower, the staff nurse has accountability and responsibility for the work that is accomplished. A staff nurse who becomes a nurse manager must transition into the new role as a generalist, orchestrating diverse tasks and getting work done through others.

A staff nurse who moves from an acute care setting to a home health agency must also undergo a role transition. Instead of balancing the needs of multiple patients, the home health nurse can focus on one client at a time. Yet, when a collegial opinion is needed during a visit, there are no readily available peers with whom to consult.

Organizations play a key role in assisting employees through role transitions. Ewens (2003) indicates that role stress can occur when the work-

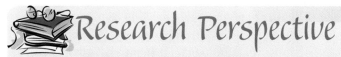

Research Perspective

Ellerton, M. L., & Gregor, F. (2003). A study of transition: The new nurse graduate at three months. *The Journal of Continuing Education in Nursing, 34*(3), 103–107.

The researchers conducted open-ended interviews with 11 nurses employed in acute care settings at 3 months following graduation. The purpose of the study was to explore the adequacy of baccalaureate nursing preparation for a staff-nurse role in a hospital setting. The nurses defined their work as a set of skills and valued knowledge they acquired from experienced staff on the unit. They were focused on tasks rather than on relationships and communication. The nurses detailed the lack of clinical practice opportunities in their academic preparation and relied on the expertise of nurses already present and working on the unit.

IMPLICATIONS FOR PRACTICE

Experienced staff nurses play a critical role in the development of clinical expertise in new graduates. Experienced nurses must be valued for the guidance they provide to new graduates emerging from academic nursing programs.

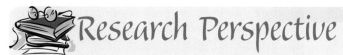

Research Perspective

Delaney, C. (2003). Walking a fine line: Graduate nurses' transition experiences during orientation. *Journal of Nursing Education, 42*(10), 437-443.

The researcher conducted a phenomenological. study investigating graduate nurses' transition experiences during orientation. Ten graduate nurses participated in 30- to 60-minute interviews with the researcher. Themes that emerged included mixed emotions, preceptor variability, the "real world" stress, culture shock, not ready for dying and death, rhythm of work, self reflection, value of nursing, and readiness to complete orientation. Stress was the most powerful common experience of the new graduates.

IMPLICATIONS FOR PRACTICE

There is a need for collaboration between academia and service to help prepare graduate nurses for the real world of nursing. Preparing students for death and dying should be woven into curricula. Preparation and selection of preceptors is vital to assisting new graduates in transition.

place does not provide the scope and flexibility for integration of new identities. The "nurse may experience frustration and disappointment and the work role becomes untenable, resulting in them either leaving or retreating back to traditional identities" (p. 224). Changes in roles can be either painful or exciting and depend largely on the work culture and support provided.

Knowing what to expect during the transformation can reduce the stress of accepting and transitioning into a new role and result in quality outcomes. Following an overview of the roles of leader, manager, and follower, this chapter describes the process of role transition, with an emphasis on strategies that can be used to ease the transition.

TYPES OF ROLES

Accepting a management position dictates accepting three roles that involve complex processes. The roles of leader, manager, and follower are complex because they involve working through and with unique individuals in a rapidly changing environment. Examples of the people with whom you interact and the processes involved in each role are shown in Table 25-1. In nursing, each of these roles relates to patients and clients.

The transition from a staff nurse role to a nurse manager leader role can occur overnight. The nurse moves from the clinical work of patient care to lead a group of employees. Arnold and Nelson (2004) indicate that the leader role has many facets, including change agent, coach, mentor, conflict manager, and management representative.

Arnold and Nelson (2004) share that an aging nursing workforce, the acuity of patient illness, the complexity of health care, and the importance of the nurse manager puts the nurse manager role in the spotlight. Strong leadership is needed at the point of care for good unit and patient-care outcomes (Srsic-Stoehr et al., 2004). Marelli (2004, p. 6) states that "the nurse manager by position and personality sets the tone for the effective completion of numerous activities. In patient care settings, the goal of these activities is a satisfied customer."

The role of follower involves respecting the authority of others and working within the system to contribute to the organizational outcomes. Managers as followers recognize their accountability to the persons above them on the organizational chart. Within a team, the manager recognizes the leadership being provided by others and supports decisions made by the group.

In the evolving healthcare environment, the nurse providing direct patient care also must function as a leader, manager, and follower. As **leader,** the nurse recognizes the uniqueness of each patient and provides feedback on clinical progress. As **manager,** the nurse links the patient to the resources to achieve clinical outcomes. Medical information is translated into a format that the patient can use to make informed decisions about treatment and self-care. Through referrals, the nurse facilitates continuity of care within the larger system. As **follower,** the nurse is accountable to the team and the

supervisor for completing the work that is assigned. The nurse as a follower practices within the policies and procedures of the organization and the standards of the profession.

Learning the leader, manager, and follower aspects of any new role can be overwhelming. Another approach to the complexity of role transition is the acronym **ROLES**, in which each letter represents a component common to all roles.

Table 25-1	LEADER, MANAGER, AND FOLLOWER ROLES: PEOPLE WITH WHOM YOU INTERACT AND PROCESSES INVOLVED IN EACH ROLE	
Role	**People with Whom Interactions Occur**	**Processes Involved in the Role**
Leader	Persons being led Peers	Listening Encouraging Motivating Organizing Problem-solving Developing Supporting
Manager	Persons being supervised Administrators Supervisors Regulating agencies	Organizing Budgeting Hiring Evaluating Reporting Disseminating
Follower	Supervisor Peers	Conforming Implementing Contributing Completing assignments

ROLES: THE ABCs OF UNDERSTANDING ROLES

Acronyms help us retain and organize information. "ROLES" (Box 25-1) is an acronym that is useful in role transition.

BOX 25-1

"ROLES" Acronym

Responsibilities
Opportunities
Lines of communication
Expectations
Support

R stands for responsibilities. What are the specified duties in the position description for the new position? What tasks are to be completed? What decisions must the person in this position make? For example, the job description for a nurse manager might include 24-hour accountability for a patient-care area (Marelli, 2004), whereas the job description for a nurse practitioner would include responsibilities to provide direct client care in a primary-care setting (Catalano, 2003). Each position has specific tasks for which the position holder is responsible.

O stands for opportunities, which are untapped aspects of the position. In the employment interview, the nurse executive may have said that the previous manager did not encourage the staff nurses to participate in continuing education. Or, while touring the unit, a manager observes that the report room is lacking in amenities. Maybe there is a new method of delivering patient care that is appropriate for the unit. These possibilities represent opportunities for a manager to influence organizational and unit goals.

L represents lines of communication. All roles involve relationships with other people (Marelli, 2004). Some of these people are above the manager on the organizational chart, others are below, still others are peers. Roles incorporate patterns of structured interactions between the manager and people in these groups. The nurse manager receives and sends messages. Being a skillful listener can be more important than being skillful in sending messages. Skill is required to communicate both the content and the intent of the message effectively. Only through practice can one develop skill. In Chapter 17, techniques of effective communication are described that are extremely important to a new manager in building the team.

E stands for expectations. Expectations vary depending on your goals. Colleagues may expect a new nurse anesthetist to be on call every weekend. Staff nurses have specific expectations of their managers and particularly want the manager to be a facilitator and a leader. The nursing executive or administrator will likely have expectations about how managers spend their time on the job—even about how much time they spend at work. Nurse executives' expectations evolve from their perspectives of the manager's accountability and duties.

Finding out in advance what the explicit and implicit expectations are of the people involved can facilitate a smoother role transition by decreasing role ambiguity (Hardy, 1978). Hardy's work with role theory suggests a strong relationship between role ambiguity (one type of role stress) and **role strain.** The major concepts of role theory are presented in the Theory Box.

There are also personal expectations related to performance as a manager. You have a mental image of the role of a manager or person in this position. The process of role transition unfolds as a new manager identifies expectations, recognizes the similarities and differences, and develops the roles of leader, manager, and follower.

S stands for support, which is closely tied to expectations about performance. All roles are shaped to some degree by the support and services others provide. The acute care nurse has peers readily available when a second opinion is needed. The same nurse may feel lost when confronted with questionable findings during a home visit. The nurse manager who must develop the unit's budget in a skilled-care facility may have no accounting department to provide services, such as a detailed analysis of the facility's expenditures. Each role has some support available. When a new position is being considered, it is important to evaluate whether support is available in areas in which a manager may lack knowledge or skill. When implementing changes in roles, the organization needs to develop support services to facilitate role transition. The two *Research Perspectives* describe the support needed by new graduates who are transitioning to the role of staff nurse.

Theory Box

HARDY'S ROLE THEORY

THEORY/CONTRIBUTOR	KEY IDEAS	APPLICATION TO PRACTICE
Hardy (1978) is credited with applying role theory to healthcare professionals. *Role* is the expected and actual behaviors associated with a position. *Role expectations* are the attitudes and behaviors others anticipate that a person in the role will possess or demonstrate. *Role stress* is a social condition in which role demands are conflicting, irritating, difficult, or impossible to fulfill. *Role strain* is the subjective feeling of discomfort experienced as the result of role stress.	Role stress is a precursor to role strain. Role stress is associated with low productivity and performance. Role stress and role strain can lead a person to withdraw psychologically from the role. Clear, realistic role expectations can decrease the role stress for a new nurse manager.	Clear, realistic role expectations can increase productivity.

■ Exercise 25-1

ROLES Assessment

Answer these questions for a position in management that you would consider.

Responsibilities

1. From the position description, what are the responsibilities?
2. For what decisions are you responsible?
3. Consider information about the management position that you learned during the interview (this may be role-played). Also consider the responsibilities of managers you have observed. Are there other responsibilities to add to your list?

Opportunities

4. What would you like to do differently from the previous manager?
5. How could your strengths or expertise benefit the people or nursing unit you would manage?
6. Dream a little (or a lot). If a person who had been a patient on the unit were describing the nursing care to another potential patient, what would you want the first patient to say? Describe the unit as you want it to be known.

Lines of Communication

7. Draw yourself in the middle of a separate piece of paper. Now fill in the people above you and below you with whom you would communicate. Draw lines from you to each person or group. On the line, identify the form of communication. For example, if

you communicate with the director of nursing through a weekly report, write on the line, "Written report."

Expectations

8. This may be the most difficult part to assess. List in short sentences or phrases the expectations each person or group may have for you in relation to your management position.

SELF	FAMILY
ADMINISTRATION	IMMEDIATE SUPERVISOR
PEOPLE YOU WILL MANAGE	

Support

9. What people do you know in the organization who could provide information that you will need to do your job?
10. What departments provide services that you could access for assistance?

Next Steps:

Now compare the lists.

Place a star next to those expectations that are held by more than one person or group. For example, you want to handle the budget of the unit efficiently, an expectation shared with nursing administration.

Circle those items that could cause conflicts.

Read the strategies section in the chapter for ideas on how to resolve these conflicts.

Save your responses to these questions to review in 3 months. You may be surprised how your own perception of your ROLES may change over time.

ROLE TRANSITION PROCESS

One way to think about the way in which someone transitions to a new role is illustrated in Box 25-2 and Table 25-2. Thinking about transitions in terms of a common social perspective may be helpful for some.

STRATEGIES TO PROMOTE ROLE TRANSITION

Becoming a manager or assuming a new role requires a transformation—a profound change in identity. Such a transformation invokes stress as the person unlearns old roles and learns the management role. Several strategies can be helpful in easing the strain and speeding the process of role transition (Box 25-3).

Internal Resources

A key strategy in promoting role transition is to recognize, use, and strengthen the internal resources of commitment, character, self-respect, and flexibility. Work commitment is a function of the fit between the role and the person's professional goals and commitments in other areas of life, such as family or church. The role of manager is not for everyone. One must consider whether personal goals and professional fulfillment can best be achieved through management. One's commitment to the challenges of managing can provide the desire to persevere during the process of role transition.

Another internal resource is character. Character is often considered synonymous with honesty and is tied to values and ethics of a person (Kouzes & Pozner, 2002). People whose characters are based on principles continue to be educated by their experiences and are service-oriented. Consistency between word and deed is used by followers to judge character. Porter-O'Grady and Malloch (2002, p. 261) indicate that character implies "the person has the moral fortitude and discipline to exemplify the highest virtues of his or her time."

Closely related to character is another internal resource—self-respect. Self-respect allows managers to weather the difficult times when there may be little external recognition. A person's value does not depend on the quality or quickness of the adjustment to the management role. Knowing what you believe in is especially important during a transition period. Writing down short statements of belief or self-affirmations and posting this information may be helpful as a visual reminder.

Halpern and Lubar (2003) relate the need for leaders to be open to unexpected outcomes. Changing circumstances in health care raise the need for flexibility. The effective leader must have the ability to learn and master new skills, translate information for staff, and adapt behavior to the situation. Halpern and Lubar (2003) indicate that the most successful leaders are open to change and adapt to new circumstances easily.

Organizational Assessment

A new manager is much like an immigrant in a new country. An immigrant learns how to access the available resources to acclimate to the new environment. Cultural practices of the new country may seem strange or odd. Such differences can be analyzed and decisions made about which aspects to incorporate into one's own culture. More subtle differences in communication patterns or group dynamics can also be identified. Understanding the nuances of social interactions is often the most difficult aspect of acclimating to a new country. The transition is smoother for the immigrant who understands herself or himself, assesses the new environment, and learns how to communicate within groups.

The new manager must also learn how to access resources in the organization. Approaching the organization as a foreign culture, the new manager can keenly observe the rituals, accepted practices, and patterns of communication within the organization. This ongoing assessment promotes a speedier transition into the role of manager. The immigrant who spends energy bemoaning the difficulties of the new country may fail to enjoy the advantages that drew the individual to the country in the first place. In the same way, the manager who focuses on the weaknesses of the organization may lack the energy to internalize the new role, a step that is critical to being an effective leader.

Role Negotiation

A strategy that is helpful during conflicting role expectations is **role negotiation**. The ROLES assessment (see Exercise 25-1) may have identified areas

BOX 25-2

Role Transition Process

Unlearning old roles while learning new roles requires an identity adjustment over time. The persons involved must invest themselves in the process. In this way, role transition can be compared with developing a relationship. The process of developing an intimate relationship with another person provides a familiar framework for considering role transition. Relationships typically move through the phases of dating, commitment, honeymoon, disillusionment, resolution, and maturity.

Role Preview

During the dating phase, the interested persons spend structured time together. Both parties present their best characteristics and dedicate a lot of energy to developing the relationship. Although both parties present their best characteristics, both also are alert to clues that the other party cannot meet their expectations. For example, one may consider the financial and emotional resources that the other person would bring to the relationship. The individuals might spend time with each other's families to get a feel for the emotional climate in which the other person grew up.

Interviewing for a management position is similar to dating. An interview involves touring the unit, visiting with people, and attempting to make a good impression. The potential employer is also attempting to make a favorable impression. The interviewee wants to find out whether this is an organization that will support his or her growth as he or she supports the growth of the organization. Questions are asked about the role of the manager, and the potential manager mentally evaluates whether the described role matches personal expectations about management. Both of these examples represent the phase "role preview."

Role Acceptance

Through the dating process, two people may decide that they want to spend the rest of their lives together and commit to the relationship. Sometimes, one or both of the people decide that they do not want to establish a long-term relationship. In a similar way, following the role preview of the interview process, both parties may agree to establish a relationship as employee and employer. Or one or more of the parties may decide not to establish the relationship. In dating, the public decision to leave other similar relationships and establish this new relationship represents a formal commitment. In role transition, the formal commitment of the employment contract implies acceptance of the management role, or "role acceptance."

Role Exploration

In new relationships, a time of dating and commitment is usually followed by a honeymoon. More than a trip to a vacation spot, the honeymoon has become synonymous with excitement, happiness, and confidence. In a new work role, people also experience a honeymoon phase. The new graduate may be relieved that the educational program was successfully completed and now a salary can be earned. When a new manager is hired, the employer is excited that the search is over. The staff is happy to have a leader, especially if staff members had input into the hiring decision. The new manager is happy, excited, and, most of all, confident in exploring the new roles involved in the management position.

Role Discrepancy

Whether by a gradual process or as the result of a particular event that serves as the turning point, eventually the honeymoon is over, and disillusionment about the relationship occurs. For example, one person may make an expensive purchase without consulting the partner. An argument is followed by a period of painful silence. Similarly, the honeymoon phase in a new employment position can be followed by a period of disillusionment.

Role discrepancy, a gap between **role expectations** and role performance, causes discomfort and frustration. Role discrepancy can be resolved by either dissolving the relationship or by changing expectations and performance. The importance of the relationship and the perceived differences between performance and expectations, the basis of role discrepancy, must be considered in light of personal values. When the relationship is valued, and the differences are seen as correctable, the decision is made to stay in the relationship. This decision requires the couple or the manager to develop the role.

Role Development

Choosing to change either role expectations or role performance or to change both is the process of **role development.** In an intimate relationship, open communication can clarify expectations. Negotiation may result in reasonable expectations. Certain behaviors

BOX 25-2

Role Transition Process—cont'd

may be changed to improve role performance. For example, one person in the relationship learns to call home to let the other know about the possibility of being late.

To reduce role discrepancy in a new management position, the same open communication and negotiation must occur. Expectations need to be clarified and stipulated by both parties. New managers evaluate management styles and techniques to determine which ones best fit them and the situation. The personal management style evolves as the individuals develop the management roles in their own unique ways. If role discrepancy can be reduced and the role developed to be satisfactory to both parties, the new manager can focus on developing the roles of the position and proceed to the phase of **role internalization.**

Role Internalization

Role internalization occurs in relationships as they mature. No longer do the persons in the relationship consciously consider their roles. They have learned the behaviors that maintain and nurture the relationship. The behaviors become second nature. The energy spent on establishing and developing the relationship can be redirected toward achieving mutual goals. In the same way, managers who have been in management positions for several years have internalized their roles. Most of the time, they do not consciously consider their roles. Managers know they have reached the stage of role internalization when they focus on accomplishing mutual goals instead of contemplating whether their role performance matches their role expectations. Managers who have internalized their roles have developed their own unique personal style of management. Table 25-2 summarizes the comparison between the phases of developing an intimate relationship and the phases of role transition to a nurse manager.

Unexpected Role Transition

Not every relationship is successful. Some relationships end in an argument, divorce, or death. When a relationship ends unexpectedly, a person goes through a griev-

ing process. In a similar way, when a person is fired, a position is eliminated, or a job description changes dramatically, the person may have to grieve before being able to engage in role transition. Health care is in a tumultuous state. Mergers, acquisitions, and reductions in force are commonplace. Focusing attention on assisting new peers, supervisors, and staff with the process is a major component of the manager's role (Marelli, 2004). To be successful, workplace restructuring must be undertaken with the same sensitivity afforded a person who has lost a relationship through death or divorce. Role transition takes time, even in reverse.

The initial response to a change in role can be shock and disbelief. The person may feel numb and unable to function. As the numbness wears off, the person may become angry. The anger fuels resistance to the change and may be directed toward those who initiated the role change. The anger may be directed internally, leading to depression. If the person is unable to acknowledge and talk about the loss, the period of grief may be extended, or emotional baggage may be created that is carried into the next role. Grieving can eventually resolve in acceptance. Lessons learned from the experience are identified and internalized. A new role is sought, and the "dating" begins again.

When a relationship is dissolved in the case of death or divorce, a legal document is prepared to formally dissolve the financial and social obligations between the persons involved. The loss of a position as a result of restructuring or a buyout should involve a similar process. The employer may offer the nurse a severance package that includes financial compensation and outplacement services. If the employer does not offer a written agreement, the nurse should formally request and negotiate reasonable compensation and assistance. Similar to signing a prenuptial agreement, a nurse may have signed a contract with the employer when hired. The terms of that agreement may require the employer to buy out (pay the salary and benefits) for the time remaining on the contract.

Written by Jennifer Jackson Gray.

of significant conflict. Writing the expectations down provides the first step in resolving areas of conflict. It is important to review the expectations listed to determine whether they are realistic. Unrealistic expectations strongly held by others may require diplomatic reeducation so that their expectations can become more realistic.

The priority of different role expectations may also require role negotiation with the person above you in the line of command. Ask for input as to which expectations have the highest priorities. Explain personal and family expectations, and clearly state the priority that meeting those expectations has. The process may have to be repeated several times before agreement on the expectations related to roles and the priority of each expectation is found. Rewriting the unrealistic expectations to be achievable can reduce three common sources of role stress—ambiguity, overload, and conflict. Each person's role makes a contribution to the end result. All individuals must understand their roles, or the team may fail.

Mentors

The process of mentoring is not a new concept. This concept has been alive since Homer's Odyssey. Odysseus leaves Ithaca to fight in the Trojan War. Before leaving, he entrusts his son to Mentor. Mentor was to develop and prepare him for his life and duties. McKinley (2004, p. 3) describes mentor as "a trusted advisor, teacher, and wise person." Dracup and Bryan-Brown (2004) indicate that mentors facilitate learning experiences and help new nurses network in a professional milieu,

---

BOX 25-3

Strategies to Promote Role Transition

- Strengthen internal resources
- Assess the organization's resources, culture, and group dynamics
- Negotiate the role
- Grow with a mentor
- Develop management knowledge and skills

Table 25-2 COMPARISON OF PHASES IN DEVELOPING AN INTIMATE RELATIONSHIP AND IN UNDERGOING ROLE TRANSITION AS A NURSE MANAGER

Phase in Developing an Intimate Relationship	Phase in Role Transition as a Nurse Manager	Characteristics of Phase
Dating	Role preview	Presentation of best characteristics to make favorable impression; both parties evaluate each other to determine likelihood of the other being able to fulfill one's expectations
Commitment to relationship	Role acceptance	Public announcement of mutual decision to initiate contract
Honeymoon	Role exploration	Experience of excitement, confidence, and mutual appreciation
Disillusionment	Role discrepancy	Awareness of difference between role expectations and role performance; reconsideration of whether to continue with contract
Resolution	Role development	Negotiation of role expectations; adjustment of role performance to approximate expectations and to find own unique style
Maturation of relationship	Role internalization	Performance of role congruent with own beliefs and individual style; achievement of mutual goals

Mentors are an important component of a nurturing environment that promotes staff retention.

Mentors can be a tremendous source of guidance and support for staff nurses and managers, serving both career functions and psychosocial functions. Career functions are possible because the mentor has sufficient professional experience and organizational authority to facilitate the career of the "mentee." Mentors nurture relationships that are mutual and equal. Dracup and Bryan-Brown (2004, p. 450) indicate that by positive modeling behaviors "the mentor is able to set a positive and constructive tone." McKinley (2004, p. 4) states that "mentoring is a fundamental form of human development where one person invests time, energy and personal knowledge to assist another person in their growth and development." The Robert Wood Johnson Nurse Executive Fellows program has identified five competencies of leaders and mentors. These include self-knowledge, strategic vision, risk-taking and creativity, interpersonal and communication effectiveness, and managing change. Box 25-4 highlights some key functions.

Sponsorship involves volunteering or nominating the mentee for additional responsibilities. A mentor can be a sponsor by creating opportunities for individual achievement and providing encouragement. The mentor may suggest the mentee be appointed to a key nursing committee or volunteer for a special assignment. Sponsorship leads to exposure or opportunities for the mentee to build a reputation of competence. With exposure, the mentor provides protection by absorbing negative feedback, sharing responsibility for controversial decisions, and teaching the unwritten rules about "how things are done around here." These unwritten rules may be more important to job success than the written rules.

Coaches provide information about how to improve performance, including feedback on current performance. **Coaching** requires frequent contact and willingness on the part of the mentee to accept feedback. Challenging assignments are given to the mentee that will stretch the limits of knowledge and skill. The mentor helps the mentee learn the technical and management skills necessary to accomplish the task, such as which numbers on the budget printout are added to achieve the total expenditures.

BOX 25-4

Functions of a Mentor

Career functions	Sponsorship
	Exposure/protection
	Coaching
	Challenging assignments
Psychosocial functions	Role modeling
	Mutual positive regard
	Counseling
	Social interaction

Modified from Kram, K. E. (1985). *Mentoring at work: Development relationships in organizational life.* Glenview, IL: Scott, Foresman.

The interpersonal relationship between the mentor and the mentee involves mutual positive regard. Because the mentee respects the career accomplishments of the mentor, the mentee identifies with the mentor's example. This role-modeling is both conscious and unconscious. The mentee with character and self-respect will evaluate the behaviors of the mentor and select those behaviors worthy of being emulated.

Counseling, as another psychosocial function of the mentor, allows the mentee to explore personal concerns. Confidentiality is a prerequisite to sharing personal information. Because the opinion of the mentor is respected, the mentor may provide guidance to the mentee. The best mentors can provide guidance while recognizing that the mentee may choose to disregard the advice.

Being mentored is a learning process. Admiration for a mentor and recognition of the mentor's commitment to self-success can provide an environment of trust in which a mentor–mentee relationship begins. Both persons develop positive expectations of the relationship, and both take the initiative to nurture the new relationship. As more of the mentor functions are experienced, the bond between the mentor and mentee grows stronger.

Relationships between mentors and mentees vary because of individual characteristics and the career phase of each. During the early phases of a career, a nurse manager is concerned about competence, and a mentor can provide valuable coaching.

As the nurse manager develops, sponsorship by a mentor can prepare the manager for a promotion. A mentor nearing the end of the work career can find fulfillment in sharing knowledge with new managers and at the same time benefit from the counsel of a recently retired colleague.

Management Education

Management performance can be hindered by a specific knowledge deficit. For example, the manager may lack business skills or knowledge about legal aspects of supervision. Most healthcare organizations have little or no management orientation. O'Connor (2004, p. 24) states that new leaders need "focused attention, education, and development." Srsic-Stoehr and colleagues (2004, p. 40) identified the elements of the nurse-manager role that required education: "assessment/addressing issues, problems, strengths; plan/set goals; make decisions; implement/manage change, develop teams; communicate/coordinate/collaborate/care; foster motivation; resolve conflict; build consensus; develop staff and self; lead; and get the big picture." Domrose (2004) indicates that hospitals are identifying, educating, and training potential leaders. Investment in education for nurse managers is an investment in the future of an organization.

Experience and education provide a firm basis for seeking additional credentials. A nursing administrator with a baccalaureate degree and 24 months of experience at a middle-management level can take an examination to become a certified nursing administrator. Nursing administrators with master's degrees and experience at the executive level can take an examination to become a certified nursing administrator, advanced. The website of the American Nurses Credentialing Center has more detailed information about certification examinations (www.nursecredentialing.org).

FROM ROLE TRANSITION TO ROLE TRIUMPH

Developing an intimate relationship can be a difficult process, but most people still value relationships enough to make the effort. Making the transition and transformation into a management role is also worth the effort. Leading lives of integrity and commitment, nurse managers set exam-

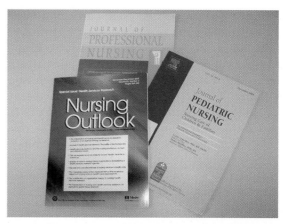

Reading professional books and journals and attending conferences are effective management and education strategies.

ples, bringing out the best in staff nurses and thereby multiplying their influence on quality patient care.

Exercise 25-2

Self-Assessment
Respond to each item using the scale. Add up your score.

1 = Strongly disagree
2 = Disagree
3 = Unsure
4 = Agree
5 = Strongly agree

1. I am responsible for my own professional development.
2. I feel confident about my ability to learn the skills I need to be an effective manager.
3. I am able to balance multiple priorities and activities.
4. I have a strong psychological desire to influence others.
5. I can develop a personal network of support.

There is no magical score that indicates your readiness for management. If you are unsure in every category, your score will be 15. A score of 20 or above indicates that you are confident that you can master the management role. If you currently have a mentor, ask that person to respond to each item to analyze your abilities. Compare those responses with your own. Do you have a realistic view of yourself?

SUMMARY

Transitions from staff nurse to charge nurse or nurse manager pose new challenges. Nurses who make these transitions with minimal discomfort are reflective of role theory in action. Although nurses today are better prepared to take on more formal leadership roles, the roles themselves are more challenging. Charge nurses and managers are responsible for mentoring and coaching new staff as they transition to the new roles they are assuming. These transition activities take time and effort to achieve the best results possible.

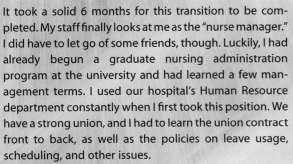

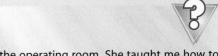

The Solution

It took a solid 6 months for this transition to be completed. My staff finally looks at me as the "nurse manager." I did have to let go of some friends, though. Luckily, I had already begun a graduate nursing administration program at the university and had learned a few management terms. I used our hospital's Human Resource department constantly when I first took this position. We have a strong union, and I had to learn the union contract front to back, as well as the policies on leave usage, scheduling, and other issues.

I have always loved providing care for our sick veterans, and it was so difficult to give that up. Even now, when the code pager goes off, it is difficult not to run. To balance this, I wear scrubs once a week and work side-by-side with my staff. It reminds me of what their day is like and keeps up my competencies, and I love it.

I also had two role models whom I relied on heavily. One was the former nurse manager of the intensive care unit (ICU), who took the nursing operations coordinator position. She showed me how to conduct the "official" business of running a unit. My mentor is the nurse manager of the operating room. She taught me how to run the ICU while "loving" my staff. I go to her when I have a difficult day, and she reminds me just how great my staff is (I already know that I am lucky to have them) and how much I have grown and where I am headed. I always feel better when I talk with her. She has taught me how to deal with difficult physicians, and we are allies. She has been my lifesaver this first year.

Taking this management position has been a life-changing experience for me. Now that I have adjusted to the role, what I enjoy most is the work I do with new graduates. I like taking young graduate nurses into the internship I created for the ICU and watching them grow into fully functioning ICU nurses. I was told it was not a good idea to take new graduates into the unit, but I have been so pleased. They are our future, and it is so exciting to watch their enthusiasm and growth!

— Robin E. Keene

 Would this be a suitable approach for you? Why?

CHAPTER CHECKLIST

Role transition is a process that takes time and energy—two scarce resources for nurse managers. Knowing what to expect and how to facilitate the process can speed role transition and minimize the expenditure of energy as the nurse manager negotiates new roles.

- Responsibilities, opportunities, lines of communication, expectations, and support are aspects common to all roles. When considering a management role, gather information about each of these aspects.

- Managers are also leaders and followers.
- Role transition is a process of unlearning old roles and learning new roles.
- The phases of role transition are as follows:
  - Role preview
  - Role acceptance
  - Role exploration
  - Role discrepancy
  - Role development
  - Role internalization
- Unexpected role transitions involve a grieving process. Financial and social obligations of the

Continued

manager and the employer may need to be formally dissolved with appropriate compensation and out-placement services.

- The phase of role preview is similar to dating in that both parties present their best characteristics to make a favorable impression.
- Commitment to a relationship is analogous to role acceptance, a public announcement of a mutual decision to initiate a contract.
- Role exploration is similar to the honeymoon phase of an intimate relationship.
- Role discrepancy has its roots in the disillusionment experienced when role expectations do not match role performance.
- Role development is a time of resolution, when role expectations are negotiated and performance is adjusted to approximate expectations.

- A maturing relationship is similar to role internalization; during role internalization, the performance of the role is congruent with one's own beliefs.
- Commitment, character, self-respect, and flexibility are internal resources that can facilitate the process of role transition.
- Role negotiation involves communicating with your supervisor to come to an agreement as to role expectations.
- Mentors can provide career and psychosocial functions, enhancing the career development of the manager.
- Educational programs provide information needed by nurses to fulfill management roles.

TIPS IN ROLE TRANSITIONING

- Role transition is a normal process. Anticipate and prepare for role changes.
- Identify the responsibilities, opportunities, lines of communication, expectations, and support for the role.
- Use your internal resources to negotiate a role that is consistent with your values and life commitments.

TERMS TO KNOW

mentor	role negotiation
role development	role strain
role discrepancy	role stress
role expectations	role transition
role internalization	ROLES

REFERENCES

Arnold, L., & Nelson, G. (2004, December). Developing the new frontline manager. *Nurse Leader, 50–53.*

Catalano, J. T. (2003). *Nursing now: Today's issues, tomorrow's trends* (3rd ed.). Philadelphia: FA Davis.

Delaney, C. (2003). Walking a fine line: Graduate nurses' transition experiences during orientation. *Journal of Nursing Education, 42*(10), 437–443.

Domrose, C. (2004). The apprentices. *Nurse Week News.* Retrieved March 29, 2005, from www/nurseweek.com/news/features/04-04/leaders_print.html.

Dracup, K. & Bryan-Brown, C. W. (2004). From novice to expert to mentor: Shaping the future. *American Journal of Critical Care, 13*(6), 448–450.

Ellerton, M. L. & Gregor, F. (2003). Changes in nursing identities: Supporting a successful transition. *Journal of Nursing Management, 11,* 224–228.

Ewens, A. (2003). Changes in nursing identities: Supporting a successful transition. *Journal of Nursing Management, 11*(4), 224–228.

Halpern, L., & Lubar, K. (2003). *Leadership presence: Dramatic techniques to reach out, motivate, and inspire.* New York: Gotham Books.

Hardy, M. E. (1978). Role stress and role strain. In M. E. Hardy & M. E. Conway (Eds.), *Role theory: Perspectives for health professionals.* New York: Appleton-Century-Crofts.

Heller, B., Drenkard, K., Esposito-Herr, M. B., Romano, C., Tom, S., & Valentine, N. (2004). Educating nurses for leadership roles. *The Journal of Continuing Education in Nursing, 35*(5), 203–210.

Kouzes, J., & Posner, B. (2002). *Leadership challenge* (3rd ed.). San Francisco: Jossey-Bass.

Marelli, T. M. (2004). *The nurse manager's survival guide: Practical answers to everyday problems* (3rd ed.). St. Louis: Mosby.

McKinley, M. (2004). Mentoring matters: Creating, connecting, empowering. *AACN Clinical Issues Advanced Practice in Acute Critical Care, 15*(2), 205–214.

O'Connor, M. (2004, October). Succession planning: A key strategy in nursing leadership education. *Nurse Leader,* 21–25.

O'Connor, M., & Walker, J. K. (2003). The dynamics of curriculum design, evaluation, and revision. Quality improvement in leadership development. *Nursing Administration Quarterly, 27*(4), 290–296.

Porter-O'Grady, T., & Malloch, K. (2002). *Quantam leadership: A textbook of new leadership.* New York: Aspen.

Srsic-Stoehr, K., Rogers, L., Wolgast, K., Chapman, T., & Douglas, R. (2004, December). Success skills for the nurse manager: Cultural debut and sustainment. *Nurse Leader,* 36–41.

SUGGESTED READINGS

Goleman, D. (2002). *Primal leadership: realizing the power of emotional intelligence.* Boston: Harvard Business School Press.

Field, D. (2004). Moving from novice to expert—the value of learning in clinical practice: A literature review. *Nurse Education Today, 24*(7), 560–565.

Thompson, S. A. (2004). The top ten qualities of a good nurse manager. *American Journal of Nursing, 104*(8), 64c–64d.

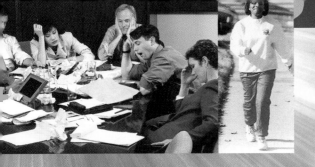

Chapter

26

Self-Management:
Stress and Time

Amy C. Pettigrew

T his chapter examines the concept of self-management—being responsible for managing and controlling your behavior so that you can accomplish the things you want with minimal personal stress. Three components of self-management are explored: stress management, time management, and meeting management. Methods for managing stress and organizing your time are introduced. Practical exercises and suggestions for stress and time management are presented that can be used for personal and professional situations to reduce stress and enhance efficiency.

Objectives

- Define self-management.
- Explore personal and professional stressors.
- Analyze selected strategies to decrease stress.
- Assess the manager's role in helping staff to manage stress.
- Evaluate common barriers to effective time management.
- Critique the strengths and weaknesses of selected time-management strategies.
- Evaluate selected strategies to manage time more effectively.

Questions to Consider

- Are you currently using self-management strategies?
- What types of activities are stressful for you?
- Can you identify ways to handle stress more effectively?
- What are your highest-priority personal and professional goals?
- Does the way you spend your time reflect your priorities?
- Are you drowning in information and paperwork?
- How does a nurse manager successfully use time to attain work goals?

The Challenge

Amy Phillips, BSN, RN
MSN Student, University of Cincinnati College of Nursing

Stress never disappears, it just sort of fluctuates! Right now is definitely a high-stress time for me. I am a full-time graduate student in midwifery, and I have a graduate assistantship, which means I work for the University (assisting teachers, doing research, etc.) in addition to my own coursework. I have a 5-year old who goes to preschool and speech therapy, and an 18-month-old who has a chronic respiratory condition. One or both of the children always has to be somewhere (school, therapy, clinic, etc.), and I still have to try to get homework done!

What do you think you would do if you were this nurse?

INTRODUCTION

How many times have you gone to bed at night feeling guilty about not having accomplished anything during the day? How many times have you stopped to wonder what you really want to be when you grow up? **Self-management** is about deciding what you want for your personal and professional self, setting life goals, developing objectives and short-term outcomes to reach the goals, and finally organizing the time and activities you undertake to reach them. Self-management is also about finding a balance among and between career, family, social activities, and self. Drucker (2000) suggests that understanding one's own strengths, articulating personal values, and knowing where one's self belongs are also important components of self-management. O'Keefe and Berger (2000) define self-management as the outcome of managing affect, behavior, and cognition.

To find this balance within ourselves, we must actively engage in taking control of our lives—no one else is going to! The three key strategies introduced in this chapter—stress management, **time management,** and meeting management—constantly interplay with our life goals. We can move in a straight line toward our personal and professional goals if stress or distractions do not interfere. When stress becomes overwhelming or others rob us of our time, the path suddenly becomes unclear. Time and stress are somewhat of a "chicken and egg" phenomenon—not enough time contributes to stress, and stress can erode efficiency and thus decrease time on task. The key lies in our ability to manage both time and stress, not only personally but also professionally. The outcome of self-management is the ability to accomplish one's high-priority professional and personal goals.

UNDERSTANDING STRESS

Nurses have learned about the effect of stress on patients and how to teach clients to manage its consequences. Nurses also need to recognize the stressors in their own lives. Everyone experiences stress—the exhilaration of a joyous event as well as the negative feelings and unpleasant physical symptoms that may be associated with a difficult life situation or even the anticipation of difficulty. Stress is the uncomfortable gap between how we would like our life to be and how it actually is. Nurses are not immune to the effects of stress. Learning what stress is, its dynamics, and some strategies to manage the distress should be part of the personal and professional maturation of nurses.

Definition

In this chapter, *stress* and *distress* are used interchangeably, although some writers regard stress as neutral and refer to the positive and negative attributes of eustress and distress, respectively. Stress management does not necessarily mean stress reduction. Rather, stress management is finding the right mix of stress and distress.

SCOPE OF STRESS IN THE WORKPLACE

Job stress has become a common and expensive problem in the American workplace. A survey completed by Barsade and Wiesenfeld (1997) reported that 29% of workers reported that they felt "quite a bit or extremely stressed at work." Smith (2000) reports that approximately 20% of a random sample of 17,000 British citizens had high or extremely high levels of stress at work. A Harris Interactive Poll conducted in 2003 indicated that 43% of American workers polled (n = 752) indicate that people in their workplace express fear or anxiety several times a week, 33% report an observed increase in anxiety or stress related physical ailments in their workplace over the past year, and 27% report an increase in personal emotional problems, such as depression, insomnia, substance abuse, or family conflicts.

Billions of dollars a year are lost to businesses from stress-related ailments. These costs include accidents, absenteeism, employee turnover, diminished productivity, direct medical, legal, and insurance costs, workers' compensation awards as well as tort judgements. According to Tangri (2002), 19% of absenteeism, 40% of turnover, 55% of employee assistant programs, 30% of short- and long-term disability, 10% of drug costs and the total cost of workplace accidents, workers' compensation claims, and lawsuits are due to stress.

SOURCES OF JOB STRESS

Job stress can be defined as the physical and emotional responses that arise when the job requirements do not match the abilities, resources, or needs of the worker. Work-related stress can lead to poor physical and emotional health and injury. There is a difference between job-related challenges (eustress), which motivate us to learn new skills and master our jobs, and distress, which can lead to exhaustion, feelings of inadequacy, and failure. If you are involved in an oral interview for a job, you will benefit from a certain amount of stress (eustress). It is stress that provides you with determination and gives you your "edge" that will help you think quickly and clearly and express your thoughts in ways that will benefit your interview process. Having your car break down on the way to the interview creates stress (distress) as you realize that you will be late for the appointment. As more is learned about the relationship of stress to physiologic changes, stressors will become even easier to identify. When one looks at job-related stressors, the stressors fall into one of two categories: external (working conditions) and internal (worker characteristics).

External Sources

Occupational stress in nursing has been well-defined and documented. Work-related stressors, such as workload, rotating shifts, high patient acuity, ethical conflicts, dealing with death and acute illness, role ambiguity, and job insecurity have all been associated with increased stress and **burnout** (Maurier & Northcutt, 2000).

Change   Nurses, as well as other healthcare providers, are still recovering from the effects of changes in healthcare financing and care delivery systems that occurred in the 1990s. Although the distress that results from change takes many forms, two underlying patterns appear to be constant. First, nurses feel trapped by conflicting expectations. They expect to furnish care, to meet patients' needs, and to be nurturing. However, organizations require nurses to be managers of patient care and of systems and value their contribution to efficiency and cost-effectiveness while simultaneously preserving quality of care. Because nurses cannot comply with both expectations, they experience considerable role conflict, frustration, and distress.

Second, the rapid required changes in work design implemented in the 1990s were changes made by administrators, often with little input from the nursing staff. Loss of autonomy, together with increases in rules and regulations, resulted in distress for nurses. They felt powerless and devalued. Nurses in some institutions have become empowered by models of shared governance. However, the processes necessary to develop such models are stressful in and of themselves, and many nurses still find themselves in systems in which they have little input to change processes.

Social   Interpersonal relations can buffer stressors or can in themselves become stressors. Outside the work setting, home can be a refuge for harried nurses; however, stresses at home, when severe, can impair work performance and relationships among staff or even result in violence that may invade the workplace.

Changes in healthcare delivery systems, as well as the current nursing shortage, have reduced the number of professional nurses, often creating situations of minimally safe staffing levels. Consequently, some nurses lose supportive, collegial relationships that may have been established over many years. Many institutions now depend on supplemental staffing with agency or "traveling" nurses, thus creating a very transient nursing staff. In other situations, nurses are reassigned or they "float" to various patient-care units, which requires that they work with unfamiliar staff. Thus, they may feel isolated or become unwillingly involved in dysfunctional politics on the unit. Such situations may also necessitate that nurses work with patients whose requirements for care may be unfamiliar, resulting in further stress related to patient-safety concerns.

Persons in management-level positions may also become stressors. Communication may come from the top down, with little opportunity for nurses to participate in decisions that affect them directly or that they may need to implement without proper training or support. Nurses may experience distress from feelings of frustration and helplessness with this lack of opportunity for input to decisions.

The Position Most student nurses entering nursing expect that caring for patients who are chronically or critically ill and for families who have experienced tragedy will be stressful. The current environment in many healthcare agencies, however, is more complex and is often characterized by **overwork,** as well as by the stresses inherent in nursing practice.

Mandatory overtime has been a controversy for several years. Nurses were expected to stay for extra shifts with little or no notice, with managers using threats of dismissal or peer pressure to ensure cooperation. Nurses, aware of and concerned about inadequate staffing, became resentful that they were carrying the stress and burden of the staffing problems that resulted from earlier changes in skill mix and care-delivery models.

Worthington (2001) discusses three main health and safety issues related to the use of mandatory overtime: prolonged exposure to hazards, fatigue, and stress. Mandatory overtime has been linked to poorer general health, increased injury rates, greater levels of illness, and even increased levels of mortality (American Federation of Teachers, 2005). By December of 2004, 10 states enacted legislation prohibiting or limiting mandatory overtime, and 15 states introduced legislation and/or regulations concerning mandatory overtime. Currently, there is movement in Congress to end mandatory overtime in hospitals, which is the first step in ending mandatory overtime for all healthcare workers (American Federation of Teachers, 2005). The research by Rogers, Hwang, Scott, Aiken, and Dinges (2004) indicates, however, that it is not so much about how one is working long hours, as in mandatory overtime, but the fact of working long hours at all that increases the risk for errors.

Role stress is an additional stressor for nurses. Viewed as the incongruence between perceived role expectations and achievement (Chang & Hancock, 2003), role stress for new graduates is related to role ambiguity and role overload. Role stress is particularly acute for new graduates, whose lack of clinical experience and organizational skills, combined with new situations and procedures, may increase feelings of overwhelming stress. Conflict between what was learned in the classroom and actual practice may add additional stress.

Gender Roles Approximately 94% of the nation's 2.9 million nurses are women (Health Resources and Services Administration, 2005), and many go home to gender-related responsibilities that may include household management, children, and aging parents. When added to the already stressful workday of the nurse, the additional responsibilities often contribute to the level of distress felt by the nurse. Erdwins, Buffardi, Casper, and O'Brien (2001) report that effectiveness in work roles is directly related to a woman's perception of fewer conflicts between work and home. They also report that the less support a woman perceives from her spouse and her direct supervisor, the more she is likely to experience work/family conflict and role strain. Kirkcaldy and Martin (2000) also found that nursing professionals perceive the home/work conflict as a major stressor. Home/work conflict was a significant predictor of decreased work satisfaction, physical health, and mental health. Age was significantly related to total stress, with older nurses reporting additional family commitments and domestic responsibility.

Evans and Steptoe (2002) examined the associations of work stress and gender-role orientation to psychological well-being and sickness-related work absences in male-dominated (accounting) and female dominated (nursing) occupations in England. They concluded that when men and women are occupationally engaged in gender-dominated occupations in which they are in the gender minority, the men and women perceived more work-related hassles, and exhibited gender-specific health effects.

Internal Sources

Personal stress "triggers" are events or situations that have an effect on specific individuals. Personal triggers might be a specific event such as the death of a loved one, an automobile accident, losing a job, or getting married. These events are in addition to daily personal stressors such as working in a noisy environment, job dissatisfaction, or a difficult commute to work. Negative self-talk, pessimistic thinking, self-criticism and overanalyzing can be significant ongoing stressors. These internal sources of stress usually stem from unrealistic self-beliefs (unrealistic expectations, taking things personally, all-or-nothing thinking, exaggerating or rigid thinking), perfectionism, or the type A personality.

An individual's ability to deal with stress may be moderated by psychological hardiness. According to Lambert, Lambert, and Yamase (2003), psychological hardiness is a composite of commitment, control, and challenge. These form a constellation that dampers the effects of stress by challenging the perception of the situation, and decreasing the negative impact of a situation by moderating both cognitive appraisal and coping. Maddi (2002), in a 12-year longitudinal study, found that individuals thriving in a stressful work environment displayed the same psychological hardiness. The commitment attitude led the individuals to be actively involved in the changes that decreased isolation. The control attitude led them to try to influence outcomes rather than sink into powerlessness and passivity. The challenge attitude led them to believe that the stressful events were opportunities for new learning.

Lifestyle choices, such as the use of caffeine, lack of exercise, poor diet, inadequate sleep and leisure time, and cigarette smoking, have a direct effect on the amount of one's stress. Most of the stress an individual has is self-generated. Recognizing that we create most of our own stress is the first step to dealing with it.

Dynamics of Stress

Stress may result from unrealistic or conflicting expectations, the pace and magnitude of change, human behavior, individual personality characteristics, the characteristics of the position itself, or the culture of the organization. Other stressors may be unique to certain environments, situations, and persons or groups. Initially, increased stress produces increased performance. However, once peak performance has been reached, additional stress results in decreased performance (Epstein, 2000).

Although some stress may be motivating and make employees more effective (eustress), distress is more often a problem that results in decreased position performance, unpleasant feelings, and illness (Rabin, 1999). Hans Selye's mid-century investigations of the nature of and reactions to stress (Selye, 1956) have been very influential. In his classic theory, Selye (1991) described the concept of stress, identified the **general adaptation syndrome (GAS)**, and detailed a predictable pattern of response (the Theory Box and Figure 26-1).

Theory Box

THEORIES APPLICABLE TO SELF-MANAGEMENT

KEY CONTRIBUTORS	KEY IDEAS	APPLICATION TO PRACTICE
General adaptation syndrome. Selye (1956) is credited with developing this theory.	The "stress response" is an adrenocortical reaction to stressors that is accompanied by psychological changes and physiologic alterations that follow a pattern of fight or flight. The general adaptation syndrome includes an alarm, resistance, and adaptation or exhaustion.	Change, lack of control, and excessive workload are common stressors that evoke psychological and physiologic distress among nurses.
The Pareto principle: Hafner, A. W. (2001)	The "Pareto principle" refers to a universal observation of "vital few, trivial many." Pareto (1848-1923) studied distribution of personal incomes in Italy and observed that 80% of the wealth was controlled by 20% of the population. This concept of disproportion often holds in many areas. Although the exact values of 20 and 80 are not significant, the observation of considerable disproportion is important to remember.	The 80-20 rule can be applied to many aspects of health care today. For example, 80% of healthcare expenditures are on 20% of the population, and 80% of personnel problems come from 20% of the staff. In quality improvement, 80% of improvement can be expected by removing 20% of the causes of unacceptable quality or performance. A nurse can also expect that 80% of patient-care time will be spent working with 20% of her patient assignment.

More recent investigations of the relationship among the brain, the immune system, and health (psychoneuroimmunology) have generated models that challenge Selye's GAS. Although Selye states that all people respond with a similar set of hormonal and immune responses to any stress, Kemeny proposes that there are two stress responses: (1) the classic GAS, contrasted with a (2) withdrawing reaction, where the person pulls back to conserve energy. Kemeny hypothesizes that people respond to the same psychological event in different ways, depending on their independent appraisal of the situation (DeAngelis, 2002).

Critical of stress research using predominately (87%) male subjects, Taylor, Klein, Lewis, Gruenewald, Gurung, and Updegraff (2000) proposed a model of the female stress response, the "tend and befriend," as opposed to the male's "fight or flight" model. The "tend and befriend" response is an estrogen and oxytocin-mediated stress response that is characterized by caring for offspring and befriending those around in times of stress to increase chances of survival.

Most nurses can easily recognize the origins of stress and its symptoms. For example, a healthcare agency may make demands on nurses, such as excessive work, that the nurses regard as beyond their capacity to perform. When they are unable to resolve the problem through overwork, with more staff, or by looking at the situation in another way, the nurses may feel threatened or depressed. They may also experience headache, fatigue, or other physical symptoms. If the stress persists, such symptoms may increase; nurses may attempt to cope by becoming apathetic or by resigning their positions. Table 26-1 gives physical, mental, and spiritual/emotional signs of overstress in individuals.

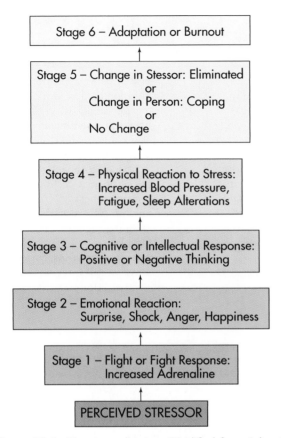

Stage 6 – Adaptation or Burnout

↑

Stage 5 – Change in Stessor: Eliminated
or
Change in Person: Coping
or
No Change

↑

Stage 4 – Physical Reaction to Stress:
Increased Blood Pressure,
Fatigue, Sleep Alterations

↑

Stage 3 – Cognitive or Intellectual Response:
Positive or Negative Thinking

↑

Stage 2 – Emotional Reaction:
Surprise, Shock, Anger, Happiness

↑

Stage 1 – Flight or Fight Response:
Increased Adrenaline

↑

PERCEIVED STRESSOR

Figure 26-1   The stress diagram. (Modified from Selye, H. [1991]. History and present status of the stress concept. In A. Monat & R. Lazarus [Eds.], *Stress and coping: An anthology* [pp. 21-36]. New York: Columbia University Press.)

In 2004, Segerstrom and Miller published a meta-analysis of research on the relationship between stress and the human immune system. They found that acute stressors (very short-term) "revved up" the immune system, preparing for infection or injury. Short-term naturalistic stressors, such as tests, tended to suppress cellular immunity while preserving humoral immunity. The immune systems of those who are older or already sick are more prone to stress-related immune system changes.

In a study of long-term care providers, Kiecolt-Glaser, Preacher, MacCallum, Atkinson, Malarkey, and Glaser (2003) found that over a 6-year period, blood tests showed that the chemical interlukin-6 (IL-6) dramatically increased in the caregivers. Overproduction of IL-6 has been associated with the development or progression of medical illnesses,

including heart disease, type 2 diabetes, certain types of cancer, osteoporosis, arthritis, and functional decline.

Epel and colleagues (2004) report that in healthy women, psychological stress, both perceived stress and stress chronicity, is significantly associated with higher oxidative stress, lower telomerase activity amd shorter telomere length, which are determinants of cell senescence and longevity. This finding has implications for understanding how stress may accelerate the onset of age-related diseases. Other researchers have found that chronic stress is correlated with undetected type 2 diabetes and visceral adiposity (Mooy, deVries, Grootenhuis, Bounter, & Heine, 2000); and Wilson, Evans, Bienias, Mendes de Leon, Schneider, and Bennett (2003, 2005) found that people who scored in the 90th percentile for proneness to distress were twice as likely to develop Alzheimer's disease as people who scored in the 10th percentile. Other physical illnesses–linked to stress include cardiovascular disease (hypertension, heart attack, and stroke), musculoskeletal disorders, psychological disorders (anxiety and depression), workplace injury, neuromuscular disorders (multiple sclerosis), suicide, cancer, ulcers, asthma, and rheumatoid arthritis. Stress can even cause life-threatening sympathetic stimulation. Wittstein et al. (2005) reported that emotional stress can precipitate severe and potentially fatal reversible left ventricular failure in patients without coronary disease, which has been labeled the "broken heart syndrome."

MANAGEMENT OF STRESS

Individuals respond to stress by eliciting coping strategies that are a means of dealing with stress to maintain or achieve well-being. These strategies may be ineffective and rely on methods such as withdrawal or substance abuse, or they may be effective in helping restore a greater sense of well-being and effectiveness. Some of these effective strategies are discussed here.

Stress Prevention

One effective way to deal with stress is to determine and manage its source. Discovering the origin of stress in patient care may be difficult because some environments have changed so rapidly that

Table 26-1 SIGNS OF OVERSTRESS IN INDIVIDUALS

Physical	Mental	Spiritual/Emotional

Physical signs of ill health:
    Increase in flu, colds, accidents
    Change in sleeping habits
    Fatigue
Chronic signs of decreased ability to manage stress:
    Headaches
    Hypertension
    Backaches
    Gastrointestinal problems
Use of unhealthy coping activities:
    Increased use of drugs and alcohol
    Increased weight
    Smoking
    Crying, yelling, blaming
	Dread going to work every day
	Rigid thinking and a desire to go by all the rules in all cases; inability to tolerate any changes
	Forgetfulness and anxiety about work to be done; more frequent errors and incidents
	Returning home exhausted and unable to participate in enjoyable activities
	Confusion about duties and roles
	Generalized anxiety
	Decrease in concentration
	Depression
	Anger, irritability, impatience
		Sense of being a failure; disappointed in work performance
		Anger and resentment toward patients, colleagues, and managers; overall irritable attitude
		Lack of positive feelings toward others
		Cynicism toward patients, blaming them for their problems
		Excessive worry; insecurity; lowered self-esteem
		Increased family and friend conflict

the nursing staff is overwhelmed trying to balance bureaucratic rules and limited resources with the demands of vulnerable human beings. In their distress, nurses may need to step back and look at the "big picture." By identifying daily stressors, the nurse can then develop a plan of action for management of the stress. This plan may include elimination of the stressor, modification of the stressor, or changing the perception of the stressor (such as viewing mistakes as opportunities for new learning) using a reframing technique.

Many of the day-to-day activities of nursing can create workplace stress. Consider the critical nature of nursing work, and the potential for serious injury to others. Staffing shortages create situations of caring for more patients with less help. Nurses may have inadequate rest because of rotating shifts or irregular schedules. Nurses are subject to significant musculoskeletal stress due to lifting, pulling, and turning patients. Nurses give physical care to those who are physically unclean or verbally abusive. Nurses watch patients and families suffer with pain and grief. These stressors are often counterbalanced by the rewards of patient appreciation, the joy of seeing a healthy baby born, or seeing the relief brought by a medication or repositioning. However, given the stressful nature of nursing, it is wise for the nurse to be alert to his or her own signs of stress, and to develop lifestyle habits that help reduce stress. Adequate sleep, a balanced diet, regular exercise, and frequent interactions with friends are excellent stress-buffering habits to develop.

According to Stoppler (2005), the top five stress-management mistakes include poor calendar habits, clutter, perfectionism, self-treatment, and following others' expectations. These may be high on your list of stress experiences. Analyze your stress experiences by completing Exercise 26-1.

Exercise 26–1

Identify what stress you experience and how you usually manage it. Create and complete the following log at the end of every day for one week. Review the log and note what situations (e.g., people, technology, values conflict) were the most common. Also identify how you most often react to stress: physically, mentally, and emotionally/spiritually. Keeping this diary for a week is helpful to determine what you respond to with stress and learn about your reactions. Ask yourself if the stress was good stress (eustress) or bad stress (distress).

DATE _____

SITUATION _____

YOUR RESPONSE _____

GOOD STRESS OR BAD _____

ACTION (How you dealt with your response) _____

_____

EVALUATION _____

Look over your week of stressors. Are there some that you encounter on a regular basis? If so, try to formulate a plan to conquer the problems. You may need to role-play, or to get continuing education to improve a specific skill. You may need to simply break a task down into smaller pieces, or to eliminate interruptions.

Symptom Management

Unpredictable and uncontrollable change, coupled with immense responsibility and little control over the work environment, produces stress for nurses and other healthcare professionals. Consequently, nurses may develop emotional symptoms such as anxiety, depression, or anger; physical alterations such as fatigue, headache, and insomnia; mental changes such as a decrease in concentration and memory; and behavioral changes such as smoking, drinking, crying, and swearing. The important factor is not the stressor, but rather how the individual perceives the stressor and what coping mechanisms are available to mediate the hormonal response to the stressor. This perception of the stressor is modulated by the baseline physiology of the individual and by earlier life experiences with stress (Rabin, 1999).

Multiple "stress-buffering" behaviors can be elicited to reduce the detrimental effects of stress. The stressor-induced changes in the hormonal and immune systems can be modulated by an individual's behavioral coping responses. These coping responses include leisure activities and taking time for self, decreasing or discontinuing the use of caffeine, positive social support, a strong belief system, a sense of humor, developing realistic expectations, reframing events, regular aerobic exercise, meditation, and use of the relaxation response.

Everyone needs to balance work and leisure in their lives. Leisure time and stress are inversely proportional. If time for work is more than 60% of awake time, or when self-time is less than 10% of awake time, stress levels will increase. Changes should be made to relieve stress, such as decreasing the number of work hours, or finding more time for leisure activities. Caffeine is a strong stimulant, and in itself a stressor. Slowly weaning oneself off caffeine should result in better sleep and more energy. Positive social support can offer validation, encouragement, or advice. There is an old saying that "a problem shared is a problem halved." By discussing situations with others, one can reduce stress. A great deal of stress comes from our belief systems, which cause stress in two ways. First is that behaviors result from them, such as placing work before pleasure. Second, beliefs may also conflict with those of other people, as may happen when clients come from different cultures. Articulating beliefs and finding common ground will help reduce anger and stress. Humor is a great stress reducer, and laughter a great tension reducer. A common source of stress is unrealistic expectations. Realistic expectations can make life feel more predictable and more manageable. Reframing is changing the way you look at things to make you feel better about them. Recognizing that there are many ways to interpret the same situation, take the positive view! Regular aerobic exercise is a logical method of dissipating the excess energy generated by the stress response, channeling the energy into healthy activity rather than turning the energy inward (Posen, 1995).

Meditation to elicit the relaxation response can be beneficial. The benefits of practicing relaxation techniques for 20 minutes daily include a feeling of well-being, the ability to learn how tension makes the body feel, and the sense that tension can be controlled. In cases of some stress-related disorders (e.g., hypertension), biofeedback may be used to monitor physiologic relaxation processes. This technique enables some individuals to better relax and to gain control over selected physiologic processes (Kuhn, 1999). Exercise 26-2 outlines one systematic relaxation technique.

Exercise 26–2

This exercise can be used in the middle of a working day, the last thing at night, or at any time you feel tense or anxious.

1. Find a place away from interruption for 10 minutes.
2. Loosen tight clothes; lie on the floor, a mat, a towel, or a couch if possible. Close your eyes, and let your body go slack.
3. Starting from the top of your body, work steadily through all your muscles, tightening and then relaxing them.

4. Lift up your head and pull it forward as far as you can, then let it fall back gently.

5. Continuing downward, press your shoulders down hard, then slowly relax them.

6. Open your fingers wide, stretch your arms out to your side, and hold them as tight and hard as you can. Then slowly let them go.

7. With your arms lying at your side, tighten your abdominal muscles as hard as you can, then relax them.

8. Lift your buttocks, tightening them as they go, and then gently let them fall back. Relax the buttocks and spine muscles, thinking consciously of the areas you are working on.

9. Do a mental check to make sure other muscles have not tightened up. Put your heels together and stretch your legs and toes as far as you can, then slowly relax them.

10. Turn on your side and lie that way for 2 to 3 minutes. Sit up slowly and recognize how you are feeling; try to keep that feeling as you go back to your activities.

Social support, in the form of positive work relationships, as well as nurturing family and friends, may be an important way to buffer the negative effects of a stressful work environment (Erdwins et al., 2001). Although friendships may be formed with colleagues, the workload and the shifting of staff from one unit to another often make it difficult to establish and maintain close relationships with peers. However, managers and co-workers who are supportive may improve morale in the workplace (Erdwins et al., 2001). The Research Perspective suggests that managing the workplace effectively also enhances retention. Nurses in a new position or in an unfamiliar geographic area must anticipate that they will benefit from the security of being part of a group that can furnish emotional support. Without easily accessible family and friends, nurses need to be intentional about seeking new, supportive personal relationships. Such efforts may help nurses cope with workplace demands that seem to exceed their capabilities. Positive coping strategies may also make nurses less likely to adopt such potentially negative coping strategies as withdrawal, lowering their standards of care, and abusing alcohol or other substances.

Burnout

Sometimes, individuals are unable to manage stress successfully through their own efforts and require assistance. Examples of behavior related to stress that feels overwhelming are found in Table 26-1. Coping strategies, such as those described previously, may furnish temporary relief or none at all. With this level of distress, one can feel overwhelmed or helpless and may be at greater risk for mental or physical illness. This constellation of emotions is commonly called *burnout*.

Burnout has been defined as a "prolonged response to chronic emotional and interpersonal stressors on the job" (Maslach, Schaufeli, & Leiter, 2000, p. 398). The sources of the stressors may

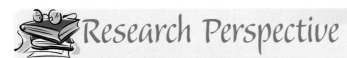

Research Perspective

Sourdif, J. (2004). Predictors of nurses' intent to stay at work in a university health center, *Nursing and Health Sciences, 6*, 59-69.

This study evaluated nurses' intent to remain employed in one Canadian university health center, and to determine the associations between intent to stay and satisfaction at work, satisfaction with administration, organizational commitment, and work group cohesion. Most of the 108 nurses completing the questionnaire planned to stay in their current job. The best predictors of intent to stay were satisfaction at work and satisfaction with administration.

IMPLICATIONS FOR PRACTICE
Given the current nursing shortage, employee retention is very important. Developing strategies that improve nurses' satisfaction with work and administration may improve retention rates. The variables in this study closely resemble many of the major workplace stressors identified by nurses.

exist in the environment, in the individual, or in the interaction between the individual and the environment. Some stressors, such as employment termination, appear to be universal, whereas other stressors, such as meeting deadlines, are more personal. For example, some nurses thrive on goals and timetables, whereas others feel constrained and frustrated and thereby experience distress. Burnout is not an objective phenomenon, as if it were the accumulation of a certain number and type of stressors. How the stressors are perceived and how they are mediated by an individual's ability to adapt are important variables in determining levels of distress.

Who is at risk for burnout? Characteristics of individuals at increased risk for burnout include perfectionism, the need for control, an exaggerated sense of responsibility, difficulty in asking for help, excessive, unrealistic guilt, suppression of feelings, and difficulty taking vacations and enjoying leisure time (Texas Medical Association, 2001).

Nurses who are burned out feel as though their resources are depleted to the point that their well-being is at risk. A self-analysis usually uncovers the characteristics of burnout. First, a feeling of physical, mental, and emotional exhaustion can be recognized. Greenglass, Burke, and Fiksenbaum (2001) found that emotional exhaustion was directly related to workload. For example, recent graduates may value total, detailed care for individuals and may have little experience in caring for more than two patients simultaneously. When confronted with the responsibility of caring for a group of six to eight acutely ill patients, they may have difficulty adapting to the realities of the workplace, and emotional exhaustion ensues.

Emotional exhaustion in turn has a direct positive effect on cynicism and somatization. A second characteristic of burnout is **depersonalization** or cynicism, a state characterized by distancing oneself from the work itself and developing negative attitudes toward work in general (Greenglass et al., 2001). Others may view this as callousness. Nurses pushed to do too much in too little time may distance themselves from patients as a means of dealing with emotional exhaustion.

A decreased sense of effectiveness (professional accomplishment and competence) is the third hallmark of burnout. Low professional efficacy has been found to be a function of higher levels of cynicism (Greenglass et al., 2001). This can lead to a

sense of failure, perceived helplessness, and finally crisis. Coping skills are no longer effective. At this point, help from others is needed.

RESOLUTION OF STRESS

Resolution of stress in its early stages can be accomplished through a variety of techniques. Nurses must be able to reach a balance of caring for others and caring for self. Table 26-2 summarizes physical, mental, and emotional/spiritual strategies.

Social Support

Peers and followers can be supportive and help reduce stress by providing assistance with problem-solving and by developing new perspectives. Family and friends can provide a safe haven and a vacation from stress. Social isolation increases stress. Social support allows one to be playful, have fun, laugh, and vent emotions.

Counseling

Persistent, unpleasant feelings, problem behavior, and helplessness during prolonged stress may suggest the need for assistance from a mental health professional. Examples of problem behaviors include tearfulness or angry outbursts over seemingly minor incidents, major changes in eating and/or sleeping patterns, frequent unwillingness to go to work, and substance abuse. In such cases, the aforementioned coping strategies afford only temporary relief; nurses with this level of distress feel overwhelmed and believe that their well-being

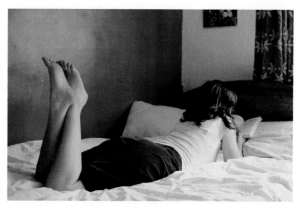

Making time for personal interests is important for personal development.

Table 26-2 STRESS MANAGEMENT STRATEGIES

Physical	Mental	Emotional/Spiritual
Accept physical limitations	Learn to say no!	Use meditation
Modify nutrition: moderate carbohydrate, moderate protein, high in fruits and vegetables, low caffeine, low sugar	Use cognitive restructuring and self-talk	Seek solace in prayer
	Use imagery	Seek professional counseling
	Develop hobbies or activities	Participate in support groups
Exercise: participate in an enjoyable activity five times a week for 30 minutes	Plan vacations	Participate in networking
	Learn about the system and how problems are handled	Communicate feelings
Make your physical health a priority	Learn communication, conflict resolution, and time management skills	Identify and acquire a mentor
Nurture yourself by taking time for breaks and lunch	Take continuing education courses	Ask for feedback and clarification
Sleep: get enough in quantity and quality		
Relax: use meditation, massage, yoga, or biofeedback		

cannot be maintained. In these stressful situations nurses may feel helpless and require professional assistance from a clinical psychologist, psychiatrist, or other mental health worker.

In some organizations, **employee assistance programs** (EAPs) provide free, voluntary, confidential, short-term professional counseling and other services for employees either via in-house staff or by contract with a mental health agency. This type of counseling can be effective because the counselors may already be aware of organizational stressors. Some nurses may have confidentiality concerns when using employer-recommended or employer-provided counseling services. Mental health professionals are bound by their professional standards of confidentiality. Nonetheless, there may be times when it is in the nurse's best interest to sign a release of information, such as when seeking employer accommodation for a certain physical or emotional problem.

Those who seek counseling outside of the workplace may be guided in their selection of mental health professionals by a personal physician, a knowledgeable colleague, or such publications as the most recent edition of *The Official ABMS Directory of Board Certified Medical Specialists 2005* (2004), which is available in many hospital libraries. When the problem underlying the distress is ethical or moral, a trained pastoral counselor may be helpful. Some clergy are certified in pastoral care or have earned a degree in another discipline such as psychology. Referrals can be obtained from hospital pastoral-care departments or churches that sponsor regional centers where certified counselors are available. When private counseling is being arranged, the health insurance contract should be checked to determine mental health benefits and the payment limitations and types of providers eligible for reimbursement.

Leadership and Management

Although social support and counseling can alter how stressors are perceived, time management and effective leadership can modify or remove stressors. Perhaps the most important stress modifier is enhancing the control that nursing staff have over their environment. First-line nurse managers have limited formal authority as individuals in most organizations, although managerial groups may be able to influence policy and resource allocation. Nurse managers can, however, control some environmental stressors on their units. First, managers can examine their own behavior as a source of subordinates' stress. A review of selected literature (Offermann & Hellmann, 1996) reveals that some leaders underestimate the influence of their behavior on subordinates' stress level and that they may attribute observed stress to the environment rather than their own behavior. This review also reported that lower performance and position satisfaction among subordinates was associated with nonparticipative, autocratic leadership styles.

In some cases, a controlling or autocratic style of management is appropriate, such as in emergency situations and when working with a large percentage of new and inexperienced employees. For the most part, however, professional nurses need and want the latitude to direct their activities within their sphere of competence. "Letting go," or delegating, means that the nurse leader trusts the personal integrity and professional competence of subordinates. It does not mean abdicating accountability for achieving accepted standards of patient care and agreed-upon outcomes.

Assistance with problem-solving is an additional way to reduce environmental stressors. Nurse leaders may provide technical advice, refer staff to appropriate resources, or mediate conflicts. Often, nurse leaders enable staff to meet the demands of their work more independently by providing time for continuing education and professional meetings to enhance competence.

Another way in which nurse leaders can reduce stress is to be supportive of staff. Support is not equated with being a friend, but rather with helping one's peers' accomplish good care, develop professionally, and feel valued personally. Leaders can ensure that the expected workload is in line with the nurses' capabilities and resources. They can work to ensure meaningfulness, stimulation, and opportunities for nurses to use their skills. Nurses' roles and responsibilities need to be clearly and publicly defined. Work schedules should be posted as far in advance as possible, and compatible with what is known about patient safety. Encouraging innovation and experimentation, for example, can motivate staff and give them a sense of greater control over their environment. Affirming a good idea or finding resources to study or implement a promising new procedure or proposal by a staff nurse is supportive. In contrast, when staff members struggle with overwork and other stressors, support is recognizing the condition and helping the nurses avoid such passive coping strategies as feeling helpless or lowering standards of care in favor of active problem-solving. Nurse leaders must be sensitive to the distress of the nursing staff and recognize it verbally without becoming counselors, which is in conflict with their role. Support may involve making nursing staff aware of resources that furnish counseling while being careful to avoid diagnostic labels and to maintain strict confidentiality. When distress relates to the personal life of subordinates, managers should focus on the effect of such situations on workplace performance, not on the events that have produced the stress.

Additionally, leaders can enhance the workplace by dealing effectively with their own stressors. Maintaining a sense of perspective as well as a sense of humor is important. Some stressors, in fact, can be ignored or minimized by posing three questions:

1. "Is this event or situation important?" Stressors are not all equally significant. Do not waste energy on little stressors.
2. "Does this stressor affect me or my unit?" Although some situations that produce distress are institutionwide and need group action, others target specific units or activities. Do not borrow stressors.
3. "Can I change this situation?" If not, then find a way to cope with it or, if the situation is intolerable, make plans to change positions or employers. This decision may require gaining added credentials that may produce long-term career benefits.

Keeping stressful situations in perspective can enable nurses to conserve their energies to cope with stressful situations that are important, that are within their domain, or that can be changed or modified.

MANAGEMENT OF TIME

There is a very close relationship between stress management and time management. Time management is one method of stress prevention or reduction. Stress can decrease productivity and lead to poor use of time. Time management can be considered a preventive action to help reduce the elements of stress in a nurse's life.

Everyone has two choices when it comes to managing time: organize or "go with the flow." There are only 24 hours in every day, and it is clear that some people make better use of time than others. It is how people use time that makes some people more successful than others. The current status of healthcare organizations, trying to do more with less, has led to more demands (stressors) being placed on care providers and care managers. The effective use of time-management skills thus becomes an even more important tool to achieve personal and professional goals. *Time management* is the appropriate use of tools, techniques, and principles to control time spent on low-priority needs and to ensure that time is invested in activities leading toward achieving desired, high-priority goals. More simply, time management is the ability to spend your time on the things that matter to you and your organization. However, it does take time to plan daily time-management strategies! By setting goals and eliminating time stealers, you will have the extra time to accomplish them.

Where Does Your Time Go?

Have you ever wasted time? Time, although a cheap commodity, is our most valuable resource. There are some commonly identified timestealers, and individuals must recognize them to guard against them. At the heart of time management is an important shift in focus. Concentrate on results, not on being busy.

Doing Too Much Do you try to do too much at once? At work, do you have three or four major projects going simultaneously? Are you a member of more than one organizational committee? Do you have to worry about what will be on the table for dinner while you are hanging an IV and planning a staff meeting? Have you ever completed a nursing intervention and realized that your mind was really somewhere else, and the patient had been ignored? If you *think* you have too much to do, you probably do! Learn to have fewer projects running simultaneously and to concentrate your efforts on one thing at a time. The first step is to be realistic and limit major commitments, then give each activity your full and undivided attention. Sometimes completing one task before starting another is the most efficient method for getting everything done. Prioritization of goals and activities each day is very helpful.

In the nursing profession, however, limiting commitments is not always possible. When you are feeling overwhelmed by the sheer volume of tasks to be completed, take the time to establish priorities

for the day. Decide what must be done versus what would be nice to do. Do not let yourself get distracted from your priority tasks. Nursing is a balancing act; priorities are always changing.

Inability to Say "No" Sometimes the smallest and simplist words are the most difficult to learn. If you are suffering from overload, you probably have gotten there by not being able to say "no." Learning to say "no" to requests is difficult, and in the process others may be displeased. If you do not say "no," however, you may end up spending a great deal of time on projects that are uninteresting or have no relationship to your personal goals and priorities. When someone asks you to do something, you need to stop and consider the request. Do you want to do the task now or sometime in the future? If not, then say so. If you wish to do the task but simply do not have the time, consider **delegation.** However, be honest with the requester—if you simply do not have the time, say so as politely as possible. If you wish to take on the task but at a later date, negotiate. Remember, accepting an assignment you will never be able to complete does not shed a favorable light on you.

Procrastination Do you put off important tasks because they are not enjoyable or because they may be difficult? Do you find excuses for not starting or completing tasks? Are you a procrastinator? By engaging in **procrastination,** or doing one thing when you should be doing something else, you give up time to complete your task and therefore limit the quality of the work you produce. There are techniques to help deal with procrastination. First, identify the reason for procrastinating. Then make that task your highest priority the next day. Reward yourself after you finish the task. Another technique is to select the least attractive element of the task to do first, and the rest will seem easy.

Some people find that they procrastinate when the task ahead is very large. The solution is to break the task down into manageable pieces and plan rewards for accomplishing each of the smaller tasks. Developing a PERT (program evaluation and review technique) chart or a Gantt chart may help in this process. PERT charts were originally developed as tools to assist in complex projects that require a series of activities, some of which must be performed sequentially, and others that can be performed in parallel with other activities.

Table 26-3 SAMPLE GANTT CHART

Task	Accountability	JAN	FEB	MAR	APR	MAY	JUNE
1. Conduct literature search	Unit CNS	———→					
2. Hold nursing practice committee meeting to review material	Chair, nursing practice committee		X				
3. Create a report for the medical staff	Chair, nursing practice committee			———	→		
4. Disseminate findings to nursing and medical staff	Chair, nursing practice committee					———	→

Envisioned as a network diagram, a PERT chart indicates all predecessor activities that must be completed before a new activity is undertaken. A Gantt chart (Table 26-3) consists of a table of project task information and a bar chart that graphically displays project schedule, depicting progress in relation to time and often used in planning and tracking a project. Both chart techniques can be used to outline how you will approach a large project. Exercise 26-3 is one way to manage procrastination.

■ Exercise 26–3

What tasks have you been putting off? Identify three tasks (1 to 3) that you really need to do—tasks that you labeled high priority, yet still have not done. For each task, write down two reasons why you have been avoiding the work (R1 and R2). Prioritize the tasks. Now break each task down into three or more manageable pieces (A, B, and C). Plan a reward to follow completion of each task.

TASKS I HAVE PROCRASTINATED ON   PRIORITY

1. _____   _____
   R1. _____
   R2. _____
   A. _____
   B. _____
   C. _____

2. _____   _____
   R1. _____
   R2. _____
   A. _____
   B. _____
   C. _____

3. _____   _____
   R1. _____
   R2. _____
   A. _____
   B. _____
   C. _____

Complaining Complaining is the act of expressing dissatisfaction or annoyance with persons, places, things, and situations. Often, the time people spend complaining about a task or a particular situation is greater than the time needed to complete the task or to deal with the issue. If you find yourself complaining repeatedly about something, stop and ask yourself what would be the ideal solution and then take the risk to act on it. If the complaint is related to another person, either take the time to talk with the person and get the problem out in the open, or sit down and write a letter to the person discussing your point of view (even if you do not mail it). If you find yourself complaining about something within the workplace, take the time to rethink the problem and generate some possible solutions, then talk to your manager. Look for solutions that are very simple or "outside the box." Go talk to your manager prepared to discuss solutions, not just your dissatisfaction or annoyance. In this way, your manager will see you as interested in contributing to the goals of the organization.

Perfectionism Perfectionism is the tendency to never finish anything because it is not yet perfect.

This approach tends to consume a great deal of time when your expected outcome is not attainable. Overcoming perfectionism takes considerable effort. However, this does not mean that you should do less than your best. Being aware of perfectionism means that you occasionally need to give yourself permission to do slightly less than a perfect job, such as buying a carryout dinner rather than preparing a four-course meal after a day at work.

Interruptions   One common distraction from priority activities is interruptions. Some interruptions are integral to the positions that you hold, but others can be controlled. A home care nurse with a large caseload can expect to be paged at any time. More commonly, however, are the numerous small interruptions by individuals who want just a "minute of your time" and take 2 minutes getting to the point! Box 26-1 identifies some specific strategies to prevent and control interruptions. The two keys to dealing with interruptions are to resume "doing it now" so that an interruption does not destroy your schedule and to maintain the attitude that whatever the interruption, it is a part of your responsibility. When you make a conscious decision not to worry about the things you cannot control, you have more energy to maintain a positive perspective and to move projects forward.

Disorganization   One of the most serious time wasters of all is disorganization. How many times have you had to spend 5 minutes trying to find something you have misplaced or misfiled? Organization can be a great time saver. Remember that the guiding principle is that organization is a process rather than the product. You can spend so much time organizing that you will never get to the task at hand (procrastination). Simple organizing guidelines include eliminating clutter, keeping everything in its place, and doing similar tasks together.

Too Much Information   The newest time waster to evolve is data proliferation. We are now in the midst of a paradigm shift in the Information Age. The technology within our workplace forces us to receive huge amounts of data and to transform these data into useful information. The computer workstation, once touted as a time-saving device, has become the driving force behind care delivery. Nurses can view the computer either as a stress-producing slave driver or as a simple tool to assist them in their daily activities.

Information overload, or "data smog," occurs when you are overwhelmed by too much information, too fast, and too often and do not have the skills to interpret the data into useful information.

BOX 26-1

Tips to Avoid Interruptions and Work More Effectively

- Chart somewhere other than in the place you will be most accessible to others.
- Ask people to put their comments in writing—do not let them catch you "on the run."
- Let the office/unit secretary know what information you need immediately.
- Conduct a conversation in the hall to help keep it short or in a separate room to keep from being interrupted.
- Be comfortable saying "no."
- When involved in a long procedure or home visit, ask someone else to cover your other responsibilities.
- Break projects into small, manageable pieces.
- Get yourself organized.
- Minimize interruptions—for example, allow voice mail to pick up the phone; shut the door.

- Keep your work surface clear. Have available only those documents needed for the task at hand.
- Keep your manager informed of your goals.
- Plan to accomplish high-priority or difficult tasks early in the day.
- Develop a plan for the day and stick to it. Remember to schedule in some time for interruptions.
- Schedule time to meet regularly throughout the shift with staff members you are responsible for.
- Recognize that crises and interruptions are part of the position.
- Be cognizant of your personal time-waster habits, and try to avoid them.

Symptoms of information overload may include a sense of inability to keep up with everything; a feeling that data keep you from accomplishing your "real job," an inability to proceed from the question or problem to fact finding; interference with sleep; a decreased ability to concentrate; irritability; and physical distress, including indigestion, heart problems, and hypertension (Murray, 2001).

Developing data and information gathering, receiving and sending skills (known as information literacy) can greatly reduce stress and improve efficiency and productivity. Gaining a new appreciation for information is important. Information is simply a tool to use to plan action or make decisions. By learning what information is important, you can learn to use it to your advantage.

Time-Management Concepts

Table 26-4 presents a classification scheme for time-management techniques. The unifying theme is that each activity undertaken should lead to goal attainment and that goal should be the number one priority at that time.

Time-Management Strategies

Goal Setting The first steps in time management are goal-setting and developing a plan to reach the goals. If determining long-term goals is difficult for you, consider setting more short-term goals—steps along the way to the long-term goal. Set goals that are reasonable and achievable. Do not expect to reach long-term goals overnight—long-term means just that. Give yourself time to meet the goals. Determine many short-term goals to reach the

long-term goal, giving yourself a frequent sense of goal achievement. Annual goals should be broken down into monthly goals, monthly goals broken down into weekly goals, and weekly goals broken down into daily goals. Give yourself flexibility. If the path you chose last year is no longer appropriate, change it. Write your goals on paper, date the page, keep it handy, and refer to it often to give yourself a progress report.

Setting Priorities Once goals are known, priorities are set. They may, however, shift throughout a given period in terms of goal attainment. For example, working on a budget may take precedence at certain times of the year, whereas new staff orientation is high priority at other times. Knowing what your goals and priorities are helps shape the "to do" list. On a nursing unit or as you work in a community setting, you must know your personal goals and current priorities. How you organize work may depend on geographic considerations, patient acuity, or some other schema.

Covey, Merrill, and Merrill (1994) identify a particular strategy to assist in prioritization. They state that people generally focus on those things that are important and urgent. By placing the elements of importance and urgency in a grid as shown in Figure 26-2, all activities can be classified, as shown.

Typically, we tend to focus on those items in cell A because they are both important and urgent and therefore command our attention. Making shift assignments is an A task because it is both important to the work to be accomplished and commonly urgent because there is a time frame

Table 26-4 CLASSIFICATION OF TIME MANAGEMENT TECHNIQUES

Technique	Purpose	Actions
Organization	Designed to promote efficiency and productivity	Organize and systematize things, tasks, and people. Use basic time-management skills
Keep focused on goals	Focuses on goal achievement	Assemble a prioritized "to do" list based on goals daily
Tool usage	Uses the right tool for planning and preparation	Use tools such as the PalmPilot
Time-management plan	Helps to refocus, to gain control, and to use information	Develop a personal time-management plan appropriately

Figure 26-2 Classification of priorities. (Modified from Covey, S. R., Merrill, A. R., & Merrill, R. R. [1994]. *First things first: To love, to learn, to leave a legacy.* New York: Simon & Schuster.)

during which data about patients and qualifications of staff can be matched. Conversely, if something is neither important nor urgent (cell D), it may be considered a waste of time, at least in terms of personal goals. An example of a D activity might be reading "junk" e-mail. Even if something is urgent but not important (cell C), it contributes minimally to productivity and goal achievement. An example of a C activity might be responding to a memo that has a specific time line but is not important to goal-attainment. The real key to setting priorities is to attend to the B tasks, those that are important but not urgent. Examples of B activities are reviewing the organization's strategic plan or participating on organizational committees.

Organization   A number of simple routines for organization can save many minutes over a day and enhance your efficiency. Keeping a workspace neat or arranging things in an orderly fashion may be a powerful time-management tool. Rather than a system of "pile management," use "file management." The adage "there is a place for everything, and everything in its place" makes for a successful workspace. A few hints include (1) planning ahead where things should go (frequently used items should be more accessible); (2) not using the top of your desk (table, computer station) for storage; (3) creating a "to do" folder; (4) creating a "to be filed" folder; and (5) having a regularly scheduled time to work your way through the folders. Everyone accumulates a pile of papers that becomes a problem over time. Take the time to sort the piles, perhaps tossing a page or two, acting on those things that are urgent, or if all else fails, filing it! The easiest way to keep a desk neat is to clean off the desk at the end of every day. After cleaning the desk, determine your priority goals for the next day and have the materials ready to work on when you start the next morning.

Time Tools   Sometimes, the real problem is that the events of the day become the driving force, rather than a planned schedule. Days may become so tightly scheduled that any little interruption can become a crisis. If you do not plan the day, you may find yourself responding to events rather than prioritized goals. If you think you are a reactor rather than a proactive time user, use a time log to list work-related activities for several days. One reason you may not be able to plan well is that you really do not have a good estimate of how long a particular activity actually takes, or you do not know how many activities can be accomplished in a given time frame.

As the nurse's role in care management increases in complexity, the need for organizational tools increases. Tracking the care of groups of patients, either as the member of a care team or in a leadership capacity, can be overwhelming. Each nurse must devise a method for tracking care and organizing time, as well as delegating and monitoring care provided by others. Although some nurses depend on a shift flow sheet or a Kardex system, others are enjoying the benefit of computerized information tracking systems. The use of handheld computer devices such as personal digital assistants (PDAs) like the PalmPilot or bar code scanners for medication administration are other methods to track information and increase safety and efficiency. The software and shareware available for the Palm Operating System can be very useful. For example, programs are available that have a drug handbook, making it possible to look up drugs, side effects, and possible interactions at the bedside. Other programs are available to calculate drug dosages, and to record patient data. The issue of client confidentiality cannot be ignored when entering data into a PDA that goes home with you at the end of your shift.

Managing Information   The first step in managing information is to assess the source. Once you have identified the sources of your data, you have a better idea of how to deal with the information. Track incoming information for a few days. Patterns will begin to emerge and will give clues as to how to deal with it. You can generally predict that, using the Pareto principle, 80% of your incoming data comes from approximately 20% of your sources, and that 80% of useful information comes from 20% of information received (see the Theory Box.)

By developing information-receiving skills, you can quickly interpret the data and convert them to useful information, discarding that which is not needed. Initially, you should reduce or eliminate that which is useless. Delete the e-mail or toss the memo in the trash. Next, monitor the information flow and decide what to do with incoming data. Find and focus on the most important pieces and then quickly narrow down the specific details you need. Identify resources that are most helpful and have them readily available. Be able to build the "big picture" from the masses of data you receive. Finally, recognize when you have enough information to act.

Once you have mastered the receiving end of information, concentrate on information-sending skills. Remember, your information is simply another person's data! Try to keep your outflow short; make it a synthesis of the information. Finally, select the most appropriate mode of communication for your message from the technology available. You may be sending your information in written (memo or report) or verbal form (face-to-face or presentation) or via telephone, voice mail, e-mail, or fax. Remember, the most important skill is to know when you have said enough. Exercise 26-4 will help you consider how you have dealt with information.

Exercise 26–4

Think of the last time you were in the clinical area. How often did you record the same piece of data (e.g., a finding in your assessment of the patient)? Remember to include all steps, from your jotting down notes on a piece of paper to the final report of the day. What information processing tools could decrease the number of steps?

MEETING MANAGEMENT

Two key time-management strategies that are critical to success are managing meetings and delegation, which are discussed in the next two sections of this chapter. Even nurses who may not have extensive management responsibilities usually are in the position of delegating tasks to less-skilled workers and can benefit from learning to make the most of meetings, either as the leader or as a group member.

Managing Meetings

Unfocused, poorly managed meetings can waste valuable time and can frustrate busy staff members. Meetings serve various purposes, ranging from creating social networks to setting formal policy. Lencioni (2004) defines four types of meetings. The daily check-in should take about 5 minutes, and it is the opportunity to check schedules and activities. This might be analogous to "touch base" meetings when we want to be sure we are all progressing as planned and that no patient-care issues are unattended. The second meeting type is weekly tactical to resolve issues. This type of meeting would be reflective of what the unit staff needs to address to ensure that they have the resources to achieve what they need to do for patients. The monthly strategic is used to address big issues that have longer term implications. These meetings are frequently standing committees of the organization on which staff serve. The quarterly off-site review is designed to analyze progress and to develop the team. It is uncommon to find that many organizations provide this frequency and intensity (Lencioni suggests this type of meeting should be 1 to 2 days) except at higher levels in the organization.

Meetings may be designed to solve problems, disseminate information, seek input, inspire the group, delegate work or authority, or create/maintain a formal power base. Unless the purpose of a meeting is to socialize, the meeting is unlikely to be effective if it is poorly managed. The following is a list of several popular techniques and strategies to enhance the productivity and effectiveness of meetings.

Tips for Managing Meetings Effectively Before scheduling a meeting, ask yourself several questions:

- Is this meeting really necessary? What would happen if the meeting never happened?
- Might a phone call or one-on-one meeting better achieve the goal?
- Is this meeting simply informational? If so, would written communication better meet the need? Would a memo or posting an announcement suffice?

• Are the people who really need to attend available to meet?

Schedule meetings right before lunch or at the end of the day. Participants will have an incentive to stick to the schedule. Set a start and stop time and reward prompt members by starting on schedule. Most of the work of the meeting is accomplished in the first hour. Try to avoid meetings lasting longer than 1.5 to 2 hours. Select an appropriate setting, where the participants are not readily accessible to interruptions. If necessary, plan the seating arrangement to prevent inappropriate behaviors such as whispering or other interruptions. If the group meets over a period of time, have group members set rules for conduct and behavior.

Distribute an **agenda.** Whenever possible, provide a written agenda to each member in advance of the meeting. Establish and make known the goal of the meeting. Attach all needed preparation reading to the agenda. The more advanced the reading or preparation that is required, the earlier members should receive agendas. Different types of agendas can be used for different purposes:

Structured agendas: If a topic is particularly controversial, consider setting a rule that requires any negative comment to be preceded by a positive one.

Timed agendas: Consider setting a specific amount of time to be dedicated to each item on the agenda. If you stick to the schedule, discussion will stay focused and you will be more likely to make it through the agenda (Box 26-2).

Action agendas: Consider submitting an agenda with a description of the needed/desired action, such as review proposals, approve minutes, or establish outcomes.

Keep the group on task. Use rules of order to facilitate meetings. Robert's Rules of Order (Robert, Evans, & Balch, 2000) may seem overly structured; however, this structure is particularly helpful when diversity of opinion is likely or important. Specifically, these rules help the person chairing the meeting by setting limits on discussion and using a specific order of priorities to deal with concerns.

Keep minutes and distribute them to participants. The minutes provide a record to refer back to if needed and also serve to convey contents to persons unable to attend.

Planning ahead for the meeting is a group leader's best strategy for a satisfactory experience. Participants must also prepare for meetings. Reviewing the agenda (or requesting one in advance if not provided), reviewing preparatory materials, and thinking through agenda items are ways that group members may assist in accomplishing the meeting goals. Meeting participants should be on time for all meetings or communicate that they will be late or unable to attend. Participants should be prepared to leave on time as well. When a meeting is poorly chaired, a committee member could volunteer to be sure that the meeting agendas and minutes are distributed. It is important to recognize

---

BOX 26-2

Sample of Timed Agenda

6 NORTH Staff Meeting

2:30 PM, September 12, 2005

Room 6224

MINUTES FOR ITEM	AGENDA ITEM	ACTION NEEDED
2	Call to Order—Unit Manager	
3	Approval of Minutes—Unit Manager	Vote
15	Introduction of new chart form for discharges— 6 North CQI Discharge Team	Approval of form—Vote
10	Discussion of pain management initiative— Pain Resource Nurses	3 unit-specific methods to improve pain management on 6 North
20	Plan for holiday staffing—Unit Manager	Approval of method—Vote

that some people deliberately avoid preparing agendas and distributing minutes in an attempt to control the meeting. Exercise 26-5 will help you understand the importance of well-run meetings.

Delegating

Delegation is a critical component of self-management for nurse managers and care managers. Appropriate delegation not only increases time efficiency but also serves as a means of reducing stress. Delegation is discussed in depth in Chapter 23, but it is also appropriate to discuss briefly as a time-management strategy. Delegation works only when the delegator trusts the delegatee to accomplish the task and to report findings back to the nurse. It does not save time for the nurse to go back and check or redo everything someone else has done. Delegation requires empowerment of the delegatee to accomplish the task. If the nurse does not

delegate appropriately, with clear expectations, the delegatee will constantly be asking for assistance or direction. Delegation can also be a means of reducing stress if used appropriately. If the nurse does not understand delegation and does not use it appropriately, it can be a major source of stress as the nurse assumes accountability and responsibility for care administered by others.

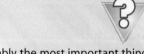

SUMMARY

Self-management is a means to achieve a balance between work and personal life, as well as a way of life developed to achieve personal goals within self-imposed priorities and deadlines. Time management is clock-oriented, and stress management is the control of external and internal stressors.

To achieve a balance in life and minimize stressors, nurses must learn to sit back and see their own personal "big picture" and examine their personal and professional goals. Personal priorities also must be established. Stressors and coping strategies need to be identified and used. By developing these techniques, nurses can gain a sense of control and become far better nurses in the process.

The Solution

I do feel I handle the stress better than I used to. Considering the increased load, I guess I must be! I definitely take better care of myself than I used to: I am vigilant about getting enough sleep, I really try to eat a balanced diet, I take my vitamin everyday, and every few days I treat myself to a really good piece of dark chocolate. I don't get as much exercise as I would like, but I am aware of it, and try to incorporate what I can (like taking the stairs instead of the elevator). I really try not to procrastinate too much, as that just increases the stress because I am thinking about the project the whole time I am putting off doing it.

My husband is really supportive, and I have a fantastic best friend. Just having somebody to vent to, or she and I will go out for ice cream or coffee, just for half an hour; that helps so much. I often take myself out for lunch when it's getting really bad, or maybe I treat myself to a massage or facial. I also meditate, and I find that really

helps tremendously. Probably the most important thing I have learned to do is really be in the present moment . . . when I am playing with the kids, I try not to fixate on how long until I can go work on whatever project, or when I'm out on Friday night I really don't think about all the stuff that just happened that week or that is coming up the next week. That helps so much, because the effect stress has is really what we do with it. So if I don't focus on all that stuff all the time my stress level is much more manageable! I think having lots of options to manage stress is important . . . not every method works for every situation, so I pick and choose what I can do at the time to get some benefit.

— Amy Phillips

 Would this be a suitable approach for you? Why?

CHAPTER CHECKLIST

Stress management and time management are two strategies for self-management. Balancing stress means caring for your emotional, physical, and mental needs. Effective delegation, using schedules and calendars and other planners, using time-management principles, and managing meetings are key strategies to be integrated into the nurse leader role. By accomplishing self-management, managers, leaders, and followers will find themselves in control of work time and stressors, as well as more confident in achieving both personal and work-related goals.

Stress and overwork are inherent in the nursing profession, and nurses can adapt and cope with stress and time pressures by learning effective ways to care for themselves and to manage time. By assessing and reducing specific stressors and time wasters, nurses can thrive within the healthcare challenges before them. Increasing skills in coping, organization, delegation, and effective time management are vital components of effective leadership. A nurse manager who can be a role model and support his or her staff in turbulent times is a true leader.

■ Stress management includes using cognitive and psychosocial activities to decrease the stress or enhance the ability to handle stress.
■ Time management includes using tools and strategies to ensure that priority goals are achieved.
■ Signs of excess stress must be heeded to prevent burnout or chronic health problems.
■ Strategies to reduce stress include the following:
  • Physical
    – Accept physical limitations.
    – Plan physical activity.
    – Maintain adequate physical health, including adequate nutrition.
    – Schedule time for breaks and relaxation.
  • Mental/emotional
    – Use problem-identification and problem-solving strategies.
    – Differentiate between perceived and objective stressors.
    – Evoke the relaxation response via meditation.
    – Recognize stress-induced behavioral changes.
    – Seek social support.
  • Management
    – Maintain awareness of the effect of behavior on others.
    – Develop a participative management style.
    – Practice a systems perspective.
    – Retain a sense of distance from stress.
■ Strategies to improve time management include the following:
  • Identification of potential time wasters
    – Too much work
    – Inability to say "no"
    – Procrastination
    – Complaining
    – Perfectionism
    – Interruptions
    – Disorganization
    – Too much information
  • Use of time-management strategies
    – Setting priorities
    – Being organized
    – Using time tools such as time logs, Kardex, shift flow sheets, and Personal Data Assistants
    – Devising a personal time management system
    – Effectively dealing with data and information
  • Appropriate delegation
    – Being willing to delegate/be delegated to
    – Giving the delegatee sufficient responsibility and authority
    – Conveying expectations clearly
    – Requiring the delegatee to be accountable
■ Strategies to improve meeting management include the following:
  • Distribute meeting agendas and minutes for reading and comments prior to the meeting.
  • Schedule meetings appropriately.
  • Use rules of order to facilitate meetings.

TIPS FOR SELF-MANAGEMENT

- Know what your high-priority goals are, and use them to filter decisions.
- Know your personal response to stress, and self-evaluate frequently.
- Make your health a priority, and use strategies that keep yourself in control.
- Use organizational systems that meet your needs; the simpler, the better.
- Simplify.
- Refocus on your priorities whenever you begin to feel overwhelmed.

TERMS TO KNOW

agenda	information overload
burnout	overwork
coping	perfectionism
delegation	procrastination
depersonalization	self-management
employee assistance program	time managment
general adaptation syndrome (GAS)	

REFERENCES

American Board of Medical Specialities (2004). *The official ABMS directory of board certified medical specialists 2005*. Philadelphia: W.B. Saunders.

Barsade, S., & Wiesenfeld, B. (1997). *Attitudes in the American workplace III*. New Haven, CT: Yale University School of Management.

Chang, E., & Hancock, K. (2003). Role stress and role ambiguity in new nursing graduates in Australia. *Nursing and Health Sciences, 5,* 155–163.

Cohen, S., & Manuck, S. (1999). Preface. In B. Rabin. *Stress, immune function and health* (pp. xi–xii). New York: Wiley-Liss.

Covey, S. R., Merrill, A. R., & Merrill, R. R. (1994). *First things first: To love, to learn, to leave a legacy*. New York: Simon & Schuster.

DeAngelis, T. (2002, June). A bright future for PNI. *Monitor on Psychology, 33*(6). Retrieved September 1, 2006, from www.apa.org/monitor/jun02/brightfuture.html

Drucker, P. F. (2000, Spring). Managing knowledge means managing one's self. *Leader to Leader, 16,* 8–10.

Epel, E., Blackburn, E., Lin, J., Dhabhar, F., Adler, N., Morrow, J., & Cawthon, R. (2004). *Proceedings of the National Academy of Science of the USA* (November 29, 2004).

Epstein, R. (2000). *The big book of stress relief games*. New York: McGraw-Hill.

Erdwins, C. J., Buffardi, L. C., Casper, W. J., & O'Brien, A. S. (2001). The relationship of women's role strain to social support, role satisfaction, and self-efficacy. *Family Relations, 50*(3), 230–238.

Evans, O., & Steptoe, A. (2002). The contribution of gender-role orientation, work factors, and home stressors to psychological well-being and sickness absence in male- and female-dominated occupational groups. *Social Science and Medicine, 54*(4), 481–492.

Fischer, J., Calame, A., Dettling, A., Zeier, H., & Fanconi, S. (2000). Experience and endocrine stress responses in neonatal and pediatric critical care nurses and physicians. *Critical Care Medicine, 28*(9), 3281–3288.

Greenglass, E., Burke, R., & Fiksenbaum, L. (2001). Workload and burnout in nurses. *Journal of Community and Applied Social Psychology, 11,* 211–215.

Hafner, A. W. (2001). *Pareto's principle: The 80-20 rule*. Retrieved July 1, 2002, from http://library.shu.edu/HafnerAW/awh-th-math-pareto.html.

Health Resources and Services Administration (2005). National sample survey of registered nurses. Retrieved May 25, 2006, from http://bhpr.hrsa.gov/healthworkforce/reports/rnpopulation/preliminaryfindings.htm.

Kiecolt-Glaser, J., Preacher, K., MacCallum, R., Atkinson, C., Malarkey, W., & Glaser, R. (2003, July 2) Chronic stress related increases in the proinflammatory cytokine IL-6. *Proceedings of the National Academy of Science of the USA.*

Kirkcaldy, B., & Martin, T. (2000). Job stress and satisfaction among nurses. *Stress Medicine, 16,* 77–89.

Kuhn, M. A. (1999). *Complementary therapies for health care providers*. Philadelphia: Lippincott Williams & Wilkins.

Lambert, V., Lambert, C., & Yamase, H. (2003). Psychological hardinessm workplace stress and related stress reduction strategies. *Nursing and Health Sciences, 5,* 181–184.

Lencioni, P. (2004). *Death by meeting*. San Fransisco: Jossey-Bass.

Maddi, S.R. (2002). The story of hardiness: Twenty years of theorizing, research and practice. *Consulting Psychology Journal, 54,* 173–185.

Maslach, C., Schaufeli, W., Leiter, M. (2000). Job burnout. *Annual Review of Psychology, 52,* 397–422.

Maurier, W., & Northcutt, H. (2000). Job uncertainty and health status for nurses during restructuring of health care in Alberta. *Western Journal of Nursing Research, 22*(5), 623–641.

Mooy, J., deVries, H, Grootenhuis, P., Bouter, L., & Heine, R. (2000). Major stressful life events in relation to prevalence of undetected type 2 diabetes: the Hoorn study. *Diabetes Care, 23* (2), 197–201.

Murray, B. (2001). *Data smog: Newest culprit in brain drain.* Retrieved from http://pespmc1.vub.ac.be/CHINNEG.html.

Northwestern National Life Insurance Complany (1992). Employee burnout: Causes and cures. Minneapolis, MN: Northwestern National Life Insurance Company.

Offermann, L. R., & Hellmann, P. (1996). Leadership behavior and subordinate stress: A 360° view. *Journal of Occupational Health Psychology, 1*(4), 382–390.

O'Keefe, E. & Berger, D. (2000) *Self-Management for College Students.* Hyde Park, N.Y.: Partridge Hill Publishers.

Posen, D. B. (1995, April). Stress management for patient and physician. *The Canadian Journal of Continuing Medical Education.* Retrieved January 28, 2005, from http://www.mentalhealth.com/mag1/p51-str.html.

Rabin, B. (1999). *Stress, immune function and health.* New York: Wiley-Liss.

Robert, H., Evans, W., & Balch, J. (Eds.). (2000). *Robert's rules of order newly revised.* Cambridge, MA: Perseus Book Group.

Rogers, A. E., Hwang, W-T., Scott, L. D., Aiken, L. H., & Dinges, D. F. (2004). The working hours of hospital staff nurses and patient safety. *Health Affairs, 23,* 202–212.

Selye, H. (1956). *The stress of life.* New York: McGraw-Hill.

Selye, H. (1991). History and present status of the stress concept. In A. Monat & R. Lazarus (Eds.), *Stress and coping: An anthology* (pp. 21–36). New York: Columbia University Press.

Segerstrom, S., & Miller, G. (2004). Psychological stress and the human immune system: A meta-analytic study of 30 years of inquiry. *Psychological Bulletim 130*(4), 601–630.

Smith, A. (2000). The scale of perceived occupational stress. *Occupational Medicine, 50*(5), 294–298.

Stoppler, M. (2005). Top five stress management mistakes. *Your guide to stress management.* Retreived January 16, 2005, from http://stress.about.com/cs/copingskills/a/mistakes_p.htm.

Tangri, R. (2002). What stress costs. *Approaching Change 3*(3), 1–14.

Taylor, S. E., Klein, L. C., Lewis, B. P., Gruenewald, T. L., Gurung, R. A. R, & Updegraff, J. A. (2000). Biobehavioral responses to stress in females: Tend-and-befriend, not fight-or-flight. *Psychological Review, 107,* 441–429.

Texas Medical Association (2001) *CME: Physician Burnout.* Retrieved February 15, 2005, from www.texmed.org/cme/phn/psb/characteristics.asp.

Wilson, R. S., Barnes, L. L., Bennett, D. A., Li ,Y., Bienias, J. L., Mendes de Leon, C. F., & Evans, D. A. (2005). Proneness to psychological distress and risk of Alzheimer disease in a biracial community. *Neurology, 64*(2), 380–382.

Wilson, R. S., Evans, D. A., Bienias, J. L., Mendes de Leon, C. F., Schneider, J. A., Bennett, D. A. (2003). Proneness to psychological distress is associated with risk of Alzheimer's disease. *Neurology, 61,* 1479–1485.

Wittstein, I., Thiemann, D., Lima, J., Baughman, K., Schulman, S., Gerstebblith, G., et al. (2005). Neurohumoral feathres of myocardial stunning due to sudden emotional stress. *New England Journal of Medicine, 352* (6), 539–548.

Worthington, K. (2001). The health risks of mandatory overtime. *American Journal of Nursing, 101*(5), 96.

SUGGESTED READINGS

Drucker, R. (1999). *Management challenges for the 21st century.* New York: HarperCollins.

Field, T., Quintino, O., Henteleff, T., Wells-Keife, L., & Delvecchio-Feinberg, G. (1997). Job stress reduction therapies. *Alternative Therapies in Health & Medicine, 3*(4), 54–56.

Lenson, B. (2002). *Good stress bad stress.* New York: Marlowe & Company.

Lyon, B. (2000). Conquering stress. *Reflections on Nursing Leadership, 26*(1), 22–23, 43.

Oncken, W., & Wass, D. (1999, November/December). Management time: Who's got the monkey? *Harvard Business Review,* reprint 99609.

Skovholt, T. (2001) *The resilient practitioner: Burnout strategies for counselors, therapists, teachers and health professionals.* Needham Heights, MA: Allyn & Brown.

Tracy, B. (2004). *Time power.* New York: AMACOM.

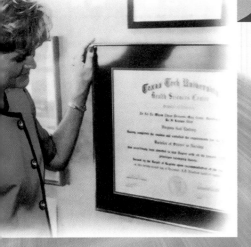

Chapter

27

Career Management: Putting Yourself in Charge

Karen A. Dadich
Patricia S. Yoder–Wise

This chapter focuses on planning and developing a professional career. These elements include identifying a career style and developing the tools needed to create career opportunities. Career development is linked to ongoing professional development. The concept of continuous lifelong learning and elements of the process of professional certification are introduced.

Objectives

- Differentiate among career styles and how they influence career options.
- Analyze person-position fit.
- Evaluate the relevance of a cover letter, curriculum vitae, and résumé as entrées to interviews.
- Use critical elements of the cover letter, résumé or curriculum vitae to develop each.
- Analyze critical elements of an interview.
- Evaluate different types of professional learning opportunities.
- Value professional expectations.

Questions to Consider

- What excites you about nursing?
- What clinical nursing experience has been most stimulating and challenging? Why?
- What excites you about leadership and management options?
- What do you want to be doing in 3 years?

The Challenge

Rebecca A. Brawley, RN, BSN
Public Health Coordinator/Prevention Manager, City of Lubbock Health Department,
   Lubbock, Texas

I began my nursing career as a licensed vocational nurse. My peers and I worked in a very relaxed environment with very effective communication among ourselves. Most of the time, the nurse manager was not included in our activities. Nor did we share information about our lives with her. With the encouragement of my husband and a close nursing colleague, I decided to return to school to complete a baccalaureate in nursing.

Following graduation, I returned to the unit where I had worked as a licensed vocational nurse (LVN) for more than 8 years and assumed the position of charge nurse on the day shift. Although I was confident that I was educationally prepared to assume this role, it never entered my mind that I would be making assignments and directing the care of my former peers. I asked myself, "How do I handle this? Do I remain a peer and a friend?

How do I keep my staff from abusing me? Will they see me as their peer and friend, or a manager? Will they do the work I assign or take it as an insult if I assign too much work?" My worst fears about each of these questions came true.

Initially, I tried to remain the friend and peer I had been before becoming the charge nurse. Clearly, that was not going to work. Quickly I discovered I was being used and abused not only by the staff who were my friends but also by staff who were new to the unit. I had to get the management of the day shift under control before it controlled me. How should I solve this problem?

 What do you think you would do if you were this nurse?

INTRODUCTION

Although taking advantage of opportunities as they develop during a **career** is important, making decisions about what you want to do in nursing and how you can go about doing it is also important. Because a nursing career can extend across a lifetime and is not institutionally based (i.e., not defined by the institution but rather by law), the options for careers in nursing are vast. Some options build primarily on experience, others build primarily on educational background, and still others require a mix of education and experience. In general, it is safe to assume that continuing to learn and to develop expertise to meet the challenges of this diverse profession is a requirement. How you reach a career goal, however, depends on what goals you set and how you manage your own development.

A FRAMEWORK

Numerous opportunities abound for nurses today. Some are in traditional roles, and some are emerging roles. But, in a few years even those roles will have evolved and other options will emerge. Historically, there was one way to become a registered nurse—a hospital-based program. Today, there are multiple ways, ranging from associate degree preparation through the nursing doctorate. In some cases, service developed the programs to answer needs they had. In others, education created the programs to serve the future needs of the country. And, in still other cases, service and education united to create programs to address an ever-increasingly complex healthcare delivery system that has what seems to be an insatiable need for registered nurses. People enter the profession with no previous experience; with previous experience in health care, but not nursing; with previous experience in nursing; and with experience in another discipline. This mix of people prepared as nurses suggests that the diversity of career options is dramatic. Although the most relevant experience and education are the most recent ones, no element of previous experience and education should be dismissed. In fact, the incorporation of elements that are distinctly yours often creates career options that might not be available to someone else.

There are several ways to develop a career. Basing career decisions on goals is a useful beginning. Some of the most notable work about careers was conducted by Friss (1989), who identified four career styles (Box 27-1). One career pathway is not better than another; rather, each is different. For example, the types of positions sought differ. *Steady state* and *linear* are the traditional career styles. The first remains at a positional plateau and becomes increasingly competent; the second moves up the hierarchy of the organization and becomes more diversified. The *entrepreneurial and transient style* is one that has fostered many nurses' creative bent. For a great deal of flexibility, and in a time of rapid changes in health care, this style fosters creative solutions to traditional problems. Finally, the *spiral* style is one seen in situations in which nurses move in and out of active practice and in situations in which nurses move in and out of a subspecialty focus, such as general pediatrics and neonatal nursing. Additionally, many nurses combine career patterns. For example, a young female may move in and out of nursing as children are born and then choose a new career style that leads to new roles.

In the midst of this complexity, thinking about careers can be either frustrating (there are too many options and too many opportunities that require specific preparation) or exciting (no better time has existed for creating one's own opportunities). There is some logic, however, to thinking about the opportunities that are available in light of what an individual wants to achieve in the profession. Figure 27-1 illustrates the fact that there is a relationship between the individual and the position. A good fit is built on strong similar goals and tolerable (or growth-producing) differences. The whole of any work situation is composed of two elements interacting in an environment where other elements influence both. That whole is symbolized by blending a person's talents with a position's expectations to create a productive whole, and simultaneously by holding positions in organizations that capitalize on a person's fit. Analyzing positions and the required skills in light of individual talents can help applicants determine positions that fit with their strengths and define gaps to be addressed. When gaps occur, they may suggest the skills development needed to form a fit or they may suggest that the position is not a good fit. The person/position fit, and how that fit evolves throughout a career, is a

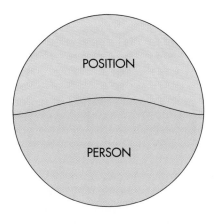

Goal: A Fit

Figure 27-1   Person-position fit.

critical consideration in appreciating positions held throughout a career. Two critical factors are evident—the person and the position.

Knowing Yourself

Being a professional holds both privileges and obligations. The legal privileges and expectations are codified in the state nursing practice acts, rules, and regulations. Because licensure is designed to provide the baseline (i.e., the minimum expectation), it does not identify or obligate any practitioner to function in a professional manner as defined by the profession itself. For example, no practice act identifies membership in a professional association as an expectation. Nor is there an expectation for community/professional service. Yet the profession, through various professional organizations, holds the expectation that nurses will belong to professional associations and provide leadership in improving communities. How to incorporate these activities in a busy, committed life can at times seem difficult. Yet, those activities and interests often enrich a career and may be very important to individuals. Knowing what is important, what is valued, and the commitment needed form the basis of understanding one's self.

Before considering any position or how to secure the best fit, consider yourself. In other words, understanding one's self helps determine what is important in a position and what kind of career to pursue. Finding a fit in the profession involves strategy. Using strategic personal planning, whether jobs are plentiful or not, always enhances the potential to secure a position that is a good fit. If

BOX 27-1

Career Styles

	EXAMPLE	DESCRIPTION	MOTIVATION AND CHARACTERISTICS	MANAGERIAL COMPLICATIONS
Steady State	Staff nurses	Constancy in position with increasing professional skill	Increasing expertise High professional identity Obligation to serve Maintenance of standards Autonomy in performance of care Preference for action Personal accountability The work itself Stability	Hold work in high esteem Decentralize Use and recognize abilities Provide feedback about patient outcomes Reward competence and tenure Provide continuing education Provide permanent assignment
Linear	Nursing service administrator	Hierarchical orientation with steady climb	Requisite authority and power Had a challenging first job Guided by internalized norms Money Recognition Opportunities for self-development	Provide management development Reward and value both education and competence Modify management selection and development systems Provide decreasing supervision
Entrepreneurial and Transient	Nurses in private practice; temporary assignments	Desire to create new service; meeting own priorities	Limited organizational commitment Opportunists Novelty/creativity Other people Achievement	Use flexibility to organization's benefit Avoid burdening them with organizational and practice decisions Provide immediate feedback
Spiral	Nurse who returns after raising a family	Rational, independent responsibility for shaping career	Novelty Prestige Intense period of employment followed by nonemployment or a different employment Care for others Opportunities for self-development Typically well paid, service-oriented recognition	Configure specific job that needs doing Be flexible about terms and length of commitment Find challenging initial assignment Negotiate Encourage creativity

Modified from Friss, L. (1989). *Strategic management of nurses: A policy-oriented approach.* Owings Mills, MD: AUPHA Press.

you are clear about your skills and abilities, you already know what you can bring to a position and what you want to achieve in order to seek the next opportunity. If you have not analyzed what your talents are, begin with the following tool. This tool is not a psychomotor skills checklist, although that might be useful for consideration too. It is a skills inventory that requires thinking on the part of the user.

■ Exercise 27-1

Using an established description of a registered nurse—for example, the one created by the Texas Board of Nursing to describe beginning competencies of new graduates (ftp://www.bne.state.tx.us/del-comp.pdf)—describe personal interests, skills, and abilities in the following areas. Consider your talents and values from the multidimensional view of nursing: communication, physical and psychological care, management, learning, teaching, scholarship, and involvement in the profession.

Professional competencies may be communicative, managerial, technical, or professional.

Provision of care: Consider abilities in the various stages of the nursing process. Is one skill more fascinating than the others? Is it more interesting to consider the outcomes and what they mean than to actually provide the care? Is the most important part about being a nurse the intimate nature of the nurse–patient relationship?

Coordination of care: Consider basic and advanced abilities. Is it a chore to work with someone assisting in providing care? Is it challenging to determine who should do what and how to schedule all the various elements of care? Is it more desirable to work within the team of nursing, or is it more desirable to work with multiple professionals? How intriguing are highly structured organizations versus ones that are less so?

Professional: Consider what being a nurse means personally. How important is being able to be involved beyond the position itself? Does what you want to be in the profession require more education? Are you willing to commit to that endeavor?

Personal: Consider how balancing a personal life and a professional life will work. What are your personal values? What is most important right now—career or family? How heavily does any college debt (student loans) weigh on you? What do you like to do for fun? Is it complementary to or at odds with your professional goals?

Synthesis: Using the above categories, create a description of how you wish to work in the next 2 to 3 years. What is important in considering any position? What is important in locale? Does the type of work setting matter? How will this work contribute to an overall career goal? What are your best strengths? How can you capitalize on them? How are they strengthened by the work you wish to pursue?

Review what you have said to determine if you have addressed issues about personal learning and teaching others; remaining competent in care and learning new skills, and involvement in the profession (member of an association, advancing nursing's knowledge and political force). Thinking about each of those areas in light of your particular interests, abilities, and skills allows you to consider the nature of your involvement in the profession. For example, if working through others and sharing knowledge are highly valued, a position as an educator might be a career goal. If working directly with patients and teaching them how to do their best in their own health care is highly valued, a position in direct practice might be a career goal. Neither is better than the other. Rather, they are different. It is the integration of your talents that creates the multiple opportunities in nursing.

Being able to describe yourself from various perspectives is useful. First, knowing your strengths tells you what you bring to a position and what you will rely on. Second, knowing your strengths helps you practice saying what they are in a succinct manner. Third, when you know your strengths and then read a particular position description, you are better able to translate your usual terminology into that of the organization. Fourth, such an analysis of your competencies allows you to see what work needs to be done to meet standards. Finally, entering into such analyses can help you see the bigger picture of your career and how what you can learn from a particular position can contribute to your overall career goals. The career styles described in Box 27-1 include the motivation and characteristics of the styles. Seeing how your self-analysis fits with the descriptors in the third column may also suggest how you see yourself approaching your career. Any type of analysis in relation to role expectations is useful in helping you to know yourself better.

Knowing the Position

No longer do most people, including nurses, assume a position and remain there forever. Exceptions commonly are found in rural areas, in faculty positions (at least once an individual is tenured), and in certain clinical specialties. So, most nurses will "rotate" through numerous positions, either by plan or by chance. Knowing that positions will change and that learning has to be fairly intense in most positions today forces candidates to manage their careers actively. The value of the work itself, not a future goal, should be considered in terms of how enticing a position is. Because of these rapid changes, each position can enrich nurses' skills and make them more competent in their current work and more desirable in prospective work. Position assessment begins with understanding the basics of an organization and evolves into the specifics that usually can be garnered only through an interview. Bolles (2005) points out that most managers look first within an organization to promote someone rather than looking broadly at the talent available. This is in contrast to how many people seek jobs. They look broadly. So, one key strategy to use is using connections and focusing on places where your talents are already known. In addition to having "inside" connections, you also have some knowledge of positions and the organization in which they exist. You also may know the manager, which research shows as the most influential factor for how staff perceive their work.

CAREER DEVELOPMENT

When you chose nursing as the focus of your professional career, you probably had no idea about the opportunities the profession would hold. The beginning of the twenty-first century reflected changes in the healthcare environment occurring at a fast and frantic pace. Solutions that resolve today's problems may not work for tomorrow's challenges. Licensure holds certain expectations about maintaining competence and living to professional standards. Legislators enact legislation based on the needs of the citizens and in relation to political pressures. When a profession is protected by legislation, others, such as consumers, insurers, regulatory agencies and employers, expect that professional standards have been and will continue to be met.

A career can be defined as progress throughout an individual's professional life. A career can be developed in several ways. Some people, including professional nurses, have a series of positions with no connection among them. Others can have divergent positions that are connected in some way. Regardless of how careers develop, the real focus is continued competence.

In today's rapidly changing society, a position that was once "a fit" may no longer work. The position is as likely to change as is the person. In this situation, a promotion may result from the expansion of a designated position. As a result, a new title/ position description is created. Another nontraditional approach to promotions occurs when a major reorganization occurs and creates different positions to meet the redefined demands. Although neither of these promotion approaches may have been a part of an individual's career plan, both are likely to happen as health care continuously reshapes itself.

Bolles (2005) suggests that there are also life-changing jobs. These can best be described as changing positions and field simultaneously. Therefore, when a charge nurse in a critical care unit assumes the role of chief nursing officer in a home health agency, a major shift has occurred. Nurses who follow a spiral career path, especially if they are second-degree students (meaning they had a different career previously), may also experience this phenomenon. Often these individuals made money in another field and now are pursuing their hearts; they may have become bored with a career that had few interactions with people; or, they may have studied in fields such as science and realized that the best application of their knowledge could occur in patient care. Because of a previous career expertise, these individuals may craft career patterns that appear very different from most others because they are using talents from two fields and trying to capitalize on them.

Irrespective of career style, core career development strategies are important. Selecting professional peers and mentors to share your development is important. Even the steady-state nurse who is not typically seeking a new position needs to develop a **curriculum vitae** (CV) or **résumé** that can document continued development of expertise. Interviewing, a two-way process, is also an important strategy to develop.

Few nurses have achieved a significant nursing career without assistance from peers and mentors. Heeding the "nay-sayers" can dampen career prospects. Having a few well-chosen peers and mentors who can respond openly with various perspectives to help with career decisions is important. For example, a nurse who seeks a career as a direct-care provider in an acute care setting could seek support from a mentor, such as a charge nurse, nurse manager, or advanced practice nurse. The mentor provides honest appraisals of an individual's career development, suggests specific strategies to enhance development, and helps with meeting the leaders in an organization. Being in a relationship with a strong role model is valuable.

Exercise 27-2

Think about an experienced nurse who serves as a role model. Would you want that person as a mentor? Ask that person to be one for you.

Table 27-1 identifies six key aspects of creating and managing a career. Although each aspect is important, one aspect that can be most useful is the who, the mentor you choose. That person can create new thinking and new opportunities and steer you to various clinical or role areas. That person can also create connections for you and help guide decisions related to timing and place. Mentors might even be able to create opportunities for you to test new approaches to clinical care or to new aspects of a position you might think of as boring.

CAREER MARKETING STRATEGIES

Although professional data can be recorded in numerous ways, the fact remains that most people do not do so in a systematic manner. Therefore, when information about one's career is needed, it is often difficult to recall. A goal of this chapter is to develop a systematic strategy for developing marketing documents that you can use throughout your professional career. Remember that Bolles (2005) indicates that the typical way an individual seeks a position is in reverse order of how employers seek to fill vacancies. For example, most employers seek to fill vacancies from within the current employee pool. Except for lateral transfers or positional promotions, most nurses, and especially new graduates, begin by using a résumé. This approach has worked well in nursing for many positions. The key is to make information distinctive in telling your professional story and in creating the appearance of a competent professional.

Data Collection

Depending on your unique background, the time spent on this activity varies considerably. The first step is to collect all previous professional information about yourself. If you are fairly new in the profession, analyze anything special you did in school, such as electives, offices held, and special assignments, and honors or special recognition that you received. If you are a second career nurse, consider all previous work and how it relates to your profession now. If you have an employment history, start with your nursing positions. Keep in mind that you will need to include other relevant information. For example, serving as a volunteer at a rape crisis center may augment a brief professional history; serving as an officer of your student organization or on the board of a voluntary association may be useful to secure a position with similar responsibilities. In addition, each of the aforementioned examples conveys a professional commitment to community life.

To begin data collection, it may be useful to start where you are and think back. If you have limited "thinking back" to do, you are in great shape for starting a systematic plan. If, however, you have been practicing nursing for a long time or had "another life" before your nursing career, you may have more difficulty compiling the information. In fact, some information may be irretrievable—do not dwell on that aspect, just record as much as you can recall. In either case, the important thing is to begin the process.

Using the categories identified in Table 27-2, compile as many facts for each category as you can recall. If you do not have information for a specific topic heading, for example, publications, create the topic heading anyway. When you publish your first article, you will have a place to record the pertinent details. Remember, the information you compile today will not have to be remembered tomorrow.

It is most useful to do this data entry on your computer. A table with headings will facilitate the

Table 27-1	KEY ASPECTS OF CREATING/ MANAGING A CAREER
Who	Mentor
What	Role and clinical options
When	"Timing is everything"; always open to opportunities; don't leave in the middle of a critical project
Where	Local or not; inpatient or outpatient
How	Proactive; your search is your job
Why	Boredom/seeking challenge/testing out ideas

Table 27-2 DATA COLLECTION

Topics	Facts Needed
1. Education	Name of school, address, phone numbers, website address, years of attendance, date of graduation, name of degree(s) received, minor earned, honors received (e.g., Dean's list), name of dean, faculty advisor, registrar's phone numbers
2. Continuing education	Date attended, places, topics and any special outcomes, type and amount of credit earned
3. Experience	Dates of employment, title of position, name of employing agency, location and phone numbers, website address, name of chief executive officer, chief nursing officer, immediate supervisor, salary range, typical duties (role description)
4. Community/institutional service	Dates of service, name of committee/task force and the parent organization (e.g., name of hospital or professional organization), your role on the committee (e.g., chairperson, secretary, member), general description of committee's functions, any unique accomplishments
5. Publications	Articles: author(s) name(s), year of publication, title, journal, volume, issue, pages; books: author(s), year of publication, title, location, and name of publisher
6. Honors	Date, description of award, special factors related to award (e.g., competitive, communitywide, national)
7. Research	Date, title of research, role in research (e.g., principal investigator, co-investigator, team member), funded/unfunded
8. Speeches/presentations given	Date, title of speech presented, place, name of sponsoring organization, nature of the presentation (e.g., keynote, concurrent session), your honorarium
9. Workshops/conferences presented	Date, title of workshop/conference presented, place, name of sponsoring group and nature of the presentation, brief description of the activity, your honorarium
10. Certification	Initial date of certification, expiration date, certifying body, area/type of certification

process. If you do not have access to a computer, the data collection process can be done using file cards with dividers for the separate categories. One card with all the required information for *each* item in a heading will make this file useful. Whether you use a computer or a file box for organizing these topic headings and all the pertinent data about yourself, this compilation of facts is for your use only. This data bank serves as your professional career memory.

■ *Exercise 27-3*

Draft an entry for your data bank. If you have sufficient time, draft a CV and résumé now. The Evolve website for this text contains an example of each. As a checkpoint for yourself, make a list of four to five professional facts/qualities that you want others to know about. You can use this list in checking your CV or résumé and in interviewing. Keep in mind that a CV or résumé serves one primary purpose—letting others know enough about you that they want to meet you, advance your career, or gain more information.

Curriculum Vitae

A CV is a listing of professional life activities. It is designed to be all-inclusive but not detailed. This document lists all your professional accomplishments without elaboration on the details of your career. It is an effective tool for listing all the facts of your professional life.

To develop a CV, simply select a logical flow of information and assemble. Information should be presented in *reverse chronologic order*. In this way, attention is drawn to your latest contributions and is a better presentation than a historic chronologic sequence. Include your name, credentials, degrees, address, phone numbers, fax number, e-mail address, and Website address (if you have one) in the heading of the document. This set of information should be distinct so that you are easy to contact. Using larger, bold type in a centered position is an example of how to distinguish this information.

Arranging the information facts by category, assemble a CV that reflects all professional involvement. The CV contains profile data about each entry; no lengthy descriptions are required. The document must be typed and appear organized. The use of subheadings for each topic facilitates development.

Exercise 27–4

If you have not done so before, create a CV from your data, and define a plan to keep the CV current.

Résumé

A résumé is a customized document developed to highlight your accomplishments and tailored to describe the way in which you can fulfill a role or meet the needs of a specific organization. Unlike the CV, the résumé is detailed. A résumé sells the individual for the specific position being sought and illustrates the fit of an individual for a specific position. For the steady-state nurse, a résumé could be used to reflect increasing skills and abilities; for others, a résumé can create specific messages about an individual's unique experiences, education, and abilities in relation to a new opportunity.

To sell yourself, you need to provide more than the facts. You need to include details. Although the information needs to be brief and to the point, it should be meaningful and reflect your experience and your accomplishments. The ideal résumé is one page, although two pages are acceptable. When detailing your accomplishments, use action words that describe your experiences. For example, if you were a volunteer for the American Diabetes Association annual "Walk for America," describing your role as a "volunteer fundraiser" is more meaningful than saying a "volunteer." This is how the rest of the world views such activities. Consider use of action words that typify activities of your career. Words such as *developed*, *created*, and *initiated* convey a powerful message in a résumé. It is important to "quantify for the organization the economic value you can potentially deliver" (Fox, 2001, p. 30).

The résumé is the best choice for selling your abilities to a potential employer. It is designed to focus on an individual's special abilities in relation to the organizational need as described in the position description. When developing a résumé, avoid fads, buzz words, and automated formats for résumé building. Using an automated format for résumé building may seem like a "quick fix," but the end product will look like all the other résumés developed in this fashion. Because your résumé will look like many others, it will be less likely to be read critically. In our world of rapid change, fads and buzz words are soon outdated. Posting a résumé on the Internet is an example of a fad whose popularity is questionable. Although many have posted their résumé on the numerous Internet sites available, few employers even look at the posted documents (Bolles, 2005).

Your customized résumé should be error-free and grammatically correct, present an accurate and articulate portrayal of your accomplishments, and be printed on high-quality paper, preferably 100% cotton bond. Electronic resumes are used by some organizations. Although this is not yet the predominant approach to applications, it is important to consider. Any attachment, such as a résumé, should be sent in Word format to ensure that the recipient can open and read the materials.

There are basically two ways to develop a résumé: a conventional or a functional approach. In either case the document should include your name, address, phone numbers, fax number, and e-mail address and web address (if you have them) at the top of the page. The conventional approach provides an optional career summary and includes position title, name and address, inclusive dates, and a succinct description of responsibilities and achievements. Education and other categories of special meaning that relate to the position sought should be included. (This information will be in your database of facts about yourself.)

The functional approach provides a career summary and identifies role functions that you have filled during your career. Those functions might include staff nurse, manager, and educator, to name a few. A functional approach is best if you are planning a sharp departure from your present position or if you had a previous career in another discipline. The focus is on your experience in diverse roles, not on the specific positions held. Education and other categories of special meaning may be added.

Exercise 27-5

Draft statements you could use in a résumé (conventional or functional, whichever would best serve your purposes) to describe one of your strengths.

Professional Letters

During your career, you will develop a series of letters to meet specific needs as you market yourself. These include a cover letter, a thank-you letter, and a resignation letter. Typically, these letters have common elements and individual characteristics that make each one unique.

All of these letters should include your name, address, phone numbers, fax number, e-mail address, and website address, if you have one, as they appear on your résumé or CV. Designating both daytime and evening phone numbers is helpful. Placing this information in a format similar to that used on your résumé or CV will make an effective package when you present your documents. Quality-bond paper reflects the image you wish to portray. Even if any of these documents is sent by e-mail or fax, the hard copy (original) should be sent as soon as possible.

Each of these letters should be no longer than one page. The date and an inside address should be included. An inside address includes the name (with credentials) of the addressee, the person's title, the name of the organization, street address, city, state, and zip code. The inside address is followed by the salutation. Usually, first names are not used. The typical salutation, "Dear Ms. Smith," for example, is followed by a colon.

Each of these professional letters usually contains three key paragraphs, which are described in the following sections. The closing follows the text of the letter; the closing is followed by your name. The usual spacing between the closing (e.g., "Sincerely") and your name is four lines. Include your full name with credentials and degrees. Sign your name as it is typed using black or blue ink. Proof all letters for layout, typographic errors, spelling, and content. If you are asked to respond by email, you can attach the cover letter as well as the CV or résumé so that the recipient has both available to share in a neat format.

Cover Letter   The cover letter is the key to getting your résumé read. It is a brief and carefully written document that is a vital source of information. The cover letter includes a statement that indicates why you are writing, why you "fit" the organization and a specific position or type of position, and how you will follow up.

Numerous positions may be advertised by an organization simultaneously. In addition, an organization may use a variety of vehicles to issue a call for applicants. Thus immediately stating why you are writing is crucial. It is often helpful to identify how you learned of the position.

Once you have stated your reason for writing, you should address the issue of "why you." The second paragraph should indicate why someone should take time to read your attached résumé. This section should state what you know about the organization and how you will fit in. Examples of competencies can be included to clarify your strengths. Reference to the enclosed résumé or CV is appropriate. Fox (2001) calls a cover letter an "impact letter" and states "a good impact letter demonstrates your potential to make an impact" (p. 49).

The closing paragraph should convey optimism—that is, you anticipate being interviewed. If you want to ensure yourself of having an additional opportunity to sell yourself, you should indicate *when* you will follow up with a phone call.

Exercise 27-6

Write a cover letter that highlights information from at least two items from your data bank. Select items that best market you and that will entice the reader to call you for an interview.

Thank-You Letter   Once again, the business format described earlier is used in a formal thank-you letter. Hand-written and sent within 24 hours of the interview, the thank-you letter may be the last chance to "sell" yourself. Even if an e-mail thank-you is used, following it with a hand-written version is important. For this reason, careful thought should be given to what you need to say in this document.

The lead paragraph should recall the interview date and purpose so that the reader can place you. If you discussed more than one position, list your preference first, and follow it with "as well as other positions" if such is true.

To help the interviewer remember you, the body of the letter should focus on elements of the interview. If a key point was described as crucial, focus your comments about your ability on that point. Use action words in describing your fit in this organization.

The closing paragraph should reference specific times identified in the interview. These times may include when you expect to hear about a position offer or when you are available. In addition, this section includes a statement of what you will do and when you will do it if you do not hear from the interviewer. This action indicates to the prospective employer that you expect to maintain control of your career.

If you have decided that the position is not a fit with your values and talents, a thank you note is still appropriate. It is possible that you will find some other position later, and you want to leave a most positive impression within the organization.

Resignation Letter   When you secure a new position, it is essential to resign effectively from your current position. A letter slipped under a manager's office door should not be the initial mechanism for notifying an organization of your intent to leave. A face-to-face meeting between you and your manager is most effective. Your resignation should be given with adequate notice. Conditions of employment will define adequate notice. Being flexible in your resignation date is often very effective in creating a positive exit strategy.

The face-to-face meeting is followed by a formal letter of resignation. Again, the business format is used. The introductory paragraph references the meeting at which you stated your intent to resign. Your date of resignation is identified, and indication of whether this date is negotiable is included.

The second paragraph highlights aspects of the employment setting that enhanced your career development. Do not use your resignation letter to offload negative feelings you may have about your current position. Keep in mind that you can always say something positive about any position you hold.

The closing paragraph concludes by asking for an exit evaluation. As you leave an organization, it is important to learn your final standing within the organization. Requesting a copy of this appraisal for your own records is also wise.

DATA ASSEMBLY FOR PROFESSIONAL PORTFOLIOS

The checklist in Box 27-2 will help you keep track of your data and assemble the facts attractively. Inclusion of these elements ensures a comprehensive view of your professional contributions and comprises a **portfolio**. Creating a professional portfolio, the basics of which are found in the citations made in your CV, can help organize one element of your professional life. Keeping notes of recognition, copies of evaluations, and pictures of your successes are examples that help round out the resource documents behind the CV data. Monsen (2005), in the preface to *Genetics Nursing Portfolios: A New Model for Credentialing*, identifies that a portfolio approach to documentation is grounded in research and "documents the clinical experience, wisdom, and expertise" of nurses (p. vii). Although this publication was developed for credentialing and the field of genetics, using it as a generic guide to creating a portfolio can help any nurse be comprehensive in summarizing important work. Although a portfolio takes time to develop and maintain, that work pays off at evaluation, promotion, and position-seeking times. Because the information addresses all aspects of professional life, the information is always available. Furthermore, because it is organized by categories, it is easy to expand information in a given area or focus on the most important work or the most recent work. In other words, this system of maintaining professional information provides the resource to respond to new or emerging opportunities.

BOX 27-2

Checklist for Constructing Marketing Documents

Data Collection

_____ 1. Data sets are used for information development.

_____ 2. Information is assembled in categoric manner.

Data Assembly

_____ 1. Discrete categories are used.

_____ 2. Assembly addresses specific position.

_____ 3. Current name, address, phone numbers, voice mail, e-mail address, and Web address are prominent (use as many as are appropriate for you).

_____ 4. Career summary (if used) (or cover letter) is prominent.

_____ 5. Key points about positions/experiences are evident.

_____ 6. A logical flow is evident.

_____ 7. Grammar, spelling, and syntax are correct.

_____ 8. Writing style is positive and direct, but not terse.

_____ 9. Action verbs are evident.

_____10. If writing in full sentences, third person and passive voice are avoided (i.e., write in the active voice).

_____11. "Canned" résumé language is avoided (e.g., "distinguished" and "all phases of . . .").

_____12. Emphasis is on competence, not years (cover letter).

_____13. Specific examples of key competencies are cited (cover letter).

_____14. The format is consistent throughout.

_____15. Personal information (e.g., health, marital status) is absent.

Appearance and Format

_____ 1. There are no typographic errors.

_____ 2. The product is "clean" (e.g., no smudges, no discrepant margins).

_____ 3. The product is readable (e.g., layout design is pleasing: white space, capitalization).

_____ 4. The paper is high-quality bond (100% cotton), white or cream.

_____ 5. The type is businesslike (no script); text is at least 10 to 12 point, and fonts are limited to one or two.

_____ 6. Emphasis is evident (e.g., centering and bold print or underlining).

_____ 7. The product is only one or two pages in length (not applicable for a curriculum vitae [CV]).

Overview

_____ 1. It is attractive, interesting, quick-reading, and competency-based.

_____ 2. The package sells you.

_____ 3. You are pleased to have it precede you.

_____ 4. Additional items are enclosed or they are assembled for personal handling at an interview.

_____ 5. If you were receiving this CV or résumé, you would want to interview this person.

THE INTERVIEW

Assuming you have used your career marketing strategies effectively, the next logical step is participating in an interview. Interviewing is a two-way proposition; the interviewee should be gathering as much information as the interviewer is. Both should be making judgments throughout the process so that if a position is offered, the interviewee will be prepared to accept, decline, or explore further. Interviews may take place with one or more individuals and may include a range of activities. To be at ease, the interviewee should wear comfortable, professional clothing. Rehearsing specific questions to ask and points to make can create comfort for these somewhat challenging situations. Be prepared to cite challenges and dilemmas you have faced and what you did and why because these types of questions are likely to be posed to you.

Do not be deluded into thinking that because you are a nurse and there is a vacancy that you will automatically secure the position. Even in times of a nursing shortage, employers are using behavioral interviewing techniques to identify the most appropriate applicant for the vacant position. Rather than being asked, "What are your weaknesses?" you may be asked, "Tell me how you handled the last mistake you made" or "How did a baccalaureate program prepare you for critical care nursing?" Applicants in some organizations are also being screened and interviewed by a panel and being asked to participate in a series of interviews. This allows more participants to have a say in the hiring process. In the business setting, many prospective employers are administering basic skills tests. You may see this practice in some healthcare settings as well. Researching the organization in advance (preferably with filing any applicant materials) can prepare you for the interview.

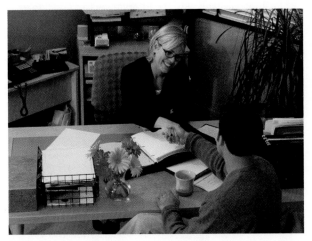

Interviewing is a two-way proposition in which both participants gather as much information as possible.

Interview Topics and Questions of Concern

During interviews, employers should ask all applicants for a given position the same questions. In addition to providing comparable information as the basis for a decision, the applicant's expectation for equal treatment is upheld. Only questions related to the position and its description are legitimate. Employers should not ask other questions (Box 27-3), and applicants should express appropriate concern if asked such inappropriate questions.

If the interviewer asks an inappropriate question, the applicant can choose not to answer the direct question by addressing the content area. For example, if asked about your spouse's employment, you might say, "I believe what you are asking is how long I will be able to be in this position. Let me assure you that I intend to be here for at least 2 years."

Each of the content areas in Box 27-3 may be acceptable, but the question is phrased inappropriately. The second column identifies approaches that are both appropriate and legal. The key to ensuring a fair interviewing process is being prepared ahead of time and knowing what can be asked legitimately and what a reasonable answer is.

Exercise 27–7

Select a partner and role-play an interview for a professional nursing position. The potential employer (manager) should focus on competencies of the prospective employee. Include questions and scenarios about common conflicts and challenges seen in the clinical setting. The interviewee (prospective employee) should highlight competencies, decision-making abilities, and critical-thinking abilities when responding to the situationally based questions.

If you have prepared well, you will know what the organization's stated beliefs are and whether they are compatible with yours. The challenge in an interview is to determine whether those beliefs are lived or merely printed words. If numerous people can relate how the mission actually is translated in a specific role, the beliefs are likely lived ones.

This chapter includes two tools designed to be used in preparing for an interview: "Checklist for Interviewing" (Box 27-4), and "Interview Goals and Content" (Table 27-3). Using the thank-you

BOX 27-3

Inappropriate and Appropriate Questions

SAMPLE OF INAPPROPRIATE QUESTIONS

1. How old are you?
2. What does your husband (wife) do?

3. Who takes care of your children?
4. Are you working "just to help out"?
5. Do you have any disabilities?

6. Where were you born?

7. What are the names of all of the organizations to which you belong?
8. What is your religious preference?

SAMPLE OF APPROPRIATE AND LEGAL QUESTIONS

1. Do you know that this position requires someone at least 21 years old?
2. This position requires that no one in your immediate family be in the healthcare field or own interests/shares in any healthcare facility. Does this pose a problem?
3. Attendance is important. Are you able to meet this expectation?
4. What are your short- and long-term goals?
5. Is there anything that would prevent you from performing this work as described?
6. This position requires U.S. citizenship. May I assume you meet this criterion?
7. What professional organizations do you belong to?

8. As you have read in our philosophy, we subscribe to a Christian philosophy. Do you understand that all employees are expected to promote this philosophy?

BOX 27-4

Checklist for Interviewing

1. Check interviewing guides, such as *What Color Is Your Parachute?*
2. Check out the new organization.
   a. Review the organization's mission, vision, and values statements before the interview (via the web or hard copy).
   b. Obtain statistics and facts.
   c. Ask about new program directions.
3. Recheck your résumé or curriculum vitae for the following:
   a. Emphasis
   b. New information
4. Practice using "action" words.
5. Decide about the following:
   a. Appearance
   b. Key points
      i. To make
      ii. To learn
   c. Tool for quick check (e.g., a file card with key points)
6. Arrive on time and alone.

7. Make a memorable entrance.
   a. Make eye contact.
   b. Shake hands.
   c. Smile.
   d. Say, "Hello, I'm [name]."
8. Position yourself with the interviewer (e.g., decide to sit at an angle).
9. Keep in mind your key points.
10. Appear interested—project competence, confidence, and energy.
11. Accentuate the positive!
12. Answer questions directly but know when not to.
13. Ask for more information.
14. Say only positive things about your present employer, but don't be untruthful.
15. Secure a time frame for notification of a position offer.
16. Thank interviewer personally.
17. Write a thank-you letter.
18. Let interviewer know your decision.
19. Put commitments in writing.

Table 27-3 INTERVIEW GOALS AND CONTENT

Interview Goals	Content
1. Personal characteristics	Describe the kind of person you are, including personality traits. Be expected to cite examples of when these traits helped or hindered you in previous situations. List situations that characterize your energy, initiative, drive, ambition, and enthusiasm. Clarify your professional values. Have a story ready that illustrates how you see yourself.
2. The work itself	Emphasize what makes you distinctive. Describe how your education and experience prepared you for this position. Describe your skills as a member of a team and a leader of a team. Prepare to address hypothetical situations that display your problem-solving, reasoning, self-confidence, knowledge, and critical-thinking. (Creates opportunity to evaluate you in action and under some stress.) Ask intelligent questions that suggest you have prepared for this interview and know something about this organization.
3. The organizational fit	Be clear about what you believe to be distinctive about this organization and how it meets your expectations for a position. Articulate your "fit" with the organization's philosophy, mission, and vision.
4. The professional betterment	Be clear about what you expect to obtain from any position you consider. Include advancement opportunities, educational support, and work/life balance.

letter described earlier in this chapter is an additional opportunity to market yourself, especially if you wish to correct or expand on an answer you provided during the interview.

The interrelationship of these strategies allows people to emphasize specialization or diversity. Each strategy leads to the next so that the potential for attaining a preferred position is enhanced. As careers progress, factors other than the specific nursing school or in-school activities take precedence in influencing career development and how an individual is seen by others. Thus updating a CV or résumé is important. Keeping a passion alive must be evident.

The Career Tips near the end of this chapter will help to keep your career vibrant.

PROFESSIONAL DEVELOPMENT

Today's employees have to manage and understand themselves, choosing work settings in which they make the greatest contributions and learning how and when to change what is done while staying mentally fit and youthful for a 50-year career (Drucker in Rosenstein, 2001). One of the keys to maintaining competence and versatility is continued learning. Learning occurs in various ways. It can occur in a conversation with colleagues, by reading an article in the general literature, or sometimes in an "ah hah" experience that provides sudden enlightenment. Although nurses could share these experiences with others, the continued learning that the profession, healthcare employers, boards of nursing, and **professional associations** (organizations) are most concerned with is formal study.

"Nursing professional development begins within the basic nursing education program, continues throughout the career of the nurse and encompasses the educational concepts of continuing education, staff development, and academic preparation" (American Nurses Association [ANA], 2000, p. 1).

A graduate degree opens numerous career opportunities and leads to new levels or areas of expertise. A graduate education may focus on a clinical area, a functional area, or a combination of both. Admission to graduate programs typically requires taking a test (often the Graduate Record Examination [GRE]), having an above-average grade point average (GPA), and graduating from a professionally accredited school of nursing.

Graduate education consists of both master's- and doctorate-level study. In some employment situations or career specialties, graduate education is required. For example, expectations for nurse practitioner preparation are centered on graduate-level preparation as opposed to the earlier certificate programs. As health care becomes more complex, persons licensed as individual practitioners, such as nurses, necessarily need more education to continue to meet the healthcare system's demands.

Exercise 27–8

Analyze the academic and clinical preparation you received in your nursing program. Do you feel confident in your knowledge base and clinical skill? Can you effectively manage multiple roles? Based on these answers, determine whether you should pursue graduate education immediately or wait until you have gained additional work experience.

Deciding to pursue graduate education may be very simple. Some applicants to baccalaureate programs already have a specific career focus in mind and the required graduate preparation is a given. New graduates are sometimes encouraged (or even required) to gain experience before seeking a master's degree or doctorate. Although experience enriches previous learning, it may not be relevant to specific graduate programs such as those entailing a major career redirection. Working while attending a graduate program may be difficult, but it is common among graduate students in nursing. Box 27-5 lists some factors to consider in selecting a graduate program.

If you are geographically bound, your fields of study may be limited. If you are not and you know what general area you want to pursue, consider the following illustration:

Example

You know you want to work with elderly patients. Your library subscribes to *The Journal of Gerontological Nursing and Geriatric Nursing.* You review the most recent year's issues of both.

You scan the masthead (i.e., the page with the editors and board members). Where are these individuals affiliated? Now you scan the articles. Are there some that are particularly intriguing? Where are the authors affiliated? Finally, look back over the lists. Are there any places emerging where the leaders in the field may be? This is a good starting place.

Distance education provides an additional option for earning an advanced degree. Although the concept of distance learning is not new (think of correspondence courses), the complex technologies used to deliver distance education is more recent. Distance educational opportunities increase access for many. Flexible scheduling and convenience permit many individuals to participate. Students may find that the increased costs (a computer with faster speed and increased memory, higher academic fees, and the potential unavailability of financial aid) associated with distance learning and the lack of face-to-face interaction are obstacles to overcome.

Exercise 27–9

Assume you are interested in graduate education.
- Talk with your local financial aid official to determine how you can learn more about financial assistance for graduate education.
- Using the Internet or the library, locate information about graduate education.
- Determine what specialties exist at the master's level.
- Determine the location of programs nearby.
- Evaluate the clinical interest of the programs of study.
- Decide if the diverse roles of the advanced practice nurse appeal.
- Consider doctoral programs. Consider those permitting entrance from the baccalaureate level.

Continuing education also contributes to professional growth. *Continuing education* is defined as "systematic professional learning experiences designed to augment the knowledge, skill, and attitudes of nurses and therefore enrich the nurses' contributions to quality health care and their pursuit of professional career goals" (ANA, 2000, p. 5).

Numerous opportunities for continuing education exist at local, state, regional, and broader levels. Selecting which opportunities to pursue may be a difficult choice. Box 27-6 lists several factors to consider in selecting any offering, but depending

BOX 27-5

Factors to Consider in Selecting A Graduate Program

Accreditation	• Does the program have national nursing accreditation (master's level)? • Is the institution regionally accredited (e.g., North Central Association of Colleges and Schools)?
Clinical/ functional role	• How closely do the descriptions of clinical/functional courses of study meet career goals?
Credits	• How many graduate credits are minimally required to complete the degree? • How many are devoted to gaining experience? • How many relate to classroom experiences?
Thesis/research	• Is a thesis required? • If not, what opportunities exist for research development? • What support is available for graduate students?
Faculty	• What credentials do faculty hold? • Are they in leadership positions in the state/national/international scenes? • Are they competent in your field of interest? • What is their reputation?
Current research	• What are the current research strengths of the institution?
Flexibility	• Do these strengths fit with your interests or is there flexibility to create your own direction? • Is flexibility present in scheduling and progress through the program?
Admission	• What is required? • Is the GRE used? • What is the minimum undergraduate GPA expected? • Is experience required? What kind? How much?
Costs	• What are the total projected costs? • What financial aid is available?

GPA, Grade point average; *GRE,* Graduate Record Examination.

on your particular goal, certain factors may be more influential than others. For example, if cost is a major factor, length and speaker may be less influential factors.

In addition to increasing your knowledge base, continuing education provides professional networking opportunities, contributes to meeting **certification** and **licensure** requirements, and documents additional pursuits in maintaining or developing clinical expertise. Sponsors of continuing education include employers, professional associations, schools of nursing, and private entrepreneurial groups.

Both types of formal professional development, graduate education and continuing education, are valuable to your professional development, and both can contribute to a specific area of career development—certification.

Exercise 27-10

Like an organization, you will develop a strategic plan for yourself. Imagine you have decided to earn a master's degree in nursing. This decision can be enhanced by a strategic plan.
- What values do you have that influence your plan?
- Are your interests in primary care, administration, or education?
- What is your target date for completion of the master's program?
- What are other factors that would interfere with your strategic plan?
- Do you have specific short-term goals or operational plans that must be attained before enrollment?

BOX 27-6

Factors to Consider in Selecting A Continuing Education Course

Accreditation/approval	• Is the course accredited/approved? If so, by whom?
	• Is that recognition accepted by a certification entity and by the board of nursing (if continuing education is required for re-registration of licensure)?
Credit	• Is the amount of credit appropriate in terms of the expected outcomes?
Course title	• Does it suggest the type of learner to be involved (e.g., advanced)?
	• Does it reflect the expected outcomes?
Speaker(s)	• Is the instructor known as an expert in the field?
	• Is the instructor experienced in the field?
Objectives	• Are the objectives logical and attainable?
	• Do they reflect knowledge, skills, attitudes, or a combination of these?
	• Do they fit a learner's needs?
Content	• Is the content reflective of the objectives?
	• Is the content at an appropriate level?
Audience	• Is the audience designed as a general or target one (e.g., all registered nurses or experienced nurses in state health positions)?
Cost	• Is it equitable with what similar nursing conferences cost?
	• Is travel required?
	• What is the actual direct expense for an individual to attend? Is it affordable?
Length	• Is the total time frame logical in terms of objectives, personal needs, and time away from work?
	• Does the time frame permit breaks from intense learning?
Provider	• Does the provider have an established reputation?

CERTIFICATION

Numerous opportunities exist for nurses to become certified (see *Research Perspective*). "Board certification signifies those nurses who have met requirements for clinical or functional practice in a specialized field, pursued education beyond basic nursing preparation, and received endorsement of their peers" (American Nurses Credentialing Center [ANCC], 2000, p. 2). It is an expectation in some employment settings for career advancement; in the field of advanced practice nursing, it is viewed as a requirement for practice and reimbursement. In many states, certification in advanced practice is the mechanism to achieve recognition as an advance practice nurse from the board of nursing.

Obtaining certification may require testing and continuing education and documented time in practice in the specialty area in addition to testing and continuing education. Recertification is a process of continued recognition of competence within a defined practice area. Many certifications require an expectation for participation in continuing education, as reported annually in the January–February issue of *The Journal of Continuing Education in Nursing.*

Certification plays an important part in the advancement of a career and the profession. In some fields, more than one examination exists; in others, there is an examination in the broad field and numerous options for very defined subspecialties. The ANCC (www.nursecredentialing.org) offers numerous certification examinations for nurse generalists, nurse practitioners, clinical specialists, nurse administrators, nurse case managers, ambulatory nurses, and informatics nurses. In addition, other certifications are offered by nursing

Research Perspective

Cary, A. H. (2001). Certified registered nurses: Results of the study of the certified workforce. *American Journal of Nursing, 101*(1), 44-52.

The work of this author reflects the outcome of the third part of the *International Study of the Certified Nurse Workforce*. A previous study indicates that registered nurses hold more than 410,000 certifications, in 134 specialties, from 67 certifying organizations, with 95 different credentials designating those certifications. This research study is the largest study of certified nurses to date. A random sample of 19,452 nurses from the registries of the 23 certifying organizations in the United States, Canada, and U.S. territories were studied to determine the certified nurses' demographic characteristics, the nature of their practice, and the benefits they attribute to certification.

Respondents came from all 50 states, the District of Columbia, Puerto Rico, the Virgin Islands, and all 12 Canadian provinces. The mean age of certified nurses was 47.2 years, with more than 39% of certified nurses aged 50 or older. Thirty-five percent held a baccalaureate degree. Ninety-five percent of respondents were working in nursing at the time of the survey, with hospitals being the most common practice site (50%), followed by community settings (17%). Forty-four percent reported working more than 40 hours per week; 41% earned $50,000 to $75,000 annually.

Registered Nurse, Certified (RN,C) was the most common credential (20%). Participants had been registered nurses for an average of 22 years and credentialed for an average of 7.8 years. Ninety-four percent practiced in the field in which they were certified; 47% provided medical-surgical nursing care.

Almost all participants (95%) reported that certification brought about at least one change in their practice; 72% reported one or more benefits.

IMPLICATIONS FOR PRACTICE

The findings of this work suggest that professional certification may provide opportunities for professional and personal growth and financial rewards. Increased confidence, competence, credibility, and control were reported. Certification has the potential for improving patient care outcomes.

specialty organizations. The Websites of these specialty organizations (or their credentialing organizations) provide specific certification requirements. Certification recognizes the competence of the nurse in a specialized area.

PROFESSIONAL EXPECTATIONS

Belonging to a professional association not only demonstrates professional leadership but also provides numerous opportunities to meet other leaders, participate in policy formation, continue specialized education, and shape the future of the profession. To learn more about an association, write to the national association and ask for information or access the Website. Requesting information should provide insight into both direct and indirect benefits of organizational membership. For example, a direct benefit may be receiving a publication or attending a meeting at reduced or no cost. An indirect benefit is knowing that your association actively lobbies on behalf of professional nurses. State boards of nursing can be contacted through the National Council of State Boards of Nursing's Website (http://www.ncsbn.org).

Depending on the type of career you want to have, belonging to a specific association may be very important because it is synonymous with leadership in the field. In nursing, the American Academy of Nursing and Sigma Theta Tau International are examples of such organizations.

Determining a logical level of involvement in an organization at the local, state, regional, or national level is important. When a bright, articulate, committed member is discovered, that individual is often asked to fulfill other expectations of the organization's work. Once again, knowing what is important to do to meet your professional goals can help you decide what level of involvement is desirable and acceptable.

Because the public places its trust in any licensed profession, there are numerous other obligations and privileges to being a professional. Some are exciting, for instance, providing testimony related to healthcare concerns. Others are troublesome, such as reporting a colleague to the state nursing board for incompetent practice. These are opportunities to improve the profession and the resultant care the general public can expect.

CAREER POTENTIAL

Traditionally, nursing has been perceived by the public as hospital-based, but that has changed dramatically. There are numerous other nursing careers, such as teacher, administrator, manager, clinical specialist, researcher, organizational executive, entrepreneur, and practitioner. These roles occur in hospitals, clinics, community and professional organizations, and the business setting. In addition, the number of clinical specialties continues to increase. Some have been a part of nursing for a long time and are experiencing major growth and recognition because of the financial and clinical impact on health care. These include such foci as occupational health, school health, and public health. Concomitantly, the traditional hospital careers are simultaneously focusing and expanding. Nurses with these focused, expert skills need to be able to function with more than one clinical population. This ability to increase expertise and flexibility will continue to be in demand. Positioning within the profession to achieve this flexibility and expertise requires career commitment, continuous self-development, a passion for nursing, and a strong foundation as a leader.

The Solution

Although I was a recent graduate and thought I knew what I needed to know, I returned to my textbooks looking for a strategy. Information on professionalism and how to handle difficult people provided a solution to my problem.

Initially, I began to pull myself away from my peers who were my friends. Long, lonely workdays were the outcome of this solution. My next strategy proved more effective. I would not assign anything to anyone that I myself would not or could not do. I became available to assist with any task, including those of the nurse aide, LVN, and other registered nurses. My knowledge and professionalism enabled the staff to begin seeing me as an integral part of the staff. Soon they began to be more open to accepting more challenging assignments.

As the days, weeks, and months passed, my relationship with the nursing staff (some of whom were my friends) blossomed into a wonderful professional relationship. Each day, I found it easier to make assignments without fear of upsetting a co-worker or a friend. We all knew what work had to be done. I recognized that I needed to treat my staff with dignity and professionalism; valuing the contribution each staff member makes was an integral part of my career development.

— Rebecca A. Brawley

 Would this be a suitable approach for you? Why?

CHAPTER CHECKLIST

Nurses must make decisions about career goals and career development. Managing a career requires a set of planned strategies designed to lead systematically toward the desired goal. The use of each strategy should be geared toward finding a good person–position fit. Career planning and development is a lifelong process focused on continual competence. Continued professional development, whether via graduate education or continuing education, is a crucial component of success as a nurse.

- Career styles contribute to the diversity of the nursing profession and reflect different ways of achieving success.
- The four career styles are as follows:
  - Steady state: characterized by constancy with increasing professional skill
  - Linear: a hierarchical orientation with a steady climb
  - Entrepreneurial/transient: focused on new services and personal priorities
  - Spiral: rational, independent responsibility for shaping the career
- Certain career control strategies are effective with every career style:
  - Selecting professional peers, mentors, and role models helps shape professional development.
  - Designing personal/professional documents that open doors for further action includes:
    - The curriculum vitae (a listing of facts) (quantitative)
    - The résumé (a sampling of the most relevant facts, with details) (qualitative)
    - Appropriate business letters that market effectively
- Interviewing at its best is a two-way interaction that enables both people to determine whether there is a good person–position fit.
- Both graduate education and continuing education contribute to a nurse's ability to provide competent care.
- Graduate education (master's- or doctorate-level study) may focus on the following:
  - A clinical area
  - A functional role area
  - A combination of both
- Factors to consider in selecting a graduate program include the following:
  - Accreditation
  - Clinical/functional role
  - Credits
  - Thesis/research requirements
  - Faculty
  - Current research
  - Flexibility
  - Admission policy
  - Cost
- Continuing-education opportunities exist at local, state, regional, national, and international levels.
- Certification is the designation of special knowledge beyond the basic licensure and is a requirement in some employment settings. Being a professional carries additional obligations and privileges to ensure that the nurse remains competent, advances the profession, and improves health care.

CAREER TIPS

- Use an expanding file to organize hard copies of your accomplishments, such as continuing-education certificates, by year so that you can report accurate data for licensure or certification.
- Update your CV at least once a year (6 months is better and 3 months is ideal) so that you always have an accurate, current set of data to share with someone should a special opportunity appear.
- Keep connected with people.
- Find a mentor; be a mentor; self-mentor.
- Learn from what you do each day: what to do differently, how to preempt errors, who to seek as a supporter.
- Focus on your strengths and build them into spectacular performances; hone the basics so that you are always prepared.
- Think about the future and what you need to be employable.

- Join two professional organizations—such as the American Nurses Association (broad professional) and the American Association of Critical Care Nurses (a specialty).
- Read professional journals and, on a regular basis, at least one other journal external to nursing to keep current with the world.
- Attend at least one professional meeting each year, especially outside of your geographic area, to network.
- Volunteer in your profession and your community.

TERMS TO KNOW

career	professional association
certification	(organization)
continuing education	portfolio
curriculum vitae	résumé
licensure	

REFERENCES

American Nurses Association (ANA). (2000). *Scopes and standards of practice for nursing professional development.* Washington, DC: Author.

American Nurses Credentialing Center. (2000*). Credentialing catalog.* Washington, DC: Author.

Bolles, R. N. (2005). *What color is your parachute?* Berkley: Ten Speed Press.

Cary, A. H. (2001). Certified registered nurses: Results of the study of the certified workforce. *American Journal of Nursing, 101*(1), 44–52.

Fox, J. J. (2001). *Don't send a résumé.* New York: Hyperion.

Friss, L. (1989). *Strategic management of nurses: A policy oriented approach.* Owings Mills, MD: AUPHA Press.

Monsen, R. B. (2005). *Genetics Nursing Portfolios: A new model for credentialing.* Silver Spring MD: American Nurses Association.

Rosenstein, B. (2001, August 20). *91-Year-old legend shares advice.* USA Today, p. 6B.

SUGGESTED READINGS

Fox, J. J. (2001). *Don't send a resume and other contrarian rules to help land a great job.* New York: Hyperion.

Hawley, C. (2001). *100+ winning answers to the toughest interview questions.* Hauppauge, NY: Barrons.

Leider, D. J., & Shapiro, D. A. (2001). *Whistle while you work: Heeding your life's calling.* San Francisco: Berrett-Koehler.

Moses, B. (1998). *Career intelligence: The 12 new rules for work and life success.* San Francisco: Berrett-Koehler.

WEBSITES

American Nurses Credentialing Center: www.nursingworld.org/ancc

American Nurses Association: www.nursingworld.org

BestjobsUSA.com: www.bestjobsusa.com

Careerbuilder.com: www.careerbuilder.com

Monster.com: www.monster.com

Sigma Theta Tau International Honor Society: www.nursingsociety.org

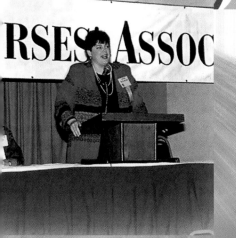

Chapter

28

Leading Through Professional Associations

Patricia S. Yoder-Wise with Sharon A. Brigher

*T*his chapter describes professional organizations and association concepts, as well as values obtained through leadership and participation in organizations. The primary focus is on the variety of opportunities and advantages that can be gained through a relationship with various professional nursing organizations. In today's changing healthcare environment, it is more important than ever for the nurse to be connected and unified with other nursing colleagues who are prepared to confront challenges and who are equipped with solutions.

Objectives

- Describe professional association concepts, such as mission statements and goals.
- Explain common structures and roles within organizations.
- Consider contributions you can make to an organization and benefits you can derive.
- Value the need for involvement in organizations and associations.

Questions to Consider

- *How will you benefit from and contribute to an organization?*
- *What is your motivation to join and/or participate?*
- *How much time do you have to devote to involvement with the organization?*

The Challenge

Howard Holsinger, RN, BSN, CNRN
National Institutes of Health Clinical Center, Bethesda, Maryland

Nurse Jane, an experienced charge nurse on the medical-surgical floor, had a reputation of constantly delegating her own work to new staff members, justifying her actions by saying she needed fewer patients because she must focus on her charge nurse duties. She claimed that being a charge nurse was stressful and that we could use the experience anyway. I had been working on this medical-surgical floor for almost a year and felt confident working with my patients and the nurses, even though I was one of the youngest and least experienced nurses on the staff. Being a team player, I rarely turned Nurse Jane down when she asked me for something, whether it was simply to page a physician, change her patient's IV bags, or call the pharmacy for a medication. I thought that she must be busy with discharge planning and would not have asked me if she did not really need the help. However, I quickly realized that she was taking advantage of her position, as well as my helpful attitude. I began to resent her when I would take her chores and she would then sit in the lounge and use that time for social phone calls, which were obviously not essential charge-nurse duties.

Before our morning shift one day, she made out the assignments and again gave herself a light assignment that consisted of two early-morning discharges, whereas the other nurse and I were given more challenging patient assignments. As the day proceeded, I was able to handle my assignment without asking for help. Nurse Jane's patients left before 11 AM without complications. After they left, she did not pick up any of our patients, and she did not have any unusual charge responsibilities on this day. I noticed that Jane seemed to take a long break after her patients were discharged, and the other nurse and I had not even stopped for lunch. Neither of her discharge patients' rooms had been cleared for housekeeping; it is the nurses' responsibility to clear before housekeeping can enter the room to prepare for more admissions.

A few hours before the shift was over, Nurse Jane came into my patient's room while I was in the middle of patient care and interrupted by saying, "Can you do me a favor?" Of course, I replied that I could. "What can I do?" Her request: "Can you clear the rooms of my discharged patients?" Frustrated, I began to think about how I would respond. How should I follow-up with Nurse Jane? Do I have to complete every task delegated from her because she is in charge? I told her that I would be out in a few minutes, and she turned around and left the room.

 What do you think you would do if you were this nurse?

INTRODUCTION

People have always been in search of others who share common interests. Networking informally can meet a part of this desire. However, associations exist to provide this opportunity, as well as to serve a purpose, such as working to improve the environment or to promote research, advocacy for seniors, and more. **Professional associations (organizations)** have been defined as groups of people who share a set of professional **values** and who decide to join their colleagues to affect change. Many nursing associations set standards and objectives to guide the profession and specialty practice. Standards can also serve as critical measurements for the profession and its practitioners. In today's changing healthcare environment, increasing num-

bers of associations are serving unique healthcare interests in society. Healthcare professionals have a plethora of associations from which to choose. Although associations have very different agendas and goals, many nursing organizations share the same motivation and long-term goal of uniting and advancing the profession.

TYPES OF PROFESSIONAL ASSOCIATIONS

Nursing students have the opportunity to become involved with the preprofessional nursing organization, the National Student Nurses Association (NSNA). NSNA provides numerous opportunities.

Through their local school chapters, nursing students can become involved, learn about policy issues, participate in leadership opportunities, and explore ways to influence the profession at an early stage in their career. For many students, NSNA has had a major impact on the direction of their careers because of the exposure to the variety of career paths and introduction to nursing leaders throughout the country. For example, an NSNA convention holds a variety of events that might include focus sessions on specific clinical or career-development topics and a panel of nurses with different roles in nursing. There are more than 75 specialty-nursing organizations that represent nurses in particular areas of the profession (Box 28-1). Some are clinically focused, such as the American Association of Critical Care Nurses, the Oncology Nurses Association, and the American Association of Neuroscience Nurses. Others are role focused, such as the American Organization of Nurse Executives and the National League for Nursing. Still others represent specific groups in nursing, such as the

---

BOX 28-1

List of Nursing Organizations

Academy of Medical-Surgical Nurses	www.medsurgnurse.org/
Air and Surface Transport Nurses Association	www.astna.org/
American Academy of Ambulatory Care Nursing	www.aaacn.org
American Academy of Nurse Practitioners	www.aanp.org
American Academy of Nursing	www.nursingworld.org/aan
American Assembly of Men in Nursing	http://aamn.org/
American Assisted Living Nurses Association	www.alnursing.org/
American Association of Colleges of Nursing	www.aacn.nche.edu/
American Association of Continuity in Care	www.continuityofcare.com
American Association of Critical Care Nurse	www.aacn.org/
American Association of Diabetes Educators	www.aadenet.org/
American Association for the History of Nursing	www.aahn.org/
American Association of Legal Nurse Consultants	www.aalnc.org
American Association of Neuroscience Nurses	www.aann.org/
American Association of Nurse Anesthetists	www.aana.com/
American Association of Nurse Attorneys	www.taana.org/
American Association of Occupational Health Nurses	www.aaohn.org/
American Association of Office Nurses	www.aaon.org/
American Association of Spinal Cord Nurses	www.aascin.org/
American College of Nurse Midwives	www.acnm.org/
American College of Nurse Practitioners	www.nurse.org/acnp/
American Holistic Nurses Association	www.ahna.org/
American Nephrology Nurses Association	http://anna.inurse.com/
American Nurses Association	www.nursingworld.org
American Nurses Credentialing Center	www.nursingworld.org/ancc
American Nursing Informatics Association	www.ania.org/
American Organization of Nurse Executives	www.aone.org
American Public Health Association	www.apha.org/
American Psychiatric Nurses Association	www.apna.org/
American Radiological Nurses Association	www.rsna.org/orgs/arna.html
American Society of Ophthalmic Registered Nurses	http://webeye.ophth.uiowa.edu/asorn/
American Society of Pain Management Nurses	www.aspmn.org/
American Society of Perianesthesia Nurses	www.aspan.org/

Continued

BOX 28-1

List of Nursing Organizations—cont'd

American Society of Plastic and Reconstructive Surgical Nurses	www.aspsn
Association of Child and Adolescent Psychiatric Nurses	www.ispn-psych.org
Association of Child Neurology Nurses	www.acnn.org/
Association of Nurses in AIDS Care	www.anacnet.org/
Association of Pediatric Oncology	www.apon.org
Association of Perioperative Registered Nurses	www.aorn.org/
Association for Professionals in Infection Control and Epidemiology	www.apic.org
Association of Rehabilitation Nurses	www.rehabnurse.org/
Association of Women's Health, Obstetrics and Neonatal Nurses	www.awhonn.org/
Case Management Society of America	www.cmsa.org
Dermatology Nurses Association	www.dnanurse.org
Development Disabilities Nurses Association	www.ddna.org
Emergency Nurses Association	www.ena.org/
Endocrine Nurses Society	www.endo-nurses.org/
Home Healthcare Nurses Association	www.hhna.org/
Hospice and Palliative Nurses Association	www.hpna.org/
Infusion Nurses Society	www.ins1.org/
International Association of Forensic Nurses	www.forensicnurse.org/
International Council of Nurses	www.icn.ch/
National Association of Clinical Nurse Specialists	www.nacns.org/
National Association of Hispanic Nurses	www.thehispanicnurses.org/
National Association of Neonatal Nurses	www.nann.org
National Association of Nurse Massage Therapists	www.nanmt.org/
National Association of Orthopedic Nurses	www.orthonurse.org/
National Association of Pediatric Nurse Practitioners and Associates	www.napnap.org/
National Association of School Nurses	www.nasn.org/
National Black Nurses Association	www.nbna.org/
National Council of State Boards of Nursing	www.ncsbn.org/
National Gerontological Nursing Association	www.ngna.org/
National League for Nursing	www.nln.org
National Nursing Staff Development Organization	http://nnsdo.org
National Organization for Associate Degree Nursing	www.noadn.org/
National Organization of Nurse Practitioner Faculties	www.nonpf.com/
National Student Nurses Association	www.nsna.org
Oncology Nursing Society	www.ons.org
Phillipine Nurses Association of America	www.pnaa03.org
Sigma Theta Tau, International	www.nursingsociety.org
Society of Gastroenterology Nurses and Associates	www.sgna.org/
Society of Pediatric Nurses	www.pedsnurses.org/
Society of Urologic Nurses and Associates	http://suna.inurse.com/
Society for Vascular Nursing	www.svnnet.org/
Transcultural Nursing Society	www.tcns.org/
Wound, Ostomy and Continence Nurses Society	www.wocn.org/

American Assembly for Men in Nursing and the National Black Nurses Association. To attract future members, many specialty organizations offer reduced membership rates to students and new graduates, which include discounted meeting and convention rates, discounts on insurance, networking opportunities, and informative publications and mailings about the association.

The "umbrella organization" that represents all nurses is the American Nurses Association (ANA), which is a full-service professional organization that represents registered nurses through its 54 constituent associations and various organizational affiliate members (www.ana.org). The ANA advances the nursing profession by fostering high standards of nursing practice. Some functions of the ANA include promoting the economic and general welfare of nurses in the workplace, projecting a positive and realistic view of nursing, and lobbying Congress and regulatory agencies on healthcare issues affecting nurses and the public (www.nursingworld.org). When the ANA was formed in 1897 and officially founded in 1901, its purpose was to protect the public from unsafe nursing care and to set standards for practice and education that could be changed and adapted over the years (Joel, 2003). Today, the ANA continues to be the voice for nursing, serving as a strong advocate and representative for the profession. Similar to the American Medical Association for physicians, policymakers look to the ANA for guidance on nursing and health-policy issues.

Exercise 28-1

Research the ANA and your state nursing organization on the Internet (www.nursingworld.org). Find the **mission** of the organization and the legislative issues of interest. Obtain/download association brochures or further information.

Unlike most professional associations that are open memberships, meaning that if you meet the basic criteria, you are eligible to be a member, Sigma Theta Tau International is an invitational association. Established in 1922, it is international and is available to nurses enrolled in baccalaureate, master's; and doctoral education programs and community leaders through a nomination process. Its mission is to create a global community of nurses who lead in using scholarship, knowledge, and technology to improve the health of the world's

people (www.nursingsociety.org). This organization is one of the primary sources for small grants to aid in beginning research and disseminates research and leadership information through various publications and meetings.

A MODEL FOR INVOLVEMENT

Few nurses graduate from their basic nursing educational program and immediately join and become involved in their professional organization. Upon graduation, nurses are focused on key aspects of professional life, such as learning basic policies and the organizational culture, evaluating peers to determine who to trust and who to avoid, and resolving numerous transitional issues, such as where to live, how to afford housing, how to manage payment of student loans, how to network with old and new friends, and how to figure out on a daily basis that they are safe practitioners learning what they need to know. Few new graduates also think about how they can benefit from professional organizational membership. Unfortunately for the individuals and for nursing as a whole, many nurses never pursue membership in any professional organization. For those who do, however, many choose to participate by only paying the membership dues. Although some nurse leaders do not see this as a valued contribution, the reality is that those who pay dues support the work of the association through a key avenue—financial. They, in essence, allow others to engage in other types of involvement. Yoder-Wise (2006) identifies involvement this way: movement occurs from a clinical focus (direct patient care) to professional (movement to policy).

STRUCTURE

Structures of organizations can vary greatly, depending on an organization's size and purpose. Many organizations are multitiered (chapter, region, national; district, state, national), designed to reach out to members in all areas of the country. For instance, the ANA is considered a three-tiered organization, with the headquarters located in the Washington, DC, area; its constituent members are the states and a federal nursing group, and local or district associations allow members to network on a grassroots level. This type of organizational structure is designed for effective information dissemination. However, it requires that all parties be communicating and responding to each other on a timely basis, which can be a challenge, particularly if an area is lacking in members. Clear lines of communication and structure are essential for associations.

The mission and goals of an association give the direction and often state the purpose for its existence. Examples of an organization's mission include striving to educate the public on healthcare issues, uniting the profession, affecting international healthcare issues, being an active player in policy and managed care, defining nursing and nursing education, developing requirements and scope of practice, and/or empowering nurses to take control of their own practices.

The organization may develop a **strategic plan,** which is a detailed map based on the mission and goals for the association's existence. Strategic plans operationalize how the organization can meet its goals and objectives. Within the strategic plan, clearly defined goals determine the organization's political agenda. The strategic plan guides the board's decisions, directs the staff's work, and informs the membership about anticipated activities.

Associations can be formally structured and are legally incorporated, yet neither is a requirement for an organization to exist. Most organizations have a set of bylaws, which refer to specific rules of order of an organization, such as accountability, authority, composition, governance, mission, and purpose. Bylaws can usually be changed by the elected body of representatives through an amendment process. The body is a part of association membership that has voting authority, thereby making decisions and electing board members to serve at the helm of the association. Officer positions vary from organization to organization. Most boards include the following: president, vice president, secretary, and treasurer. The board functions at its best when the individual officers experience a sense of teamwork. The entire board must collectively work together to be as productive and efficient as possible.

Parliamentary Procedure, guided by Robert's Rules of Order (2000), is the method used to conduct most association business for board or the elected body meetings. This body can pass motions, resolutions, and amendments. It can also create goal or policy statements or alter the bylaws. The board is elected by the membership to carry out the directives of the membership and to function on their behalf between meetings. The board can establish subgroups, or committees, to carry out specific functions and tasks for the associations. Examples of committees may include governmental relations, practice, membership recruitment and retention, and convention planning. Committees encourage participation by members with different levels of interest and passion. The members are the volunteers who pay membership dues and contribute their time, play active roles in the organization, and help carry out the mission of the organization. Collectively, the different entities coordinate efforts to have an extraordinary effect within the professional and personal realm of nursing.

Another important part of the organizational structure is the executive staff, which may consist of an executive director and support staff, who are typically salaried and located at the association headquarters, which is usually based in a large, urban city. The association headquarters and size of the staff will vary according to available financial resources and the mission. The staff provides general support and disseminates information to the members through phone calls, mailings, and listservs. They coordinate conventions and meetings while serving as a constant point of information and resource for members. Some organizations hire outside consultants to perform specific tasks, such as strategic planning and financial or organizational restructuring. Consultants are typically nonbiased, professional individuals who can offer suggestions that make an association more efficient without getting involved in the politics of the organization. Because many organizations have strong political agendas, registered lobbyists are commonly employed to work closely with the state and/ or federal members of Congress.

Connecting With an Organization

The size of an organization can be misleading. Bigger is not necessarily better. The size of the group is not so important as how the group is organized and who is leading it. Therefore, it is extremely important to do some research before making a commitment through membership. In today's world of high-speed Internet access, it is easy to access an abundance of information through the computer, rather than spending time calling and requesting membership applications and brochures. In addition, reading about the officer and membership composition of the organization is important. Most associations have a website that lists information regarding leader contact and biographical information, locations of their next meetings or activities, current policy issues and their positions, election information, and other valuable resource links. Some organizations permit e-mail subscriptions so that you are notified on a regular basis about evolving events.

Exercise 28-2

Attend a local district meeting in your association, observe the dynamics, and network with the members.

Expectations of Membership

Upon joining a nursing organization, you may receive information on the history of the organization, future meetings and current activities, officer contact information, and local contacts. One of the most important things that you can do is connect with your local organization so that you can immediately begin networking. Decide how much time you can allocate to the organization. There are several different ways to be involved, all of which carry different time commitments. Do not assume that a certain role or committee position entails a set amount of time. The fact remains that most associations are composed of volunteers, all of whom have very busy schedules and different motivations for becoming involved. Taking time to talk to an officer or attend a local meeting and observe the group and the dynamics before deciding to make commitments will help ensure that you make an informed decision. Some members enter into the organizational experience with unreal expectations and quickly become disenchanted and disappointed with the organization, which results in completely pulling away from the organization. To maximize your experience, you owe it to yourself to do your homework, research the organization, talk to the members, determine the sense of the group dynamics, and assess what you want to derive from the experience and how you can contribute to the organization. Look at your strengths and talents and see if there is a need or a fit within the organization. Finally, remember that the organization is composed of humans who are volunteering their time; therefore, you should not expect a "perfect" organization. Every organization has its struggles, but you can gain tremendous benefits, both personally and professionally, from your involvement.

Exercise 28-3

While you are at an association meeting, challenge yourself to speak to at least two members and find out about their work setting and their nursing role. Make sure to get contact information or a business card from at least two individuals whom you can call in the near future. On the back of the business card, write something about that person that will help you remember them for the future (e.g., long black hair, nurse manager on the neurology unit at Methodist Hospital). It is also helpful to have a date and the name of meeting so you can "place" the person in your mind. You may use these cards in the future when you are looking for a job or need a specific question answered, and they will serve as an invaluable resource.

Joining/Reasons for Involvement

Motivation to join an organization can vary a great deal. Organizational membership has become an integral part of one's career development. The average nurse may hold membership in a variety of social and professional organizations, devoting more time to one particular area of interest. For example, nurses may choose to belong to one or more organizations. Nurses who define themselves as leaders and who want to have greater influence than their place of work should join at least one professional association. Some reasons for joining organizations may include a sense of responsibility to the profession or the hope that they are contributing to the greater good of the profession. Other reasons might include the desire to enhance their résumé and marketability purposes. The nurses' employer may encourage membership and even pay for the employees' membership fee. Some nurses may join because they want to promote their profession, have particular legislative interests, or have other social reasons. A common belief among nurses is that their organization of choice can help improve conditions and care for their patients. In addition, there are those who choose to be active participants by joining committee work, running for office, or taking on other leadership roles. Organizations need all types of members, both active and passive participants, so that they can carry out their missions and conduct activities and business. In addition, organizational involvement, like any socialization process, can improve nursing morale. Being around others who take pride and celebrate the nursing profession is contagious, and you will inevitably spread that attitude. Whatever your personal preference for level of involvement, you are contributing greatly to your profession by simply joining and becoming a member, but active involvement within an association can guarantee a world of opportunities.

Some nurses choose to belong to their state nurses association because they want to protect their licensure status and affect health care through legislative endeavors. Others choose to belong because of specific benefits such as liability insurance and education.

Some individuals belong to professional organizations because they are required to do so. In some cases, employment contracts make it mandatory for the nurse to join a union and pay dues to receive a paycheck. Many state associations have instituted a workplace advocacy program, which provides the nurse with communication and conflict resolution tools.

Exercise 28–4

Think about what motivates you to join or not join the state nurses' organization. Make a list of your strengths (communication, organization, budgeting, legislative interests). Look at positions within the organization that interest you. On a separate list, write out reasons why you would want to be a part of the association.

What You Can Gain from Participating in an Organization

In today's rapidly changing environment of health-care delivery and services, nurses must remain active and involved in the decision-making process that affects the nursing profession. Policy makers will proceed with making decisions that affect nursing practice if nurses do not ensure that they are at the table with input and guidance. Nursing organizations recognize this reality and are taking on a more vital role than ever by participating in discussions that range from local and state to national levels.

Organizations provide members with a variety of ways to lead and relate to others. A common misconception is that you must take on an officer or committee position to be "involved." However, even just paying dues is involvement because it is an investment of money in your future. Participation can occur at a variety of levels; it is important to know just what you want to attain from organizational involvement. Assessing your own motivations and goals before joining and making time commitments within the organization is important. Participation is a personal decision and is guided by one's personal commitment and time limits. If you want to strengthen or develop an attribute, such as public speaking, you should seek out positions and opportunities within the organization that would enable you to develop that skill. Likewise, if you wish to become more politically knowledgeable about current legislation and the political process, you could seek involvement in legislative affairs activities. After you have had time to observe the group structure and its working dynamics, it is extremely important to verbalize your interests to the officers and chairs of committees. Often, the voluntary organizations are eager to receive assistance and may take it upon themselves to make your activity assignments for you. You should not hesitate to reject any assignments and start by communicating effectively from the beginning. Take control by vocalizing your time limitations, interests, and objectives. This proactive action will prevent frustration and miscommunication and ensure that you will have a productive, fulfilling experience.

Personal Benefits Some associations offer substantial scholarships for nurses who are pursuing higher education and certifications. They might also offer scholarships to attend policy meetings, such as the Nurse In Washington Internship, organized by the National Federation for Specialty Nursing Organizations, or the Annual Health Policy Institute, conducted by the Center for Health Policy, Research, and Ethics of George Mason

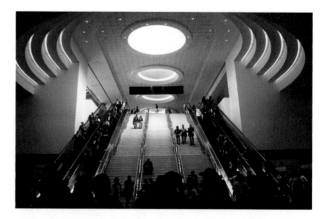

Networking at national meetings provides ways to share practice information and to create career opportunities.

University. These two internships are examples of opportunities through which nurses can learn about legislative issues, the political process, health-care advocacy, and how to be more effective on local, state, and national levels. Another benefit of membership is the opportunity to travel for conventions and meetings. Most organizations rotate their regular convention meeting sites so that members throughout the country will have an opportunity to attend.

With ever-increasing time demands on individuals today, volunteering for activities outside of work and family has become increasingly difficult. Because volunteers comprise the majority of members within an organization, associations are aware that traditional incentives for member participation may not be enough to draw new members. However, there are benefits that are not advertised. For example, networking and exposure to different opportunities within the nursing profession are two of the most valuable benefits of belonging to an organization. Some nurses may stop working for a time because of family or educational priorities. Organizational membership can help these nurses stay connected to professional issues and colleagues through meetings and publications so that the transition back into practice will not be as difficult. Given these possibilities, membership in nursing organizations can provide a continuous source of professional colleagues for today's nurse to draw upon for invaluable advice and collective support.

With the abundant opportunities in nursing, nurses rarely remain in the same position for an extended period. Chances are that most nurses will work in a variety of settings over the course of their career. Therefore, today's nurse needs to socialize with nurses in different career paths within nursing. This socialization can take place through district meetings or state or national conventions. For example, many organizations have conventions at which they might feature a nurse panel representing a variety of innovative positions within the field, which will expose the member to new and emerging fields. Such meetings also provide members with a potential contact for nurses who hope to transition into that particular area of nursing.

In addition to networking, the professional organization can serve as an additional training ground through which nurses can build skills and gain wonderful experiences. They also provide opportunities for leadership development through committees or in officer positions, which can provide invaluable skills training (Box 28-2). Villarruel and Peragallo (2004) found involvement in professional associations to be a training ground for leadership skills (see the Research Perspective).

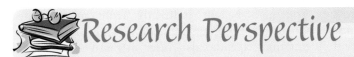

Research Perspective

Villarruel, A. M. & Peragallo, N. (2004). Leadership development of Hispanic nurses. *Nursing Administration Quarterly, 28*, 173-180.

A descriptive study involving officers and chapter presidents of the National Association of Hispanic Nurses produced a small, but meaningful number of responses to eight (8) open-ended questions about leadership. Ethnic diversity was evident among the respondents: Hispanic, Mexican/Mexican American, Puerto Rican/Cuban and nurses from Central and South America. The mean age of respondents was 44.6 years, most were engaged in practice, and most held a master's degree. The key theme was that they "glued" diverse people with a common goal. Comments tended to indicate limited differences about leadership based on ethnicity; however, not having had a mentor who was Hispanic was a challenge. Volunteer activities, including nursing professional organizations, were seen as an essential source for developing leadership abilities.

IMPLICATIONS FOR NURSING PRACTICE

For nurses interested in developing leadership abilities, participation in professional organizations is essential. Now that we know how important mentors "like me" (gender, ethnicity, socioeconomic, etc) are, all nurse leaders should be willing to serve as leaders and to support professional development of those eager to be leaders.

BOX 28-2

Skills Learned from Organizational Involvement

- Conflict resolution
- Interpersonal communication
- Public speaking
- Mentoring
- Conducting meetings
- Creating agendas
- Facilitation
- Delegation
- Consensus-building
- Strategic-thinking
- Team-building
- Political advocacy
- Legislative work/lobbying
- Problem-solving

Members of nursing associations learn first-hand about diversity among patient populations, as well as within the profession. Clinical issues that affect practice on local, state, and federal levels are addressed. Opportunities to work as a group to influence and educate policymakers are also evident. The organization and members' ability to influence health care in a policy arena is one of the most significant benefits of membership. On the most basic level, nurses can influence legislation for their profession by simply becoming a member and adding strength through numbers. For further involvement, nurses can participate on a legislative committee and become involved in their local, grassroots politics. By being acquainted with the political players in their area, nurses can ensure that they are at the table for discussions on health-care and policymaking decisions. Nurses' ability to advocate for their patients is not confined to the bedside. Nurses must learn to use advocacy in the political arena as well. Nursing organizations are tremendous advocates and can have great political strength (Mason, Leavitt, & Chaffee, 2002). Consistently, the Harris poll reports that the public trusts information about health care provided by registered nurses. This powerful information reinforces the fact that nurses must be involved in healthcare discussions and decision-making policies.

Whether you are a new or experienced nurse, you will encounter ethical or professional dilemmas. Members of a nurses association can be non-biased, safe colleagues to ask for advice about your situation. They can provide feedback options for your situation, based on their experience, especially when you may not want to discuss it with co-workers who could be directly involved. They also may be connected to the experts in the field and serve as a connection for further dialog.

Professional Benefits You can benefit directly from belonging to an organization. Associations can serve as a springboard for your career. If you are networking within an organization, you will inevitably meet members who work in your field or even one that you hope to enter. Becoming acquainted with these men and women and working with them on association activities provides potential job opportunities or other benefits. How many times have you said to yourself, "What a small world!" after bumping into someone that you haven't seen in a while or finding out that you have a connection with someone with whom you have been talking? Well, the nursing world is even smaller, and you could enter an interview or board meeting and find an ally on your side by simply previously meeting or working with them in an organization. Other disciplines use association membership as a key base for position referrals. You also benefit indirectly from membership. Coalition building, unification, and advancing of nursing's agenda also offer attractive reasons to belong. Politically, nurses are so much stronger if they have one unified voice that speaks to Congress on the profession's behalf. Members of Congress and their staff have voiced concerns about the inconsistency of nursing's message, specifically if a specialty nursing organization pushes its individual agenda without connecting it into the common message that pertains to all nurses. This occurrence can be prevented if the profession organizes messages in advance. Specialty nursing organizations have an extremely important role that is enhanced when tied to communicating and collaborating with the other nursing entities. The American Medical Association has been masterful at coordinating their general legislative message with the specialty medical associations, as well as stating their membership benefits upfront (Box 28-3).

BOX 28-3

Tangible Benefits from Organizational Involvement

- Substantial discounts on continuing education
- Certifications
- Credentialing
- Group insurance plans for professional liability, hospitalization, and disability
- Travel services, such as auto rentals, hotel stays, and restaurant visits
- Quick access to staff experts on practice advocacy
- Legal, legislative, and educational issues
- Professional standards
- Discounts on professional journals

CONCLUSION

Professional associations and organizations are powerful influences on the nursing profession and health care in general. For the individual nurse, the personal and professional opportunities are endless. You can enhance your career development while seizing the opportunity to make a tremendous impact on the profession. When a nurse invests time, passion, and energy into an association, the individual, patient, and nursing profession will all benefit. You owe it to yourself to learn more about nursing organizations that might interest you and to get involved. It can change your life and your career path and take you to unbelievable places. After all, what do you have to lose? If you decide that you are not happy with an organization after joining, you have only benefited by experiencing the people and purpose. You should feel confident in searching for one that is a better fit. Meanwhile, be assured that your membership dues allow other nurses and the association to work behind the scenes for the profession's best interest. That is a comforting thought in today's fast-paced environment. Just knowing that there are nurses who are monitoring the issues, ready to respond on behalf of the profession, is quite an empowering thought! In the words of Henry Ford, "Coming together is a beginning, keeping together is progress, and working together is success." Nurses embrace this teamwork spirit more than any other profession. Choose to make a difference, and join your association. It is truly a win-win experience!

The Solution

During the previous week, I had asked the advice of an experienced nurse colleague who had served as a charge nurse for several years. This colleague was also an active leader in his professional nursing organization. He knew that I wanted to keep a professional work environment with Nurse Jane, but I was tired of feeling that she was taking advantage of me. He advised me with specific communication tools that worked for him, which was to talk with the individual in a nonconfrontational manner while communicating my feelings directly and without emotion. I decided to follow his advice.

After I finished my direct patient care, I took a few minutes to calm down and later approached her, asking to speak with her in private in the lounge. I started the conversation by praising her expertise and telling her I recognized that being charge nurse can be stressful at times. I explained that I respected our professional working relationship and that is why I wanted to address a serious concern. I told her that I did not appreciate being asked to complete tasks for her when she would turn around and use that time for social interaction or sitting in the lounge. Therefore, I was not willing to clear her rooms for her, given that there were 2 more hours on the shift. I was firm with my communication and concluded that I wanted to continue being a team player and being helpful to her, but I would not tolerate being "used" when she would have plenty of time to do those tasks on her own. I explained that I would be setting guidelines for myself, gauging when I felt it would be appropriate to help her, depending on my own individual assignment. I encouraged her to try to complete the tasks independently, but if it was not possible, I would then be more than happy to help her. I felt she was receptive and she explained that she would try to be more sensitive to me and other co-workers and would make

Continued

The Solution—cont'd

an honest effort to complete the task before requesting my help.

By setting those guidelines and covering the communicating techniques with my nurse colleague beforehand, I felt I was able to handle the situation without destroying our working relationship. In the end, it proved to create a stronger working relationship with Nurse Jane. Shortly thereafter, my co-workers began to see a change in Nurse Jane's efforts to complete her assignment. My communication with Nurse Jane was much easier from that point forward, and eventually Nurse Jane approached me and expressed her appreciation for my honest feedback and appreciated the fact that I went to her directly to resolve the situation without going to the nurse manager.

— Howard Holsinger

Would this be a suitable approach for you? Why?

CHAPTER CHECKLIST

Professional development can take place in a variety of ways. However, involvement in professional associations can open doors to opportunities that would never have been possible otherwise. Levels of participation in the organization can vary from paying your dues to holding an officer position on the board of directors. Assessing your individual strengths, motivations, and goals before making a commitment to an organization is important. Many nurses find that the membership association can help develop professional skills and provide them with goals that they can achieve. When you are seeking your first job, look to members of the state nurses' association to get acquainted with colleagues and find out about their job and workplace environment. Aside from the networking benefits, the opportunity to get involved in the professional nurses association is a chance to make a difference in the profession, for your patients and for future nurses.

- Numerous organizations exist in health care.
  - The American Nurses Association and numerous specialty organizations focus on improving the profession itself and the care patients receive.
  - Most associations have both volunteers and employed staff to accomplish the organizational goals.
- Connecting with an association produces numerous benefits.
  - Involvement levels vary based on personal situations.
  - Strengths and talents should guide selection of involvement.
  - Some nurses are covered by employment contracts via union activities.
  - Workplace advocacy strategies help nurses interact on an individual or group basis in the employment situation.
- Nurses can make various contributions to the profession through association involvement.
  - Networking is facilitated.
  - Associations provide the input to policymakers who determine policies and legislation affecting the practice of nursing and patient rights and benefits.
  - Attendance at meetings provides valuable contacts and different points of view.
  - Work to reverse the workforce shortage in nursing is being led by the professional associations.

TIPS FOR PROFESSIONAL DEVELOPMENT AND ORGANIZATIONAL INVOLVEMENT

- Create an individual mission statement.
- Research and create a file of educational programs of interest.
- Research and create a file of potential future professional opportunities.
- Read nursing journals and attend conventions to keep up on the latest within your profession.
- Participate/volunteer for a grassroots political activity that relates to your professional interests (e.g., city council races, PTA elections).

TERMS TO KNOW

committee
mission
professional association (organization)
strategic plan
values

REFERENCES

American Medical Association. Web site/membership services. Retrieved July 13, 2002, from www.ama-assn.org.

Cronin, S. N., & Becherer, D. (1999). Recognition of staff nurse job performance and achievements: Staff and manager perceptions. *Journal of Nursing Administration, 29*(1), 26–31.

Joel, L. (2003). *Kelly's Dimensions of professional nursing* (9th ed.). New York: McGraw-Hill.

Marquis, B., & Huston, C. (2000). *Leadership roles and management functions in nursing: Theory and application* (3rd ed.). Philadelphia: Lippincott.

Mason, D., Leavitt, J., & Chaffee, M. W. (2002). *Policy and politics in nursing and health care* (4th ed.). Philadelphia: Saunders.

Robert III, H. M., Evans, J. W., Honemann, D. H., & Balch, T. J. (Eds.). (2000). *Robert's rules of order newly revised* (10th ed.). Cambridge, MA: Perseus Book Group.

Villarruel, A. M., & Peragallo, N. (2004). Leadership development of Hispanic nurses. *Nursing Administration Quarterly, 28,* 173–180.

Yoder-Wise, P. S. (2006). Professional issues: Creating the challenge. *Annual Review of Nursing Education,4,* 67–83.

SUGGESTED READINGS

Covey, S. R. (1991). *Principle-centered leadership.* New York: Fireside.

Lindell, A. R. (2000). Insights and inquiry: Why would one want to be president of a major association? *Journal of Professional Nursing, 16*(3), 131.

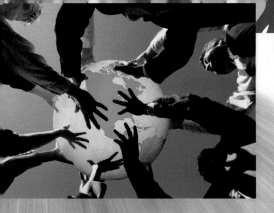

Chapter

29

Thriving for the Future

Patricia S. Yoder-Wise

T his chapter explores the potential for the future and how the changes we face can be maximized to our benefit—organizationally and personally. Key leadership skills are presented, as are strategies for visioning activities about the future. Projections for the future and their implication for nursing are included.

Objectives

- Value the need to think about the future while meeting current expectations.
- Ponder two or three projections for the future and what they mean to the practice of nursing.

- Determine three projections for the future that have implications for individual practice.

Questions to Consider

- How will the future of nursing differ from what you see in practice today?
- How will you be prepared to manage the changes that will occur?
- Where will you learn about the projected changes to incorporate into your own work?
- What life changes do you believe will occur that will in turn affect your professional role?

The Challenge

Sara McCumber, APRN, BC, MSN
Adult/Family Nurse Practitioner, Duluth Clinic, Duluth, Minnesota

I had been working for several years and had just accepted a position as a correctional nurse working with high-risk adolescents and adults. I pictured my job of completing physical assessments and managing the medication-delivery system. Over time, I learned that I was working with a population that was poor, had high-risk health behaviors, lacked access to health care, and often had physical and mental health problems. They often were returned to the community with many of the same problems. As the only nurse and health advocate in the facility, I realized that I had to search out and develop innovative solutions to the multitude of unmet health needs. I also knew I didn't have the skills or experiences to develop effective interventions. I also figured out that there were no likely changes in the future that would improve the care for this population.

 What do you think you would do if you were this nurse?

INTRODUCTION

Leading and managing in nursing constitute a consistent challenge. Even nurses who expect to be followers find that new demands call for continuous leadership and increased self-management skills. More important, the work of the future is being accomplished in teams, and a strong team does not emerge from weak members. You may have heard President Harry S. Truman's often-quoted phrase, "The buck stops here." But Michael Hammer, author of *Beyond Reengineering*, in the videotape "The Secrets of Shared Leadership," says, "The buck stops everywhere!" The point is we are all accountable for something, and unless our part in the overall scheme is inconsequential, which it usually is not, we must lead when we have the insight, the ability, or the skill that is needed to move a situation forward. Sometimes, merely articulating the problem and posing solutions demonstrates leadership (Fagin, 2000). Thus, every nurse has some leadership role to execute in practice.

LEADERSHIP DEMANDS FOR THE FUTURE

Nurse administrators and leaders consistently say that the characteristic they are most seeking in tomorrow's professional nurse is leadership. In probing what that means, we often find themes that relate to our activities that may have serendipitous outcomes. We shape the public's view of the profession, the organization in which we work, and health care in general. We influence interdisciplinary views of what it is to be a professional, and we create the expectations about what the profession's potential can be. All of those examples form some of the leadership potential that exists for the future.

If we think about the world as a loose web, we know that every element has the potential to influence every other element. This connectivity with each other, whether within our profession or within the team, means that we influence others all of the time. This influence molds our practices and beliefs as we move health care forward and also changes how we influence others subsequently.

LEADERSHIP STRENGTHS FOR THE FUTURE

Six leadership strengths seem to be what are needed for the future (Lipman-Blumen, 2000). Box 29-1 provides a summary. Any one of these strengths is valuable to an organization, but the combination

Six Leadership Strengths for the Future

Ethical political savvy: knowing how to effect change and use resources from an ethical, altruistic perspective

Authenticity and accountability: being committed to the group rather than self, which leads to credibility; to be open in decisions

Politics of commonalities: ensuring an environment that allows as many stakeholders as possible to achieve at least a part of their respective agendas

Thinking long-term, acting short-term: committing to what is best for the future and acting in the present to move toward that goal, including developing the future leadership to succeed current leaders

Leadership through expectation: encouraging others through expectations rather than through micromanagement

Quest for meaning: leaving a legacy through guiding others

From Lipman-Blumen , J. (2000, Summer). The age of connective leadership. *Leader to Leader, 17,* 39-45.

strength in inclusivity (politics of commonalities). This is in contrast to what many of us face in our everyday work of not capitalizing on thinking long-term and acting short-term. Much of the work of the Institute for Healthcare Improvement (www.ihi.org), for example, is built around the fact that change is slow and cumbersome. When we are faced with the pressures of providing care to patients versus changing the system, we often remain focused on the patient, thus losing the opportunity to change an issue for many patients. Clearly, to be effective in the future, we must embrace the opportunities to think longer term so that more people are affected by our actions. Again, perhaps because of our history of attention to details, we may need to challenge ourselves in developing our ability for leadership through expectation. Moving from micromanagement to focusing on setting expectations for those for whom we are accountable may feel uncomfortable. Yet, it is that movement that reinforces our ability to deal with longer term issues. Additionally, the quest for meaning suggests that our actions today create the foundation on which future leaders will build. Thus, if we fail to capitalize on today's opportunities, we are diminishing the place at which future leaders will start their careers. It is incumbent on us to raise expectations about what comprises good, safe, quality care, and how nurses contribute to those expectations.

These abilities are ones that develop over time, but the key is that the foundation is present. As Porter-O'Grady, Igein, Alexander, Blaylock, McComb, and Williams (2005) indicated, critical thinking allows us to build and renew the necessary foundation. (See the *Literature Perspective.*) Our foundation begins with our concern for and advocacy about patient care. That foundation is fairly well-engrained in professional nurses' beliefs. The movement from focusing on the nurse-patient relationship to the big picture of nursing (politics and public or health policy activities) may take several years, but the foundation is there (Fagin, 2000). What we do in our professional lives is the legacy we leave for future generations.

of all makes a leader invaluable. Ethical, political savvy can be based on the Code of Ethics for Nurses (American Nurses Association [ANA], 2001), the Scope and Standards for Nurse Administrators (ANA, 2004), and Fagin's work (2000). Basing our actions on ethical principles to affect the political system that influences the availability of healthcare (and other) resources allows us to demonstrate the trust the public places in us. Most of us have capitalized on our authenticity and accountability to demonstrate our concern for others, whether through collective action, crying with families, or listening carefully to what our colleagues and clients say. Because so much of nursing's work is accomplished in teams, we have considerable

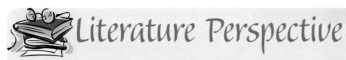

Literature Perspective

Porter-O'Grady, T., Igein, G., Alexander, D., Blaylock, J., McComb, D., & Williams, S. (2005). Critical thinking for nursing leadership. *Nurse Leader, 3*(4), 28-31.

Eight authors were cited in a table exemplifying 18 attributes of critical-thinking. Of the attributes cited, only analysis, evaluation, and judgment were cited by all 18 authors. "The organization and discipline of critical process becomes increasingly important in the requisites for good thinking, especially in times of great change" (p. 29).

The authors define critical-thinking as a disciplined process of reflection and thinking so that actions are based on substantive information. Although critical-thinking has been emphasized in nursing education programs, it has not always been tied to leadership practices. The authors see the process of critical-thinking as comprising interpretation of data and circumstance; analysis to determine relationships; inference for conclusions, evaluation, and explanation about the con-clusions; and self-regulation in reflecting on the process to determine that best efforts were made. The leader's key task is then to saturate the organization with the process so that all employees are doing their best.

"Leaders create context. A part of creating context in the clinical environment is the generation of a *spirit of critical thinking*" (p. 31). This means that our obligation is to create the environment in which critical-thinking flourishes.

IMPLICATIONS FOR PRACTICE
Nurses are well-prepared in the skill of thinking critically. The urgency of the immediate cannot become the tyranny of quality. Rather, nurses must think critically for themselves and foster an environment in which such activity is highly valued, as both a clinical and a leadership skill.

Exercise 29-1
Using the six strengths cited previously, write a description of what you believe your strengths to be. Provide as much detail as possible so that the description helps you see your best strengths.

Nurses who seek leadership opportunities will find that there are many available—in the employment setting, in professional organizations, and in voluntary, community organizations. Balancing the multiple demands in an era of rapid changes and the resultant new expectations becomes an even greater challenge. Merely being employed is no longer sufficient; we must be *employable*. This suggests that we must constantly be focused on competence, on learning, on what the future holds, and on what patients want and need. Failure to do so will make us unemployable and will make the profession undesirable. To be valued in the future, we need to know what the future might encompass. In fact, in 2000 Sigma Theta Tau International identified that one of the eight skills needed for career success was to become a "futures thinker" (Sigma Theta Tau, 2000).

VISIONING

Whether you are a leader, a follower, or a manager, being able to visualize in your mind what the ideal future is becomes a critical strategy. A **vision** can range from that of an individual to that of a group or to a whole organization. No matter how we engage in this visioning activity, we must be open and honest about what we think for the future. Creating our own circle of advisors or brain trusts (those who do not necessarily think as we do, but who are creative thinkers) allows us to test ideas so that we enhance our own thinking and performance to higher levels. Peter Senge, author of *The Fifth Discipline: The Art and Practice of the Learning Organization* (1990), says that all leadership is really about is people working at their best to create the future. And, that, in reality, is what we do everyday.

This chapter is designed to share some views about the future so that you can think about them in relation to what it means to lead and manage. This "thinking about" the future, like visions, is further enriched through sharing in open dialogues.

Select a group of three or four peers and brainstorm about what you think the future of nursing will be. Consider how technology will affect what we do; consider where our primary place of service will be and how we will deliver care. Think about the changes in society and the political pressures for effective health care and what those might mean for nursing. Create a list of ideas to share with others.

Although no one knows the future for certain, there are many entities that engage in formal discussions and predictions. These range from structured groups, such as the World Future Society (http://www.wfs.org), to regular reports and books. Although not everyone is a futurist, each of us needs to be aware of trends. Thinking about the future should be mind expanding; it is the most nonstereotypical thinking you can do. In everyday practice, you can ask yourself and others, "what if" questions. We take for granted that certain practices have remained unchanged. Yet, technology *and* creative thinkers and investigators prove us wrong on a regular basis.

If the future is about teams and group work (which it is), there are many implications for nursing. Skills related to working with others and facilitating their work and ways to reach decisions about practice and the workplace will be crucial. If the work is group-based, how will evaluations and compensation be structured in the future? Will you receive favorable reviews because the group you work with is productive? Will a group receive a bonus or merit salary increase? If you are not a team player, will you be useful to the organization at all? This is one example of how to rethink the future.

■ *Exercise 29–3*

Consider the above questions and suggest how compensation will be formed in the future.

SHARED VISIONS

The concept of **shared visions** suggests that several of us buy into a particular view. If we think of a familiar concept, stress, and what Selye (1976) described as eustress and distress, we have a continuum.

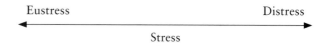

Again, if you think about stress, you recall that each of us views an event differently and that having no stress results in death. Comparably, we can think about how society is evolving currently. Stability and total **chaos** are the ends of a continuum. Moving in some way between those two ends suggests that we live in a constant state of disequilibrium in which we strive toward stability while recognizing we experience chaos. The figure below suggests that in times of great stability, society makes little progress (but life probably seems serene). In times of great chaos, in contrast, society may transform itself (and life may seem uncontrollable). Thus it is even more important to think about the projections for the future. As one example for most of us, think what we were doing, thinking, believing, and valuing on September 10, 2001. Then think about each in relation to September 11, 2001. We moved from some point on that continuum closer to chaos no matter where we were in the world.

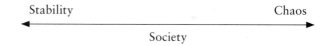

As we move from "traditional" practices to evidence-based ones, we can assume that we might experience more chaos. The comfort of the known is gone; rather practices are evaluated on a regular basis and changes are incorporated so that we are all doing the latest "best" for patients. As the Research Perspective illustrates, many nurses are ill prepared to function in the evolving evidence-based practice environment. Yet, it is our ability to retrieve information and analyze and evaluate it that influences our currency with practice expectations. We seem to value the need for shared visions, which include the idea of operating from a rich data-based approach. To be able to do so, however, we also need to hone our skills in projecting for the future so we know where practice is headed.

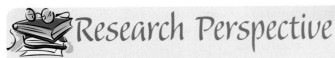

Research Perspective

Pravikoff, D.S., Tanner, A.B., & Pierce, S.T. (2005). Readiness of US nurses for evidence-based practice. *American Journal of Nursing, 105*(9), 40–51.

This is a descriptive, exploratory survey that was mailed to a geographically stratified random sample of 3000 registered nurses in the United States; 760 clinical nurses responded. The distribution was reflective of the distribution of nurses within the defined regions in the United States. The survey tool consisted of 93 items that had various response formats. Some items were direct response (e.g., yes); others were rank-order responses. Key findings included: 58% of the respondents said that they did not use research reports at all; 82% indicated they never used the hospital library; only 46% of the respondents said they were familiar with the term "evidence-based"; 57% said their organization did not have a library; 83% said they considered themselves somewhat (or better) successful in Internet searches, but only 19% felt successful in using CINAHL and 36% in using MEDLINE. Additionally, 83% never or rarely sought a librarian's assistance; 82% did not use the library (where one existed); and 77% had not received instruction in the use of electronic resources. Only 36% said they had access to electronic databases at work; only 40% had unit based access to journals. In the ranking section (lack of time was cited in the survey and excluded from the options due to the previous studies indicating that this was always the first choice response), lack of value for research in practice was the number one ranking item!

IMPLICATIONS FOR PRACTICE

Nurse respondents in this study indicated that they knew they needed knowledge to perform adequately, yet they often did not take advantage of services (if such were available) and defined that the resources were not available. Dramatic changes must occur in clinical areas, preferably at the unit level, to link nurses with the knowledge they need to effect quality care.

PROJECTIONS FOR THE FUTURE

If you watch future reports on television or read *Trend Letter* or *The Futurist* (The World Society publication) or current books (such as *The World is Flat: a Brief History of the Twenty-First Century* by Thomas L. Friedman), you will find comparable themes about the future. The following are some forecasts for the future that will affect nursing; it is possible to ask the "what if" questions with each:

- Knowledge will change dramatically, requiring that we all be dedicated learners.
- Knowledge will evolve from the intensity of the current information evolution so that we will access content with meaning and applicability for our work.
- A power shift will occur toward health care because of the intensity of the developing knowledge and its use in making cost-effective decisions about care.

- The healthcare system will have to change in order to remain financially viable and as employers limit healthcare coverage and genetics allow us to know more about how an individual would respond to treatment, a shift toward eliminating the current disparities is more likely to occur.
- The world will be seen increasingly as a continuum without borders that prevent trade and inventions, including those related to health care.
- Technology will continue to revolutionize health care.
- Increasing diversity will result in:
  - More people who are older.
  - More people moving to different parts of the country or the world.
  - A greater need for speaking two or three languages.
- People no longer will be satisfied with service; they will want an experience.
- There will be increased violence and simultaneously an increased expectation for civility.

- Stores will be either very small or huge.
- Macromarketing (targeting masses) will be out; micromarketing (targeting specific populations) will be in.
- Job security will be out; career options will be in.
- Competition will be out; cooperation will be in.
- Work will be sporadic.
- More people will be living with chronic diseases.
- More people will be overweight and consequently experience various related diseases.
- Bioengineering will make possible interventions that currently do not exist.
- Emphasis on prevention will redirect care efforts.
- Work will be accomplished by teams.
- Everyone will need to be a leader.

Exercise 29-4

Review the list of projections and consider how each might affect what you envision as your career. Make a note of one or two phrases that are the top implications. Look at the list again, and evaluate each of the items to determine which ones you believe will be most important to you. Rank order the top five. Compare your list with two or three colleagues' lists, and offer your rationale for your selection. After you hear other viewpoints, consider if you would change your own rankings.

IMPLICATIONS

So should we be concerned with these forecasts? Are they likely to come true? Historically, Cornish (1997) analyzed the predictions from the February

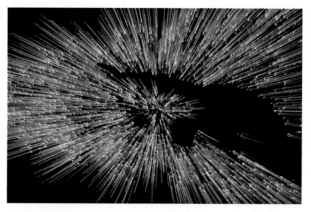

The future explodes with potential.

1967 issue of *The Futurist*. Of the 34 forecasts that could be judged, 23 were accurate, and 11 were not. However, some of the 11 were accurate trends that did not meet the targeted date, often because of shifting national priorities, such as funding. If this is true historically, we might assume that forecasting, which becomes better refined each year, will continue to be a valuable tool for the future.

CONCLUSION

Numerous changes will occur throughout our lifetimes. It is only a matter of time before we say (if we haven't already), "when I was young . . .". Our description might be of something that today is considered fairly advanced. For those who want to thrive, the future forecasts are like the gold ring on the merry-go-round. If you risk and reach far enough, you can grasp it! Lead on . . . ¡Adelánte!

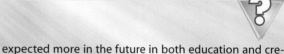

The Solution

I joined the professional organization for correctional health professionals and reviewed nursing publications to identify some of the possible options that were viewed as currently successful or likely to happen in the near future. I networked with colleagues at local and state meetings and identified that a graduate degree in public health nursing would help me develop the skills to address the health needs of my population. I also decided to pursue the Clinical Nurse Specialist in Community Health Nursing certification. I was clear that society

expected more in the future in both education and credentials. Additionally, I believed that I had the skills to develop community programs and research studies to help me address the high-risk needs of my client population.

— Sara McCumber

Would this be a suitable approach for you? Why?

CHAPTER CHECKLIST

This chapter addresses the need to think about the future, and what that means for current practice involvement by all nurses is what is needed to keep the profession relevant to the constantly emerging future.

   Six leadership strengths are needed for the future.

- Ethical political savvy
- Authenticity and accountability
- Politics of commonalities
- Thinking long-term, acting short-term
- Quest for meaning
- Visioning irrespective of your role in the profession.

   Shared visions are important.
   Numerous projections for the future can shape what our individual and collective practices will be.

TERMS TO KNOW

chaos
shared vision
vision

REFERENCES

American Nurses Association (ANA). (2001). *Code of ethics for nurses with interpretive statements.* Washington, DC: The Association.

ANA. (2004). *Scope and standards for nurse administrators* (2nd ed). Washington DC: The Association.

Cornish, E. (1997, January/February). The Futurist forecasts 30 years later. *The Futurist, 31,* 45–48.

Fagin, C. (2000). *Essays on nursing leadership.* New York: Springer.

Lipman-Blumen, J. (2000, Summer). The age of connective leadership. *Leader to Leader, 17,* 39–45.

Porter-O'Grady, T., Igein, G., Alexander, D., Blaylock, J., McComb, D., & Williams, S. (2005). Critical thinking for nursing leadership. *Nurse Leader, 3*(4), 28–31.

Pravikoff, D. S., Tanner, A. B., & Pierce, S. T. (2005). Readiness of US nurses for evidence-based practice. *American Journal of Nursing, 105*(9), 40–51.

Selye, H. (1976). *The stress of life.* New York: McGraw-Hill.

Senge, P. (1990). *The fifth discipline: The art and practice of the learning organization.* New York: Doubleday Currency.

Sigma Theta Tau International. (2000). Eight skills for a healthy career. *Reflections, 26*(1), 20–21.

SUGGESTED READINGS

Begun, J. W., & White, K. R. (1995). Altering nursing's dominant logic: Guidelines from complex adaptive systems theory. *Complexity and Chaos in Nursing, 2*(1), 5–15.

Rubin, H. (2000, March). Here are the 10 commandments of leadership that I carried down from the mountaintop. *Fast Company,* 276–280.

Glossary

Absenteeism The rate at which an individual misses work on an unplanned basis. (Ch. 24)

Accommodation An unassertive, cooperative approach to conflict in which the individual neglects personal needs, goals, and concerns in favor of satisfying those of others. (Ch. 22)

Accountability The expectation of explaining actions and results. (Ch. 23)

Accreditation Process by which an authoritative body determines that an organization meets certain standards to such a degree that the organization is able to meet the standards as a whole and without ongoing monitoring of each aspect of performance. (Ch. 6)

Acknowledgment Recognition that an employee is valued and respected for what he or she has to offer to the workplace, team, or group; acknowledgments may be verbal or written, public or private. (Ch. 17)

Active listening Focusing completely on the speaker and listening without judgment to the essence of the conversation; an active listener should be able to repeat accurately at least 95% of the speaker's intended meaning. (Ch. 17)

Activity or productivity report A report typically including units of service provided, number of beds, number of occupied beds, number of patients typically cared for per day, and average length of stay. (Ch. 13)

Advocate One who proactively speaks for another to ensure certain needs or wishes are met. (Ch. 21)

Agenda A written list of items to be covered in a meeting and the related materials that meeting participants should read beforehand or bring along. Types of agendas include structured agendas, timed agendas, and action agendas. (Ch. 26)

Allocation of scarce resources Distribution of resources needed for care but which may exceed budget levels. (Ch. 22)

Apparent agency Doctrine whereby a principal becomes accountable for the actions of his or her agent; created when a person holds himself or herself out as acting on behalf of the principal; also known as *apparent authority*. (Ch. 4)

Associate nurse A licensed nurse in the primary care model who provides care to the patient according to the primary nurse's specification when the primary nurse is not working. (Ch. 12)

At–will employee An individual who works without a contract. (Ch. 18)

Autocratic An authoritarian style that places control within one person's position. (Ch. 5)

Autonomy Personal freedom and the right to choose what will happen to one's own person. (Ch. 4)

Average daily census (ADC) Average number of patients cared for per day for a reporting period. (Ch. 13)

Average length of stay The number of patient days in a specific time period divided by the number of discharges in that same time period. (Ch. 13)

Avoiding An unassertive, uncooperative approach to conflict in which the avoider neither pursues his or her own needs, goals, and concerns nor helps others to do so. (Ch. 22)

Bar coding systems/bar code technology Systems that encode data electronically into a format of bars and spaces that represents letters or numbers. (Ch. 10)

Barriers Factors, internal or external to the change situation, that interfere with movement toward a desirable outcome. (Ch. 16)

Benchmarking Best practices, processes, or systems identified by a quality improvement team to be compared with the practice, process, or system under review. (Ch. 19)

Beneficence Principle that states that the actions one takes should promote good. (Ch. 4)

Biomedical technology The use of machines and implantable devices to provide physiological monitoring, diagnostic testing, drug administration, and therapeutic treatments in patient care. (Ch. 10)

Budget A detailed financial plan, stated in dollars, for carrying out the activities an organization wants to accomplish within a specific period. (Ch. 11)

Budgeting process An ongoing activity of planning and managing revenues and expenses to meet the goals of the organization. (Ch. 11)

Bureaucracy Characterized by formality, low autonomy, a hierarchy of authority, an environment of rules, division of labor, specialization, centralization, and control. (Ch. 7)

Burnout Disengagement from work characterized by emotional exhaustion, depersonalization, and decreased effectiveness. (Ch. 26)

Capital expenditure budget A plan for purchasing major capital items, such as equipment or a physical plant, with a useful life greater than 1 year and exceeding a minimum cost set by the organization. (Ch. 11)

Capitation A reimbursement method in which healthcare providers are paid a per-person-per-year (or per-month) fee for providing specified services over a period of time. (Ch. 11)

Care MAP Abbreviation for a Multidisciplinary Action Plan, which combines a nursing care plan with a critical path. The purpose is to expedite patient care by improving the expected outcome during a designated hospital day. (Ch. 12)

Career Progressive achievement throughout a person's professional life. (Ch. 27)

Case management A person-oriented service that reflects multidisciplinary cooperation and coordination. (Ch. 3)

Case-management model A model of delivering patient care based on patient outcomes and cost containment. Components of case management are a case manager, critical paths/critical pathways, and unit based managed care. (Ch. 12)

Case manager A baccalaureate or master's degree-prepared clinical nurse who coordinates patient care from preadmission through discharge. (Ch. 12)

Case method A model of care delivery in which one nurse provides total care for a patient during an entire work period. (Ch. 12)

Case mix The volume and type of patients served by a healthcare provider. (Ch. 11)

Cash budget A plan for an organization's cash receipts and disbursements. (Ch. 11)

Centers for Disease Control and Prevention (CDC) The main federal agency protecting the health and safety of people in the United States. (Ch. 18)

Certification Designation of special knowledge beyond basic licensure. (Ch. 27)

Chain of command The hierarchy depicted in vertical dimensions of organizational charts. (Ch. 7)

Change agents Individuals with formal or informal legitimate power whose purpose is to initiate, champion, and direct or guide change. (Ch. 16)

Change management The overall processes and strategies used to moderate and manage the preparation for, effect of, responses to, and outcomes of any condition or circumstance that is new or different from what existed previously. (Ch. 16)

Change outcome The end product of a change process. (Ch. 16)

Change process The series of ongoing efforts applied to managing a change. (Ch. 16)

Change situations The field comprised of various factors and dynamics within which change is occurring. (Ch. 16)

Chaos A condition of disorder or confusion. (Ch. 29)

Chaos theory Theoretical construct defining the random-appearing, yet deterministic, characteristics of complex organizations (see *Nonlinear change*). (Ch. 16)

Charge nurse A registered nurse responsible for delegating and coordinating patient care and staff on a specific unit. A resource person for all staff; there is usually one charge nurse each shift per unit. (Ch. 12)

Charges The cost of providing a service plus a markup for profit. (Ch. 11)

Chemically dependent A psychophysiological state in which an individual requires a substance, such as drugs or alcohol, to prevent the onset of symptoms of abstinence. (Ch. 24)

Clinical guidelines Statements of practice expectations developed by a group of healthcare practitioners to guide the clinical management of patients. (Ch. 20)

Clinical Nurse Leader An evolving role of the professional nurse being developed by the American Association of Colleges of Nursing (AACN). (Ch. 12)

Closed shop A collective bargaining situation that requires membership (or at least dues-equivalent payment) (as opposed to open shop). (Ch. 28)

Coaching The strategy a manager uses to help others learn, think critically, and grow through communications about performance. (Ch. 14)

Coalitions Groups of individuals or organizations that join together temporarily around a common goal. This goal often focuses on an effort to effect change. (Ch. 9)

Collaboration Conjoint, interdisciplinary problem solving from an equal power base on the patient's behalf; also, an assertive, cooperative approach to conflict in which the individual is able to work creatively and openly with others to find the solution that best achieves all important goals. (Ch. 22)

Collective action A mechanism for achieving professional practice through group decision making. (Ch. 18)

Collective bargaining Mechanism for settling labor disputes by negotiation between the employer and representatives of the employees. (Chs. 4, 18, 28)

Commitment A state of being emotionally impelled; feeling passionate about and dedicated to a project or event. (Ch. 17)

Committees A small group of appointed or elected individuals to serve an express function or to accomplish a specific goal for the organization (e.g., advisory committee, policy and agenda committee). (Ch. 28)

Common law System of jurisprudence that is derived from principles rather than rules and regulations and that consists of comprehensive principles based on justice, reason, and common sense. (Ch. 4)

Competing Assertive, uncooperative approach to conflict in which the individual pursues own needs at the expense of others. (Ch. 22)

Complexity theory Requires leaders to expand and respond to engaging dynamic change and focus on relationships rather than on prescribing and approaching change as a lock-step, pre-prescribed method. Traditional organizational hierarchy plays a less significant role as the "keeper of high level knowledge" and replaces it with the idea that knowledge applied to complex problems is better distributed among the human assets within an organization, without regard to hierarchy. Leaders try less to control the future and spend more time influencing, innovating and responding to the many factors that influence health care. (Ch. 1)

Compromising Moderately assertive, cooperative approach to conflict in which the individual's ability to negotiate and willingness to give and take results in conflict resolution and fulfillment of priorities for all involved. (Ch. 22)

Computerized prescriber order entry (CPOE) System that uses computers for creating orders for care to be made electronically and to coordinate with other elements of an individual's care and record so that one entry performs multiple functions. (Ch. 10)

Confidentiality Right of privacy to the medical record of a patient; also, a respect for the privacy of information and the ethical use of information for its original purpose. (Ch. 4)

Conflict A perceived difference among people and a four-stage process including frustration, conceptualization, action, and outcomes. (Ch. 22)

Consolidated systems A group of healthcare organizations that are united based on common characteristics of ownership, regional location, or mutual performance objectives for the purpose of optimizing utilization of their resources in achieving their missions. (Ch. 6)

Consumer focus Centering of action or attention on the participant or user as a whole. (Ch. 21)

Continuing education Learning activities intended to build on educational and experiential bases of the professional nurse for enhancement of practice, education, administration, research, or theory development to improve public health (ANCC, 1991). (Ch. 27)

Continuous quality improvement (CQI) A comprehensive program designed to continually improve the quality of care. Often used interchangeably with total quality management, quality management, quality improvement, and performance improvement. (Ch. 19)

Contractual allowance A discount from full charges. (Ch. 11)

Coping The immediate response of a person to a threatening situation. (Ch. 26)

Corporate liability The condition of being responsible for corporate loss related to acts performed and not performed in meeting obligations to operate legally and judiciously. (Ch. 4)

Cost The amount spent on something; the national healthcare costs are a function of the price and utilization of healthcare services; a healthcare provider's costs are the expenses involved in providing goods or services. (Ch. 11)

Cost–based reimbursement A retrospective payment method in which all allowable costs are used as the basis for payment. (Ch. 11)

Cost center An organizational unit for which costs can be identified and managed. (Chs. 11, 13)

Creativity Conceptualizing new and innovative approaches to solving problems or making decisions. (Ch. 5)

Critical Path/Critical Pathway A component of a care MAP that is specific to diagnosis-related group reimbursement. The purpose is to ensure patients are discharged before insurance reimbursement is eliminated. (Ch. 12)

Critical-thinking A composite of knowledge, attitudes, and skills; an intellectually disciplined process. Also, the ability to assess a situation by asking open-ended questions about the facts and assumptions that underlie it and to use personal judgment and problem-solving ability in deciding how to deal with it. (Ch. 5)

Cross–culturalism Mediating between and among cultures. (Ch. 8)

Cultural competence The process in which the healthcare provider continuously strives to achieve the ability to effectively work within the cultural context of a patient (Camphina-Bacote, 1999). This includes attitudes, behaviors, and policies that allow people to work together effectively in cross-cultural situations. (Chs. 8, 21)

Cultural diversity A vast range of cultural differences related to institutional, ethnic, gender, religious, or other variables that convey a set of beliefs or values that have become factors needing attention in living and working together. It is often applied to an organization that seeks to deal with the interface of people who are different from each other (Simons et al., 1993). (Ch. 8)

Cultural imposition Tendency of an individual or group to impose their values, beliefs, and practices on another culture (Leininger, 2002b). (Ch. 8)

Cultural marginality Situations and feelings when people exist between two different cultures and do not yet perceive themselves as belonging to either one (Choi, 2001). (Ch. 8)

Cultural sensitivity Capacity to feel, convey, and react to ideas, habits, customs, or traditions unique to a group of people. (Ch. 8)

Culture A way of life. It is developed and communicated by a group of people, consciously or unconsciously, to subsequent generations. It consists of ideas, habits, attitudes, customs, and traditions that help create standards for a group of people to coexist. It makes a group of people unique (Simons et al., 1993). (Chs. 8, 18)

Curriculum vitae A listing of professional life activities. (Ch. 27)

Cybernetic theory Regulation of systems by managing communication and feedback mechanisms. (Ch. 16)

Data Discrete entities that describe or measure something without interpretation. (Ch. 10)

Database A collection of data elements organized and stored together. (Ch. 10)

Decision–making Purposeful and goal-directed effort using a systematic process to choose among options. (Ch. 5)

Deeming authority A power granted by one with power so that the recipient acts in his or her place. (Ch. 6)

Delegatee The individual who becomes accountable for performing delegated activities. (Ch. 23)

Delegation Achieving performance of care outcomes for which an individual is accountable and responsible by sharing activities with other individuals who have the appropriate authority to accomplish the work. (Chs. 23, 26)

Delegator The individual with authority to share activities with another. (Ch. 23)

Democratic A leadership style that places control within the group at large where shared authority leads to decisions. (Ch. 5)

Depersonalization Inability to become involved in human relationships and interactions. (Ch. 26)

Differentiated Nursing Practice A model of care that recognizes the difference in the level of education and competency of each registered nurse. The differentiation is based on education, position, and clinical expertise. (Ch. 12)

Diffusion of innovation Process by which ideas spread through a culture. (Ch. 20)

Disease management Continuous, coordinated processes to manage the progression of care over the course of a disease. (Ch. 12)

Dualism An "either/or" way of conceptualizing reality in terms of two opposing sides or parts (right or wrong, yes or no), limiting the broad spectrum of possibilities that exists between. (Ch. 17)

E–learning Learning supported by the use of a Web-based electronic format. (Ch. 10)

E-mail A telecommunications system in which a computer user can exchange messages with other computer users via a network. (Ch. 10)

Effective communication A process that leads to positive outcomes for senders and receivers in terms of clarity, usefulness, and efficiency. (Ch. 17)

Electronic medical record (EMR) Computer-based patient record that capitalizes on the features of electronic processes. (Ch. 10)

Electronic medication administration record (e–MAR) Electronic format of the centralized information pertaining to medications administered to a patient. (Ch. 10)

Emancipated minor Person under the age of adulthood who is no longer under the control and regulation of parents and who may give valid consent for medical procedures; examples include married teens, underaged parents, and teens in the armed services. (Ch. 4)

Emerging workforce The so-called twenty-something generation that was born between the years of 1965 and 1985. (Ch. 2)

Emotional intelligence Monitoring emotions in a situation to guide actions and inform thought processes. (Ch. 1)

Employee assistance programs Programs designed to provide counseling and other services for employees through either in-house staff or a contracted mental health agency. (Ch. 26)

Empowerment A sharing of power and control with the expectation that people are responsible for themselves; also, the process by which we facilitate the participation of others in decision making within an environment where there is an equitable distribution of power. (Chs. 9, 14, 18)

Entrenched workforce Employed persons over the age of 35 who are thought of as the Baby Boomer generation. (Ch. 2)

Ergonomics Science of fitting the job to the worker. (Ch. 4)

Ethics Science relating to moral actions and moral values; rules of conduct recognized in respect to a particular class of human actions. (Ch. 4)

Ethics committee Group of persons who provide structure and guidelines for potential healthcare problems, serve as an open forum for discussion, and function as patient advocates. (Ch. 4)

Ethnicity One's migratory status, race, language, and dialect and sense of distinctiveness (Spector, 2000). (Ch. 8)

Ethnocentrism Using the culture of one's own groups as a standard for the judgment of others, or thinking of it as superior to other cultures that are merely different (Simons et al., 1993). (Ch. 8)

Evidence–based practice The integration of individual clinical expertise, built from practice, with the best available clinical evidence from systematic research applied to practice. (Chs. 10, 20)

Expected outcomes The result of patient goals that are achieved through a combination of medical and nursing interventions with patient participation. (Ch. 12)

Expert system A program that mimics the inductive and deductive reasoning of a human expert. (Ch. 10)

Expert witness Person testifying who has special knowledge about a given subject; knowledge of expert witnesses must generally be such that it is not normally possessed by the average person; contrasts with a lay witness. (Ch. 4)

Facilitators Factors, internal or external to the change situation, that promote movement toward a desired outcome. (Ch. 16)

Factor evaluation system A patient classification system that incorporates specific elements or critical indicators and rates patients on each of these elements. Each indicator is assigned a weight or numerical value. (Ch. 13)

Failure to warn Newer area of potential liability for nurse managers that involves the responsibility to warn subsequent or potential employers of nurses' incompetence or impairment. (Ch. 4)

Fee-for-service A system in which patients have the option of consulting any healthcare provider, subject to reasonable requirements that may include utilization review and prior approval for certain services but does not include a requirement to seek approval through a gatekeeper. (Ch. 6)

Fidelity Keeping one's promises or commitments. (Ch. 4)

Fixed costs Costs that do not change in total as the volume of patients changes. (Ch. 11)

Fixed FTEs Full-time equivalent roles that do not fluctuate based on patient care demands. (Ch. 13)

Flat organization Characterized by decentralization of decision-making to the level of personnel carrying out the work. (Ch. 7)

Follower Person who contributes to a group's outcomes by implementing activities and providing appropriate feedback. (Ch. 3)

Followership Those with whom a leader interacts; involves assertive use of personal behaviors in contributing toward organizational outcomes while still acquiescing certain tasks to the leader or other team members. (Chs. 1, 18)

For-profit organization An organization, such as a hospital, that is operated to create excess income (profit) for the benefit of owners or stockholders. (Ch. 6)

Forecast The process of making decisions about the future based on multiple sources of data. (Ch. 13)

Foreseeability Concept that certain events may reasonably be expected to cause specific consequences; third element of negligence/malpractice. (Ch. 4)

Full-time equivalent (FTE) An employee who works fulltime, 40 hours per week, 2080 hours per year. (Chs. 11, 13)

Functional nursing A method of providing patient care by which each licensed and unlicensed staff member performs specific tasks for a large group of patients. (Ch. 12)

Functional structure Arrangement of departments and services by specialties. (Ch. 7)

Gatekeeper Liaison between the consumer and the healthcare market. (Ch. 21)

General adaptation syndrome (GAS) A pattern of response to stress (Selye, 1956). (Ch. 26)

Governance System by which an organization controls and directs formulation and administration of policy. (Ch. 18)

Group A number of individuals assembled together or having a unifying relationship. (Ch. 17)

Halo or recent behavior bias effect Only positive (halo) or recent (recency) performances are acknowledged. (Ch. 14)

Health Insurance Portability and Accountability Act (HIPAA) An act mandating a centralized data base and assuring the public of confidentiality about their health care. (Ch. 10)

Health (medical) literacy An individual's capacity to obtain, process, and understand health information needed to make appropriate health decisions. (Ch. 21)

Healthcare consumer Patient/customer who uses healthcare provider resources. (Ch. 21)

Healthcare provider Agencies, insurers, physicians, nurses, and allied health people providing health-related business to consumers. (Ch. 21)

Hierarchy Chain of command that connotes authority and responsibility. (Ch. 7)

High tech Mechanistic perspective that relates to the use of technology in the diagnosis and treatment of disease. (Ch. 21)

High touch Caring, humanistic perspective that relates to the use of human skills in the care and treatment of patients. (Ch. 21)

High-complexity change A complicated change situation characterized by the interactions of multiple variables of people, technology, and systems. (Ch. 16)

Horizontal integration The condition that results when two (or more) organizations with similar services come together. (Ch. 6)

Horn effect Only negative performances being acknowledged. (Ch. 14)

Hybrid Possessing characteristics from several types of organizational structures. (Ch. 7)

Indemnification Obligation resting on one person to make good any loss or damages another has incurred because of the person's actions or inactions; refers to the total shifting of the economic loss to the party chiefly responsible for that loss. (Ch. 4)

Independent contractor One who makes an agreement with another to perform a service or piece of work and retains in himself or herself control of the means, method, and manner of producing the result to be accomplished; sometimes called an *independent practitioner*. (Ch. 4)

Influence The process of using power; may range from the punitive power of coercion to the interactive power of collaboration. (Ch. 9)

Informal change agent Persons without designated authority who advance the change among a group of people. (Ch. 16)

Informatics The use of knowledge technology. (Ch. 10)

Informatics competencies The integration of knowledge, skills, and attitudes in the performance of various nursing activities that involve data, information, and knowledge within prescribed levels of nursing practice. (Ch. 10)

Information Communication of reception of knowledge, consisting of interpreted, organized, or structured data. (Ch. 10)

Information overload A state of stress brought about by a lack of information-processing skills. (Ch. 26)

Information technology The use of computer hardware and software to process data into information to solve problems. (Ch. 10)

Informed consent Authorization by patient or patient's legal representative to do something to the patient. (Ch. 4)

Internet The worldwide network of computers communicating via an agreed-upon set of protocols. (Ch. 10)

Interpersonal conflict Conflict that occurs between or among people. (Ch. 22)

Intrapersonal conflict Conflict that occurs within an individual. (Ch. 22)

Justice Principle that persons should be treated equally and fairly. (Ch. 4)

Knowledge Information that is combined or synthesized so that interrelationships are identified. (Ch. 10)

Knowledge technology The use of expert and decision support systems to assist in making decisions about patient care delivery. (Ch. 10)

Knowledge worker An individual who performs nonrepetitive, nonroutine work consuming considerable levels of cognitive activity and judgment. (Ch. 10)

Labor cost per unit of service A comparison of budgeted salary costs per budgeted volume of service with actual salary costs per actual volume of service. (Ch. 13)

Labor law Examples of these federal mandates include the 1935 Wagner Act, which established election procedures for collective bargaining representatives, and the 1947 Taft-Hartley Act, which placed curbs on some union activity and excluded employees of not-for-profit hospitals from coverage. (Ch. 18)

Labor union Association of workers that exists for the purpose of bargaining, either in whole or in part, on behalf of the workers with management about the terms of employment. (Ch. 4)

Law Sum total of rules and regulations by which a society is governed; rules and regulations established and enforced by authority or custom within a given community, state, or nation. (Ch. 4)

Leader Person who demonstrates and exercises influence and power over others. (Ch. 3)

Leadership The use of personal traits to constructively and ethically influence patients, families, and staff through a *process* in which clinical and organizational outcomes are achieved through collective efforts. (Chs. 1, 2)

Learning organization The designation of a type of organization in which continual learning as an expectation permeates all levels to promote adequate responses required by dynamic, accelerated change. (Ch. 16)

Liability Refers to one's responsibility for his or her own conduct; an obligation or duty to be performed; responsibility for an action or outcome. (Ch. 4)

Liable Refers to one's responsibility for his or her actions or inactions. (Ch. 4)

Licensure A right granted that gives the licensee permission to do something that he or she could not legally do absent such permission; the minimum form of credentialing, providing baseline expectations for those in a particular field without identifying or obligating the practitioner to function in a professional manner as defined by the profession itself. (Ch. 27)

Line function A function that involves direct responsibility for accomplishing the objectives of a nursing department, service, or unit. (Ch. 7)

Low-complexity change An uncomplicated change situation characterized by the interactions of the limited influences of people, technology, and systems. (Ch. 16)

Magnet recognition A distinction granted by the American Nurses Credentialing Center for quality nursing services. (Chs. 1, 12)

Malpractice Failure of a professional person to act in accordance with the prevalent professional standards or failure to foresee potential consequences that a professional person, having the necessary skills and expertise to act in a professional manner, should foresee. (Ch. 4)

Managed care Care purchased through a public or private healthcare organization whose goal is to promote quality healthcare outcomes for patients at the lowest cost possible through planning, directing, and coordinating care delivered by healthcare organizations that it may own, have contractual agreements with, or have authority over by virtue of the fact that it reimburses the organization for services provided its patients. This model rewards providers for low utilization of care that is relatively low in cost; also, a system of care in which a designated person determines the services the patient uses. (Chs. 3, 6, 11)

Management The activities needed to plan, organize, motivate, and control the human and material resources needed to achieve outcomes consistent with the organization's mission and purpose. (Chs. 1, 2)

Management theory The theory related to the activities described in management. (Ch. 1)

Manager A person who directs a team of workers. (Ch. 3)

Marketing Analysis, planning, implementation, and control of programs for the purpose of meeting organizational objectives. (Ch. 15)

Master staffing plan The overall plan for allocating numbers and types of personnel, taking into consideration numerous factors that predict these factors. (Ch. 13)

Matrix structure An organizational structure influenced by dual authority, such as product line and discipline. (Ch. 7)

Mediation A process using a trained third party to assist with conflict resolution. (Ch. 22)

Mentor An experienced person who helps a less experienced person navigate into expertise. (Chs. 2, 18, 25)

Meta-analysis Statistically combines similar studies on a particular issue to determine if the findings are significant across settings. (Ch. 20)

Mission Statement of an organization's reason for being. (Chs. 7, 28)

Modular Nursing A modified team nursing model focused on the geographic location of patient rooms and assignment of staff members. (Ch. 12)

Motivation The instigation of action based on various factors, both intrinsic and extrinsic. (Ch. 1)

Multiculturalism Maintaining several different cultures. (Ch. 8)

Near miss A clinical situation that resulted in no injury, but that highlights the need for action (i.e. attempted suicide, last minute cancellation of surgery on wrong patient). (Ch. 19)

Negative feedback Information indicating a correction is needed. (Ch. 16)

Negligence Failure to exercise the degree of care that a person of ordinary prudence, based on the reasonable person standard, would exercise under the same or similar circumstances; also known as *ordinary negligence*. (Ch. 4)

Negotiating Conferring with others to bring about a settlement of differences. (Chs. 9, 22)

Networks Resources of colleagues upon whom you can draw for advice; formal systems to provide services. (Chs. 6, 9)

Nonlinear change Change occurring from self-organizing patterns, not human-induced ones, in complex, open system organizations. (Ch. 16)

Nonmaleficence Principle that states that one should do no harm. (Ch. 4)

Nonproductive hours See *Nonproductive time.* (Ch. 11)

Nonproductive time Benefit time such as vacation or sick time. (Ch. 13)

Nonpunitive discipline A disciplinary measure, usually verbal, describing existing standards and goals to which the parties agreed; pay is not withheld; employee either agrees to adhere to the standards in the future or to be terminated. (Ch. 24)

Nurse practice act Legal scope of practice allowed by state legislation and authority. (Ch. 4)

Nursing care delivery model The method used to provide care to patients. (Ch. 12)

Nursing Licensure Compact The mutual recognition model among states that agree to allow a nurse to hold licensure in one state and to practice in other states. (Ch. 3)

Nursing minimum data set (NMDS) Uniform standard for collecting comparable essential patient data. (Ch. 10)

Open shop A contract situation that allows but does not require members to join. (Ch. 28)

Operating budget A financial plan for day-to-day activities of an organization. (Ch. 11)

Optimizing decision Selecting the most ideal solution or option to achieve goals. (Ch. 5)

Organizational chart A chart that defines organizational positions' responsibility for specific functions. (Ch. 7)

Organizational conflict Conflict that occurs when a person confronts an organization's policies and procedures for patient care and personnel and its accepted norms of behavior and communication. (Ch. 22)

Organizational culture The attitudes, behaviors, and policies evident in an organization that create the ambiance and operation of the workplace. (Chs. 3, 7)

Organizational structure A framework that divides work within an organization and delineates points of authority, responsibility, accountability, and non–decision-making support. (Ch. 7)

Organized delivery system (ODS) Network of healthcare organizations, providers, and payers who provide a comprehensive package of healthcare services at a competitive price. (Ch. 11)

OSHA Occupational Safety and Health Administration. (Ch. 18)

Outcome criteria The result of patient goals that are expected to be achieved through a combination of nursing and medical interventions. (Ch. 12)

Outcomes Anticipated or actual effects of program activities and outputs. (Ch. 20)

Overwork A situation in which employees are expected to become more productive without additional resources. (Ch. 26)

Participative Comparable to democratic style; involves others in making decisions. (Ch. 5)

Partnership model A method of providing patient care when an RN is paired with an LPN/LVN or an unlicensed assistive person to provide total care to a number of patients. (Ch. 12)

Paternalism Principle that allows one to make decisions for another; often called *parentalism.* (Ch. 4)

Patient–care outcome A measurable end result of patient care. (Ch. 19)

Patient–focused care A model in which staff functions become centralized on a unit to reduce the number of staff required; emphasizes quality, cost, and value. (Ch. 12)

Patient outcomes See *Expected outcomes.* (Ch. 12)

Patient satisfaction Measurement, frequently by an external service, of patient perception about care and services; frequently presented in reports or ratings and often compared with a prior time period and comparable service. (Ch. 21)

Payer mix The volume and type of reimbursement sources for a healthcare provider. (Ch. 11)

Payers Sources of healthcare financing or payment for health services; includes government, private insurance, and individuals (self-pay). (Ch. 11)

Percentage of occupancy The patient census divided by the number of beds on the unit. (Ch. 13)

Perfectionism The tendency to never finish anything because it isn't quite perfect. (Ch. 26)

Performance appraisal Individual evaluation of work performance. (Ch. 14)

Performance improvement (PI) The application of quality improvement principles on an ongoing basis. Often used interchangeably with total quality management, continuous quality management, quality improvement, and quality management. (Ch. 19)

Personal digital assistant (PDA) Handheld device that contains data such as addresses and schedules; this device may also be web-enabled. (Ch. 10)

Personal liability Serves to make each person responsible at law for his or her own actions. (Ch. 4)

Philosophy Values and beliefs regarding nature of work derived from a mission and the rights/responsibilities of people involved. (Ch. 7)

Planned change Change expected and deliberately prepared beforehand by using systematic directional processes to develop and carry out activities to accomplish a desired outcome. (Ch. 16)

Polarities Situations involving two interdependent opposites between which a shifting of emphasis naturally occurs. (Ch. 22)

Policy A consciously chosen course of action (or inaction) directed toward some end (Kalisch & Kalisch, 1982). (Ch. 9)

Politics A process of human interaction within organizations. (Ch. 9)

Portfolio A professional assemblage of materials that represent the work of the professional. These materials include such elements as evaluations, letters of recommendation or appreciation, certificates of accomplishment, copies of articles, documentation of projects (research, clinical changes, and management projects are examples), additional educational achievements (continuing education and degree achievement). (Ch. 27)

Position description A general overall description of the duties and responsibilities of the employee. (Ch. 14)

Power The ability to influence others in the effort to achieve goals. (Ch. 9)

Primary care First access to care. (Ch. 6)

Primary nurse One who delivers autonomous care. (Ch. 12)

Primary nursing A model of patient care delivery whereby one registered nurse functions autonomously as the patient's main nurse throughout the entire hospital stay. (Ch. 12)

Principlism Emerging theory of ethics that incorporates existing ethical principles and attempts to resolve conflicts by applying one or more of the ethical principles. (Ch. 4)

Privacy The right to protection against unreasonable and unwarranted interference with one's solitude; the right of an individual to be left alone. (Ch. 4)

Private non-profit (or not-for-Profit) organization Organization that has funds redirected to maintenance and growth rather than as dividends to stockholders. (Ch. 6)

Problem–solving Using a systematic process to solve a problem. (Ch. 5)

Process of care The desired sequence of steps that have been designed to achieve clinical standardization. (Ch. 1)

Procrastination Doing one thing when one should be doing something else. (Ch. 26)

Productive hours Paid time that is worked. (Ch. 11)

Productive time Time an employee actually works. (Ch. 13)

Productivity The ratio of outputs to inputs or, in nursing terms, of services to resources used to provide services. (Ch. 11)

Professional association (organization) An alliance of practitioners within a profession that provides opportunities for its members to meet leaders in the field, hone their own leadership skills, participate in policy formation, continue specialized education, and shape the future of the profession. (Chs. 27, 28)

Profit An excess of revenues over expenses. (Ch. 11)

Progressive discipline A step-by-step process of increasing disciplinary measures, usually beginning with an oral warning, followed by a written warning, suspension, and termination, if necessary. (Ch. 24)

Prospective reimbursement A method of payment in which the third-party payer decides in advance the flat rate that will be paid for a service or episode of care. (Ch. 11)

Prototype evaluation system System of classifying in broad categories. (Ch. 13)

Providers See *Healthcare provider.* (Ch. 11)

Public institution Providing health services under the support and direction of local, state, or federal government. (Ch. 6)

Quality assurance (QA) A process that focuses on the clinical aspects of a provider's care, often in response to an identified problem. (Ch. 19)

Quality improvement (QI) An ongoing process of innovation, prevention of error, and staff development used by an organization that has adopted a quality management philosophy. Often used interchangeably with total quality management, continuous quality management, quality improvement, and quality management. (Ch. 19)

Quality indicators Measurable elements of quality that specify the focus of evaluation and documentation. (Chs. 3, 21)

Quality management (QM) A corporate culture emphasizing customer satisfaction, innovation, and employee involvement in quality improvement activities. Often used interchangeably with total quality management, continuous quality management, quality improvement, and performance improvement. (Ch. 19)

Quantum theory A physics theory stating that energy is not a smooth-flowing continuum, but rather bursts of energy that are related. (Ch. 3)

Radio Frequency Identification (RFID) Wireless systems allowing for non-contact reading; capable of tracking movement. (Ch. 10)

Randomized clinical/controlled trial (RCT) Study where patients are assigned by chance to one of the groups defined in the study. (Ch. 20)

Redesign Technique to analyze tasks to improve efficiency. (Ch. 7)

Reengineering A complete overhaul of an organizational structure. (Hammer & Champy, 1993). (Ch. 7)

Research A systematic investigation to determine the truth or falsehood of a hypothesis. (Ch. 20)

Research utilization Process of synthesizing, discriminating, and using research-generated knowledge to make an impact or change in existing practices. (Ch. 20)

Respect for others The highest ethical principle, respect for others acknowledges the right of individuals to make decisions and to live by those decisions. (Ch. 4)

Respondeat superior A doctrine by which the employer is given accountability and responsibility for an employee's negligent actions incurred during the course and scope of employment. (Ch. 4)

Responsibility The condition of being reliable and dependable and being obligated to accomplish work. (Ch. 23)

Restructuring Technique to enhance organizational productivity. (Ch. 7)

Résumé A summary of professional abilities and facts designed for specific opportunities. (Ch. 27)

Revenue Money earned by an organization for providing goods or services. (Ch. 11)

Right-to-work Refers to nonunion workplaces. The employer gives the employee the option to join a union or professional association. The nurse is responsible for direct communication with the employer. (Ch. 28)

Risk management Integrated into a quality management program as a process of developing and implementing strategies that will minimize risks and mitigate the impact of adverse effects. This includes preventing patient injury, minimizing financial loss after a problem/error occurs, and preserving agency reputation. (Ch. 19)

Role Expected or actual behavior, determined by a person's position or status in a group. (Ch. 3)

Role ambiguity A condition in which individuals do not have a clear understanding about performance and evaluation. (Ch. 14)

Role conflict A condition in which individuals understand the role but are unwilling or unable to meet the requirements. (Ch. 14)

Role development Choosing to change role expectations and/or role performance. (Ch. 25)

Role discrepancy A gap between role expectations and role performance. (Ch. 25)

Role expectations The attitudes and behaviors another anticipates a person in the role will possess or demonstrate. (Ch. 25)

Role internalization Stage at which a person has learned behaviors that maintain a role so thoroughly that the person performs them without consciously considering them; energy once spent on establishing these behaviors can be redirected to other goals. (Ch. 25)

Role model A person who enacts a role, typically in a positive way, so that others can follow the example. (Ch. 18)

Role negotiation Resolving conflicting expectations about personal management performance through communication. (Ch. 25)

Role strain The subjective feeling of discomfort experienced as a result of role stress; may manifest through increased frustration, heightened emotional awareness, or emotional fragility to situations. (Chs. 24, 25)

Role stress A social condition in which role demands are conflicting, irritating, or impossible to fulfill. (Chs. 24, 25)

Role theory A framework used to understand how individuals perform within organizations. (Chs. 3, 14)

Role transition The process of unlearning an old role and learning a new role. Transforming one's identity from being an individual contributor as a staff nurse to being a leader as a nurse manager. (Ch. 25)

ROLES An acronym used to identify the components of a role: *r*esponsibilities, *o*pportunities, *l*ines of communication, *e*xpectations, and *s*upport. (Ch. 25)

Root–cause analysis The process used to identify all possible causes of a sentinel event and all appropriate risk-reduction strategies. (Ch. 19)

Satisficing decision Selecting an option that is acceptable, but not necessarily the best option. (Satisfy + suffice = satisfice.) (Ch. 5)

Scheduling The implementation of the staffing plan by assigning unit personnel to work specific hours and days. (Ch. 13)

Secondary care Disease restorative care. (Ch. 6)

Self–management The ability of individuals to actively gain control of their lives; components include stress management, time management, meeting management, and the ability to delegate. (Ch. 26)

Sender–receiver The two required participant roles in the communication process. (Ch. 17)

Sentinel event A serious unexpected occurrence involving death or injury, such as suicide, infant abduction, or wrong site surgery. (Ch. 19)

Service In a healthcare context, the interaction between a consumer and the system to the extent needs are addressed. (Ch. 21)

Service line A functional unit of management in which all related concepts of medical care are grouped. (Chs. 7, 21)

Shared governance A term used to describe a flat type of organizational structure with decision making decentralized. (Chs. 7, 18)

Shared vision Agreement among a team of people working toward a common end; concurrence on what the desired state in the future will be. (Ch. 29)

Significance Condition in research when the finding exceeds or equals the criteria set for a chance occurrence. (Ch. 20)

Smart card Credit card–like devices that store data. (Ch. 10)

Staff function Function that assists those in line positions in accomplishing primary objectives. (Ch. 7)

Staff mix The proportion of RNs to LPNs/LVNs to UAPs in a specific setting. (Ch. 12)

Staffing The function of planning for hiring and deploying qualified personnel to meet the needs of patients for care and services. (Ch. 13)

Staffing model The conceptual approach of accomplishing the work to be done on a given unit. (Ch. 13)

Staffing regulations Licensing regulations required by the state department of health, usually related to the minimum number of professional nurses on a unit at a given time. (Ch. 13)

Standard of care Level of quality considered adequate by a profession; skills and learning commonly possessed by members of a profession; also written at a minimum level. (Ch. 4)

Statute Rule/regulation created by elected legislative bodies; also known as *statutory law*. (Ch. 4)

Strategic plan The operationalization of an organization's mission, goals, and objectives. (Ch. 28)

Strategic planning A process designed to achieve goals through allocation of resources. (Ch. 15)

Strategies Approaches designed to achieve a specific purpose. (Ch. 16)

Structure Formal systematic arrangements that are elements of the whole. (Ch. 7)

Structured nursing language A standardized and organized set of concepts and relationships that nursing informatics research has shown to be useful in representing the nursing domain. (Ch. 10)

Subculture Element of a main culture that has formed its own culture that differs in some way. (Ch. 18)

Synergy A phenomenon in which teamwork produces extraordinary results that could not have been achieved by any one individual. (Ch. 17)

Synergy Model A model of care delivery adopted by the American Association of Critical Care Nurses which matches the needs and characteristics of the patient with the competencies of the nurse. Seven characteristics are unique to every patient and each nurse has varying levels of ability which are categorized into eight competencies. When the knowledge, skills, and competencies of the nurse are utilized to meet the complex needs of the patient and family, the care is optimal. (Ch. 12)

Teaching institution An academic health center and affiliated hospital. (Ch. 6)

Team A number of people associated together in specific work or activities. (Ch. 17)

Team nursing A small group of licensed and unlicensed personnel, with a team leader, responsible for providing patient care to a group of patients. (Ch. 12)

Telehealth Use of modern telecommunications and information technologies for provision of health care to individuals at a distance and transmission of information to provide that care; involves use of two-way interactive video-conferencing, high-speed phone lines, fiberoptic cable, and satellite transmissions. (Ch. 10)

Tertiary care Rehabilitative or long-term care. (Ch. 6)

Third–party payers Private and public agencies that contract with an individual to assume responsibility to pay under defined conditions for specified healthcare services. (Ch. 6)

Time management The use of tools, techniques, strategies, and follow-up systems to control wasted time and to ensure that the time invested in activities leads toward achieving a desired, high-priority goal. (Ch. 26)

Total patient care See *Case method*. (Ch. 12)

Total quality management (TQM) A comprehensive program designed to achieve perfection in quality of care. Often used interchangeably with continuous quality management, quality management, quality improvement, and performance improvement. (Ch. 19)

Transactional leadership The act of using rewards and punishments as part of daily oversight of employees in seeking to get the group to accomplish a task. (Ch. 2)

Transculturalism Bridging significant differences in cultural practices. (Ch. 8)

Transformational leadership An act of encouraging followers to follow the leader's style and change their interests into a group interest with concern for a broader goal. (Ch. 2)

Unit of service A measure of the work being produced by the organization, such as patient days, patient or home visits, or procedures. (Chs. 11, 13)

Unlicensed assistive personnel Healthcare workers who are not licensed and who are prepared to provide certain elements of care under the supervision of a registered nurse (e.g., technicians, nurse aides, or certified nursing assistants). (Ch. 12)

Utilization The quantity or volume of services provided. (Ch. 11)

Values Inner forces that influence decision making and priority setting. (Chs. 1, 4, 28)

Variable costs Costs that vary in direct proportion to patient volume or acuity. (Ch. 11)

Variable FTEs Those full-time equivalent positions that depend on the demand for care, typically staff positions. (Ch. 13)

Variance Anything alters a patient's progress through a normal care path. (Chs. 11, 12)

Variance analysis Budget-control process to determine differences between income and expense, projected and actual costs. (Ch. 11)

Variance report A report defining the difference between the actual and projected staffing or budgeting. (Ch. 13)

Veracity Principle that compels the truth be told completely. (Ch. 4)

Vertical integration Alignment of organizations to provide a full array or continuum of services. (Ch. 6)

Vertical organization A linear structure that describes hierarchal responsibility of positions. (Ch. 7)

Vicarious liability Imputation of accountability upon one person or entity for the actions of another person; substituted liability or imputed liability. (Ch. 4)

Vision The desired future state. (Chs. 1, 7, 29)

Voice technology Control of computer by vocal input. (Ch. 10)

Whistleblower A person who makes public a serious wrongdoing or danger concealed within an organization when internal actions have failed to correct or make public a situation. (Ch. 18)

Wireless (WL) messaging An extension of an existing wired network that uses radio-based systems to transmit data signals through the air without any physical connections. (Ch. 10)

Workload The amount of work distributed to a person or unit for a given time period. (Ch. 13)

Workplace advocacy Refers to acting on or in behalf of another who is unable to act for himself or herself to effect change about workplace conditions. (Ch. 18)

World Wide Web (WWW) Set of standards and communication protocols that allow information to be shared across the Internet regardless of the user's platform. (Ch. 10)

Application Activities

CHAPTER **1** APPLICATION ACTIVITY

Managing, Leading, and Following

INTRODUCTION

Effective managers focus efficiently on objectives, tasks, procedures, and policies. Recently, however, the emphasis has been on leaders who provide vision, inspiration, and empowerment. Exactly what do these terms mean? Who should lead, manage, or follow, and when? The activities in this section are designed to help you recognize the differences among leading, managing, and following and to recognize how and why these behaviors are essential for organizations to move forward.

ACTIVITY 1-1

1. What words come to mind when you think of *leader?*

2. What words come to mind when you think of *follower?*

3. Analyze the differences between the two lists. Do you think of leaders in different ways than you think of followers?

4. Recall pairs of leaders-followers from politics, science, education, the media, or personal experience. As you recall these pairs of individuals, what made one the "leader" and the other the "follower"? How did the leader contribute to the follower's success? How did the follower contribute to the leader's

success? Were there times when the leader functioned more as the follower? Were there times when the follower functioned more as the leader? What does this analysis tell you about the nature of leader-follower relationships?

ACTIVITY 1-2

Write a short analysis of the similarities and differences between managers and leaders on a unit of a hospital with which you are familiar. Discuss these similarities and differences with others (staff nurses, nurse managers, and other students).

ACTIVITY 1-3

1. In the spaces below, write a list of the positive consequences (beneficial outcomes) that occur when one manages well, when one leads well, and when one follows well.

Beneficial Outcomes or Consequences

Managing Well	Leading Well	Following Well
a. Orderly, organized unit	a. Progressive, creative unit	a. Balanced teamwork
b.	b.	b.
c.	c.	c.
d.	d.	d.
e.	e.	e.
f.	f.	f.

2. Write any observations, questions, and/or conclusions you have about the lists you created.

3. Write a list of the negative consequences/outcomes of (or difficulties caused by) overemphasizing managing to the exclusion of leading and then of overemphasizing leading to the exclusion of managing.

Negative Outcomes or Consequences

Overemphasizing Managing	**Overemphasizing Leading**
a. Limited freedom for staff	a. Out of touch with reality
b.	b.
c.	c.
d.	d.
e.	e.

List negative outcomes of ineffective or passive followership.
a. Waits for others to assume responsibilities
b.
c.
d.
e.

4. Write any questions, observations, and/or conclusions you have about the three lists you have created.

5. Discuss with at least one other person the benefits and negative results (all lists) of leading and managing. List specific ways you could (or have seen others) shift emphasis between leading and managing.
   a. What behaviors, policies, procedures, and so forth facilitate a shift of emphasis from managing to leading and back again in the institution(s) you have chosen for Activity 1-2?

   b. What behaviors, policies, procedures, and so forth block this shifting emphasis in the institution(s) you have chosen?

   c. What new behaviors, policies, procedures, and so forth would produce an effective shifting in the future in the institution(s) you have chosen?

ACTIVITY 1-4

Read at least three articles concerning managing and leading. Notice the degree to which the articles focus on the benefits of either leading or managing and the consequences of the other. When this occurs, the article tends to be a "crusade" for one side of this dilemma as though the author's favored approach is the solution to a particular problem. By overemphasizing the favored side, you could eventually experience its negative consequences, just as walking on top of a seesaw will at some point make it tip downward (refer to the negative consequences you listed). Do any of your articles call for leading and managing together, or mix them into a "superperson" profile? This may lead to clouding the distinctions and ignoring the need to emphasize leading or managing when appropriate.

1. What do the articles recommend about shifting focus?

2. With what level of certainty do the authors speak about the most needed behaviors?

3. What recommendations could you use in your clinical or work setting?

4. Why?

ACTIVITY 1-5

1. Team up with another student in your class. Separately, compile a list of what you each believe are leadership behaviors. Try to list at least 10.

   1.   6.

   2.   7.

   3.   8.

   4.   9.

   5.   10.

2. Review your lists and mark your initials beside each behavior that you believe describes some of your own behaviors. Do this without input from anyone else. Using the same lists, mark your partner's initials beside those behaviors you have observed in the other student. Do this activity without any input from the other student. When finished, compare lists.

3. What do you both notice about the differences in how you view yourselves and how you view one another?

4. What did you learn about yourself?

5. Do others see you as having more or fewer leadership traits than you believe you have? Why?

CHAPTER 2 APPLICATION ACTIVITY
Developing the Role of Leader

INTRODUCTION

This section contains three activities that will help you identify your own leadership priorities. Leadership is a privilege that is earned and maintained at the pleasure of followers. Without followers, there is no need for a leader. These exercises should give you an opportunity to explore your own leadership potential.

ACTIVITY 2-1

Fill in the following survey according to the directions.

What Nurses Value in Their Leaders

For *each* of the four clusters of traits, do the following:

Circle the three most important traits in the leader you want to follow.

Mark each circled trait in order of importance by placing a 1 next to the most important trait in your leader, a 2 by the second most important, and a 3 by the third most important.

Place an "X" next to the least important trait in your leader.

Attitudes

Caring	Optimistic	Supportive	Approachable
Cooperative	Respectful of subordinates	Inspirational	Personable
Hard work ethic	Cheerful	Positive attitude	Flexible
Reasonable	Fair	Calm	

Intrinsic Qualities

Dependable	Dignified	Strong willed	Motivated
Dedicated	Detail oriented	Loyal	Wise
Trustworthy	Nonjudgmental	Understanding	Integrity
Reliable	Creative	Intelligent	Honest

Acquired Skills

Business sense	Professional	Decisive
Good reasoning skills	Risk taker	Available
Advocate	Practical knowledge	Clinical competence
Good people skills	Good communicator	Career experience
Assertive		

Personal

Motivator of others	High energy	Empowering
Interested in quality	Friendly	Visionary
Sense of humor	Communicator	Team player
Responsive to people	Mentoring attitude	Receptive to people and ideas

Now compare your responses with the top 10 responses of more than 100 young nurses and nursing students from throughout the United States.

Top 10 desired traits in a leader:
1. Receptive to people (personal skill)
2. Team player (personal skill)
3. Honest (intrinsic skill)
4. Good communicator (acquired skill)
5. Positive attitude (attitude skill)
6. Good people skills (acquired skill)
7. Approachable (attitude skill)
8. Knowledgeable (acquired skill)
9. Motivates others (personal skill)
10. Competent (acquired skill)

Least desired traits in a nurse manager:
1. Risk taker
2. High energy
3. Cheerful
4. Creative
5. Detail-oriented and Inspirational (tied)

Compare yourself to these young nurses. Notice which of their desired traits are listed in the acquired skills section. Can you think of ways that a leader could improve these skills? How many of your responses were listed in the acquired skills section? What about attitude? Can you change your attitude? The one intrinsic quality listed by the national sample was "honest." What would you do with a leader who was not honest? Do you think that national and global leaders are basically honest? Why is it so important that nursing leaders be seen as honest?

ACTIVITY 2-2

How do you make good followers? Can you be a good leader if you have never been a good follower? Separate into groups of five people. Respond to the following two questions, then regroup and see if you can come to some consensus on these questions.

What are the two most important features of a good follower?

1. _____

2. _____

Which one of each pair of words is more important for an effective follower? (Circle the more important word.)
　　Creative or Passive
　　Steady or Flexible
　　Trusting or Questioning
　　Doer or Thinker
　　Discuss the merits of each word with your group. Now, decide which one word is the most important in describing a follower.

　　Write the word here: _____

How did you decide on this word? Did you vote? Did someone urge the others to accept his or her word? If it was not your word, did you feel like you lost? A good leader makes even the losers feel like winners. If you followed someone else's lead, did you exhibit the qualities embodied in the word you used to describe a good follower? Sometimes leaders are followers, and sometimes followers are leaders. The key is to do both well to be effective.

ACTIVITY 2-3

Leader Observation Activity or "Watch and Learn"

Attend a professional nursing meeting. Identify the president or chairperson. Watch that person interact with other members.
- Is there anything consistent that he or she does during these interactions?
- Watch the leader's eye contact. What is he or she looking at during the meeting?
- What does the leader do after the meeting?
- Is there someone else at the meeting who seems to be the unofficial leader? What makes you think so?

Questions you might want to ask include the following:
1. What kind of preparation does the president/chairperson have to fulfill this role?
2. What percentage of the membership is present at this meeting?
3. Was this a typical meeting?
4. What kinds of issues does this group deal with? What is the most pressing issue currently?
5. Is this a growing organization or a stable one?
6. How long has the leader been a member?
7. Why does he or she belong?
8. What advice does the leader have for you to become a part of the leadership team?

CHAPTER **3** APPLICATION ACTIVITY

Developing the Role of Manager

INTRODUCTION

Does the role of nurse manager intrigue you? Do you think you would like to be nurse manager? It is the best of times for nursing because this era of health care calls for creativity, flexibility, and tenacity—three attributes that students often possess. The exercises you are about to complete should elevate these attributes to higher peaks of excellence. Try them with your peers, share them with your peers, and most importantly, learn from them with your peers.

ACTIVITY 3-1

Role-play the following scenario in a group of 9 to 12 peers. Use your experience in clinical settings as the basis for your knowledge.

Roles: Nurse manager of a home health agency, 3 to 4 staff nurses, and 5 to 8 home health aides

Scenario: The agency needs to develop a new care delivery model based on the influence of evidenced-based practice care. Work as a group to develop different roles for this new model. Do not limit yourselves to what you currently see in practice. For each new role, identify assets and liabilities, such as costs inherent in each role (e.g., recruitment, education, benefits).

ACTIVITY 3-2

In what ways can technology be used by a home health agency in a home setting? For example, list client data that might be computer-based for entry or retrieval at a home site. What teaching aspects for health promotion/disease prevention can be done with your client using computer technology? Are you willing to use PDAs for data storage/retrieval?

ACTIVITY 3-3

You are about to downsize your hospital unit. You have been told that your role as nurse manager will expand to cover more patient care areas and that the staff for each shift on your present unit will be reassigned. How can you prepare yourself and your staff for this change? Consider small staff meetings to let people talk about the new changes. Also, consider your own and your staff's adaptability traits. Write down a tentative plan for addressing the downsizing and staff relocation.

ACTIVITY 3-4

You have been repeatedly asked to change the continuous quality program so that it reflects evaluation of outcomes. You have changed the program at least twice, yet your supervisor is not satisfied with the quality outcomes, especially in relation to cost containment. What other strategies can you use to meet management and customer expectations? Write a paragraph that reflects your plan and your ability to maintain objectivity and sustain the demands of the job. Consider research strategies, collaboration with others, exploration of root cost analysis (in and out of the institution), and patient care standards.

CHAPTER 4 APPLICATION ACTIVITY

Legal and Ethical Issues

INTRODUCTION

The increasing demands in health care for cost containment and quality in patient care services, combined with increasing technology, pose escalating legal and ethical questions. As the healthcare scene changes, so do the questions that are posed to staff nurses and managers. This section presents dilemmas that can assist in heightening your awareness of legal and ethical issues prominent today. The exercises are representative of current examples of common dilemmas that nurses may encounter.

ACTIVITY 4-1

The Required Request law has been enacted in a majority of states. Essentially, this law requires that after all deaths, all families must be made aware of the possibility of donation of organs and tissues. The nurse manager or his or her representative, at the time of death or immediately before the patient's death, may be expected to request the organs.

1. Identify the ethical principles underlying the Required Request law by giving specific examples of how these principles are used by nurses when requesting organs after death.

2. Review the three ethical theories presented in the text. Which theory most guides your position regarding the Required Request law? State three reasons to support your position.
   Position:

   a.

   b.

   c.

ACTIVITY 4-2

You are the nurse manager on a busy intermediate coronary care unit. You have just received a request from the admitting department for a bed on your unit, but there are no beds available. You inform the admitting department and request more information on the patient. The information you receive is that the patient is a 73-year-old woman with severe congestive heart failure who needs to receive intravenous

(IV) medications. The physician has requested that she be on a monitored bed while receiving the medication. There are no telemetry beds available.

After reviewing all of the patients on the unit, the director decides to transfer a 48-year-old man who had a myocardial infarction 2 days earlier. The patient is transferred, and you receive the woman with congestive heart failure. The next day you find out that during the night the patient who was transferred was found in complete arrest when the nurse on the other unit made rounds at 2 AM. The man was resuscitated but is now in intensive care with brain damage resulting from the anoxia that occurred before he was resuscitated.

1. Was the decision to transfer the patient out of the intermediate care unit appropriate? Given the outcome of the situation, should you have refused to take the elderly female patient and kept the younger male patient in your unit? Provide a rationale for your answer.

2. Use the MORAL model discussed in the text to review this ethical dilemma.

   M   Massage the dilemma; identify and define the issues in the dilemma.

   O   Outline the options.

   R   Resolve the dilemma.

   A   Act by applying the chosen option.

   L   Look back and evaluate the entire process.

ACTIVITY 4-3

As a nurse manager, you are responsible for review of all incidents that occur on your unit to determine whether they were reported according to protocol and if appropriate follow-up has been completed.

On the previous day, one patient received injuries to her hand while ambulating when an IV controller slipped on the IV pole and pinned her hand between the controller and a platform designed to be used as a flat surface to hold equipment while working with the IV. The incident report states: "Patient was ambulating to bathroom at 10:30 PM and used the IV pole to stabilize herself while walking. The controller fell down the pole and pinned her right hand to the small table beneath it. Injury evident to right hand. Hand immediately began to swell, and patient had acute pain. X-ray film revealed a fracture of the third and fourth metacarpal of the right hand. Physician notified, responded, and orthopedic consult ordered."

The nurse's note in the chart states: "Patient ambulating to bathroom using IV pole to stabilize herself. IV controller fell, pinning hand, resulting in injury. This would not have happened if I had been present to help her. She stated that she turned on her light but no one answered because the unit was very busy at the time. Physician notified and responded. Incident report filed."

1. Identify and examine potential liability from this incident.

2. How does the note made in the chart affect the potential liability for (a) the nurse involved, (b) the nurse manager, and (c) the institution?

   a. Nurse:

   b. Nurse manager:

   c. Institution:

3. Rewrite the nurse's note so that you could advise someone in a similar situation about documentation.

CHAPTER **5** APPLICATION ACTIVITY

Making Decisions and Solving Problems

INTRODUCTION

Because proper problem identification is key to effective problem-solving and decision-making, the exercises in this section provide an opportunity to enhance your skills in this area. Activity 5-1 involves use of a "gap analysis" technique to differentiate a problematic state from the ideal state. Activity 5-2 provides an opportunity to collaborate with a colleague to reflect on the possible causes of a problem and possible remedies to solve it.

ACTIVITY 5-1

Gap Analysis

A gap analysis is another way of envisioning problem solving. Select a professional problem and a colleague who is familiar with the problem. Describe the elements of the problem under the heading "Description of Present Undesired State/Conditions," then identify the desired future state/conditions that would ideally solve the problem.

Description of Present   Description of Desired
 Undesired State/Conditions   Future State/Conditions

ACTIVITY 5-2

Problem Definition

There are many different ways to define a problem, starting with the way different people perceive it. One method is to answer the four questions that follow. Select a problem, choose a partner who is familiar with the problem, and answer the following questions. As you formulate and write problem definitions, you can reflect about the following:

1. Who and what are affected in what "problematic ways"? Consider these possibilities: How many people, and who specifically, are negatively affected? What other things are affected and how?

   Who (as you see it):   Who (as your partner sees it):

   What (as you see it):   What (as your partner sees it):

2. Who and/or what is causing it? What people are causing this problem, especially in the ways they are interpreting the circumstances and what is happening?

   Who (as you see it):   Who (as your partner sees it):

   What (as you see it):   What (as your partner sees it):

3. What type of a problem is being confronted? What is this problem really about: Is it missing resources; a lack of training/skills; power struggles; inaccurate, inadequate, or superfluous communication; a lack of clarity of mission, priorities, roles, or norms; poor performance and results; misunderstandings; unethical actions; poor public relations, etc.? Is this really a conflict over information, goals, means, or values/standards rather than a problem to solve? Is it a dilemma that has been mismanaged, or treated like a solvable problem?

   _____

   The type of problem (as you see it):   The type of problem (as your partner sees it):

4. What are the intended goals/specific results to remedy the situation? What are the specific goal(s) and intended result(s) to remedy this situation?

   Goal(s):

   Intended result(s):

   How would the situation look if this problem were completely solved? What will be the same and what will be different?

Specific goals/results (as you see it):   Specific goals/results (as your partner sees it):

Modified from Jung, C., Pino, R., & Emory, R. (1973). *Research utilizing problem solving.* Portland, OR: Northwest Regional Educational Library.

ACTIVITY 5-3

Adapt the format of the Decision Grid below to a personal or professional decision you are currently trying to make. Examples of decisions might include what type of car to purchase, where to go on vacation, which school to submit applications to, vendor selection decisions, and type of nursing care delivery system to use, just to name a few.

You can provide weights to the variables under consideration by rank ordering them from lowest (0) to highest importance (X) (this should be the number that represents all the variables influencing your decision. In the example, it is 4).

Score the options under consideration in each of the variable columns from 0 (poor) to 3 (good). Multiply the score by the weighting factor.

Options under Consideration	Time	Cost	Legal/Ethical Issues	Equipment Needed

After completing the grid, respond to the following questions:

1. Did using the Decision Grid assist you in weighing the pros and cons between each option?

2. Which option had the highest score after multiplying the weighting factors and the scores?

3. Is the option with the highest score your desired option? If not, what other factors should you consider in making the decision?

CHAPTER **6** APPLICATION ACTIVITY

Healthcare Organizations

Introduction

Changes in the healthcare system, its organizations, and its financing are bringing about rapid developments in the modes and sites of care delivery. As acute care facilities become more focused on the acutely ill, community facilities that focus on people who are less acutely ill are being developed. No longer are people who are ill or who need surgery cared for in acute hospitals. They are in intermediate care agencies, in clinics, and at home. These activities focus on how the community is changing its healthcare facilities, on changes in healthcare delivery that have occurred in the past 5 years, and on the emerging trends.

ACTIVITY 6-1

Form a group with three to five of your classmates who identify themselves as highly committed and productive. Assume that you have been charged with the responsibility to provide the local health planning community with definitive information that they can use for future planning.
1. Scan community publications (e.g., newspapers, magazines, brochures) to develop a scenario of what the healthcare scene in your community was like 3 years ago and how it has changed in yearly increments. Write your description of the agencies and services available in the space below.
   What health care was like 3 years ago:

   2 years ago:

   1 year ago:

   Today:

2. Answer the following questions.
   How many new agencies have been established? What are they?

How have existing agencies been modified by adding programs, redesigning facilities for different services, combining with others, and so forth?

Describe the patients (clients) served then and now, using the following questions as guidelines: How has acuity changed?

How have census and access changed?

How has professional nursing staffing changed?

How have patients' healthcare demands changed?

How have reimbursement systems (e.g., insurance, HMOs) changed, expanded, and/or declined?

3. Using your answers to the questions in item 2, develop a visual representation (e.g., form, grid, mindmap, graph, chart, table) to depict the changes in the agencies.

4. Based on the information you have gathered, what are your conclusions? What trends can you identify?

5. Using the information you have gathered and keeping in mind the trends you just described, write a scenario that predicts the future. You already have all the data you need to do so. Keep in mind that nurse-owned and nurse-managed organizations may be essential components of networks in the evaluation. Use a separate sheet of paper for your forecast.

ACTIVITY 6-2

1. Collect news articles, magazine articles, photos, advertisements, brochures, and so forth regarding local healthcare services or services in some identifiable region. List your article titles.

2. Organize these items into time frames or developmental stages. Highlight new agencies and services within the time periods you select.

3. Identify geographic areas with the newest developments and expansions, perhaps with a creative visual or map.

4. On a poster board, create a visual collage that displays the historical trends in healthcare delivery in the areas you have selected.

5. Present your collage to others.

CHAPTER **7** APPLICATION ACTIVITY

Understanding and Designing Organizational Structures

INTRODUCTION

A primary factor to be considered in designing organizational structures is the amount of autonomy required in decision-making. For example, in settings where patients' conditions are unstable and unpredictable, structures are needed that provide for a great deal of independence in decision-making. Flexibility and independence in decision-making is required in settings where access to higher levels for decision-making is not available.

Making decisions at the level that patient care is occurring provides many advantages to patients and their nurses. When decision-making is delegated to this level, there has to be some means of ensuring that patients are treated equally and that one patient is not provided with advantages that are not granted to another. Agency guidelines for care, established by the nurses providing the care, are one method of ensuring that all clients are treated equally.

ACTIVITY 7-1

Obtain at least two organizational charts. Compare them in terms of their missions. For each organization, describe the following:
1. The placement, authority, and reporting levels for nursing

2. How decisions about nursing issues are likely to be made

3. The decisions that staff nurses are encouraged to make

ACTIVITY 7-2

Describe the characteristics of a typical decentralized organization.
1. List the positive factors of working in such an organization.

2. Describe the requirements to achieve efficiency and effectiveness within this structure.

3. Consider that the organization is completely decentralized. Describe the challenges of working in such an organization. What methods could be used to overcome these challenges?

ACTIVITY 7-3

The new chief nursing officer for the Cady Institute is reviewing several theories and philosophies in preparation for implementing one that can carry the organization through the twenty-first century. In perusing the literature, it became apparent that the concept of shared governance was most appealing because it seemed consistent with the mission of the institution as well as that of the nursing division. You have been appointed to the new committee that has been formed to review the requirements to be considered before this change. As a responsible member of this committee deliberating the proposed change, you have been requested to review the literature and cite at least three advantages and three disadvantages for this proposal.

Advantages of Shared Governance

1.

2.

3.

Disadvantages of Shared Governance

1.

2.

3.

Having completed this assignment, you report your findings to the committee at large. The committee then requests that you make a recommendation on the adoption of such a model.

Your recommendation:
I recommend that shared governance be/not be (select one) adopted. My recommendation was based on the following considerations (please describe each in one or two sentences):
1. How does the educational level of staff affect the decision?

2. What style(s) of managerial leadership are preferred?

3. How will nursing staff members demonstrate autonomy?

CHAPTER **8** APPLICATION ACTIVITY

Cultural Diversity in Health Care

INTRODUCTION

The purposes of the exercises in this section are to (1) help you examine your own cultural attitudes to determine how they influence your behavior and (2) compare and contrast your cultural beliefs and practices with those of others who come from a different cultural background.

ACTIVITY 8-1

Cultural Diversity Exercise: Cultural Awareness

1. Describe the differences among the terms *culture*, *race*, and *ethnicity*.

2. List at least six common characteristics usually associated with the middle-class American culture.

    1.

    2.

    3.

    4.

    5.

    6.

3. Describe common characteristics found in the culture of Western scientific medical practice (e.g., belief in medical model, germ theory).

4. Identify the four most prominent cultural groups in your area.

   1.

   2.

   3.

   4.

   Choose two groups for an in-depth study. Identify the groups in relation to their health beliefs/customs in the areas of birth and death, and their use of folk healers or folk medicines.

5. Determine four similarities and four differences between the "folk medicine" and "Western, scientific medicine" systems. (You may need to think broadly.)

Similarities   **Differences**

a.   a.

b.   b.

c.   c.

d.   d.

ACTIVITY 8-2

Cultural Values Checklist

The following is a short checklist regarding culturally determined values, attitudes, and beliefs, especially as they pertain to health care. Read each statement carefully and then place the number that most closely reflects your beliefs regarding each statement. You must choose 1 (mostly agree), 2 (somewhat agree), 3 (neutral), 4 (somewhat disagree), or 5 (mostly disagree) for each statement as it is written. This requires that you be as introspective as possible to determine where you stand on each of the issues presented. Please remember that there is no right or wrong answer, just individual attitudes and beliefs. By answering as honestly as possible, this exercise will help you be more conscious of your own culturally determined beliefs.

_____   1. Infants with severe handicaps ought to be left out to die.
_____   2. Extraordinary medical treatment is always indicated.
_____   3. My role as a nurse is to always resuscitate patients who could benefit from it, no matter what has been decided previously.
_____   4. I must follow physician's orders.
_____   5. Older patients should be allowed to die with dignity.

_____   6. Medical technology has advanced the quality of life.

_____   7. Children should not be involved in giving consent for treatments.

_____   8. Families ought to make decisions about life-or-death situations without involving the patient.

_____   9. Children should participate in human experimentation that is not harmful, even if it has no benefit to them.

_____   10. Prisoners should participate in scientific experiments to repay society for their wrongdoings.

_____   11. Women should seek medical care from female physicians to avoid potential discrimination.

_____   12. Children whose parents refuse to have them receive medical care should be removed from their families through court action.

_____   13. Research using fetuses should be pursued vigorously.

_____   14. Life support systems should be discontinued after several days of flat electroencephalogram.

_____   15. Health professionals are a scarce resource in many parts of the country.

_____   16. Nursing is a subservient profession, especially to the medical profession.

_____   17. As a nurse, I must relinquish my personal philosophy to support the philosophies of others.

_____   18. All patients, regardless of differences, should be treated in a humanistic way.

_____   19. I should give mouth-to-mouth resuscitation to a derelict if he needs it.

_____   20. A child who is disabled has value.

_____   21. All forms of human life have value.

_____   22. I should be involved in decision-making regarding ethical issues in practice.

_____   23. Committees should decide who receives scarce resources, such as kidneys.

_____   24. Patients' individual rights should be more important than the rights of society at large.

_____   25. A person has the right to make a living will.

_____   26. Underdeveloped countries should be given health and financial support from developed countries.

_____   27. I should support all the positions on ethical issues taken by my professional association.

_____   28. The care component of nursing practice is not as important as the cure component of medical practice.

_____   29. The nurse's primary role in decision-making on ethical issues is to implement the selected alternative.

_____   30. I feel afraid when caring for a patient who is dying.

_____   31. Children who have disabilities should be institutionalized.

_____   32. Patients in mental health institutions and prisons should be given behavior modification therapy to make them conform to society.

_____   33. Personal possessions of patients should be removed to guarantee safekeeping during hospitalization.

_____   34. Patients should have access to their own health information.

_____   35. Withholding health information fosters patient's recovery.

_____   36. A patient with kidney failure is always able to get kidney dialysis when needed.

_____   37. Society should bear the cost of extraordinary medical interventions.

_____   38. Confidentiality is an important part of the nurse's role.

_____   39. As a nurse, I should value responsibility.

_____   40. Nurses have a right to withhold information to facilitate nursing research on human subjects.

_____   41. The patient who refuses treatment should be dropped from the health supervision of an agency or professional.

_____   42. Transplantations should be done whenever needed.

Personal Application

1. Add the number of 1s, 2s, 3s, 4s, and 5s that you have.

2. How many statements do you have clear ideas (1s and 5s) about?

3. Do these outweigh the number of ambivalent (neutral) statements you listed?

4. Look at the statements that you agree with (1s and 2s). Is there a relationship between the statements that influenced your responses (e.g., age of patient, patient acuity)?

5. Look at the statements that you disagree with (4s and 5s). Is there a relationship between these statements that influenced your responses?

6. Analyze the cluster of statements below. Is there any consistency in the way that you rated these statements? What variables influenced your decision?

Cluster 5, 8, 14, 25, and 30: Relates to issues pertaining to death
Cluster 3, 4, 16, 17, 22, 27, 28, 29, and 38: Relates to the profession of nursing
Cluster 2, 6, 14, 36, 37, and 42: Relates to issues raised by advanced technology
Cluster 1, 7, 9, 12, 20, and 31: Relates to children
Cluster 9, 10, 13, and 40: Relate to human experimentation
Cluster 3, 7, 8, 11, 12, 18, 19, 21, 24, 25, 33, 34, 35, 38, and 41: Relates to patients' rights
Cluster 9, 10, 24, 26, 32, and 37: Relates to society's rights
Cluster 15, 23, and 36: Relates to allocation of resources
Cluster 3, 4, 17, 18, 19, 22, 27, 29, and 39: Relates to perceptions of obligations

From Wagner, K. D., Johnson, K., Kidd, P. S. (2006). *High acuity nursing* (4th ed.), p. 23. Adapted with permission of Pearson Education, Inc., Upper Saddle River, New Jersey.

ACTIVITY 8-3

One responsibility of a family is to provide health care for its members by helping them stay well and taking care of members who are ill. Health promotion activities and care given during illness vary greatly among families. Each function is very much influenced by the family's cultural orientation. Friedman (1992) describes six stages of family health/illness interactions that greatly influence each individual's response to health care. These stages are health promotion, illness recognition, care seeking, healthcare system, acute response, and adaptation to illness/recovery.

It is important to note that the family will not make contact with the healthcare delivery system until at least the fourth stage of this interaction continuum. Therefore the family may have engaged in various health activities before they ever have contact with anyone in a professional setting.

The Family Health/Illness Practices Inventory is designed to increase awareness of family and cultural values that shape health and illness practices. It is a tool that can increase self-awareness of the cultural factors that shape your current approach to health care. When used as an interview tool, it can increase awareness of other cultural perspectives regarding health care.

Complete your own Family Health/Illness Practices Inventory. Try to remember what it was like for you as a child growing up and answer the questions based on what your family did before you became a nurse.

Family Health/Illness Practices Inventory

1. Health promotion
Cite three health promotion/disease prevention activities done by your family.

1.

2.

3.

Did you consider your parents to be healthy, frail, sickly? What about your siblings?

How did your family define *health?*

2. Illness recognition

Who was the primary person in the family responsible for determining whether a family member was ill?

Who was primarily responsible for determining what should be done about the illness?

Who in the family was seen as the "health expert"?

3. Care-seeking

Who did the family turn to for information regarding the illness if the family was unable to resolve the problem on its own?

Did the family discuss the problems with extended family members, neighbors, or friends, or go straight to a health professional?

4. Healthcare system

Did the family use folk practitioner/healers?

Where was the initial contact with the healthcare delivery system made (e.g., healer, private physician, clinic, hospital)?

Who in the family was responsible for deciding where to seek help?

5. Acute response

What did it mean to be "sick" in your family?

What behaviors were expected of the sick person and of other family members in relation to the sick member?

If it was a serious illness or crisis, how did the family cope? Who was seen as the leader in times of crisis?

What happened if the traditional leader was sick?

6. Adaptation to illness/recovery

Did anyone in the family have a chronic illness?

How did that affect the other family members?

Who did the family depend on for support (physical, emotional)?

After completing your own Family Health/Illness Practices Inventory, interview someone from a different cultural background. Explain that you are trying to learn more about how different cultures and families view health and illness. Assure the person that the information will be kept confidential, or seek out a classmate whose cultural background is different from yours and mutually compare and discuss your responses.

Friedman, M. (1992). *Family nursing: Theory and practice* (3rd ed.). Norwalk, CT: Appleton & Lange.

CHAPTER 9 APPLICATION ACTIVITY

Power, Politics, and Influence

INTRODUCTION

Who would you say is the most important person at your place of employment? Give it some thought before you respond! Is it the president or chief executive officer? Is it the person who makes the most money? Is it the person who supervises the most employees? Is it the person who has the authority to fire or demote you? Is it the physician with the most influence? Is it the patient who threatens to sue you? This chapter examines the nature, impact, and uses of power in nursing management.

ACTIVITY 9-1

1. Review the definitions of power in the Theory Box (Types of Power) in the chapter. Write a short personal example fitting each definition.
   a. Personal:

   b. Expert:

   c. Position:

   d. Perceived:

   e. Information:

   f. Connection:

2. Now reread the above introduction. Who is the most powerful person at your hospital? Explain why the most powerful person could be you, the nurse.

ACTIVITY 9-2

Read the case below, considering the different types of power. Reflect on the behaviors listed for Chris, the emergency department charge nurse in the case.

Clinical Case Study

Chris Starr (RN, BSN, CEN), the charge nurse in a very busy emergency department, was exhausted at the end of a 12-hour shift. Sixty-six patients had been triaged, assessed, cared for, counseled, educated, admitted, transferred, and/or discharged. One patient died. Some of the nursing responsibilities/behaviors carried out by Chris on this shift included:

_____ a. Took/gave shift report every 4 hours.
_____ b. Assigned staff to patient care responsibilities.
_____ c. Aassigned staff to nonnursing responsibilities such as ordering supplies, room checks, and testing emergency equipment.
_____ d. Oriented two new medical students to department protocols and expectations.
_____ e. Requested assistance from the nursing supervisor to obtain ICU beds for two critical patients.
_____ f. Called the children's protective agency to request emergency placement for three abandoned children brought in by the police.
_____ g. Yelled over the phone at a newspaper reporter who insisted on obtaining details of a recent accident.
_____ h. Assisted a staff nurse to support very distressed family members whose elderly parent had just died.
_____ i. Talked to the coroner for 10 minutes by phone.
_____ j. Cared for five patients whose nurse left for a dinner break.
_____ k. Assisted three staff members who were restraining an out-of-control, intoxicated patient.
_____ l. Intervened between a staff nurse and physician who disagreed about a patient care issue.
_____ m. Promised to talk privately to an angry unit secretary later in the shift if there was time.
_____ n. Gathered all staff together at 11 PM to thank them for their hard work and good care.

Write out short responses to the following questions about the case.

1. Cite all of the bases of power that Chris exhibited. (Place the number of the power base that she used at the left side of each statement above.) Label each one according to the chapter definition: 1 (expert), 2 (information), 3 (position), 4 (personal), 5 (perceived), and 6 (connection).

2. How did this nurse empower the staff? Cite two ways.
   a.

   b.

3. Cite two missed opportunities for empowerment that you saw.
   a.

   b.

4. Visualize this nurse and write your description of this nurse.
   What does Chris look like?

   How does Chris speak to people?

What values does Chris embody?

What influential person in your life does Chris remind you of?

ACTIVITY 9-3

Empowerment as defined in Chapter 9 is the process by which we facilitate the participation of others in decision-making and taking action in an environment where there is an equitable distribution of power. Empowerment is power-sharing and a form of feminine leadership. All of the following can be powerful attributes of a professional nurse. Rank them in order of importance to you by numbering them in the blanks provided (1 being most important).

_____ Professional knowledge, specialized knowledge
_____ Technological competence
_____ Professional experience
_____ Problem-solving skills
_____ Comfort with conflict resolution
_____ Ability to communicate clearly with colleagues
_____ Commitment to organizational philosophy and mission
_____ Above-average financial compensation
_____ Sense of humor
_____ Positive feelings of work satisfaction

Give this same list to a nursing colleague and to a nonnursing colleague and ask them to rank these items. Compare all three rankings. What similarities and differences exist?

Similarities:

Differences:

ACTIVITY 9-4

1. Meet in groups of three or four. Discuss the responses you wrote for the questions about the case in Activity 9-2 featuring Chris Starr, RN.
2. What "power tools" were most effective in this example?
   a.

   b.

   c.

   d.

3. Describe the "coalition building" behaviors Chris demonstrated.
   a.

   b.

   c.

4. Discuss the following assertion and its implication for your future in nursing and in nursing management: "Collegiality demands mutual respect, not friendship!" Are friendships and being a respected manager mutually exclusive? Why or why not? Is friendship with colleagues essential to you for effective working relationships? Why or why not?

ACTIVITY 9-5

Meet in groups of five or six. Combine your group rankings from Activity 9-3 (or make arrangements to combine the entire class's rankings).

1. What conclusions can you draw from this exercise? Identify, describe, and explain differences that exist among the rankings by nurses.
   a.

   b.

   c.

2. What can you conclude?
   a.

   b.

   c.

3. Do differences exist between the nurse rankings and the nonnurse rankings? Discuss specific similarities, differences, and conclusions.
   Similarities:

   Differences:

   Conclusions:

ACTIVITY 9-6

Complete this exercise in a group of 4 to 6 people. You are committed to the concept of health care for all. A bill is proposed in your state legislature to extend limited healthcare benefits, a combination of low-cost insurance and Medicaid, to the working poor who do not have access to healthcare insurance through their employers. Identify three powerful behaviors that you can utilize to support the passage of this bill that will operationalize an important aspect of health policy.

1.

2.

3.

CHAPTER **10** APPLICATION ACTIVITY

Managing Information and Technology: Caring and Communicating with Computers

INTRODUCTION

These exercises will help you use the information presented in the chapter. The first activity can be used to help you think about your current practice from an information perspective. This exercise should help you understand the process to develop an evidence-based practice.

The second activity helps you subscribe to the student nurse listserv. Other list addresses are also provided for you. Try a few of them; they all provide valuable information for students and nurses in practice.

The third activity will help you find information on the Internet. A list of search engines and instructions for accessing them is provided. Be sure to use the help function to learn more about using these engines.

ACTIVITY 10-1

Evidence-Based Practice

Think about a specific patient population you work with often. Choose a problem or condition that you encounter in that population for which you do not know what therapy the evidence suggests (i.e., what the literature recommends for effective treatment). Go to the library's online reference databases and enter the Cochrane Library Database. (If you need assistance, talk with the librarian at the reference desk in the library.)

First-Time Users

The Cochrane Library contains databases, records, documents, Medical Subject Headings (MeSH), and search history screens. Review any content that you would like by placing your cursor over the highlighted text and clicking once. When you are finished, click the Back button on your browser (as many times as needed) to get to the screen containing the Cochrane Databases.

All Users

1. In the search term box, enter the problem or condition (keep the terms concise) for which you want to know the effective treatment recommended by the literature and then click the Search button. The number of "hits" will be listed. Click on the highlighted text. Read through your list of "hits." Click on one or more pertinent reviews and find the recommended therapies. Print out key reviews if you would like. If the "hits" are too broad, you can try narrowing your search (see the search techniques under the Help option).

2. The next time you are in the clinical setting, find an expert clinician and ask about his or her experience with whatever the recommended therapy was for the selected problem or condition. Does actual practice vary from recommended research evidence? If they differ, ask the clinician if he or she has tried the recommended approach and what the clinician's assessment of actual and recommended practices is. Reflect on what you have heard and read. Developing expertise comes from the integration of theoretical and practical knowledge.

ACTIVITY 10-2

Using a Listserv

Using one of the search engines in Activity 10-3, enter the term "SNURSE-L" to link to the site and to subscribe to the SNURSE-L listserv. Be sure to save the instructions returned to you by email. They explain how to unsubscribe to the listserv when you are finished using it. Read the messages for a few days to see what other students are saying. This is called *lurking*. You will notice that there are many responses and additions to a topic of interest. These messages become a "thread." When you are comfortable and have something to contribute, you may send a message to the list by clicking the reply button. Do *not* use all capital letters in your reply; this is considered to be shouting (and rude). Keep your messages short and to the point.

1. Did you have problems subscribing to the listserv? Were you able to find help?

2. Once you were subscribed, what information did you find useful for you? What information did you provide that was interesting and informative for others?

3. Did the listserv members respond to you?

4. Click on the Print button to make a copy of your latest message.

Listserv Addresses

Remember to send subscribe and unsubscribe commands to the server address. Send the command message to the designated address. Be sure to type the commands "subscribe" or "unsubscribe" (see the Example screen) in your message.

ACTIVITY 10-3

The Internet contains so much information that sometimes you may be unable to find what you are looking for. Search engines were developed to search through millions of websites to find exactly what you need. Following is a list of some common search engines and their functions.

Search Engine	Address (URL)	Description
AltaVista	www.altavista.digital.com	Fast searches; indexes every word on millions of pages; if information is on the web, you'll find it here
Just Ask	www.ask.com	Can ask questions in "plain language"
Google	www.google.com	Comprehensive access; rated highly by users

Lycos	www.lycos.com	Unique options will work around misspellings; is a useful older site
Webcrawler	www.webcrawler.com	Handles searches in an orderly and logical manner; reviews and recommends the best websites; not as fast as some others
Yahoo	www.yahoo.com	Well-organized categories; easy-to-find, useful information, finds only keywords; a good place to start

1. Access your browser and enter the address (called the *uniform resource locator* or *URL*) of one of the search engines listed previously. Search for information that you need for patient education or for a paper that you are writing. What did you find? Was there too much information? Try searching for the keyword diabetes or cystic fibrosis. What did you find? Click the print icon on the tool bar to print and keep your findings.

2. Use the Internet to access the Centers for Disease Control and Prevention (CDC). Type the URL for the CDC in the address bar: www.cdc.gov/. When the CDC home page opens, click on an icon (picture) or underlined topic and follow the links. Use the Back and Forward buttons on the toolbar to move between the pages.

3. Check some of the statistics. Find information that might be useful in writing a paper about HIV or diabetes. Find health information for travelers.

4. Do you know how to write a reference for information that you find on the Internet? Check with your library for the latest APA format for citing electronic information because this is now an accepted form of reference. You can also access the website containing this information. The URL is www.nyct.net/~beads/weapas.

CHAPTER **11** APPLICATION ACTIVITY

Managing Costs and Budgets

INTRODUCTION

This section provides additional opportunities to consider in how to manage both costs and budgets.

ACTIVITY 11-1

1. You are a staff nurse in an ambulatory care clinic that is making a transition from fee-for-service reimbursement to capitation. Review the incentives for cost control in both methods of reimbursement. How are they different? How will this change affect the nursing practices in the clinic? What will be the important considerations when caring for patients under capitation?

2. Torrell Medical Center (TMC) grants all full-time employees 10 paid holidays and 12 paid vacation days annually. In addition, the Nursing Department experiences 6.4 average annual sick days and 1.6 other paid and nonpaid days off (e.g., bereavement, jury duty, education) per employee.
   a. How many productive hours are worked per full-time employee?

   b. One of TMC's medical-surgical units is expanding its capacity from 38 to 45 beds. The average daily census is anticipated to increase by 4 patients. The unit's average patient care standard is 5.4 hours of nursing care per patient day. How many *additional* full-time equivalents (FTEs) will be needed as a result of the proposed expansion?

3. How is productivity measured on the unit or at the agency where you practice? What is the process for monitoring productivity? What is the role of staff nurses in monitoring and improving productivity?

4. For the past 3 months, nursing salaries have exceeded the budgeted amount by 10%. Is this a positive or negative variance? How would you begin to investigate this variance? What factors might contribute to it? Which factors are controllable by the nurse manager? Are unfavorable or negative variances always a problem? Why or why not?

ACTIVITY 11-2

Do this exercise with a partner. Develop charts or other graphic ways to illustrate the following activities.

Scenario: Expansion!

You have been informed that because of your statistical justification efforts, administration has recognized the need for more monitored beds. This means that your department will expand from its current 11 monitored beds to 20 such beds. As a nurse manager, you are initially very pleased about this expansion, but then you feel dismay because you will have a lot of work to do and only a little time in which to accomplish it. You also have an additional 12 FTEs to add to your current 20.5 FTEs. The current staffing mix is as follows:

RN FTEs = 12 (10 full-time and 4 part-time)

LPN (LVN) FTEs = 3.5 (2 full-time and 3 part-time)

Nursing assistant FTEs = 1.5 (6 work every other weekend and 1 works the Friday along with her weekend)

Nursing aide FTEs = 1.0 (full-time, but works only Monday to Friday)

Unit clerk FTEs = 2.5 (2 full-time, working 9 to 5:30 during the week and every other weekend, and 1 part-time, working 6 PM to 10 PM Monday through Friday)

The additional 12 FTEs include all support personnel (unit clerks, nursing assistants, and aides as well as RNs and LPNs [LVNs]).

Establish the following:

1. List three goals for the new expanded unit. Include patient outcomes such as discharge criteria, acuity level, and patient teaching.

    a.

    b.

    c.

2. Make a list that differentiates the allocation of FTEs of caregivers and support personnel. Some of the support personnel may also be listed as caregivers, such as nursing assistants and/or unit clerks who are cross-trained as nursing aides. Consider the following when doing the allocation:
   a. There are nine more patients who require care.
   b. There are times when there is no unit clerk available, and the daytime clerks have to work overtime to cover the period from 5:30 to 6:00 PM.
   c. Who will be observing nine additional monitors? Would you want to consider a monitor tech or cross-training for some of the other available personnel?

   d. Consider patient outcomes. Will your patients be on the monitor during their entire stay in the unit and when the monitor is discontinued they are transferred, or will they remain on the unit until discharge and require a lower level of care?

   e. Currently the acuity level is higher than the original staffing plan was designed for, which is resulting in the nursing staff working overtime on a daily basis.
3. Decide how many part-time versus full-time positions you will need to accomplish the goals set forth previously. Remember that when a part-time person works overtime, it is not usually paid at time and a half and they frequently are asked to contribute more to receive benefits.

4. Determine the minimum number of staff necessary for all three shifts. Keep in mind that the staffing ratio on your unit is currently one RN or, in some cases, LPN (LVN) to four patients. Take into account that full-time staff on your unit currently work 12-hour shifts and every third weekend.

5. Discuss with your partner and develop a clear rationale to demonstrate your understanding of over-budgeted hours and overtime.

CHAPTER **12** APPLICATION ACTIVITY

Care Delivery Strategies

INTRODUCTION

Healthcare delivery has been significantly impacted by many factors. The nursing shortage, managed care, and financing reforms will continue this rapid transformation in models of care delivery. Identifying characteristics, strengths, and liabilities of each system will enable the nurse to match the care delivery strategy with the agency's philosophy, goals, and organizational and financial structure.

ACTIVITY 12-1

You are the charge nurse on a 10-patient subacute care unit. There are two RNs, one LPN/LVN, and one nursing assistant working today. Each care delivery strategy has different functions for care providers (e.g., in primary care, RNs have different functions than in the functional method). Describe the role of each care provider in each of the care delivery strategies below.

Case Method

RN #1 role:

RN #2 role:

LPN/LVN role:

Nursing Assistant role:

Functional Method

RN #1 role:

RN #2 role:

LPN/LVN role:

Nursing Assistant role:

Team Nursing
RN #1 role:

RN #2 role:

LPN/LVN role:

Nursing assistant role:

Primary Nursing
RN #1 role:

RN #2 role:

LPN/LVN role:

Nursing Assistant role:

Nurse Case Management
RN #1 role:

RN #2 role:

LPN/LVN role:

Nursing Assistant role:

ACTIVITY 12-2

As a nurse manager, you know that each care delivery model has advantages for the manager, staff, patient, and family. For each care model, describe two advantages and two disadvantages for the nurse manager, the staff nurse, and the patient and family.

ACTIVITY 12-3

As a baccalaureate prepared nurse, which model for nursing care delivery would you be satisfied to work in? State a rationale for your selection, including characteristics of the model that appeal to you. What if you were an associate-degree nurse? Which model for nursing care delivery would your chief financial officer favor? Why?

CHAPTER 13 APPLICATION ACTIVITY

Staffing and Scheduling

INTRODUCTION

Staffing any nursing division is complex and challenging. Calculating staffing needs includes many factors, all of which are compounded whenever the number of staff and the appropriate mix are challenged, such as during a time of high demand for nurses. Some key factors are the average census, length of stay, complexity of care, legal and accreditation expectations, and staff qualifications. Balancing the needs of a given division in terms of the care needed with the needs and expectations of staff is a challenge all managers face. Institutional policies and contracts and state laws, rules, and regulations influence decisions.

ACTIVITY 13-1

You are the manager of a medical-surgical unit. The unit has 32 beds and an occupancy rate of 75%. The desired staffing mix consists of four RNs, two LPNs/LVNs, and two nursing assistants on the 7 AM to 3 PM shift; three RNs, one LPN/LVN, and two nursing assistants on the 3 PM to 11 PM shift; and two RNs, one LPN/LVN, and one nursing assistant on the 11 PM to 7 AM shift. Using the formulas from Chapter 13, determine how many FTEs of each category of employees will be necessary to cover the staffing expectations. Remember, this division will operate 24 hours every day, including weekends and holidays.

Key Factors
The employment benefits include the following:
    7 holidays per year
    10 sick days per year
    15 vacation days per year
    Every other weekend off
Determine the following:
    Number of RN FTEs needed:

    Number of LPN/LVN FTEs needed:

    Number of nursing assistant FTEs needed:

Using this same staffing pattern, determine what percentage of staff is allocated to each shift.

    Allocated to 7 AM to 3 PM: _____%

    Allocated to 3 PM to 11 PM: _____%

    Allocated to 11 PM to 7 AM: _____%
    TOTAL: 100%

ACTIVITY 13-2

Using the 32-bed unit just described, determine to what average daily census (ADC) a 75% occupancy rate equates. Now assume that the actual patient days in the past month were 836. Using the formula in Box 13-4 of the text, calculate the real ADC. Finally, assume that during the past month there were 102 discharges. Determine the average length of stay.

ACTIVITY 13-3

You have called a staff meeting and have encouraged the staff to bring concerns regarding staff satisfaction. The focus of this meeting is to consider a new approach of self-scheduling. Before looking at how such an approach could actually be implemented, you want staff to consider the pros and cons of the current approach (a managerial function) with the pros and cons of the potential approach (a self-scheduling approach). Complete the following chart to illustrate and clarify the dilemmas, benefits, issues, and problems associated with each.

Positives to Self-Scheduling
1. Staff control over schedule

2.

3.

4.

5.

Negatives to Self-Scheduling
1. Peer negotiation regarding the schedule

2.

3.

4.

5.

Positives to Managerial Scheduling
1. Efficiency

2.

3.

4.

5.

Negatives to Managerial Scheduling
1. Staff complaints

2.

3.

4.

5.

Now assume that you and your group decide to initiate self-scheduling on a trial basis. Before initiating this new approach, you will need to write some guidelines for self-scheduling. Review the chart above for ideas.

Guidelines for Self-Staffing (Proposed)

1. May only schedule Friday or Monday off, with a weekend off one time per month.

2.

3.

4.

5.

CHAPTER **14** APPLICATION ACTIVITY

Selecting, Developing, and Evaluating Staff

INTRODUCTION

The following exercises provide an opportunity for you to identify personal preferences for various types of appraisals, as well as the strengths and weaknesses for methods commonly used. You may wish to critique an appraisal from a system in which you are currently employed or in which you have had clinical experience. Finally, you may develop and critique typical dialogues among professionals. Behaviors that foster empowerment and disempowerment, whether verbal or nonverbal, should be identified.

ACTIVITY 14-1

Design a performance appraisal process that you believe would help you grow professionally. Which of the performance appraisal types listed would be a part of your preferred process? In the spaces that follow, identify the strengths and limitations of each. State a rationale for each regarding how the process could help you professionally.

a. *Graphic rating scales* provide feedback that can:
Strengths:

Limitations:

b. *Forced distribution* provides feedback that can:
Strengths:

Limitations:

c. *Peer review* provides feedback that can:
Strengths:

Limitations:

d. *Management by objectives* provides feedback that can:
Strengths:

Limitations:

e. *Behaviorally Anchored Rating Scales* provide feedback that can:
Strengths:

Limitations:

State three performance criteria that should be included in your process.
1.

2.

3.

Meet with one to three peers to construct a performance appraisal form incorporating each of the performance criteria that you have identified. Do this on a separate sheet of paper.

Share the group process that has been developed with a person responsible for appraising you, or someone who would. Will that person agree to use your process to assist you to grow professionally? Remember, because your organization uses a particular system does not preclude the use of an *additional* system!

ACTIVITY 14-2

Assess the state of performance appraisal in a clinical organization (setting) by using the checklist below.

_____ 1. Does your organization have a formal performance appraisal system? (If "no," see last item on this list.)
_____ 2. Does it use graphic rating scales?
_____ 3. Does it use forced distribution?
_____ 4. Does it include peer review?
_____ 5. Is it based on management by objectives?
_____ 6. Are the objectives based on a strategic plan?
_____ 7. Does it include a behaviorally anchored rating scale?
_____ 8. Does it influence compensation?
_____ 9. Does it serve as the basis for discipline?
_____ 10. Is it used to determine training needs?

_____ 11. Does it increase role clarity?
_____ 12. Do appraisal meetings occur at least quarterly?
_____ 13. Is the system based on up-to-date position descriptions/criteria?
_____ 14. Is there a clearly defined training process for appraisers?
_____ 15. Every organization has an appraisal process! If your organization has no formal process, you can be sure that an informal process exists. Your performance is assessed!

Cite three examples of criteria used in the informal system in the organization.

1.

2.

3.

What is your opinion regarding the workings of the informal system of appraisal in your organization?

How does the informal system of performance appraisal reflect the values, climate, or culture of the setting? Cite two ways.

1.

2.

ACTIVITY 14-3

Examine and analyze typical dialogues among nurses, managers, and other healthcare professionals. Cite three instances of both empowering and disempowering behaviors.

Empowering behaviors:

1.

2.

3.

Disempowering behaviors:

1.

2.

3.

CHAPTER 15 APPLICATION ACTIVITY

Strategic Planning, Goal-Setting, and Marketing

INTRODUCTION

In Chapter 15, you learned the importance of planning strategically, developing clear goals and objectives, implementing in a disciplined manner, and marketing concepts in the field of health care. You also considered the critical importance of integrating the planning, targeting, implementing, and marketing functions. This section provides processes to enable you to develop skills in performing these functions.

ACTIVITY 15-1

1. To identify the marketing strategies of a healthcare organization, obtain a copy of at least one marketing brochure or plan for your own organization or one with which you are familiar.
2. Analyze the completeness and effectiveness of your brochure or plan according to the following criteria:
   a. Is the market for each product or service clearly defined?
   b. Are organization resources (capacity to deliver the product or service) quantified for each product or service?
   c. What are the marketing objectives? Are they realistic, specific, measurable, and mutually consistent?
   d. Are specific market segments identified for increased penetration?
   e. Is the planned mix of products and services clearly defined or will the mix be reactive to market requirements?

ACTIVITY 15-2

Select a healthcare organization and assess its current state with regard to the planning, targeting, implementing, and marketing functions. You can conduct this type of assessment by reviewing such relevant documents in the organization as mission statements, strategic plans, tentative budgets, and so forth. In reviewing documents to assess the current state, what would you use as review criteria? List those criteria below. Determine how well each criterion was met by checking one of the columns for meeting each criterion.

Reviewing the Strategic Plan

Review Criteria	Not Met	Partly Met	Fully Met
1.	_____	_____	_____
2.	_____	_____	_____
3.	_____	_____	_____

Reviewing Goals and Objectives

Review Criteria	Not Met	Partly Met	Fully Met
1.	_____	_____	_____
2.	_____	_____	_____
3.	_____	_____	_____

Reviewing the Marketing Plan

Review Criteria	Not Met	Partly Met	Fully Met
1.	_____	_____	_____
2.	_____	_____	_____
3.	_____	_____	_____

ACTIVITY 15-3

Create a small group discussion with students outside of class.
1. The case study in Chapter 15 of the online resources lists four forthcoming changes and develops a strategic planning document that responds to those changes. With your group members, discuss how the plan would have to be altered if the changes included the following, rather than those mentioned in the case:
   a. The advisory committee was composed mainly of healthcare professionals.
   b. The marketing plan was targeted to lower socioeconomic groups only.
   c. The health promotion expectations were divided among existing agencies.
   d. Costs and outcomes were the only basis for evaluation.

2. What are the main principles inherent in the concepts of budget reductions and increased regulation?

ACTIVITY 15-4

Planning is a critically important function. Without plans, we cannot sustain long-term initiatives. However, planning must exist within a context of spontaneity, just as spontaneity must exist within a context of planning. To value one and eliminate the other will lead to system dysfunction!

1. List the benefits of planning.

2. List the problems associated with planning. Think about the problems that would occur if everything were planned and people were prohibited from taking any spontaneous action.

3. List the benefits associated with spontaneous action.

4. List the problems associated with spontaneous action. Think about the problems that would occur if no one in the organization did any planning.

ACTIVITY 15-5

Planning requires effective vision, goals, and objectives. The text discusses guidelines for effective goals. Using these guidelines and examples, on a separate sheet of paper, write some specific short-term, medium-range, and long-term goals for a department or team. Discuss them with another student and revise them as needed.

CHAPTER 16 APPLICATION ACTIVITY

Leading Change

INTRODUCTION

This section contains one application activity that asks students to propose a plan for an actual or hypothetical change in a nursing situation. Guidelines and a sample plan will guide the development of the plan. The best outcome for this activity is for students to implement their plans in actual healthcare organizations. The ultimate outcome is the development of effective change management skills by further enhancing students' conceptual foundations about roles and approaches in leading change.

ACTIVITY 16-1

The use of planned change models for less complex, low-level change can be effective. Most organizational change, however, takes place in groups, units, and departments responsive to influences outside and inside (open system). Thus, managing the influencing factors of a change situation in conjunction with a plan's elements for the change can lead to creative results.

Using the guidelines for planning a change, the change planning worksheet, and the sample of a plan for a hypothetical change, develop a plan for a change. Select a change situation, either an actual or a hypothetical one, and follow the problem-solving format of the planning worksheet to (1) assess the change situation, (2) develop an activity plan for implementation supported by sound change theories and principles, and (3) decide on methods to evaluate the change process and outcomes. The activity plan should reflect several potentially feasible outcome scenarios to work toward and specifically identified resources, timelines, responsible parties, and strategies to achieve each outcome. Discuss your proposed plan with your peers, instructors, and individuals in the change situation.

The following worksheet provides a general framework for planning low-level change. The worksheet headings and sections outline essential points to consider. The guidelines explain the completion of the worksheet section by section.

Guidelines

Section I: Situational Assessment and Analysis

Developing an appropriate plan for a change requires an accurate assessment of the situation needing the change. Effective assessment results in accurate identification of the key elements operating in the situation, not to be confused with symptoms of the need. The elements may be human, technological, system, or other. The need may be a problem needing resolution, a need requiring innovative action, or a measure improving quality.

Part A
Describe the actual situation needing change, naming and briefly describing the who, what, when, where, why, and how elements.

Part B
Using your initial assessment data in Part A, identify current and anticipated facilitators and barriers operating in the change situation. Using a numerical weighting system, rate each factor's strength or potential to either promote (+1 is low and +5 is high) or hinder (−1 is low and −5 is high) the change process. Choose strategies that have the most potential to increase the influences of facilitators and reduce or eliminate the effects of barriers.

Part C
Analyze all factors assessed. State whether you will proceed with the plan. If the weight of the barriers outweighs the strength of the facilitators, reconsider the feasibility of initiating the change.

Section II: Implementation Plan

Write acceptable change outcomes/goals and corresponding objectives and evaluation methods. State predictable unexpected occurrences.

Part A
Describe several desired outcomes using specific, concrete terms. Although broad in nature, the outcomes are used to measure change progress throughout and at the end of the change.

Part B
Objectives are specific descriptions of the processes needed to achieve change outcomes. State objectives in terms of needed resources (materials, space, finances, staff) and desired timelines for each outcome/goal. List objectives in the approximate order in which they will occur. Define accountable parties and what evaluation methods will be used.

Part C
Unexpected occurrences and circumstances will probably affect the change process. Try to predict these and designate potential strategies to respond to them if they do happen.

Part D
Various methods exist for collecting information throughout and at the end of the change process. Choose appropriate methods as needed to measure attitude, behavior, or knowledge during the change and after the change; the influences or concerns hampering the implementation process; or the degree to which objectives are met and the outcomes achieved.

Section III: Evaluation and Revision

It is important to judge the effectiveness of the plan for change and its implementation. Both the processes and outcomes of the change should be evaluated for effectiveness to project what could be improved in future endeavors.
1. State to what degree outcomes were met.

2. Indicate ways to improve the change process or outcome quality.

Part A

1. Describe the actual situation in terms of who, what, when, where, how, and why.

2. Complete a force field analysis by identifying the facilitators and barriers in the change situation. Numerically, rate their potential strength (+1, low to +5, high; −1, low to −5, high). For each facilitator or barrier, indicate strategies appropriate for managing the influences of the factors. Focus on information, relationships, and possible alterations in the pool of outcome scenarios. Use strategies to reduce the effects of barriers and foster the effects of facilitators.

Facilitators (+/Pro)	Strength Rating	Strategies	Barriers (−/Anti)	Strength Rating	Strategies
a.			a.		
b.			b.		
c.			c.		
d.			d.		

3. State how influences of the facilitators and barriers are equal to or different from each other based on your assessment of their strength. State whether you will proceed with the plan.

Part B

1. State at least three desirable outcomes/goals for proposed change in specific, measurable terms.

   a.

   b.

   c.

2. State and sequence outcomes in terms of specific resources, time frames, strategies, and responsible parties for each outcome. Use the table on the next page.

3. Identify unexpected occurrences and potential strategies to manage them.

   a.

   b.

4. State methods for measuring the progress and outcome of the change process.

Ongoing/Process	**Outcome/Summative**
a.	a.
b.	b.
c.	c.

Section IV: Conclusion

1. State to what degree outcomes/goals were met.

2. Indicate ways to improve the change process or outcome/goal quality.

Outcome/Goal	Resources	Time Frame	Strategies	Responsible Parties
a.				
b.				
c.				

CHAPTER **17** APPLICATION ACTIVITY

Building Teams Through Communication and Partnerships

INTRODUCTION

Teamwork is the name of the game these days. In almost every type of institution there is an emphasis on building and maintaining effective teams. Despite this focus on teamwork, many of us still have old habits and beliefs about being effective individuals. Remember all those times you decided, and others encouraged you, to, "Do it yourself" or "Be strong and handle it alone!" Now the emphasis has changed to cooperating and collaborating. These activities aim to increase your understanding of what produces high-performing teams. You will learn the power of focusing your attention on commitment to a particular task. You will also discover how to maintain the cohesiveness of a group and how individualist behaviors affect groups.

ACTIVITY 17-1

1. List at least five criteria for effective teamwork.

    a.

    b.

    c.

    d.

    e.

2. Recall a team you have observed. Identify what was missing from the team's performance. Apply criteria to your observations and experience in the group.

3. Based on your reading of Chapter 19 and various articles, list three specific ways to enrich team performance.

    a.

b.

c.

4. Identify and commit to at least two new actions you could take to improve your role as a team member. Write them down and set deadline dates.

a. I will _____ by _____.

b. I will _____ by _____.

ACTIVITY 17-2

Examine a work group that you are familiar with, either currently or from the past. Select two people you have worked with: one person with whom you enjoyed working and one with whom you were very reluctant to work. For each person, list two behaviors that are characteristic of that person's interactions with others.

Person I Enjoyed Working with

1.

2.

Person I Was Reluctant to Work with

1.

2.

Next, respond to the following:

Do you demonstrate behaviors from either list?	YES	NO
Would you fall exclusively in one list or the other?	YES	NO

Cite two examples of your behavior to support your answer.
1.

2.

In considering the person you were reluctant to work with, cite two positive behaviors for him or her:
1.

2.

In what ways could you encourage growth and expansion of those behaviors?
1.

2.

What could this person contribute to a team?
1.

2.

ACTIVITY 17-3

Make a list of your strengths and limitations as a team member and as a team leader.

Team Member Strengths
1.

2.

3.

Team Leader Strengths
1.

2.

3.

Team Member Limitations
1.

2.

3.

Team Leader Limitations
1.

2.

3.

Now examine each of these and determine how each enhances or interferes with the team process.

CHAPTER **18** APPLICATION ACTIVITY

Collective Action

INTRODUCTION

These activities ask you to reflect on those skills that will contribute to your success in collective action within the practice of nursing. Activity 18-1 begins with the Personal You and will influence your performance within the Professional You context. The remaining activities give you an opportunity to consider your role within nursing practice.

ACTIVITY 18-1

1. You have developed many interpersonal skills within your life. List three interpersonal skills that are essential for nurses to achieve collective action.

   a.

   b.

   c.

2. In the space provided, describe activities that will help you refine these skills.

3. Identify other skills that you think will assist you in collective action within your nursing practice.

ACTIVITY 18-2

Eden Valley is a community hospital. That is, it is an institution that operates solely within the community in which it is located. It is experiencing financial pressures. The options being considered include selling to a national company, joining a multihospital group in the surrounding area, or trying to preserve its identity. Employees, including nurses, are experiencing stress related to the uncertainty. Employees in other job categories are unionized. Several nurses believe that it is a good time to consider organizing a staff union. They contact the constituent member association (CMA) to discuss their concerns.

1. What factors will influence the establishment of a union?

2. What factors will be a barrier to the establishment of a union?

3. Identify other strategies the nurses might consider before formalizing action to create a union.

4. What criteria are important in the selection of a union?

ACTIVITY 18-3

Obtain a copy of a collective bargaining contract between nurses and their employer. (If there are no contracts for nurses in your area, obtain a copy of a collective bargaining [union] contract used by another group.) Identify three features of the contract that are important to you. Identify any features of the contract that are objectionable to you.

Features Important to You	Features Objectionable to You
1.	1.
2	2.
3.	3.

ACTIVITY 18-4

Nurses can no longer ignore or be uninformed about the business side of healthcare delivery. Knowledge of the facilities in which you practice and trends in the industry are necessary to make informed decisions. Imagine you have been informed that the hospital must decrease the number of registered nurses because of new business practices designed to reduce costs and thus approximate insurance payment levels. From your perspective and those of your nurse colleagues, the hospital is doing fine. Identify three sources of public information related to an organization's financial health. Who would you contact to assist you in obtaining the information?

ACTIVITY 18-5

Read two articles or two Websites about nurses working together to effect change. (Examples might include www.centerforamericannurses.org and www.nursingadvocacy.org.) Identify how this collective action empowers nursing to meet the work of the profession.

ACTIVITY 18-6

Identify three subcultures within your current practice setting. The subcultures may be in nursing or not, or within your unit or not. Describe three characteristics of each subculture.

1.

   a.

   b.

   c.

2.

   a.

   b.

   c.

3.

   a.

   b.

   c.

CHAPTER **19** APPLICATION ACTIVITY
Managing Quality and Risk

INTRODUCTION

Total quality management (TQM) and continuous quality improvement (CQI) programs must be fully integrated into an organization's culture to be effective at improving the quality of care. Every member of the healthcare team, particularly those providing direct patient care, must be actively involved in quality management, including preventing errors before they occur and identifying and correcting adverse events. Managing quality and risk focus on increasing safety and maximizing quality outcomes.

ACTIVITY 19-1

1. Form groups of four. Each group member will conduct his or her own interview with a healthcare professional regarding quality improvement. Select interviewees from the institutions in which you work or have clinical experience. Ask the interviewees to address quality improvement in their institution. You will want to interview people at different levels of the organization to gain a broad perspective of everyone's understanding of the process. Suggested people to interview include the nurse manager, staff nurse, unit secretary, physician, director of quality improvement, and people from other departments.
2. After interviewing these people, reflect on and answer the following questions:

   a. Did each person give you a similar picture of the quality improvement process? Why or why not?

   b. If there were differences, were they significant? Why or why not? (If the differences are significant, they can affect how well the quality improvement process works.)

   c. Discuss the interviews in your groups and determine what similarities and differences you found.

ACTIVITY 19-2

Use the following steps to apply quality improvement principles to your own practice. Use a separate sheet of paper for your responses.
1. Identify a process or procedure that you perform routinely and wish to improve.

2. Using a flowchart, delineate each step of the procedure.
3. Collect data that show your present ability to do this process or procedure.
4. Set a measurable standard of excellence for this procedure. Use established standards if available, but remember to also determine what your customers value and expect.
5. Develop a plan to improve your practice to meet this standard. This could include further reading, education, or consultation with peers.
6. Collect data to document your improvement in this procedure.
7. Disseminate your findings.

ACTIVITY 19-3

Obtaining information from your customers is very important when assessing quality of care. Ask five patients about quality of care. (Be certain to obtain the nurse manager's permission first.) The following are some suggested questions to use in your interview:
1. What was most satisfying about the care you have received?
2. What was least satisfying about the care you have received?
3. Have there been any delays in the care that was provided (e.g., pain medication delayed, meal tray served late, call light not answered)?
4. Who was most attentive to your specific needs (e.g., physician, nurse, nursing assistant, housekeeper)?
5. What would you like to see changed?
6. What would you like to see stay the same?
7. Would you recommend this institution to others?
8. Is there anything else you would like to share regarding the quality of care you have received?

ACTIVITY 19-4

Obtain a copy of the form used in an institution to report incidents or occurrences. Review the related policy and procedure. Interview a staff nurse regarding the policy and procedure. Does the nurse's understanding match what is written in the policy and procedure manual?
1. What happens to the incidence report after it is completed by the reporting individual?
2. What types of incidents are to be reported (internally and externally)?
3. What is the most frequently occurring incident?
4. How is corrective action taken after an occurrence has taken place?

CHAPTER **20** APPLICATION ACTIVITY

Translating Research into Practice

INTRODUCTION

Nurses are increasingly expected to incorporate research evidence into practice. While healthcare organizations are called upon to create an infrastructure that supports the use of research evidence, nurse managers and leaders need to create a work environment culture that promotes the identification and implementation of research-based solutions to practice problems. These activities are designed to increase your understanding of evidence-based practice, how you can promote positive attitudes toward research, and how to facilitate the implementation of research-based practices.

ACTIVITY 20-1

This activity complements Exercise 20-1. Select a research study that is related to the area of interest identified in Exercise 20-1. You will need to locate a study that has positive results. This can usually be determined by reading the abstract.

1. Would the results of this study be applicable to the patient population on your unit? Why or why not?

2. Identify two practice changes that you would consider making as a result of reading this study.
   a.

   b.

3. How do you think your patients' preferences and values might be related to the practice changes that you would consider making? (Consider that for some interventions, your patients would of course want you to institute the change. For example, patients would want you to institute a skin assessment protocol if they were at risk for pressure ulcers.)

ACTIVITY 20-2

This activity involves using the study that you found in the research column in a clinical nursing journal for Exercise 20-3. Read the research study and answer the following questions:

1. What is the patient population or the setting?

2. What is the intervention or area of interest for this study?

3. What interventions are being compared in this study? Is a treatment or a risk factor being considered?

4. How was the study outcome measured?

5. What are the results?

6. Put the answers to the above questions into the PICO format: patient, intervention (interest), comparison, and outcome. Use the PICO terms to do a search in PUBMED. Did your search yield similar studies?

    P:

    I:

C:

O:

7. Select one study and compare the results with your original study. How are these two studies similar or different?

ACTIVITY 20-3

Mrs. Williams was recently diagnosed with breast cancer. She will be receiving radiation and chemotherapy once she recovers from her surgery. She is worried that she will be extremely tired from the chemotherapy and won't be able to continue working to retain her health benefits. Mrs. Williams wonders if starting a walking program would reduce her fatigue while she is on her chemotherapy protocol. For this scenario, identify the patient population, intervention (interest), comparison, and outcome.

Patient population:

Intervention (interest):

Comparison:

Outcome:

ACTIVITY 20-4

A hospital's quality assurance committee wants the nursing department to add a falls risk assessment to the nursing admission form. Since the patient population on this particular clinical unit consists primarily of older adults and falls have increased in the last year, the nurse manager is recommending that a more comprehensive evidence-based falls prevention program be instituted. This exercise will consist of role-playing using the above situation. The nurse manager is discussing the implementation of an evidence-based falls prevention program with the staff, which consists of:

1. A new graduate with 3 months of experience who is worried about being able to organize care and learn new skills and competencies. She is a baccalaureate graduate who had a research course that focused on using research evidence for practice.

2. A staff nurse with 10 years of experience who has never had a research course and is not interested in going back to school or learning new knowledge. This nurse is apt to be characterized as a "laggard" in terms of innovation adoption as described by Rogers (2005).

3. A staff nurse with 15 years of experience. This person worked in a large medical center with an active research program before taking a job at the community hospital, and she is most likely to be characterized as an "early adopter." This nurse had a research course 5 years ago when she returned to school for a bachelor's degree; however, it did not include much about evidence-based practice.

Role-players should address concerns related to implementing such a program and address issues that need to be dealt with in order to make the evaluation and implementation of such a program successful. Be sure to focus on how to capitalize on the strengths of the organization, as well as realistically focus on difficulties that might be encountered. At the conclusion of this exercise, identify five elements of a strategic plan for the implementation of a research-based program for falls prevention.

1.

2.

3.

4.

5.

List three things that the administration must consider before implementation.

1.

2.

3.

Define a measurable outcome for the implementation of a falls prevention program.

ACTIVITY 20-5

Understanding and using research evidence requires specific knowledge and skills, including an understanding of how innovations are adopted and an understanding of your particular organization's culture. Complete the following self-assessment. Identify your strengths and limitations, as well as a strategy to address a limitation for each of the following areas:

1. Understanding how to read and interpret research studies

Strength:

Limitation:

Strategy for improvement:

2. Skill in using search engines and databases to locate research evidence

Strength:

Limitation:

Strategy for improvement:

3. Understanding the process for the adoption of innovations
Strength:

Limitation:

Strategy for improvement:

4. Understanding organizational culture and requirements for implementing evidence-based practice
Strength:

Limitation:

Strategy for improvement:

ACTIVITY 20-6

Implementing an evidence-based practice program in an agency requires an understanding of key stake-holder concerns. For a specific evidence-based practice problem identified in Exercise 20-1, identify three key stakeholders who should be involved in the discussion of how to address this particular practice problem in your clinical agency. (Use titles or positions, not names.) Include an assessment of what you think that person's or group's most important concern about the particular practice problem might be.

Stakeholder	Concern
1.	
2.	
3.	

What would be important to address for each of these stakeholders in implementing an evidence-based solution to your identified practice problem?
1.

2.

3.

CHAPTER 21 APPLICATION ACTIVITY

Consumer Relationships

INTRODUCTION

An awareness of how consumer relations affect the provision of nursing care is essential. Consumers are faced with many changes in the healthcare delivery system. When patients enter the healthcare system, they lose a significant amount of control. Their families may be experiencing stress due to changes in their relationships with their loved ones and the burden of additional responsibilities. The following exercises are designed to help you identify how nurses can promote positive experiences with health care.

ACTIVITY 21-1

Mr. Smith, who is 82 years old, has a history of chronic obstructive pulmonary disease and a had a coronary artery bypass graft 6 months ago. He developed a sternal infection that took a long time to resolve after discharge. Two weeks ago, Mr. Smith developed pneumonia and was admitted. Subsequently, he went into respiratory failure, was placed on a ventilator, and was transferred to intensive care. When it became apparent that weaning from the ventilator was going to take an extended time, Mr. Smith was transferred to a medical-surgical unit. Mr. Smith has generally been able to communicate some of his basic needs to the staff and follow commands.

Mr. Smith's son is a physician who practices in another state. He was extremely angry about the transfer and has been complaining that the nursing staff is not competent to manage ventilated patients. The nursing staff has been diligent in providing care for Mr. Smith and ensuring that the weaning protocols are followed. However, they suspect that Mr. Smith's son has been adjusting the ventilator settings, making it more difficult for them to wean Mr. Smith from the ventilator.

You are the nurse manager of the unit and today is the first day that you are back from vacation. When you return from a meeting, you have a message to call the vice president for nursing regarding a patient complaint. When you call, you are told that Mr. Smith's son has called the hospital administrator and demanded that a nurse on the unit be fired; he is also putting pressure on Mr. Smith's physician to join in the demand. Mr. Smith's physician is convinced that not all of the nurses have been following the weaning protocol. Although the nurses have reported their suspicions about the son changing the ventilator settings to Mr. Smith's physician and the nursing supervisor, no one has spoken directly to Mr. Smith's son. You are asked to investigate the situation.

Upon investigation, you find that Mr. Smith's son is very upset because he was not consulted before his father was transferred to your unit. He also believes that the nurses are not carrying out his father's weaning protocol correctly. He believes that his father's physician and the nurses have been dismissive of his advice and concerns. The staff nurse is a recent graduate and is fearful of being fired. No one has attempted to talk with Mr. Smith's son about his concerns.

Review the textbook pages promoting successful consumer relationships: service, advocacy, teaching, and leadership. Then answer the following questions.

1. How can your staff effectively provide services for Mr. Smith? List four ways.
    a.

b.

c.

d.

2. If Mr. Smith's son refuses to collaborate with the staff in the plan of care, cite three effective ways to support the nursing staff regarding his demands.
   a.

   b.

   c.

3. How are you going to respond to the vice president for nursing and to the hospital administration?
   a.

   b.

   c.

4. How will you handle Mr. Smith's son's demand that the staff nurse be fired? Cite your approach and give a supportive rationale for your selection.
   Approach:

   Rationale:

5. How will you be an advocate for Mr. Smith?
   Approach:

   Rationale:

6. How will you be an advocate for Mr. Smith's son?
   Approach:

   Rationale:

ACTIVITY 21-2

Some institutions have designated patient representatives who act as ombudsmen (advocates) for the hospital and the patient. Sometimes the hospital's risk manager serves in this role. They are often first in line and highly skilled in handling patient complaints. Consider how a person in such a position may effectively respond to the concerns of Mr. Smith's son. Make a list of at least three possible actions the patient representative could take and the rationale for each.

Action   **Rationale**

1.

2.

3.

Compare your responses with those of at least two other classmates. Were your responses the same? Different? How would you modify your actions?

ACTIVITY 21-3

Refer to Activity 21-1. This activity involves role-playing, with a time limit of 3 to 5 minutes.

1. Divide into small groups of five to seven students. Two students will role-play while the others observe. For the role-players for Mr. Smith's son and the staff nurse, don't be afraid to express feelings of anger, fear, disappointment, and so forth. Think about how you would respond (both in words and in feelings) if you were the person. Observers should make notes about what is said, what may be said differently, and the body language of the role-players.

2. Discuss what was observed. Be open to making and receiving recommendations regarding the nurse role-play from your peers. This is your chance to receive nonthreatening feedback from your peers before confronting this possible situation clinically.

3. After completing one role-play, two other members of the group rotate roles and complete the same process. Everyone should have the opportunity to have played at least one role, either as the nurse or as Mr. Smith's son.

   Other possible role combinations include the following: Mr. Smith's son and the hospital administrator; the nurse manager and the vice president for nursing; Mr. Smith and the nurse manager; Mr. Smith's son and the nurse manager; the nurse manager and the staff nurse; the nurse manager and Mr. Smith's physician; or the ombudsman (from Activity 21-2) and any one of the aforementioned persons.

4. Identify how it would feel to be in the role you are assigned. For example, as the patient, you want to make your own decisions; as the family, you want to be sure your loved one receives excellent care; and as the staff nurse, you feel concerned because you know the family's behavior may be detrimental to the patient.

   I felt:

5. Discuss the feelings that were identified as a group. For example, as the nurse manager, you felt defensive while you were discussing the situation with the vice president for nursing. List five suggestions generated by the group to avoid defensiveness.

   a.

   b.

   c.

d.

e.

6. Consider what response would have made you feel better. For example, you become angry while talking to Mr. Smith's son and tell him you are going to have his father's doctor talk to him. With the assistance of the group, list five ways that this might have been said differently.
   a.

   b.

   c.

   d.

   e.

ACTIVITY 21-4

It is the practice of some institutions to have patient care conferences. The goals of these conferences are to handle case management services, solve problems that may occur, and design a plan to provide quality care for the patient. It is also a good time to support your peers who may be having difficulties in providing care when there are problems.

You are responsible for leading a patient care conference and outlining a plan of care for Mr. Smith. Outline your plans for the conference. How will you involve Mr. Smith and his son in decisions regarding the provision of care. What role should his son have in this process? Would you invite Mr. Smith's son to attend the conference? Why? (Provide a rationale.)

How will you involve Mr. Smith in his care in the future? Identify five ways.

1.

2.

3.

4.

5.

How will you handle Mr. Smith's son's desire to be involved in his father's care? Provide a rationale.

Approach:

Rationale:

Compare your responses to those of two of your classmates. What are areas of difference and areas of similarities in your responses?

ACTIVITY 21-5

Obtain a copy of a frequently used patient education brochure, handout, or standardized consent document. Scan a page of the document into a word processing program and use the word processor tools menu to determine the reading level of the document. If the reading level is at more than a sixth-grade level, make recommendations for simplification. If the reading level is at a high level, what strategies would you use for recommending changes?

CHAPTER **22** APPLICATION ACTIVITY

Conflict: The Cutting Edge of Change

INTRODUCTION

The following activity assumes you have completed and scored the Conflict Self-Assessment in Chapter 22 and responded to the questions in Boxes 22-5, 22-7, 22-9, 22-11, and 22-13. Effective conflict resolution and polarity management lead to effective leadership for change.

ACTIVITY 22-1

After you have read Chapter 22, complete and score the Conflict Self-Assessment in the text. Next, on a separate sheet of paper, write out your responses to the self-assessment questions for each of the five approaches to conflict (avoiding, accommodating, competing, compromising, and collaborating), focusing only on conflicts in your professional life. (If you are not yet in a professional position, you might instead focus on conflicts during your "career" as a student.) Use the Conflict Reflection Form that follows to focus your thinking. What new behaviors have you committed to for the future?

Conflict Reflection Form

Look at your scores on the Conflict Self-Assessment and responses to the five sets of self-assessment questions in the textbook. Reflect on how you act during conflict (professional and/or personal). Be honest with yourself without being critical.

1. How do you tend to balance the following polarities related to conflict?
   a. Unassertiveness and assertiveness?

   b. Uncooperativeness and cooperativeness?

   c. Avoidance and involvement?

   d. Escalation and minimization of any conflict?

   e. Rigid control and loose improvisation?

   f. Revelation and concealment of information?

   g. Intellectual and emotional reactions?

2. Which two approaches to conflict resolution do you tend to underemphasize? Why?
   a.

   b.

3. Which two do you tend to use most often? Why?
   a.

   b.

4. How might you be overemphasizing some approaches? Are they situation specific, or are they just the ones you rely on? Why?

5. When and how might you be matching approaches effectively to the particular nature of conflicts in which you are involved?

6. When and how might you be matching approaches ineffectively with the particular nature of conflicts in which you are involved?

ACTIVITY 22-2

Playing Twenty Questions: Conflict Analysis

Reflect on past and present conflicts in which you have been directly involved. Choose one conflict to focus on, particularly if it seems to be reappearing with the same or with other people. Check the text to determine whether it is a polarity. If it is, choose another conflict that is not a polarity. Then write out your responses to each of the 20 questions below.

Defining the Conflict

1. Who was the conflict between? How were they affected?
   Who:

   How:

   Who:

   How:

2. Who else was affected and how?
   Who:

   How:

3. What was the actual conflict? What were the perceived incompatibilities?

Conflict Process Analysis

Frustration Stage

4. What did you feel at the beginning and in the early stages of the conflict?

5. Why did you feel this way?

6. How did you act as a result of these feelings?

7. What do you think the other people felt at the beginning and in the early stages of the conflict?

8. Why do you think they felt this way?

9. How did they act as a result of these emotions?

10. After the conflict moved into the conceptualization stage (see the following), what other emotions or changes in your initial emotions occurred? Why?

Conceptualization Stage

11. What did you think the real conflict (or issue, fight, disagreement, and so on) was? Why?

12. What do you now believe that the other people believed the conflict (or issue, fight, disagreement, and so on) was? Why?

13. Where did you and others have serious differences: facts and information, goals and objectives, means and methods of action, and/or standards and values?

14. Describe why you had the following differences:
    a. Exposure to different data?

    b. Different interpretations of the information?

    c. Differences in your roles and position?

    d. Different values and beliefs?

    e. Cultural differences?

    f. Different directions from someone else?

15. After the conflict moved into the action stage, what new views of the conflict (conceptualizations) were created by those involved? Why?

Action Stage

16. How did you act specifically (and which of the five approaches to conflict were tried)? Why?

17. How did the other people act? Why?

18. After the conflict clearly was in the outcome stage, were there any new actions by anyone that were aimed at resolving this conflict or in changing any of the outcomes that follow?

Outcomes Stage

19. What happened to the quality of task accomplishment and efficiency of action as a result of the actions taken? Why?

20. What happened to the quality of the relationships among those involved?

ACTIVITY 22-3

Imagine that you will be in a conflict in the future similar to the one you just analyzed in Activity 22-2. Knowing what you do about this past conflict, your tendencies in approaching conflict (review the self-assessments in Chapter 22), and the five different approaches to conflict, write out a short scenario below (including all four stages of the process) describing how you could act to resolve the conflict.

CHAPTER **23** APPLICATION ACTIVITY

Delegation: An Art of Professional Practice

INTRODUCTION

Delegation is a critical strategy for nurses to accomplish their work. It requires that nurses know many facts about patients, other workers, legal and ethical implications, and what the research suggests. Chapter 23 provided key information for making appropriate delegation decisions. Once you understand the basics, skills can be developed for determining assignments from two perspectives. The first requires knowing about specific patients in terms of some criteria, and the second requires hypothesizing what to anticipate in an unknown patient population. The following activities are designed to help you apply what you have learned in the chapter.

ACTIVITY 23-1

Arrive for your next clinical assignment 1 or 2 hours early. Using the actual patients on your unit (or in your population actively served) and the projected staffing, apply the factors for delegation for the antici-pated tasks. Complete this assignment for at least five patients who have multiple tasks to be accomplished. After that, use Table 23-2 as a screening activity to determine whether your original conclusions were consistent with the answers you provided to the questions from Table 23-2. Which elements of the criteria and the questions were most difficult to assess? Why? When the assignments are actually made, compare your decisions about care with those actually made. Finally, ask the nurses responsible for those five patients how a decision was reached about delegation. If the nurses do not address factors such as how long the delegatee has worked with the nurses, be sure to ask. Also ask if the nurses know the type of training the delegatee has had. Finally, ask what one factor is the most important to each individual in deciding what to delegate.

ACTIVITY 23-2

Select a partner. Each of you should choose an uncommon (and preferably previously unstudied) chronic disease condition. In the space provided, identify the condition and your literature source. Next, identify what tasks you believe would be typical for a patient with that condition. Then list what care tasks you would delegate to a new nursing assistant. Identify what to ask. Provide a rationale and a method of evalu-ating your decision. In your rationale statement, include how intense the supervision is likely to be.

Condition:

Source:

Delegated tasks:

Questions:

Rationale:

Method of evaluation:

CHAPTER **24** APPLICATION ACTIVITY

Managing Personal/Personnel Problems

INTRODUCTION

Successfully managing personal/personnel problems is a crucial element of the role of a nurse manager. To master this role function requires that the manager be able to accurately identify personnel problems, develop intervention strategies, implement those strategies, and then evaluate the effectiveness of the interventions. The exercises in this section will help you develop the assessment and intervention skills necessary to successfully manage personnel problems.

ACTIVITY 24-1

Personal/Personnel Problems: Chemical Dependency

1. Review the following documents:
   a. Your state board of nursing's policy and procedures regarding chemically impaired nurses
   b. The American Nurses Association *Code of Ethics for Nurses*
   c. A healthcare agency's policy and procedures regarding chemically dependent employees
   d. A healthcare agency's policy regarding employee drug screening

2. Define the differences between substance dependence and substance abuse.
   Substance dependence is:

   Substance abuse is:

3. List three factors leading to substance abuse in employees.
   a.

   b.

   c.

4. List five of the most common types of abused substances.

   a.

   b.

   c.

   d.

   e.

5. Describe four signs and symptoms of dependence/abuse that may be evident in a chemically impaired employee.

   a.

   b.

   c.

   d.

6. Write a short paragraph either supporting or contesting the following statements regarding chemically impaired healthcare employees. Use a separate sheet of paper.
   a. Substance dependence/abuse is a disease and therefore not fully under the control of the affected person. Substance abusers should be treated, not punished.
   b. Nurses and other healthcare professionals, with their knowledge about drugs and their social contract with patients, should be held to higher standards than the general population.

7. Obtain a copy of personnel policies from an agency in which you have clinical experience. Analyze the policy in relation to the following factors, recording your answers in the space provided.
   a. Is the *Diagnostic and Statistical Manual* (DSM-IV) definition used to define substance dependence/abuse in the agency policy?

   b. Is there a policy for reporting suspected or known impaired employees? If so, what is the role of the nurse manager? Of the staff nurse?

   c. Does the policy include plans for intervention and treatment? Is an employee assistance program (EAP) provided for employees? What is the manager's role in intervention?

d. Does the policy include a notification procedure? If so, who within the agency administration is to be notified? What is the policy for notifying the state board of nursing if the impaired worker is a nurse?

e. List three key elements that you think should be included in an "ideal" agency policy.

f. Does the return-to-work section of the policy identify how the recovering nurse will be monitored?

g. Are there conditions within the policy to address how a relapse will be handled?

ACTIVITY 24-2

Personal/Personnel Problems: Mandatory Drug Testing for Healthcare Professionals

1. Review a copy of the following documents:
   a. An agency's policy and procedure regarding chemically dependent employees
   b. An agency's policy regarding employee preemployment and on-the-job drug screening
   c. Your state board of nursing's policy and procedures on reporting suspected chemically dependent nurses
   d. The American Nurses Association *Code of Ethics for Nurses* (determine their policy statement regarding substance abuse)
   e. An agency's policies on nondiscrimination in employment under the Americans with Disabilities Act

2. Prepare to debate the issue of mandatory drug testing for healthcare employees. Read the following debating statement. Prepare five key points to argue for each side (pro and con) of the issue, drawing support for your arguments from the list of readings given previously: *Approximately 70% of all cases handled by state boards of nursing are related to chemically impaired nurses, and nurses have entered into a social contract with their patients to provide safe care; therefore, mandatory random drug testing should be done on all practicing nurses.*

Pro	**Con**
a.	a.
b.	b.
c.	c.
d.	d.
e.	e.

ACTIVITY 24-3

1. Read about the legal, regulatory, and ethical issues related to termination of an employee. Refer to the following reading as a guide. Curtin, L. (1996). Ethics, discipline, and discharge. *Nursing Management,* 27(3), 51-52.
2. Review an agency's policies and procedures for terminating employees.
3. Read the following scenario. Carefully weigh the pros and cons of each termination decision, considering the legal, ethical, and personal factors that enter into your decision.

Downsizing Scenario

You are a nurse manager in an agency that is experiencing financial difficulties, and this problem affects more than just your agency. You are located in a county that is economically depressed, and unemployment is high. You have just received the budget for the next financial year and note that you have lost one full-time position, meaning you must lay off one of your full-time nurses. Because of a poor economic situation, it is not possible to transfer within the agency and the layoff will most likely be a permanent one. Also, no other agencies in the area are hiring, although some jobs may be available through a staffing pool or on a contingency basis. You must decide which of the following three employees to lay off. This is a nonunion agency, each of the nurses has the same number of years of service with the hospital, and all three have had very similar performance evaluations for the last 3 years.

Nurse A: Nancy is 50 years old and entered nursing later in life after raising a family of four. She is married to the hospital's chief of staff, and some of the younger nurses on the unit resent her "country club" attitude. They think she is not really serious about nursing and only works to escape being bored. Nancy does a good job, but she does have some difficulty working with other staff nurses. You personally like Nancy a great deal. She is closer to you in age and life experience than the other staff nurses, and you find yourself turning to her for advice and support. Nancy has confided in you that she really enjoys her newfound career. She says that for the first time in her life, she has an identity of her own instead of always being somebody's daughter, spouse, or mother. Nancy has missed 4 days of work in the last 6 months: 2 days to take her mother to the doctor for evaluation of Alzheimer's disease, 1 day because her husband unexpectedly told her that she had to accompany him to an important hospital social event, and 1 day for calling in sick.

Nurse B: John is 35 years old and the only male nurse on your unit. He has suffered a number of personal crises and losses in the past 2 years. His 2-year-old son has Down syndrome, and his 10-year-old son was killed in an automobile accident last year. About 6 months ago, his father died unexpectedly from a heart attack. John has confided in you that he is really struggling with these personal losses. He is especially having difficulty with losing his son because he says he will never be able to do all the "father and son things" with his 2-year-old son that would have been possible with the older son. John says he just doesn't feel the same kind of bond with either his 2-year-old son or his 6-year-old daughter. John also states that he's having difficulty with his wife. Their relationship is very strained and stressful. He's not sure if the marriage will survive. He says that he has been very depressed over all of these crises and has sought professional counseling. He also tells you in confidence that the psychiatrist has him on antidepressants to help him cope. John has missed 4 days of work in the last 6 months. All of them have been on Mondays. He says that the depression has at times made it difficult for him to start another week.

Nurse C: Carrie is 33 years old and very well liked by her peers. She is an informal leader in the group. You personally don't like Carrie very much. She was working on the unit before you became manager, and she has constantly challenged you since you arrived. She is argumentative and resistant to change, but she always ends up doing what you ask her to do. You worry about the effect that she has on unit morale, yet none of the staff nurses has ever reported having difficulties working with her. About 9 months ago, Carrie seriously injured her back when a patient she was ambulating started to fall. Carrie saved the patient from injury, but she was on medical leave for 6 weeks because of the incident. Her recovery may have been hindered by the fact that she is 40 pounds overweight. Because of her back injuries, she often requests that she be assigned to charge (desk) duty. Other staff nurses have offered to give her their charge duty or volunteered to help her with patient care if she needs any assistance. Carrie has missed 4 days in the past 6 months: 2 days on two separate instances, both for complaints of back pain.

Which nurse will you lay off?

List two reasons to terminate or retain each of the nurses.
Nancy
1.

2.

John
1.

2.

Carrie
1.

2.

Indicate one personal, ethical, and legal issue that may be raised in terminating each of the three nurses.
Nancy
Personal:

Ethical:

Legal:

John
Personal:

Ethical:

Legal:

Carrie
Personal:

Ethical:

Legal:

CHAPTER 25 APPLICATION ACTIVITY

Role Transition

INTRODUCTION

Roles in health care are changing rapidly. Are you in the midst of a role transition, or are you anticipating the transition from nursing student to "real nurse"? No matter which situation you are in, Activities 25-1 and 25-2 can provide valuable insight. Thoughtful responses to the questions will help you clarify the roles of a nurse manager, your strengths, and your areas needing improvement.

ACTIVITY 25-1

1. Read Chapter 25 and complete the Roles Assessment. In that assessment, you are asked to analyze job responsibilities, opportunities to contribute and grow professionally, lines of communication, and expectations of others around the nurse manager. Talk to two staff nurses and ask each of them, "What are the two most important roles that a nurse manager must fulfill?"

Nurse #1   **Nurse #2**
a.   a.

b.   b.

Ask a nurse manager, "What are the two most important roles that you must fulfill?"
a.

b.

Compare the responses of the staff nurses and the nurse manager.
Similarities:

Differences:

Conflicts:

Share your impressions with two or three peers. Synthesize the information each of you has received from the staff nurses and managers. Identify as a group the similarities and differences in how staff nurses and nurse managers view the manager role. What conflicts exist between these perspectives?

Similarities:

Differences:

Conflicts:

Discuss responses with your peers and others (managers, staff) and have them assist in clarifying the multiple roles and expectations.

2. What roles and responsibilities excite you? Why?

3. Which ones seem to demand a "risk and stretch" for you? Why?

4. Which roles and responsibilities would you rather not have? Why?

◼ ACTIVITY 25-2

Complete the self-assessment in Chapter 25. As requested in the assessment, talk with a mentor of yours and compare your perspective of yourself with the mentor's perspective. You also could use some of the sentence completions that follow as additional items on which to focus.

1. One recent example of my success in providing leadership is:

2. I am especially proud of my ability to:

3. The part of my work I especially like is:

4. I believe in my capability to manage difficult:

5. I am very responsible in relation to:

6. A goal I have met in the past year of which I am most proud is:

7. I think my supervisor would evaluate my effectiveness as:

8. My colleagues would describe me as:

9. I accomplish the most when I:

10. One thing I am more successful with this year is:

CHAPTER **26** APPLICATION ACTIVITY

Self-Management: Stress and Time

 INTRODUCTION

The following activities afford the reader opportunities to put the principles described in Chapter 26 into action. The first activity invites you to analyze how stress and time management are related. Identifying your own coping skills and seeking more positive ways of managing stress are the focus of the second activity. The third exercise invites you to use your time management skills to plan a successful meeting.

 ACTIVITY 26-1

Self-Management

1. Consider your last clinical day. On a separate sheet of paper, complete a time log for the entire day, from rising in the morning to going to sleep at night. Include the approximate amount of time you spent on each nursing task during the clinical day.
2. Identify those activities that took longer than expected by underlining those items.
3. Analyze the description in terms of the time management skills of goal setting, prioritization, organization (O), use of time tools (T), and dealing with information (I). Label each with the corresponding letters.
4. Identify periods of the day that were stressful by bracketing the time.
5. Analyze the stressful activities in relation to why they were stressful (S) and how you dealt with the stress. Label stressful items with an "S," and to the right, describe how you responded.
6. Analyze the appropriateness of a peer's stress management strategies.
7. Review the principles of self-management in Chapter 26 and identify how the day might have been made to be less stressful.

ACTIVITY 26-2

Stress

Use the following questions as a guide to understanding how you perceive stress, respond to it, and attempt to gain mastery over it.
1. Think about a recent situation in which you experienced a high level of distress. Indicate how you responded.
   Emotionally:

Behaviorally:

Physically:

Review what you have written and identify whether your coping strategies were negative (N) or positive (P), labeling each accordingly.

Consider an alternative approach for those coping strategies you have identified as negative.

2. Describe a situation in which you were in conflict with another person. How was that situation influenced by your expectations and behavior? Could the conflict have been avoided or resolved differently?

ACTIVITY 26-3

Meeting Management

Examine the Tips box on how to manage a meeting at the end of Chapter 26. Given the list of agenda items below, organize a 2-hour meeting to address them all. On a separate sheet of paper, list them in an agenda with specific time limits for each item. Be prepared to give the rationale for the specific order you choose. When would you hold this meeting? What site might you choose for this meeting?

Agenda Items

a. Discuss how to make team meetings more effective.
b. Decide on a new schedule format.
c. Share the news.
d. Discuss new possibilities for continuous improvement on the unit.
e. Decide when to hold a shift party.
f. Review the last meeting's minutes.
g. Revise a report form.
h. Discuss agenda items for the next meeting.
i. Give out assignments.
j. Answer questions.

CHAPTER **27** APPLICATION ACTIVITY

Career Management: Putting Yourself in Charge

INTRODUCTION

Career management takes thought, time, and energy. The alternative to managing your own career is to experience whatever comes your way and hope for the best. Developing your career is related not only to securing a "good" position but also to planning your career in the way that you wish to proceed to meet your short- and long-term goals. It means being proactive for yourself.

Chapter 27 identified specific strategies to launch a career and to keep it on a positive trajectory. The following activities are designed to use the elements presented in the chapter to create commonly used documents to market yourself in a manner that will enable you to "stand out among the rest."

ACTIVITY 27-1

You are in the last days of your undergraduate nursing program, with many career options open to you. You have had diverse opportunities throughout your educational program that make you marketable for a variety of positions. Using the facts that you have compiled in your data collection system, create a résumé for each of the positions you are considering: (1) staff nurse in a surgical intensive care unit that accommodates many trauma patients, (2) staff nurse for a high-risk perinatal unit that cares for indigent patients who have had minimal prenatal care, and (3) staff nurse in an ambulatory surgery center that admits patients in the morning and discharges them later in the day after their surgery.

ACTIVITY 27-2

It is 6 months since your graduation from your nursing program. Update your data collection system, entering elements that have occurred since graduation. Complete a curriculum vitae (CV), which you are required to submit with your graduate school application.

ACTIVITY 27-3

Your nurse manager has selected you as a candidate to be interviewed for one of the mentorship positions on your unit. She tells you that the organization is developing a mentorship program for nursing service. The intent of this program is to mentor new staff as they join the organization. It is an honor to be considered for this position, and you must interview with a panel of nursing staff, nurse administrators, and nurse educators. If you are selected to be a mentor, you will attend mentor development classes and receive an adjustment to your base salary. You have been asked to submit a cover letter as a means of introducing yourself to the committee. Prepare your cover letter and practice interviewing for the position with one of your classmates.

CHAPTER **28** APPLICATION ACTIVITY

Leading Through Professional Associations

INTRODUCTION

Leaders can be found in a variety of settings, including clinical, policy, research, and management settings. That an individual is a good manager does not necessarily mean that the individual would be a good leader. Leadership traits are acquired in a variety of ways. How can nurses learn leadership skills? Professional associations provide opportunities to engage in leadership activities and encourage professional growth. The activities here are designed to assist you in developing the necessary skills.

ACTIVITY 28-1

1. How do you define or describe a professional association? An organization? Are there any differences? Similarities?

2. Do you know faculty or coworkers who are members or officers of an association? Who? Which associations?

3. Have you explored opportunities within your local, state, and national student nurses' association (www.nsna.org)?

ACTIVITY 28-2

1. In the space provided, make a list of benefits that you might receive by joining your nursing association.

2. Create a brief outline of your 1-year and 5-year goals and career plan.
   1-year:

   5-year:

   What barriers have you identified that you think may prevent you from accomplishing the goals you have identified?
   1-year:

   5-year:

   Write a list of goals that you have for personal and professional development (e.g., make a public speech, write an article, hold an officer position, conduct research, be a manager).

   Do you have any concerns about getting involved in a professional association? If so, what (e.g., fear that the organization will require too great of a time commitment)?

   Speak with faculty members and/or coworkers about their ideas and what they value and the benefits they receive through membership.

ACTIVITY 28-3

1. Read at least two articles concerning professional nursing organizations. Using the Internet, access the American Nurses Association at www.nursingworld.org.
2. Research at least one specialty nurse organization on the Internet and attend a meeting (e.g., Emergency Nurses Association).
3. Find out when a local association meeting is and attend one. Check the dates of the state conventions because there are invaluable opportunities for new graduates and they are often offered to students at special, reduced rates. List specific opportunities. Designate whether a reduced rate is available for students and/or new graduates.

CHAPTER **29** APPLICATION ACTIVITY

Thriving for the Future

INTRODUCTION

Being so busy on a day-to-day basis, including the planning of personal and work activities, seems to consume the majority of our days. Still, successful people actively think about the future and what the implications of the future are for what needs to be done now. Whether that requires refocusing your career or gaining new skills, the key is not to be caught unaware and unprepared.

ACTIVITY 29-1

1. Review the strengths for the future listed in Box 29-1. Write a short self-evaluation of your skills within each of the six areas.
   Ethical political savvy:

   Authenticity and accountability:

   Politics of commonalities:

   Thinking long term, acting short term:

   Leadership through expectation:

   Quest for meaning:

Now write a personal goal statement to improve one area. This should focus on becoming better prepared for the future in nursing.

ACTIVITY 29-2

Go online to the World Future Society (WFS) (www.wfs.org) and determine what the "hot topics" are. Then go to three online newspapers such as the Washington Post, the New York Times, and your local paper. Scan the articles there to see if you find current articles that relate to the predictions and issues determined through the WFS. If you see relationships, list three of the topics here. If you don't see any such relationships (which may relate to the current stories of the day), think about what the WFS said and what you see in health care and create a list of three topics here. Include a rationale for why you think each has importance for health care in the future.

a.

b.

c.

Using those three topic areas, consider what you need to do to be better prepared in one of the areas. List at least two activities you could begin within the next month.

ACTIVITY 29-3

1. Consider the following statement: The healthcare system will have to change to remain financially viable, and as employers limit healthcare coverage and genetics allow us to know more about how an individual would respond to treatment, a shift toward eliminating the current disparities is more likely to occur.

2. Go online and search for the term "health disparities," then determine a profile of the populations that are most disparate in their health care. List the characteristics of that profile.

Compare this description with how you would describe the client population in your primary clinical agency. List any differences here.

In one short paragraph, describe what you as an individual nurse could do to reduce health disparities in your client population.

Index

Page numbers followed by *b, t,* or *f* indicate boxes, tables, or figures, respectively.